LAURA

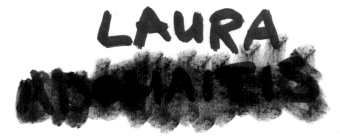

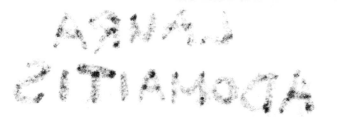

Pathophysiology of the Motor Systems

Principles and Clinical Presentations

Pathophysiology of the Motor Systems

Principles and Clinical Presentations

Edited by:

Christopher M. Fredericks, PhD
Professor
Department of Physiology
Medical University of South Carolina
Charleston, South Carolina

Lisa K. Saladin, BMR (PT), MSc
Director and Assistant Professor
Physical Therapy Education Program
Department of Rehabilitation Sciences
Medical University of South Carolina
Charleston, South Carolina

F. A. DAVIS COMPANY • Philadelphia

F. A. Davis Company
1915 Arch Street
Philadelphia, PA 19103

Printed in the United States of America

Last digit indicates print number: 10 9 8 7 6 5 4 3 2 1

Publisher: Jean-François Vilain
Senior Allied Health Developmental Editor: Ralph Zickgraf
Production Editor: Nancee A. Vogel
Cover Designer: Louis J. Forgione

As new scientific information becomes available through basic and clinical research, recommended treatments and drug therapies undergo changes. The author(s) and publisher have done everything possible to make this book accurate, up to date, and in accord with accepted standards at the time of publication. The authors, editors, and publisher are not responsible for errors or omissions or for consequences from application of the book, and make no warranty, expressed or implied, in regard to the contents of the book. Any practice described in this book should be applied by the reader in accordance with professional standards of care used in regard to the unique circumstances that may apply in each situation. The reader is advised always to check product information (package inserts) for changes and new information regarding dose and contraindications before administering any drug. Caution is especially urged when using new or infrequently ordered drugs.

Library of Congress Cataloging-in-Publication Data

Pathophysiology of the motor systems : principles & clinical
    presentations / edited by Christopher M. Fredericks, Lisa K.
Saladin.
        p.   cm.
    Includes bibliographical references and index.
    ISBN 0-8036-0093-3 (hardcover)
    1. Musculoskeletal system—Pathophysiology.   2. Neuromuscular
diseases—Pathophysiology.   3. Musculoskeletal system—Physiology.
4. Motor learning.   I. Fredericks, Christopher M., 1944-   .
II. Saladin, Lisa K., 1962-
RC925.6.P38   1995
616.8'3—dc20   95-37900
                                                                                    CIP

Dedication

—■—

*T*his book is dedicated to the clinicians, researchers, and students who seek to understand the causes and to ameliorate the consequences of motor dysfunction.

Preface

—■—

The education of physical therapy, occupational therapy, and other students preparing for careers in the rehabilitative health sciences must contain adequate exposure to normal human anatomy and physiology, as well as human pathophysiology. Courses considering this material generally constitute the bulk of the basic science content of these programs. Ultimately, much of the clinical work of these professionals will specifically revolve around rehabilitation of disability resulting from disturbance of somatic function. It is thus particularly important that students develop an in-depth understanding of normal somatic function, as well as its dysfunction and the resultant deficits that this may produce. Such an understanding provides a basis for insight into the etiologies and presentations of the clinical problems to which these students will ultimately be exposed as therapists, as well as a basis for their treatment.

In many educational programs, a natural but counterproductive schism develops between the basic and clinical elements of the curriculum. Students are exposed, on the one hand, to basic science courses (often with a minimal clinical content, presented by instructors with little understanding or concern for the actual utility of this information), and, on the other hand, to applied clinical courses. Often little success is achieved in establishing the interrelationship between the two. This results in an artificial separation of basic and clinical sciences in the minds of students. The basic sciences are not motivating and are difficult to learn; moreover, clinical understanding is impeded by a lack of insight into the pathogenesis of various somatic diseases and the underlying rationales for treatment.

The purpose of this text is to provide the student with an integrated discussion of the motor systems that includes consideration of both normal and disturbed motor function.

Specifically, this text discusses somatic activity in an orderly fashion, beginning with the individual components (cells and tissues) of the motor system and progressing to motor control at the level of the spinal cord and ultimately to the complex control exerted at supraspinal levels. While necessary neuroanatomical correlates are described at each level, emphasis is placed upon functional considerations and how these processes are reflected in the characteristics of normal and abnormal motor activity. Overall motor control is discussed both in terms of traditional hierarchical models of control and in terms of more behaviorally oriented systems and dynamic control models currently under exploration.

Following discussion of the normal operation of the somatic systems, the text introduces pathoclinical topics by describing the primary signs and symptoms arising from motor dysfunction. Basic disease families (e.g., myopathies, neuropathies, cerebellar disorders) are covered in detail. We have emphasized recognition of the most characteristic signs and symptoms of each disorder and understanding of how disordered function has created these clinical features (i.e, pathogenesis). In each group, specific syndromes are presented as examples. While extensive discussion of treatment per se is beyond the scope of this text, in some instances discussion of treatment approaches is used to clarify the pathogenesis of a disorder.

Finally, the book closes with a discussion of the far-reaching functional consequences of immobilization. Morbidity and mortality accompanying locomotor dysfunction seldom arise directly from inadequate neuromuscular activity itself but rather from the impact that this disordered function has on other physiologic systems. Therefore, it is important that therapists who focus on somatic function consider the implications of motor dysfunction for the overall health of the individual.

Christopher M. Federicks
Lisa K. Saladin

Acknowledgments

———■———

The authors would like to thank Katy Egan, Diane Collins, and Wendy Linder for their tireless efforts in the face of endless requests for word processing, editing, and research. Recognition and appreciation are also due Diane E. Raeke (BFA) for her careful and thoughtful rendering of many of the illustrations in this text.

We also want to thank the following reviewers for their close reading of and insightful comments on the various stages of manuscript: Leonard Elbaum, Associate Professor and Director of Research, Physical Therapy Department, Florida International University; Paul C. Leavis, Senior Scientist, Muscle Research, Boston Biomedical Research Institute; Deborah S. Nichols, Associate Professor, Physical Therapy, School of Allied Health Profession, The Ohio State University; Jan F. Perry, Associate Professor and Chairman, Physical Therapy Department, School of Allied Health, Medical College of Georgia; and R. Scott Ward, Professor, Co-Director, Division of Physical Therapy, University of Utah.

Finally, we would like to express our sincerest appreciation for the understanding and support offered throughout this project by our loving families.

Contributors

———■———

Patricia A. Burtner, PhD
Lecturer of Occupational Therapy
Department of Orthopaedics
School of Medicine
University of New Mexico
Albuquerque, New Mexico

Christopher M. Fredericks, PhD
Professor
Department of Physiology
Medical University of South Carolina
Charleston, South Carolina

Robert J. Morecraft, PhD
Assistant Professor
Department of Anatomy and Structural Biology
School of Medicine
University of South Dakota
Vermillion, South Dakota

Diane E. Nicholson, PT, NCS, PhD
Assistant Professor
Director, Movement Dysfunction Laboratory
Division of Physical Therapy
College of Health
University of Utah
Salt Lake City, Utah

James G. Phillips, PhD
Lecturer
Department of Psychology
Monash University
Clayton, Victoria, Australia

Lisa K. Saladin, BMR (PT), MSc
Director and Assistant Professor
Physical Therapy Education Program
Department of Rehabilitation Sciences
Medical University of South Carolina
Charleston, South Carolina

George E. Stelmach, EdD
Professor
Department of Exercise Science and Physical Education
Arizona State University
Tempe, Arizona

Gary W. Van Hoesen, PhD
Professor of Anatomy and Neurology
Department of Anatomy
University of Iowa
Iowa City, Iowa

Marjorie H. Woollacott, PhD
Professor
Department of Exercise and Movement Science
Institute of Neuroscience
University of Oregon
Eugene, Oregon

Contents

—■—

BASIC COMPONENTS OF THE MOTOR SYSTEM

The Cells and Tissues

Overview

In the final analysis, the fundamental properties of the locomotor system are determined by the cells and tissues of which it is composed. Accordingly, any understanding of normal motor behavior must begin with an understanding of the characteristics of these cells and tissues. The purpose of the chapters in this section is to introduce these properties and to demonstrate the ways in which they influence motor activity.

The entire motor system is composed of nerve and muscle cells, all of which are specialized cells called **excitable cells.** Although these cells share the basic structural and biochemical features possessed by all animal cells, they differ from other cells in their fundamental electrical properties. These cells, because of their specialized plasma membranes, can be "excited" to produce action potentials. Neurons are specialized for transmitting these action potentials (impulses) rapidly and accurately throughout the nervous system. In addition, they have extensive interconnections with one another, which provides a mechanism for sorting and processing this information. These capabilities permit the timely initiation and coordination of motor responses undertaken by the motor system.

Skeletal muscle, on the other hand, is specialized to respond to the impulses (commands) of the somatic nervous system with a motor response. The motor system is capable of highly varied and complex motor activities, and much of this flexibility resides in the unique structural and functional properties of the muscles themselves. As will be discussed, skeletal muscle is capable of contractions varying tremendously in force, duration, and precision. Moreover, muscle is a highly adaptable tissue that can respond to functional demands placed on the motor system, with dramatic alterations in muscle size, strength, and endurance.

It should be emphasized that the overall motor system has both afferent and efferent components. Sensory and motor (effector) mechanisms are both anatomically and functionally intertwined. Continuous, detailed sensory input is required for most normal motor activity. Sensory information both triggers volitional and reflex motor behaviors and allows them to be efficiently and accurately carried to completion. Disruption of basic sensory mechanisms may contribute directly to the distortion or loss of motor capabilities.

Although the capabilities inherent in these cells and tissues are the source of the power and diversity of our motor repertoire, they also constrain it. There are distinct limits, for example, on how fast neurons can conduct impulses and how frequently they can be stimulated. In addition, the different skeletal muscles have distinct limits in the force, speed, and duration of contractions that they can produce. The form and complexity of all our motor activities are ultimately defined by the functional limits of these cells.

CHAPTER 1

■

Excitable Cells: Their Morphology and Physiology

Christopher M. Fredericks, PhD

- *Basic Membrane Properties*
- *The Membrane Potential*
- *Electrical Properties of Excitable Cells*
- *Morphology of Excitable Cells*
- *Cell-to-Cell Communication: The Synapse*
- *Disturbances of Excitability and Synaptic Transmission*

*T*he locomotor system is composed of neurons and muscle fibers, all of which are specialized cells called excitable cells. These cells differ from other cells in their fundamental electrical properties. As we shall see, the unique capabilities of these cells equip them to participate in the acquisition, transmission, and processing of information, as well as in the contractile activity on which locomotor activity is based. To understand the functioning of the motor system in all its complexity, it is necessary to have a basic understanding of the electrical properties of the cells of which it is composed.

In the following discussion of these electrical properties, emphasis is placed on the characteristics of neurons. A detailed discussion of muscle follows in Chapter 2.

Basic Membrane Properties[1-6]

The electrical properties of nerve and muscle that are so fundamental to the functioning of the somatic system are rooted in the basic membrane processes present in all animal cells. An understanding of these basic properties is a necessary first step in the understanding of locomotor activity.

The fundamental electrical properties of all cells are determined by the distribution of ions across the cell membrane. This distribution reflects two basic aspects of membrane function: selective permeability and specialized transport proteins.

Selective Permeability

Although the cell (plasma) membrane may seem at first glance to be a very simple structure, it is actually a complex biologic system playing many important roles in overall cell function. The cell membrane not only regulates the passage of substances to and from the cell but also detects signals from the cellular environment and forms physical attachments to other cells. All cell membranes consist of a double layer (bilayer) of lipid molecules in which a variety of proteins are embedded (Fig. 1–1).[5,6] Some of these proteins span the entire membrane and are termed **transmembrane proteins**. Others do not cross the entire membrane but perform functions that are localized to one side of the membrane. The lipid bilayer prevents the passage of most molecules through the membrane, whereas the transmembrane proteins provide discrete pathways for the transfer of certain substances through this lipid barrier.

Cell membranes vary tremendously in the ease with which various substances pass through them. Cell membranes are largely impermeable to intracellular proteins and other organic molecules that make up most of the intracellular anions. The permeability to smaller molecules is more variable, depending on the ability of these substances to penetrate the lipid component of the membrane or to pass through the membrane via various transport proteins embedded in it. The membrane is highly permeable to water. Its permeability to other substances depends on their size, lipid solubility, and charge. Small, uncharged, nonpolar molecules such as carbon dioxide and urea diffuse rapidly through the membrane, whereas large, uncharged, polar molecules such as glucose diffuse much more slowly. **The diffusion of charged particles (i.e., ions) across the membrane is extremely slow.**

Transport Proteins[1–10]

More rapid movement of ions is made possible by their interaction with membrane transport proteins incorporated into the membrane. Some transport proteins are simply channels with an aqueous center that permit ions to diffuse into or out of the cell (Fig. 1–2). Some of these channels are continuously open; others open and close intermittently (i.e., are "gated"). Some are opened or closed by alterations in the membrane potential **(voltage-gated channels)**; others do so by binding to a specific molecule or ligand **(ligand- or substrate-gated channels)**. Such ligands include hormones and neurotransmitters. Typical voltage-gated channels are the sodium or potassium channels; a typical ligand-gated channel

Cell Membrane

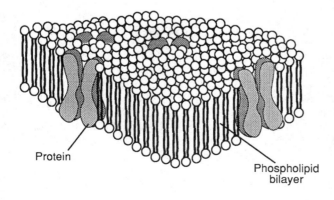

Protein

Phospholipid
bilayer

Figure 1–1. Cell Membrane. All cell membranes consist of a double layer of lipid molecules in which a variety of proteins are embedded.

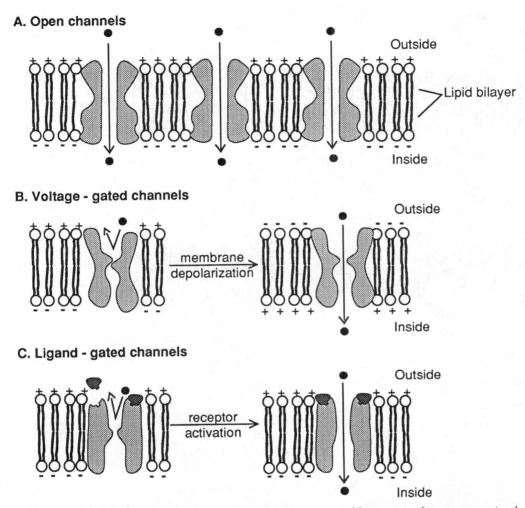

Figure 1–2. *Membrane Transport Proteins.* Cell membranes are traversed by a variety of transport proteins that provide channels for the movement of materials across those membranes. Such channels may (*A*) be continually open or be intermittently opened (*B*) by membrane potential changes or (*C*) by binding with certain substances called ligands.

is the acetylcholine receptor. **Other transport proteins are carriers** that bind ions and other molecules, then by changing their configuration move the bound molecules from one side of the cell membrane to the other (Fig. 1–3). When carriers move substances along their electrical or chemical gradients, no energy is required and the process is called **facilitated diffusion.** When substances are transported against their electrical and chemical gradients, energy is expended and the process is termed **active transport.** In animal cells, energy for active transport is almost always provided by hydrolysis of adenosine triphosphate (ATP), with the carrier molecules themselves having ATPase activity. Perhaps the most important of these systems is the Na^+–K^+ ATPase, which is also known as the Na^+–K^+ pump.[11–13] Na^+–K^+ ATPase is found throughout the body. Active transport of Na^+–K^+ is, in fact, a major energy-consuming process, accounting for about one third of the energy used by cells. In neurons, it accounts for 70% of energy consumption.

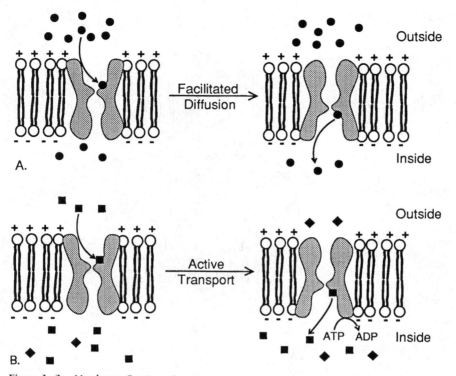

Figure 1–3. *Membrane Carriers.* Carriers are transport proteins that can bind specific molecules and transport them from one side of the membrane to the other. Carriers are required for both (*A*) facilitated diffusion and (*B*) active transport.

The Membrane Potential

Most living cells maintain an electrical potential difference across their plasma membrane (Fig. 1–4).[1] In other words, the membrane is somewhat polarized, the inside being slightly more negative than the outside. **This polarity, termed the** *membrane potential,* **can be measured.** By convention, the polarity of the membrane potential is described in terms of the sign of the excess charge on the inside of the cell. The membrane potential at rest varies from about −5 to −90 mV. In excitable cells it ranges from −60 to −90 mV (e.g., motor neuron, −70 mV; skeletal muscle, −90 mV). In excitable cells, the membrane potential may undergo dramatic changes during excitation, changes that do not occur in nonexcitable cells.

Resting Membrane Potential[1,14–18]

The resting membrane potential is the term used to describe the baseline level of membrane polarization that exists when a cell is at rest. Two transport proteins are fundamental to the generation and maintenance of this potential: a K^+ leak channel that permits K^+ to diffuse out of the cell; and the Na^+–K^+ pump that moves Na^+ out of the cell and K^+ back into the cell (Fig. 1–5). In a normal resting cell, potassium ion diffuses out of the cell along its concentration gradient through the K^+ channels. At the same time, sodium ion diffuses into the cell. However, since the permeability to K^+ is much greater (50 to 100 times) than it is to Na^+, the passive K^+ efflux is much greater than the passive Na^+ influx.

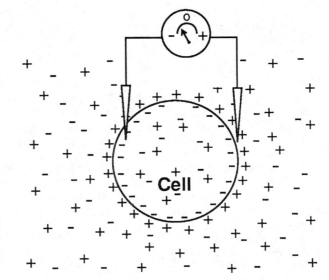

Figure 1–4. *The Membrane Potential.* In most living cells, the cell membrane is somewhat polarized. This reflects a slight excess of positive charge along the outer surface of the cell and a slight excess of negative charge along the inner surface. This polarity can be measured and varies from about –60 to –90 mV in muscle and nerve cells.

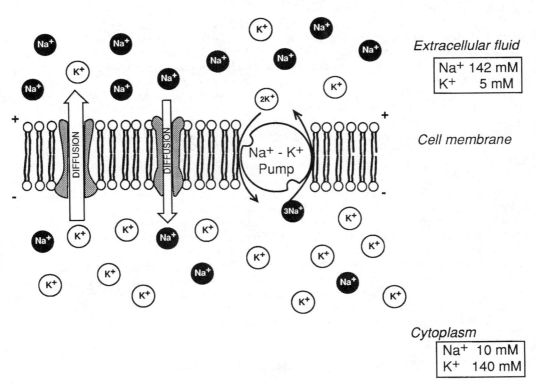

Extracellular fluid

Na⁺	142 mM
K⁺	5 mM

Cell membrane

Cytoplasm

Na⁺	10 mM
K⁺	140 mM

Figure 1–5. *Origins of the Resting Membrane Potential.* The membrane potential results primarily from an unequal distribution of Na^+ and K^+ across the cell membrane. This distribution reflects the varying permeabilities of the membrane to K^+, Na^+ and their associated anions, as well as the ongoing activity of the $Na^+–K^+$ pump. (Adapted from Marieb, EN: Human Anatomy and Physiology, ed 2. The Benjamin/Cummings Publishing Company, Inc., Redwood City, CA, 1992, p 75.)

Because the membrane is impermeable to most of the anions in the cell, the K$^+$ efflux is not accompanied by an equal efflux of anions. In this way, **the membrane is maintained in a polarized state, with the inside negatively charged compared with the outside.** The Na$^+$–K$^+$ pump indirectly contributes to the resting membrane potential by maintaining the concentration gradients down which the ions diffuse to produce most of the charge separation. The pump also makes a small direct contribution to the membrane potential because it pumps three Na$^+$ out of the cell for every two K$^+$ it pumps in. The size of the resting membrane potential is a function of the ionic concentrations present at the cell membrane and can be predicted by the Nernst and Goldman equations. As these mathematical expressions suggest, a change in either ion permeability or ion concentration will alter this potential.

The actual number of ions responsible for the resting membrane potential is a minute fraction of the total number present. The imbalance of positive and negative ions that constitutes the membrane potential is concentrated along the inner and outer surface of the cell membrane. The bulk of the intracellular and extracellular fluid is electrically neutral.

It is important to remember that the resting membrane potential is ultimately dependent on active, energy-requiring processes. Energy is consumed by the Na$^+$–K$^+$ pump, which transports Na$^+$ and K$^+$ across the cell membrane against their respective concentration gradients. Cells obtain energy for this transport from ATP. If the metabolic requirements of these cells are not met, whether it is because of anoxia, ischemia, or some enzymatic defect, ATP production will be impaired and the cell will be unable to generate and maintain a resting potential. As described in later chapters, this can seriously impair both neuronal and muscular activity.

Although calcium ion does not directly contribute to the membrane potential of nerve and muscle, it strongly influences the overall electrical activity of these cells. The concentration gradient of calcium ions across the cell membrane is similar to that of sodium ions, but because of its low permeability, calcium does not share directly in the generation of the charge separation across the membrane. Calcium is, however, bound to the external surface of the membrane, where it influences the membrane responses that occur during activation of the cell. **In general, calcium ions tend to reduce or limit changes in sodium conductance, thereby "stabilizing" the membrane.**[14]

Calcium ions also play a role in the release of neurotransmitter substances that occurs at both neuron-to-neuron synapses and at the neuromuscular junction. Calcium ions may also be involved in the conduction of action potentials in certain dendrites.

The membrane permeability of most cells to chloride is relatively high, and many membranes do not contain Cl$^-$ pumps. In these cells, chloride is distributed according to the charge distribution created by the sodium and potassium interactions previously described, resulting in a greater Cl$^-$ concentration outside the membrane than inside. The concentration difference in chloride across the membrane is thus generated passively by electrical forces, rather than by active pumps, as is the case for sodium and potassium. Chloride ions make no direct contribution to the magnitude of the membrane potential. In cells that do actively transport Cl$^-$, Cl$^-$ diffusion does contribute to the magnitude of the membrane potential. Certain neurons, for example, actively pump Cl$^-$ out of the cell, and the net diffusion of Cl$^-$ back in contributes to the excess negative charge inside the cell; that is, it increases the magnitude of the membrane potential.

Electrical Properties of Excitable Cells

Most cells have a resting membrane potential that is maintained within rather narrow limits. **Excitable cells are distinguished from ordinary cells by the characteristic alterations that occur in their membrane potential when they are stimulated.**[1,14–16,19] These alterations are of two basic types: local graded potentials and action potentials.

Local Graded Potentials[1,14-17,19]

Graded potentials are transient, localized shifts in membrane potential. These may occur in response to various stimuli and may have either a hyperpolarizing or a depolarizing effect. They are called "graded" potentials because the size of the potential change varies with the intensity of the stimulus (Fig. 1-6). These graded potential changes remain relatively localized, restricted to the area of the cell in which they are generated. They do not spread throughout the entire cell. Local potentials of different magnitudes and even different directions can be summated and integrated by single cells and are, therefore, an important contributor to the processing of information within the locomotor system. **Graded potentials include receptor potentials, synaptic potentials (both excitatory and inhibitory), and muscle end-plate potentials.**

Although all graded potentials are analogous to the extent that they arise from localized changes in the permeability of the membrane to one or more ions, they differ in the specifics of these changes. Essentially, four basic mechanisms account for local potential changes:

1. An increase in conductance of potassium increases K^+ efflux from a cell, which results in a hyperpolarization.
2. An increase in conductance of sodium increases Na^+ influx into a cell, which results in a depolarization.
3. An increase in conductance of both sodium and potassium increases Na^+ and K^+ flux in opposite directions, which results in a depolarization but to a lesser extent than in #2.
4. An increase in conductance of chloride increases Cl^- influx into a cell, which results in a hyperpolarization.

As discussed in more detail later, synaptic potentials may involve all these mechanisms. Generator and end-plate potentials involve the third mechanism.

Decremental Conduction

Graded potentials are highly localized, because they are only poorly conducted away from the initial site of stimulation (Fig. 1-7). Whenever a local change in membrane potential occurs, a current will flow between this region and the adjacent regions of the cell membrane. The greater the potential change, the greater the current flow. This local current flow removes positive charges from the nearby regions along the outside of the membrane and adds positive charges to adjacent sites along the inside of the membrane. In this way, the current flow produces depolarization (a decrease in the amount of charge separation) of the adjacent membrane. Because of ions leaking back and forth across the membrane, however,

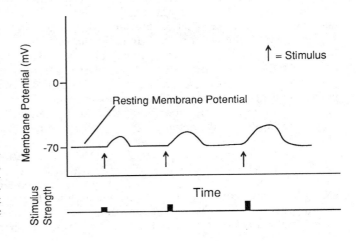

Figure 1-6. *Graded Potentials.* A variety of stimuli may induce transient, localized shifts in the membrane potential of excitable cells. These potential changes are "graded" to the extent that they vary in magnitude with the intensity of the stimulus.

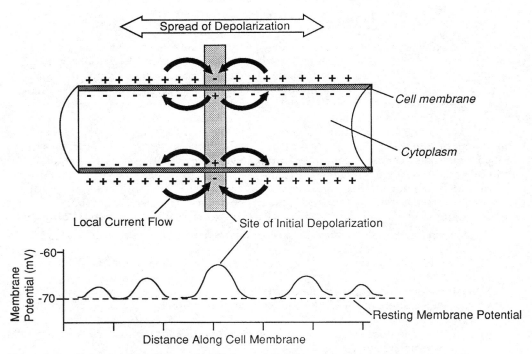

Figure 1–7. *Decremental Conduction of Graded Potentials.* Although graded potentials are conducted by local current flow away from the site in the membrane at which they are initially stimulated, this conduction is not very effective and is highly decremental. Such potentials are highly localized and seldom spread more than a few millimeters from their point of origin.

the magnitude of the current quickly decreases with distance away from the initial site of potential change. In other words, this spread is highly decremental. In fact, local currents and hence graded potentials almost completely die out within a few millimeters of their point of origin. **Accordingly, graded potentials can function as signals over only very short distances** (a few millimeters). Nonetheless, they play very important roles in the integration of signals by excitable cells, especially nerve cells.

Temporal and Spatial Summation

Multiple stimuli and the local graded potential changes that they produce can summate to produce a combined effect. The summation of similar potential changes is additive, whereas hyperpolarizations and depolarizations tend to cancel each other out.

Summation can occur both temporally and spatially (Fig. 1–8). Local potentials are not instantaneous; rather, they develop and subside over intervals of a few milliseconds. Local potentials, therefore, outlast their stimuli. The occurrence of a second stimulus at the same site during the course of the first local potential will summate with any portion of the first potential change that remains. This summation of local potentials that occur near each other in time is **temporal summation.** Different graded potentials have different time courses. The longer the duration of the potential, the more likely temporal summation is to occur. By means of temporal summation, the cell can integrate signals that are arriving at different times.

Although these graded potentials by their very nature remain localized within the region of the cell within which they originate, they do influence by local current flow some adjacent cell membrane. As described previously, the potential will spread, though decrementally, over a finite distance in the membrane (usually a few millimeters). A second stimulus near the first, but not at the same site, will result in summation of the membrane effects in the areas of overlap of the two stimuli; this is **spatial summation.**

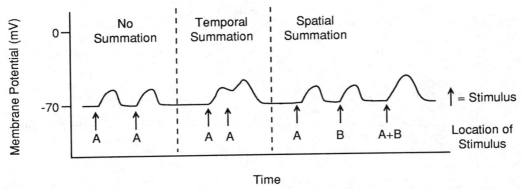

Figure 1–8. *Summation of Local Potentials.* When local potentials are stimulated in rapid succession they may overlap in time, creating an additive effect called *temporal summation.* Similarly, when local potentials are stimulated simultaneously at two different areas in the cell membrane they may overlap spatially, creating *spatial summation.* Summation is critical to the integration of information throughout the locomotor system.

By summating the effects of many stimuli, the membrane of the cell may integrate information arriving from a variety of different sources, impinging on the membrane at different sites and at different moments in time. As we shall see, **temporal and spatial summation are critically important for the processing of both sensory and motor information** within the locomotor system.

Action Potentials[1,14–17,19–23]

Action potentials are rapid alterations in the membrane potential, during which the polarization of the membrane may change from its resting membrane potential (i.e., –60 to –90 mV) to +30 mV and back again in less than 1 msec (Fig. 1–9). Action potentials differ in many respects from local, graded potentials, including their capacity to be propagated over long distances. In fact, only by the propagation of action potentials is the nervous system able to transmit information throughout the locomotor system.

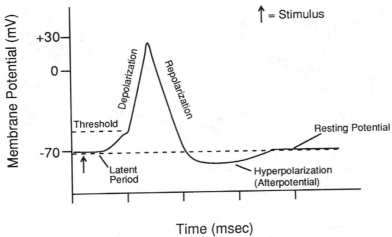

Figure 1–9. *The Action Potential.* This graph shows various components of the action potential defined in terms of the membrane potential.

In the resting state, the membrane ion channels that are open are predominantly those that are permeable to K^+ and Cl^-. Almost all the Na^+ channels are closed. A slight decrease (depolarization) in the resting membrane potential will lead to an automatic redistribution of ions that will restore that potential. Increased K^+ movement out of the cell and simultaneous movement of Cl^- into the cell will result in net movement of positive charge out of the cell with the consequent restoration of the resting membrane potential. These processes occur in all polarized cells and tend to keep the resting membrane potential relatively constant.

In excitable cells, however, reduction of the membrane potential may trigger marked changes in ion permeabilities, which result in the dramatic alterations in membrane electrical characteristics that make up the action potential. In nerve and muscle, when membrane depolarization exceeds some critical threshold value (about 7 mV) above the resting membrane potential, voltage-sensitive sodium channels begin to open, ultimately increasing the membrane permeability to Na^+ up to several thousand-fold.[15,24,25] This allows Na^+ to rush into the cell, along both concentration and electrical gradients (Fig. 1–10). During this period, more positive charges in the form of Na^+ enter the cell than are leaving in the form of K^+. The membrane potential thus decreases and eventually reverses polarity, becoming positive on the inside and negative on the outside of the membrane. This constitutes the **depolarization phase** of the action potential. Once a membrane depolarization begins to activate the sodium channels, the sodium influx intensifies. This causes a further depolarization of the membrane, which actuates more sodium channels, causing even more influx of Na^+, and so on. In this way, the depolarization phase of the action potential is self-accelerating and accounts for the rapidity with which the action potential occurs. The increase in sodium conductance, however, is short-lived, lasting only a fraction of a millisecond. The sodium channels are rapidly closed by the rising membrane potential, accompanied by voltage-stimulated opening of potassium channels. These two events lead to K^+ diffusion out of the cell that is greater than Na^+ diffusion into the cell, returning the membrane potential to its resting level (the **repolarization phase**). The opening and closing of the potassium channels is somewhat slower and more prolonged than that of the sodium channels and explains the persistence of hyperpolarization (**positive afterpotential**), which concludes the action potential.

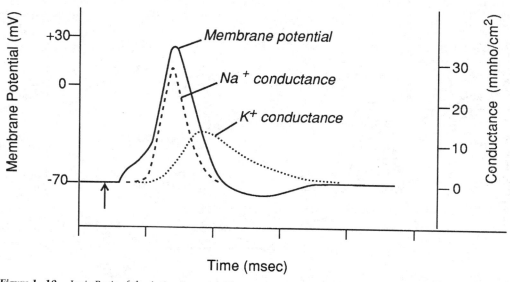

Figure 1–10. *Ionic Basis of the Action Potential.* The action potential is caused by characteristic alterations in the membrane permeability and hence conductance of Na^+ and K^+. In general, Na^+ influx depolarizes, whereas K^+ efflux repolarizes or hyperpolarizes the cell.

The threshold depolarization that triggers the action potential in the first place may be reached by a single local potential or by summating multiple local potentials. This depends on the types of stimuli involved (i.e., at a sensory receptor) or on the types of excitable cells interacting with one another (i.e., at a synapse). **Once the threshold for excitation of a given cell is reached, action potentials will occur with a constant amplitude and form, regardless of the strength of the stimulus. The action potential is therefore described as "all or none" in character.**

The amounts of Na^+ and K^+ that actually move across the membrane during the action potential are extremely small relative to the total numbers present. Nonetheless, if this tiny number of ions crossing the membrane with each action potential were not eventually moved back across the membrane, the concentration gradients of Na^+ and K^+ would gradually disappear and action potentials could no longer be generated. Cellular accumulation of Na^+ and a loss of K^+ is prevented, however, by the continuous action of the Na^+–K^+ pump. Normally, action potentials do not change ion concentrations enough to result in any changes in the resting membrane potential. Significant changes in ion concentrations can be measured only after prolonged, repeated stimulation. Actually, in nerve cells, hundreds of action potentials can occur even after the Na^+–K^+ pump is stopped experimentally.

Excitability[1,14–16,19–25]

The *excitability* of a cell is the ease with which the cell may be stimulated to produce an action potential. During the action potential, characteristic changes occur in the excitability of both nerve and muscle. In nerve, for example, as a local depolarization develops (which ultimately may trigger the action potential), excitation becomes easier as the action potential threshold is approached. Once the action potential is initiated, the ease of stimulation declines. During the rising phase and much of the falling phase of the action potential, the cell is less sensitive to stimulation; it is refractory. An **absolute refractory period** corresponds to the period from the time the threshold is reached until repolarization is partially completed. During this interval, the sodium channels become inactivated, and no amount of excitatory input can reopen them. The only condition that will reopen them is for the membrane potential to return to close to the original resting level. Following the absolute refractory period is a shorter **relative refractory period**, during which a larger than normal stimulus is required to produce an action potential. This relative refractoriness is due both to some sodium channels remaining inactivated and to potassium channels being wide open. After the relative refractory period, while the membrane is still somewhat depolarized and hence closer to threshold, excitability is increased. This is the **supernormal period**. Finally, during the hyperpolarization of the afterpotential, larger stimuli are required. This is the **subnormal period**. Similar changes occur in the muscle cell during excitation. The exact duration of these periods of altered excitability varies appreciably among excitable cells and must be determined empirically for each specific cell type.

The refractoriness of nerve and muscle cells has important implications for their overall function. The absolute refractory period, for example, sets an upper limit on the maximum firing frequency for an axon. This period for large myelinated nerve fibers, for example, is about 1 msec. Therefore, most large mammalian nerves cannot conduct impulses at a frequency higher than about 1000 per second. The refractoriness of the membrane behind an advancing action potential also plays a major role in preventing impulses from reversing their direction.

As we have seen, the excitability of nerve and muscle reflects the distribution of ions across the cell membrane. **Changes in the extracellular concentration of various ions may** effect this distribution and thereby **alter excitability,** possibly with clinical consequences. Because the sodium permeability at rest is so low, changing the external sodium concentration has little effect on the resting membrane potential, although this may change the size of the action potential. Changing extracellular potassium, on the other hand, may markedly alter the membrane potential. Reduced extracellular potassium (hypokalemia) by promoting the efflux of K^+ increases the resting membrane potential, thereby making nerve and muscle cells more difficult to excite (i.e., to depolarize to action potential threshold). Clinically, hypokalemia is often manifested as muscle weakness. Increased external potassium (hyper-kalemia) acts to decrease the membrane potential, bringing it closer to the threshold for excitation. Although not directly involved in establishing the membrane polarity, either at rest or during the action potential, calcium influences excitability by virtue of its role in "stabilizing" or controlling ion channels. The extracellular concentration of Ca^{2+} affects the voltage level at which the sodium channels are activated (opened). When Ca^{2+} is deficient in the extracellular fluid, the amount of membrane depolarization necessary to initiate the changes in Na^+ conductance that produce the action potential is reduced. A nerve fiber may therefore become highly excitable, sometimes discharging spontaneously and repetitively. In this way, hypocalcemia may be manifested clinically as hyperirritability of peripheral motor neurons, which causes excessive, involuntary muscle activity called tetany. Increased Ca^{2+} concentrations, on the other hand, decrease the excitability of muscle and nerve.

Certain chemical agents disturb the cellular processes underlying excitation and are used to purposely alter excitability. Among these substances are a variety of local anesthetics (e.g., cocaine, procaine, and tetracaine) that act directly on the sodium channels, making it more difficult for these gates to open, thus reducing membrane excitability. Local anesthetics can disrupt excitation and impulse conduction in both sensory and motor neurons, as well as affect muscle directly.

Propagation[1,14–16,19–25]

One of the most important characteristics of the action potential is its capacity to propagate itself over long distances. An action potential initiated in any region of a nerve or muscle fiber will spread to all other regions of that cell in a nondecremental fashion. This characteristic permits the nervous system to transmit information throughout the body.

When an area of the membrane is depolarized during an action potential, ionic currents flow both across and along that membrane (Fig. 1–11A). In the area of the depolarization, Na^+ flows inward across the membrane carrying positive charges (current). Current also flows longitudinally for several millimeters along both the inside and the outside of the membrane. This flow of positive charges tends to depolarize adjacent regions of the membrane. In normal tissue, this depolarization is sufficient to shift the membrane to threshold, thereby activating sodium channels and generating an action potential in the immediately surrounding membrane. In this way, **an action potential can spread in all directions away from its site of initiation until the entire membrane of an axon or muscle fiber has been depolarized.** Because of its refractory period, the potential cannot reverse and spread back into an area just depolarized and will only be conducted away from its origin.

Unlike local potentials, action potentials are conducted so effectively that their amplitude does not diminish during their propagation. This is *nondecremental conduction.* In this way, no distortion occurs as propagation takes place along the membrane; the action potential arriving at the end of the cell is identical with the initial one. Occasionally, in an abnormal fiber the action potential may reach a point on the membrane at which it does not generate sufficient voltage to stimulate the adjacent areas of the membrane. At this point, its propagation stops.

Action potentials in skeletal muscle cells are initiated near the middle of the cell and propagate toward the two opposite ends. In most nerve cells, on the other hand, action potentials are initiated at one end of the cell and propagate toward the other end. In addition, the zone of refractoriness trailing behind each action potential prevents the impulse from reversing direction (Fig. 1–12). In this way, physiologic impulses normally pass along axons in one direction, the **orthodromic** direction, arising at synaptic junctions or receptors, to be propagated to the other end of the neuron. Conduction in the opposite direction is called **antidromic.** Since chemical synapses, unlike axons, permit conduction in one direction only, any antidromic impulses that arise will fail to pass the first synapse they encounter. Axons can be artificially stimulated along their length to conduct impulses in both directions. Although this is not natural, antidromic conduction can be used in studies of conduction velocity.

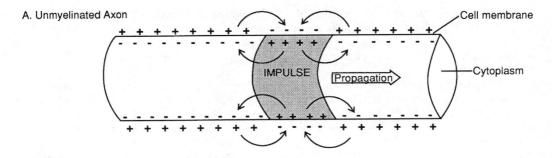

A. Unmyelinated Axon

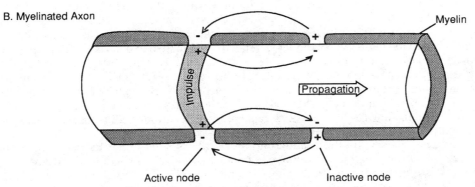

B. Myelinated Axon

Figure 1–11. *Action Potential Propagation.* Action potentials are conducted along excitable cell membranes by local current flow (movement of positive charges) that depolarizes adjacent areas of the membrane. The region of electronegativity (the impulse) provides a sink for this current flow as indicated by the curved arrows. (*A*) In unmyelinated fibers, the impulse is propagated as a continuous wave of depolarization spreading along the cell. (*B*) In myelinated fibers, the impulse "jumps" from node to node, a process called *saltatory conduction.*

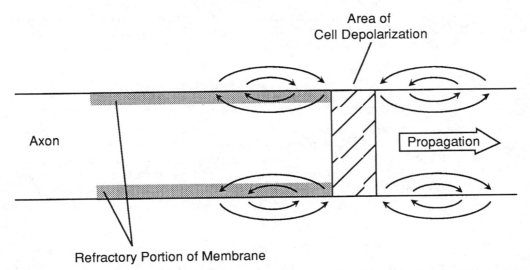

Figure 1–12. *Membrane Refractoriness.* The refractoriness of the membrane behind an advancing action potential prevents the impulse from reversing its direction, thus maintaining the unidirectionality of propagation. (Adapted from Smith, CUM: Neurobiology, ed 2. Oxford University Press, New York, 1988, p 300.)

In neurons, the rate of conduction of the action potential along the membrane depends on fiber diameter and on whether or not the fiber is myelinated. The larger the fiber diameter, the faster the action potential is propagated. A large fiber offers less resistance to longitudinal current flow, and thus adjacent regions of the membrane are brought to threshold faster.

Many axons in the central and peripheral nervous system, especially within the locomotor system, demonstrate increased conduction velocity because they are insulated with a fatty substance called *myelin*. A myelinated axon is fully sheathed in myelin except at areas called the *nodes of Ranvier*. Since the insulator, myelin, makes it more difficult for current to flow across the membrane, action potentials do not occur in the sections of membrane protected by myelin; they occur only at the nodes of Ranvier where the myelin is interrupted. An action potential at one node produces sufficient longitudinal current flow to depolarize adjacent nodes to threshold, thereby propagating the action potential, skipping from one node to the next (see Fig. 1–11*B*). This is saltatory conduction. *Saltatory conduction* causes a more rapid conduction of the action potential than occurs in nonmyelinated fibers of the same axon diameter, with myelinated axons conducting up to 50 times faster than the fastest unmyelinated fibers. Conduction velocities range from about 0.5 m/s for small-diameter unmyelinated fibers to more than 120 m/s for large-diameter myelinated fibers. Saltatory conduction is also beneficial to the extent that it conserves energy for the axon. Since only the nodes of Ranvier depolarize, much less energy is expended reestablishing the sodium and potassium concentration differences across the membrane after a series of nerve impulses.

The largest, most rapidly conducting nerve fibers are found in the peripheral locomotor system carrying motor commands to skeletal muscle. As will be discussed later, this capacity for high-velocity conduction is fundamental to the function of the motor system, allowing rapid transmission of information over the long distances that intervene between the information processing areas of the central nervous system and the skeletal muscle out in the periphery. When conduction velocities are pathologically slowed, motor function is impaired. Measurement of peripheral conduction velocities is a useful diagnostic tool, with many pathologic processes producing detectable changes in velocity. In multiple sclerosis, for example, pathologic destruction of myelin in the central nervous system results in delayed or blocked conduction in a variety of pathways.

It is important to remember that **action potential (impulse) conduction** along an axon, or muscle fiber for that matter, is not a passive process as occurs with the conduction of electricity through a wire. It **is an active process requiring that the basic structure and function of the cell membrane be normal.** As will be discussed in later chapters, all kinds of locomotor disturbances can arise when these processes are disturbed.

Morphology of Excitable Cells

The locomotor system is composed of excitable cells. These cells have a highly specialized morphology, which allows them to efficiently carry out specific types of activities within the locomotor system. Neurons are specialized for the processing and transmission of information, whereas muscle cells are specialized for responding to excitation with contraction. The structure of neurons is described here, whereas that of muscle is considered in Chapter 2.

Nerve Cells[25–30]

The basic functional unit of the nervous system is the individual nerve cell or neuron. Neurons, which have evolved from primitive neuroeffector cells, are excitable cells that are specialized for the processing and transmission of information. As previously described, this

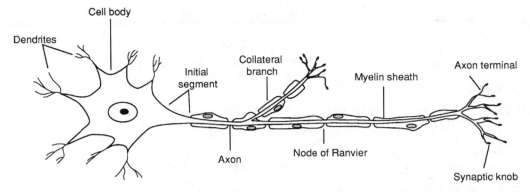

Figure 1–13. *General Structure of a Neuron.* In this case, a somatic spinal motoneuron is used to illustrate the characteristic morphologic features of neurons.

information is coded in the form of different types of electrical activity, ranging from local, graded potentials to action potentials.

Neurons occur in a diverse assortment of specialized shapes and sizes, but most have the same fundamental structure. The basic morphologic features of the neuron are well illustrated by the typical spinal motor neuron (Fig. 1–13). The spinal motor neuron, like most neurons, consists of three basic parts: (1) the cell body, (2) the dendrites, and (3) the axon. The **cell body, soma,** or **perikaryon** contains a well-defined nucleus and nucleolus surrounded by granular cytoplasm. Within the cytoplasm are typical cellular organelles such as lysosomes, mitochondria, and Golgi complexes. Active neurons also contain a well-developed rough endoplasmic reticulum (Nissl bodies), which functions in protein synthesis, and a system of microtubules and neurofibrils, which functions in cell transport. The cell body is the metabolic center of the cell, where, under the control of the nucleus, proteins and other metabolically important substances are produced. The **dendrites** are highly branched outgrowths of the cell body. Like the cell body, they typically contain endoplasmic reticulum, mitochondria, and other cytoplasmic organelles. A spinal motor neuron usually has five to seven main dendrites, which themselves are extensively branched. Dendrites serve as the chief receptive apparatus for the neuron and conduct impulses toward the cell body. The **axon** is a long, single process extending from the cell body that conducts nerve impulses away from the soma. It originates from a somewhat thickened area of the cell body, the axon hillock. The first portion of the axon is the initial segment, which is the region of the axon at which the action potential is usually initiated. Along the length of the axon, there may be small side branches called collaterals. The axon and its collaterals terminate by branching into many fine filaments called axon terminals or telodendria. Each of these ends in a bulblike synaptic knob or bouton. The cytoplasm of the axon contains mitochondria and neurofibrils but, unlike the cell body, does not contain the ribosomes and rough endoplasmic reticulum required for protein synthesis. The synaptic knobs are notable for their numerous granules or vesicles in which are stored the synaptic transmitters secreted by the neuron.

Many axons, including those of spinal motor neurons, are covered by a multilayered sheath made of myelin, a fatty material formed by the plasma membranes of specialized cells that are closely associated with the axons.[31] The myelin sheath envelops the axon except at its terminus and at the nodes of Ranvier that are about 1 mm apart. In the periphery, the myelin sheath is formed by Schwann cells. In the central nervous system, many neurons are also myelinated, but the cells that form the myelin are oligodendrogliocytes rather than Schwann cells. Myelin sheaths are first laid down during the latter part of fetal development and during the first year of life. The amount of myelin increases with growth and development, and its presence greatly increases the speed of nerve impulse conduction. Since myelination is still progressing during infancy, an infant's responses to stimuli are not

Table 1–1. *Basic Classes of Neurons*

Afferent Neurons

Function—Transmit impulses arising in sensory receptors into the CNS.
    Each neuron, including its cell body and long peripheral axon, is outside the CNS.
    Only a relatively short axonal process enters the CNS.

Efferent Neurons

Function—Transmit impulses from the CNS to effector cells (muscles or glands) in the periphery.
    The cell body, dendrites, and a short segment of axon are within the CNS.
    Most of the axon is outside the CNS.

Interneurons

Function—Connect neurons within the brain and spinal cord for processing and integration of information.
    They account for about 99% of all neurons.
    All are located within the CNS.

---

as rapid or coordinated as those of an older child or an adult. Some mammalian nerve cells are not myelinated at all, but are simply surrounded by Schwann cells.

Neurons exist in many shapes and sizes. **Regardless of their form, neurons can be divided functionally into three basic types:** afferent neurons, efferent neurons, and interneurons (Table 1–1). Portions of afferent and efferent neurons lie outside the central nervous system, whereas interneurons lie entirely within the central nervous system. **Afferent neurons** are specialized for "sensing" or responding to changes in their environment. At their peripheral endings, afferent neurons have sensory receptors that are designed to be excited by special types of stimuli, such as light, sound, heat, and pressure. As a result of their stimulation, afferent neurons send impulses *to* the central nervous system. **Efferent neurons,** on the other hand, transmit impulses *from* the central nervous system to effector cells (muscle or gland) in the periphery. **Interneurons,** which account for about 99% of all nerve cells, connect cells within the brain or spinal cord and function in the processing and integration of information.

Neurons can also be classified structurally on the basis of the number of processes that extend from the cell body (Fig. 1–14). **Bipolar neurons,** for example, have two processes, one at either end. This type is found in the retina of the eye. **Multipolar neurons** have several dendrites and a single axon extending from the cell body. In mammalian systems, this is by far the most common type of nerve cell. Motor neurons are good examples of multipolar neurons. Within this category, the morphology of different cells varies greatly. Differences among multipolar cells are largely due to variations in the number and length of the dendrites and in the length of the axon. The number and extent of the dendritic processes in a given cell correlate with the number of synaptic contacts that other neurons make on that cell. The length of the axon (which may vary from a few millimeters to more than 1 m) reflects the signaling function of a neuron. Neurons with long axons carry information from one region of the central nervous system to another or to and from the periphery. Neurons with short axons primarily process information within a small limited region of the nervous system. These cells serve as local interneurons in various nuclei of the brain and in reflex pathways. Many other differences in structure exist as well.

Pseudounipolar neurons have a single short process emanating from the cell body that divides like a T to form a longer process. Many sensory neurons are pseudounipolar, with one end of the long process receiving sensory stimuli and the other synapsing with cells within the central nervous system. Located along the middle of the axon, sensory neuron cell bodies may be better protected from injury than if they were situated way out in the periphery along with the receptor structures. Regardless of where the cell body is located, the basic receptive function of the dendrites and the transmission function of the axon are the same.

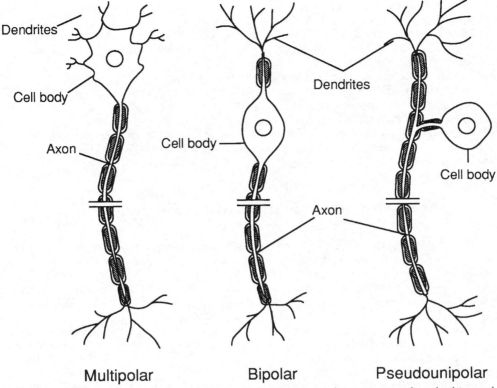

Figure 1-14. *General Structural Types of Neurons.* Multipolar neurons have numerous short dendrites and one long axon; bipolar neurons have one axon and one dendrite; pseudounipolar neurons have one short branch that bifurcates to form an axon and a dendrite. (Adapted from Rhoades, S and Pflanzer, P: Human Physiology. Saunders College Publishing, Philadelphia, 1989, p 217.)

Because the axon and nerve terminals lack ribosomes and the rest of the cellular apparatus necessary for the synthesis of proteins and other essential cellular constituents, these materials must be synthesized elsewhere in the neuron and transported to axonal sites of utilization. All necessary proteins and other cell components are synthesized in the endoplasmic reticulum and Golgi apparatus of the cell body and carried along the axon by specialized axonal transport systems.[30-33] There are two basic types of axonal transport. Slow transport is unidirectional, carrying cytosolic proteins from the cell body down the axon at a rate ranging from 0.2 to 2 mm/d. Constituents transported in this manner include microtubules and neurofilaments used in renewal of the cytoskeleton and various enzymes catalyzing the reactions of intermediary metabolism. In contrast, the fast-transport system is a bidirectional system that functions in the antegrade transport of both membrane and secretory proteins as well as in the retrograde retrieval of material from the synaptic milieu. For example, while synaptic vesicles are extensively recycled in the terminal membrane, some used vesicles are carried back to the cell body and deposited in lysosomes. Moreover, some of the materials taken up at the nerve ending by endocytosis (e.g., nerve growth factor) are carried back to the cell body. The rate of transport is 250 to 400 mm/d.

As discussed in more detail in Chapter 15, recent research has shown that defects in axonal transport are central to the pathogenesis of many neuronal disorders. Inadequate rates of delivery and delivery of abnormal materials may impair the maintenance of axonal structure and function. When severed from the cell body, a neuron process quickly degenerates. In addition, abnormal retrograde transport may provide undesirable toxic and biologic agents access to the cell body. Tetanus toxin, as well as polio, rabies, herpes, and other viruses, may reach the central nervous system by this route.

Note that **only about 10% of the cells in the nervous system are neurons; the remainder are glial cells, or neuroglia.** These cells, which are generally smaller than neurons, form a supportive network for neurons and line the ventricles of the brain and the central canal of the spinal cord. Specialized glial cells also produce myelin, whereas others scavenge microbes and other debris from the central nervous system by phagocytosis. Glial cells have a membrane potential that varies with the external K^+ concentration but do not generate propagated potentials. These cells may produce substances that are trophic to neurons. Glia are of particular clinical interest because they are a common source of tumors (gliomas) of the nervous system. Gliomas may account for 40% to 50% of brain tumors and are highly invasive.

Cell-to-Cell Communication: The Synapse

Throughout the locomotor system, excitable cells communicate with one another. This communication is accomplished through cell-to-cell interactions termed synapses.[19,22,34–40] Synapses provide a mechanism not only for the transmission of excitation from one cell to the next but also for the extensive processing of that information. Even the simplest examples of motor activity involve many muscle fibers, neurons, and synapses.

Synapses within the locomotor system may occur between neurons or between a motor neuron and a muscle cell. The latter are discussed in Chapter 3. Neuronal synapses most often occur between the axon terminal of one neuron, and the cell body or dendrites of a second neuron. In certain regions, synapses may also occur between dendrites, between a dendrite and a cell body, or between an axon terminal and a second axon terminal. **A neuron conducting impulses toward a synapse is called a** *presynaptic neuron,* **whereas neurons conducting signals away from a synapse are** *postsynaptic neurons.* In a multineuronal pathway, a single neuron can be postsynaptic to one group of cells and simultaneously presynaptic to another.

A postsynaptic neuron may have thousands of synaptic junctions on the surface of its dendrites and cell body, so that signals from many presynaptic neurons converge on it. A single spinal motor neuron, for example, probably receives about 10,000 synaptic endings. Neurons in other parts of the spinal cord and brain may receive presynaptic terminals ranging from only a few to more than 150,000. These differences make neurons in different parts of the nervous system react differently to incoming signals and therefore perform different functions. In the case of the neuromuscular junction, one neuron synapses with each muscle cell.

There are two types of synapses—electrical and chemical (Fig. 1–15).[34,35] At **electrical synapses,** the plasma membranes of the presynaptic and postsynaptic cells are joined together by gap junctions that allow the local currents accompanying an action potential in the presynaptic neuron to flow directly into the postsynaptic neuron, inducing a postsynaptic action potential. Most of the synapses in the human nervous system, however, are **chemical synapses** and depend on presynaptically released chemicals called **neurotransmitters** to stimulate the postsynaptic neuron. Although electrical synapses have the advantage of rapid transmission without delay, chemical synapses provide many more inherent opportunities for adjustment and control of signal transmission. As we shall see, this capacity is fundamental to all aspects of motor control.

Figures 1–15*B* and 1–16 illustrate the structure of a typical **chemical synapse.** The basic features of different chemical synapses are relatively constant. The terminal filament of the presynaptic neuron ends in a swollen terminal called the synaptic knob or bouton. These terminal knobs contain abundant mitochondria and synaptic vesicles. **A narrow gap or synaptic cleft** (usually 200 to 300 Å wide) **separates the presynaptic and postsynaptic**

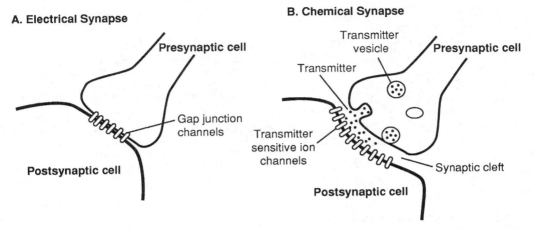

A. Electrical Synapse

Presynaptic cell

Gap junction channels

Postsynaptic cell

B. Chemical Synapse

Transmitter vesicle

Transmitter

Presynaptic cell

Transmitter sensitive ion channels

Synaptic cleft

Postsynaptic cell

Figure 1–15. Comparison of Electrical and Chemical Synapses. (A) In electrical synapses, signal transmission from one excitable cell to another is accomplished by direct electrical coupling through gap junctions. (B) In chemical synapses, transmission is accomplished through the liberation of a chemical transmitter from the presynaptic cell that alters the membrane potential of the postsynaptic cell. (Adapted from Patton, HD, et al: Textbook of Physiology, ed 21. WB Saunders, Philadelphia, 1989, p. 131.)

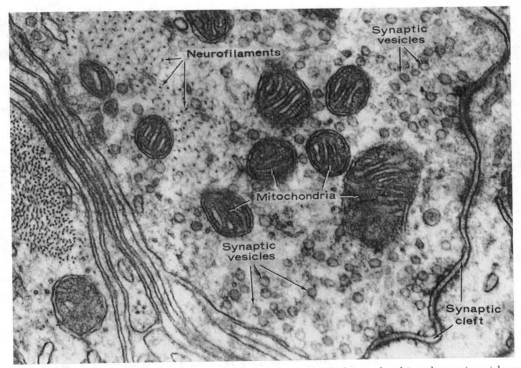

Neurofilaments

Synaptic vesicles

Mitochondria

Synaptic vesicles

Synaptic cleft

Figure 1–16. Electron Micrograph of a Typical Chemical Synapse. Multiple mitochondria and synaptic vesicles are evident in the nerve filament, and a typical synaptic cleft is visible between the presynaptic and postsynaptic membranes. (From Fawcett, DW: A Textbook of Histology, ed 11, p 349, with permission. Copyright © 1986 Chapman & Hall, New York.)

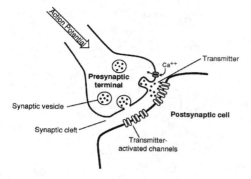

Figure 1–17. *Major Steps in Neurochemical Transmission.* The presynaptic neuron terminal contains many small vesicles containing neurotransmitter. With the arrival of an action potential at the neuron terminal, many of these vesicles fuse to the presynaptic membrane and release their contents into the synaptic cleft. This release is associated with increased Ca^{2+} flux across the presynaptic membrane. The liberated transmitter diffuses across the synaptic cleft, binding with postsynaptic receptors and opening ligand-gated channels. Alterations in ion fluxes and in the postsynaptic membrane potential follow.

neurons and prevents the direct propagation of current from the presynaptic neuron to the postsynaptic cell. **Signals are transmitted across the synaptic cleft by means of a neurotransmitter** substance released from the presynaptic axon terminal (Fig. 1–17). This transmitter substance is stored in the vesicles of the terminal. When an action potential arrives at the end of the axon and depolarizes the terminal membrane, small quantities of the neurotransmitter are released from the presynaptic terminal into the synaptic cleft. Specifically, depolarization of the synaptic terminal causes voltage-sensitive calcium channels in the terminal membrane to open and calcium to diffuse inward across the presynaptic membrane. This influx of calcium causes some of the presynaptic vesicles containing transmitter to fuse with specific release sites on the inner surface of the plasma membrane and to release their contents into the synaptic cleft by a process called **exocytosis.** Often, several hundred vesicles release their transmitter into the cleft following a single action potential. Having released their transmitter contents, the vesicles are pinched off from the membrane to be reused or replaced. Although the neuron terminals are capable of manufacturing some substances, such as the neurotransmitter acetylcholine, they depend on the delivery of many materials, such as enzymes, neuropeptides, and membrane components, from the neuron cell body where they are synthesized.

Once released from the axon terminal, the transmitter molecules diffuse across the cleft and bind to specific receptor sites on the postsynaptic membrane. Combination of the transmitter with the receptor site opens specific ion channels in the postsynaptic cell membrane. These ligand-gated channels are normally closed and open only as a result of binding with a specific neurotransmitter. There is a slight delay between the arrival of the impulse at the presynaptic terminal and the onset of the postsynaptic response. This pause lasts less than 1 msec and is called the **synaptic delay;** it results mainly from the time required for the release of transmitter from the axon terminal. The time required for the transmitter to diffuse across the synaptic cleft is negligible.

After a transmitter is released into the synaptic cleft, it binds with and activates (opens) almost immediately the ion channels with which it specifically interacts. These channels, however, remain open only briefly and quickly close. The reason for this is that **the transmitter is rapidly removed from the synaptic cleft** and hence from its receptor sites. Removal of transmitter is accomplished by (1) **diffusion** of the transmitter out of the cleft, (2) **enzymatic destruction** of the transmitter within the cleft, or (3) **active transport** of the transmitter back into the presynaptic axon terminal to be reused. This is called reuptake. The degree to which each of these methods of removal is used is different for each type of synapse and transmitter.

Because transmitter is stored and released only on the presynaptic side of the synaptic cleft and the receptor sites are on the postsynaptic side, **chemical synapses operate in only one direction.** This one-way transmission imposes a directionality on the flow of information within the nervous system. Action potentials can move along a given multineuronal pathway in one direction only. This is critical to the orderly processing and transmission of information.

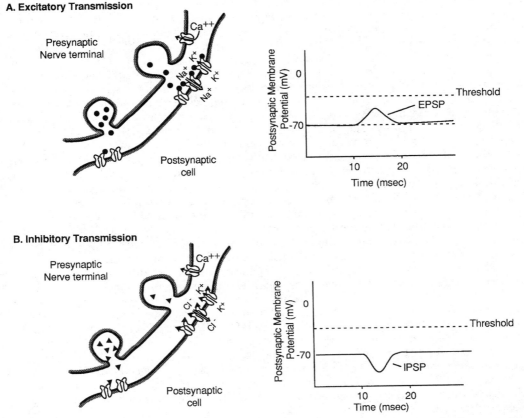

Figure 1–18. *Comparison of Excitatory and Inhibitory Synaptic Transmission.* (A) In an excitatory synapse, the postsynaptic response to the neurotransmitter is depolarization (produced, for example, by opening Na^+ and K^+ channels), which moves the postsynaptic membrane potential closer to the action potential threshold. (B) Activation of an inhibitory synapse results in postsynaptic hyperpolarization (produced, for example, by opening Cl^- channels), which reduces the likelihood of a postsynaptic action potential.

Neurotransmitters can cause both excitation and inhibition, depending on the nature of the transmitter and the type of receptor present on the postsynaptic membrane. In some cases, a single transmitter may cause excitation or inhibition, depending on the type of postsynaptic receptor. In other instances, the same postsynaptic cell may be excited or inhibited, depending on the type of transmitter present. More than 30 different substances have been implicated in neurotransmission. It is believed that each neuron releases only one type of transmitter and that it releases the same transmitter from all of its separate terminals.

The following discussion of synaptic function focuses on the characteristics of nerve-to-nerve interactions; details of nerve to muscle communication are discussed in Chapter 3.

Excitatory Synapses[19,34–40]

At an excitatory synapse, the postsynaptic response to the neurotransmitter is depolarization, bringing the membrane potential closer to the threshold for generation of an action potential (Fig. 1–18A). Here the effect of the transmitter binding to its receptor site is to simultaneously increase the permeability to both sodium and potassium. These ions are then free to move according to the electrical and chemical gradients present across the membrane. Because both the electrical and chemical gradients promote flux of sodium into the cell and because in the case of potassium the electrical gradient is opposed by the concentration gradient, the opening of these channels results primarily in Na^+ rushing to the inside of the membrane. There is thus a net movement of positive ions into the neuron, slightly depolarizing the postsynaptic membrane. **This depolarization is termed the** *excitatory postsynaptic potential* (EPSP). The magnitude of the EPSP is proportional to the amount of transmitter released. The size of the EPSP tends to increase in "steps," reflecting the fact that transmitter is released in discrete packets or quanta corresponding to the contents of individual synaptic vesicles. The release of the contents of a single presynaptic vesicle does not ordinarily increase the postsynaptic potential to threshold. Instead, an increase of this magnitude requires the discharge of many vesicles at the same time or in rapid succession and summation of their effects. An estimated discharge of about 70 presynaptic vesicles is required for the activation of a single spinal motor neuron.

The EPSP differs in many respects from the action potential. First, **the EPSP is a local, graded potential that functions to bring the postsynaptic membrane potential toward its threshold.** Unlike the action potential, it is neither all or none nor propagated along the neuron (or muscle cell). Second, the increases in permeability to sodium and potassium that produce the potential change are simultaneous rather than sequential, as occurs in the action potential. Third, the EPSP is not followed by a refractory period. It is usually necessary for numerous EPSPs to summate in order to evoke an action potential. If the EPSP had a refractory period, summation of successive EPSPs would be more difficult.

After the postsynaptic membrane is depolarized to threshold, an action potential occurs. The action potential, however, does not arise on the somal membrane adjacent to the excitatory synapses. Instead, **it begins in the initial segment of the axon** (see Fig. 1–13). The soma has relatively few voltage-gated sodium channels in its membrane, which makes it difficult to open the number of channels necessary for eliciting the action potential. On the other hand, the membrane of the initial segment of the axon has a much greater concentration of voltage-gated sodium channels and therefore can much more readily generate an action potential. Once the action potential begins, it travels both outward along the axon and backward over the soma. It may also travel backward into some of the dendrites, but not into all of them because they, like the soma, have very few voltage-gated sodium channels.

When excitatory synapses are repeatedly stimulated at a rapid rate, the rate of discharge of the postsynaptic cell eventually declines because of fatigue of synaptic transmission. Fatigue is an important characteristic of synaptic function. When an area of the nervous system becomes overexcited, fatigue ultimately curtails this excessive activity. Synaptic fatigue is, for example, a major contributor to the waning of convulsions and to muscle fatigue following extremely intense motor activity. Synaptic fatigue is mainly due to exhaustion of neurotransmitter. Progressive inactivation of postsynaptic receptors and an accumulation of Ca^{2+} inside the postsynaptic cell may also be involved.

Inhibitory Synapses[19,34–40]

Activation of an inhibitory synapse produces changes in the postsynaptic membrane that reduce the likelihood of the cell generating an action potential (see Fig. 1–18B). **At an inhibitory synapse, binding of the neurotransmitter to its receptor sites on the postsynaptic membrane usually opens potassium or chloride channels or both.** Since the equilibrium potentials for both Cl^- and K^+ in neurons are usually more negative than the resting membrane potential, **these permeability changes lead to a hyperpolarization of the membrane.** This hyperpolarization is called *an inhibitory postsynaptic potential* (IPSP). The IPSP moves the membrane potential away from the threshold for excitation and thus makes the stimulation of an action potential less likely. Like EPSPs, IPSPs can summate both spatially and temporally. Simultaneous EPSPs and IPSPs tend to nullify each other.

In cells in which the equilibrium potential for Cl^- is equal to the resting membrane potential (i.e., those in which Cl^- are not actively transported), a rise in Cl^- permeability will not generate an IPSP, but will still decrease the likelihood that the cell will reach threshold during excitatory input. This is because it increases the amount of sodium current necessary to displace the membrane potential away from the resting potential. In some synapses, IPSPs are elicited not by opening potassium or chloride channels but by closing sodium channels.

Postsynaptic inhibition serves to moderate motor activity. Certain substances can prevent this from occurring. A toxin produced by the tetanus bacterium, for example, blocks inhibitory interneurons from impinging on motor neurons to skeletal muscle. This reduces the inhibitory input to these neurons and leaves the excitatory inputs unchecked, resulting in grossly exaggerated muscle activity. Extremely powerful muscle spasms and convulsions result (tetanus). The chemical, strychnine, has very similar effects.

Presynaptic Inhibition[19,34-40]

At any specific synapse, inhibition can be asserted at both presynaptic and postsynaptic sites. Postsynaptic inhibition (discussed previously) refers to a hyperpolarization of the postsynaptic membrane that acts to reduce the effectiveness of any synaptic input to that neuron. **In presynaptic inhibition, inhibitory neurons form synaptic connections with a presynaptic neuron** (Fig. 1–19). The effect of this presynaptic input is to decrease the influx of Ca^{2+} into the nerve terminal that would normally accompany the presynaptic action potential. **This causes a reduction in the amount of transmitter it releases** and thus reduces the postsynaptic potential. In this way, presynaptic inhibition is selective, inhibiting only certain presynaptic terminals and leaving other inputs to the postsynaptic neuron unaffected. Presynaptic inhibition also encompasses a different time frame than does postsynaptic inhibition. Presynaptic inhibition requires many milliseconds to develop and can last minutes or even hours. Postsynaptic inhibition, as might occur at a spinal motor neuron, lasts for only 10 to 15 msec. Presynaptic inhibition is critically important for imposing a degree of restraint on the motor system. In its absence, motor activity may become intolerably intense.

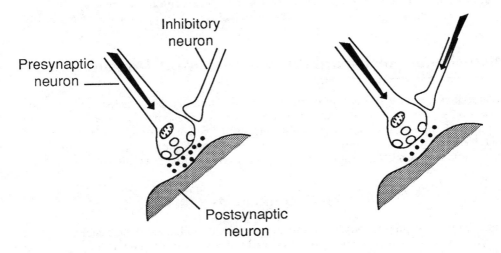

a) **Presynaptic inhibitory neuron inactive**

b) **Presynaptic inhibitory neuron active**

Figure 1–19. *Presynaptic Inhibition.* Presynaptic inhibitory neurons reduce the amount of transmitter released by decreasing the influx of Ca^{2+} associated with the presynaptic action potential.

Presynaptic Facilitation

Presynaptic synapses may also result in facilitation of synaptic transmission. In this instance, presynaptic influx of Ca^{2+} is enhanced. This is possibly brought about by prolongation of the action potential causing more persistent Ca^{2+} influx, and hence, prolonged transmitter release.

Integrative Function of the Synapse[19,22,39-41]

The synapse is not only the site at which communication occurs between excitable cells, it is also the site at which information flowing between these cells is processed. Most postsynaptic neurons receive inputs from many presynaptic cells. Moreover, these presynaptic neurons may themselves be influenced by other neurons impinging upon their axon terminals. The generation of a postsynaptic action potential is the net consequence of the influences exerted by all of these participating cells. As discussed previously, the postsynaptic cell may be both excited and inhibited by neurotransmitters, producing EPSPs and IPSPs, respectively. On balance, this cell will be influenced to the extent that these **EPSPs and IPSPs summate** both temporally and spatially. In other words, the excitatory and inhibitory influences impinging upon the postsynaptic membrane are "integrated" **to yield a net inclination or disinclination to fire.** The synaptic output (impulse pattern) is thus an integrated summary of all the synaptic inputs. For example, as we shall see, motor commands traveling to skeletal muscle in the form of spinal motor neuron action potentials are the result of thousands of complementary and conflicting influences converging on the anterior horn cell. The integration that occurs at all levels of the central nervous system is necessary for the control of motor activity.

The synapse between nerve and skeletal muscle is in many respects simpler than that of many neuron-to-neuron contacts. Only one presynaptic terminus communicates with each postsynaptic membrane (end plate), using only one excitatory neurotransmitter (acetylcholine) acting on one type of excitatory postsynaptic receptor. Consequently, relatively little processing of information occurs at the neuromuscular junction. The processing required for motor control has already been accomplished within the central nervous system. The simplicity of this synapse permits rapid, discrete activation of skeletal muscle fibers.

Disturbances of Excitability and Synaptic Transmission

Neuronal excitability and synaptic transmission are complex phenomena, and there are many ways by which they can be disturbed, whether it is in response to disease, drugs, or injury. Some of these disturbances are mild and short-lived, resulting from the expected consequences of variations in physiologic activity. Others are more severe, are considered pathologic, and may result in serious, even life-threatening, clinical manifestations.

Ion Concentrations

Disturbances in the ion concentrations on which the fundamental electrical properties of the cell are based **can significantly alter cellular excitability.** The resting potential depends primarily on **potassium** concentrations. Changes in the extracellular concentration of potassium can alter the resting membrane potential and hence excitability. Decreases in extracellular potassium lead to hyperpolarization of the cell, making it less excitable. In patients who have lost potassium because of disease or medication, this may be manifested as impaired motor activity (weakness or paralysis). Increased extracellular potassium leads to a lower resting potential. These cells are more excitable and generate action potentials in response to smaller stimuli or may fire spontaneously. An extremely high concentration may maintain the membrane potential at a level above threshold, preventing further excitation. In this way, increased extracellular potassium may produce manifestations of either heightened or depressed activity in neurons or muscle fibers. **Sodium ions** are of primary importance in the generation of action potentials, and interference with the flow of Na^+ can block impulse generation. A decrease in extracellular sodium may lower spike potential amplitude to the extent that it may not generate sufficient local current in adjacent membrane to be propagated. Nerve conduction block may result. Increased sodium tends to increase the size of the action potential but has little clinical effect. Calcium ions bind to ion channels and acts to stabilize the membrane potential. Hypocalcemia results in a decreased resting potential and increased excitability and may lead to spontaneous neuronal and muscular activity (tetany). Even moderate hypocalcemia may be manifested by tingling or muscle twitching. An excess of calcium tends to block action potential firing and enhance synaptic transmission, but produces demonstrable effects only at very high concentrations. It is interesting that divalent cations such as magnesium and cobalt can interfere with the influx of Ca^{2+} associated with presynaptic terminal depolarization, thereby reducing the Ca^{2+}-dependent release of neurotransmitter.

Hydrogen Ion Concentration (pH)

Excitable cells are highly responsive to changes in the pH of the surrounding extracellular fluid. **Alkalemia** greatly increases neuronal excitability. For example, the relative small rises in arterial pH that are caused by hyperventilation can trigger signs of excessive motor activity. A rise in arterial pH from the normal of 7.4 to about 7.8 often causes convulsions. **Acidemia,** on the other hand, greatly depresses neuronal activity. A fall in pH from 7.4 to less than 7.0 usually causes a comatose state. For instance, in very severe diabetic or uremic acidosis, coma always develops. The cellular effects of changes in H^+ concentration are complex, but partly reflect changes in the availability of Ca^{2+} for binding to the cell membrane.

Hypoxia

Excitable cells are highly dependent on an adequate supply of oxygen. Impaired oxygen delivery to these tissues, whether it is due to environmental deficiency, inadequate blood flow, or some other defect, quickly compromises the metabolic processes necessary for the maintenance of appropriate concentration gradients, protein synthesis, and axonal transport. For example, cessation of oxygen supply for only a few seconds can cause complete inexcitability of neurons.

Drugs

Most drugs that act on the nervous system do so by altering synaptic mechanisms. Such agents may have presynaptic or postsynaptic effects, blocking or distorting receptor/transmitter interactions, impairing transmitter synthesis, storage or release, and impeding transmitter reuptake or degradation. Neuronal and muscle cell activity may be enhanced or inhibited. Many such agents have useful applications in the treatment of locomotor disorders, whereas others distort motor activity as an undesirable side effect.

A number of drugs are used to improve skeletal muscle function through their actions on synaptic activity in the central nervous system.[42] One group acts primarily on the basal ganglia. These agents exert either dopaminergic or anticholinergic effects, and are useful for the treatment of Parkinson's disease and related disorders. A second group is used to treat spasticity and acute muscle spasms. One of these agents, baclofen, is particularly effective in reducing the frequency and severity of flexor or extensor spasms in spinal-cord–injured patients. Baclofen is believed to exert this effect by depressing synaptic transmission in the spinal cord. **A whole group of drugs is also used to both increase and decrease skeletal muscle activity through effects on the neuromuscular junction or on the muscle itself** (see Chapters 2 and 3). A powerful toxic agent is strychnine, which by blocking the action of certain inhibitory transmitters unleashes spinal motor neurons, leading to unbridled, convulsive motor activity. A detailed discussion of the many agents that affect synaptic function in the locomotor system is beyond the scope of this text.

Level of Utilization

Many of the functional characteristics of the synapse are affected by the extent to which the synapse is actually used. Adequate levels of activity are necessary for maintenance of the health of the synapse. With inadequate utilization, deleterious changes may occur in both the presynaptic and postsynaptic cells. Presynaptic cells may lose the ability to produce adequate amounts of neurotransmitter. Postsynaptic cells may atrophy and change in their sensitivity to neurotransmitter. Cells that lose their innervation often become much more sensitive to transmitters, a phenomenon called **denervation hypersensitivity.** These kinds of changes are particularly evident at the junction between somatic motor neurons and skeletal muscle. The implication is that when motor function is disrupted, for whatever reason, destructive changes may occur in inactive neuronal pathways and muscle cells, compounding the initial defect.

RECOMMENDED READINGS

Aidley, DJ: The Physiology of Excitable Cells, ed 3. Chapters 3–6. Cambridge University Press, Cambridge, 1990.

Alberts, B, et al: Molecular Biology of the Cell, ed 2. Chapters 6 and 19. Garland Publishing, New York, 1989.

Brinley, FJ, Jr: Excitation and Conduction in Nerve Fibers. Chapter 2. In Mountcastle, VB. (ed): Medical Physiology, ed 14. CV Mosby, St. Louis, 1980.

Darnell, J, Lodish, H, and Baltimore, D: Molecular Cell Biology, ed 2. Chapters 13, 14, and 20. Scientific American Books, New York, 1990.

Guyton, AC: Basic Neuroscience, ed 2. Chapters 5–7. WB Saunders, Philadelphia, 1991.

Junge, D: Nerve and Muscle Excitation, ed 3. Chapters 1–3. Sinauer Associates, Sunderland, MA, 1992.

Kandel, ER, Schwartz, JH, and Jessell, TM (eds): Principles of Neural Science. Parts I and III, ed 3. Appleton & Lange, Norwalk, CT, 1991.

Krueger, BK: Toward an Understanding of Structure and Function of Ion Channels. FASEB J 3:1906, 1989.

Levitan, B and Kaczmarek, LK: The Neuron: Cell and Molecular Biology. Oxford University Press, New York, 1991.

Nicholls, JG, Martin, AR, and Wallace, BG: From Neuron to Brain: A Cellular and Molecular Approach to the Function of the Nervous System, ed 3. Chapters 2–5, 7. Sinauer Associates, Sunderland, MA, 1992.

Patton, HD, et al (eds): Textbook of Physiology, vol 1, ed 21. Excitable Cells and Neurophysiology, Chapters 1 to 5, 11. WB Saunders, Philadelphia, 1989.

Shepherd, GM: Neurobiology, Section I. ed 2. Oxford University Press, New York, 1988.

Siegel, GJ, et al (eds): Basic Neurochemistry: Molecular, Cellular and Medical Aspects, ed 4. Chapters 1–4, 6, and 9. Raven Press, New York, 1989.

Stein, WH: Channels, Carriers, and Pumps: An Introduction to Membrane Transport. Academic Press, San Diego, 1990.

REFERENCES

1. Hille, B: Introduction to Physiology of Excitable Cells. Chapter 1. In Patton, HD, et al (eds): Textbook of Physiology, ed 21. WB Saunders, Philadelphia, 1989.

2. Guyton, AC: Basic Neuroscience, ed 2. Chapter 5. Transport of Ions Through the Cell Membrane. WB Saunders, Philadelphia, 1991.

3. Kutchai, HC: Cellular Membranes and Transmembrane Transport of Solutes and Water. Chapter 1. In Berne, RM and Levy, MN (eds): Physiology, ed 3. Mosby-Year Book, St. Louis, 1993.

4. Alberts, B, et al: Molecular Biology of the Cell, ed 2. Chapter 6. The Plasma Membrane, Garland Publishing, New York, 1989.

5. Albers, RW: Cell Membrane Structure and Functions. Chapter 2. In Siegel, GJ, et al (eds): Basic Neurochemistry: Molecular, Cellular, and Medical Aspects, ed 5: Raven Press, New York, 1994.

6. Darnell, J, Lodish, H, and Baltimore, D: Molecular Cell Biology, ed 2. Chapter 13. The Plasma Membrane. Scientific American Books, New York, 1990.

7. Siegelbaum, SA and Koester, J: Ion Channels. Chapter 5. In Kandel, ER, Schwartz, JH, and Jessell, TM (eds): Principles of Neural Science, ed 3. Appleton & Lange, Norwalk, CT, 1991.

8. Unwin, N. The Structure of Ion Channels in Membranes of Excitable Cells. Neuron 3:665, 1989.

9. Stein, WH: Channels, Carriers, and Pumps: An Introduction to Membrane Transport. Academic Press, San Diego, 1990.

10. Catterall, WA: Structure and Function of Voltage-Sensitive Ion Channels. Science 242:50, 1988.

11. Hille, B: Transport Across Cell Membranes: Carrier Mechanisms. Chapter 2. In Patton, HD, et al (eds): Textbook of Physiology, ed 21. WB Saunders, Philadelphia, 1989.

12. Albers, RW, Siegel, GJ, and Stahl, WL. Membrane Transport. Chapter 2. In Siegel, GJ, et al (eds): Basic Neurochemistry: Molecular, Cellular, and Medical Aspects, ed 5. Raven Press, New York, 1994.

13. Kaplan, JH and Deweer, P (eds): The Sodium Pump: Structure, Mechanism, and Regulation. 44th Symposium of the Society of General Physiologists. Rockefeller Press, New York, 1990.

14. Guyton, AC: Basic Neuroscience, ed 2. Chapter 6. Membrane Potentials and Action Potentials, WB Saunders, Philadelphia, 1991.

15. Hille, B and Catterall, WA: Electrical Excitability and Ionic Channels. Chapter 4. In Siegel, GJ, et al (eds): Basic Neurochemistry: Molecular, Cellular, and Medical Aspects, ed 5. Raven Press, New York, 1994.

16. Koester, J: Membrane Potential. Chapter 6. In Kandel, ER, Schwartz, JH, and Jessell, TM (eds): Principles of Neural Science, ed 3. Appleton & Lange, Norwalk, CT, 1991.

17. Shepherd, GM: Neurobiology, ed 2. Chapter 5. The Membrane Potential. Oxford University Press, New York, 1988.

18. Nicholls, JG, Martin, AR, and Wallace, BG: From Neuron to Brain. Chapter 3. Ionic Basis of the Resting Potential. Sinauer Associates, Sunderland, MA, 1992.

19. Alberts, B, et al: Molecular Biology of the Cell, ed 2. Chapter 19. The Nervous System. Garland Publishing, New York, 1989.

20. Berne, RM and Levy, MN (eds): Physiology, ed 3. Chapter 3. Generation and Conduction of Action Potentials, Mosby-Year Book, St. Louis, 1993.

21. Hille, B: Membrane Excitability: Action Potential Propagation in Axons. Chapter 3. In Patton, HD, et al (eds): Textbook of Physiology, ed 21. WB Saunders, Philadelphia, 1989.

22. Darnell, J, Lodish, H and Baltimore D: Molecular Cell Biology, ed 2. Chapter 20. Nerve Cells and the Electric Properties of Cell Membranes. Scientific American Books, New York, 1990.

23. Shepherd, GM: Neurobiology, ed 6. Chapter 6. The Action Potential. Oxford University Press, New York, 1988.

24. Koester, J: Voltage-Gated Ion Channels and the Generation of the Action Potential. Chapter 8. In Kandel, ER, Schwartz, JH, and Jessell, TM (eds): Principles of Neural Science, ed 3. Appleton & Lange, Norwalk, CT, 1991.

25. Nicholls, JG, Martin, AR, and Wallace, BG: From Neuron to Brain, ed 3. Chapter 4. Ionic Basis of the Action Potential. Sinauer Associates, Sunderland, MA, 1992.

26. Jungqueira, LC, Carniero, J, and Kelly, RD: Basic Histology, ed 7. Chapter 9. Nerve Tissue. Appleton & Lange, Norwalk, CT, 1992.

27. Peters, A, Palay, SL, and Webster, H de F: The Fine Structure of the Nervous System, ed 3. Oxford University Press, New York, 1991.

28. Barr, ML and Kiernan, JA: The Human Nervous System: An Anatomical Viewpoint, ed 6. Chapter 2. Cells of the Central Nervous System. JB Lippincott, Philadelphia, 1993.

29. Raine, CS: Neurocellular Anatomy. Chapter 1. In Siegel, GJ, et al (eds): Basic Neurochemistry: Molecular, Cellular, and Medical Aspects, ed 5. Raven Press, New York, 1994.

30. Shepherd, GM: Neurobiology, ed 2. Chapter 3. The Neuron. Oxford University Press, New York, 1988.

31. Morell, P, Quarles, RH, and Norton, WT: Myelin Formation, Structure, and Biochemistry. Chapter 6. In Siegel, GJ, et al (eds): Basic Neurochemistry: Molecular, Cellular, and Medical Aspects, ed 5. Raven Press, New York, 1994.

32. Hammerschlag, R, Cyr, JL, and Brady, ST: Axonal Transport and the Neuronal Cytoskeleton. Chapter 27. In Siegel, GJ, et al (eds): Basic Neurochemistry: Molecular, Cellular, and Medical Aspects, ed 5. Raven Press, New York, 1994.

33. Ochs, J and Brimijoin, WS: Axonal Transport. Chapter 21. In Dyck, DJ and Thomas, PK (eds): Peripheral Neuropathy, ed 3. WB Saunders, Philadelphia, 1993.

34. Shepherd, GM Neurobiology, ed 2. Chapter 4. The Synapse, Oxford University Press, New York, 1988.

35. Kandel, ER, Siegelbaum, SA, and Schwartz, JH: Synaptic Transmission. Chapter 9. In Kandel, ER, Schwartz, JH, and Jessell, TM (eds): Principles of Neural Science, ed 3. Appleton & Lange, Norwalk, CT, 1991.

36. Erulkar, SD: Chemically Mediated Synaptic Transmission: An Overview. Chapter 9. In Siegel, GJ, et al (eds): Basic Neurochemistry: Molecular, Cellular, and Medical Aspects, ed 5. Raven Press, New York, 1994.

37. Detwiler, PB and Crill, WE: Synaptic Transmission. Chapter 11. In Patton, HD, et al (eds): Textbook of Physiology, ed 21. WB Saunders, Philadelphia, 1989.

38. Nicholls, JG, Martin, AR, and Wallace, BG: From Neuron to Brain. Chapter 7. Principles of Synaptic Transmission, ed 3. Sinauer Associates, Sunderland, MA, 1992.

39. Berne, RM and Levy, MN (eds): Physiology, ed 3. Chapter 4. Synaptic Transmission, Mosby-Year Book, St. Louis, 1993.

40. Guyton, AC: Basic Neuroscience, ed 2. Chapter 7. Organization of the Central Nervous System: Basic Functions of Synapses and Transmitter Substances. WB Saunders, Philadelphia, 1991.

41. Shepherd, GM: Neurobiology, ed 2. Chapter 7. Synaptic Potentials and Synaptic Integration, Oxford University Press, New York, 1988.

42. Cedarbaum, JM and Schleifer, LS: Drugs for Parkinson's Disease, Spasticity, and Acute Muscle Spasms. Chapter 20. In Gilman, AG, et al (eds): Goodman and Gilman's The Pharmacologic Basis of Therapeutics, ed 8. McGraw-Hill, New York, 1993.

CHAPTER 2

■

Skeletal Muscle: The Somatic Effector

Christopher M. Fredericks, PhD

- *Structure*
- *Molecular Basis of Contraction*
- *Muscle Performance*
- *Muscle Metabolism (Provision of Energy)*
- *Adaptive Response of Muscle to Exercise*
- *Hormone-Induced Effects on Muscle*
- *Skeletal Muscle and Aging*

*T*he somatic nervous system innervates skeletal muscle. As such, this **muscle is the effector tissue of the motor system.** In other words, it is the means by which efferent motor commands from the somatic nervous system produce a motor effect. The motor system is a tremendously flexible system capable of highly varied and complex motor activities. Much of this flexibility resides in the unique structural and functional properties of muscle itself. As discussed later in the chapter, skeletal muscle is capable of contractions varying tremendously in force, duration, and precision. Moreover, skeletal muscle is a highly adaptable tissue, the characteristics of which can change markedly in response to demands placed on the motor system.

Skeletal muscle is the largest single tissue in the body, making up about 40% of the total body weight. Most skeletal muscle is attached to the bony skeleton, on which it exerts forces that either move components of the skeleton or fix them in a particular position. In addition, a few groups of skeletal muscle are more involved with certain visceral activities. These muscles are the diaphragm, the extraocular muscles, the muscles of the middle ear, the sphincters of the gastrointestinal and urogenital tracts, and fibers in the tongue, larynx, and upper esophagus. It should be remembered that motor disorders can adversely affect both groups of muscle.

Structure[1-8]

More than 400 anatomically distinct whole muscles exist in the human body, each defined by a thick connective tissue sheath, called the **epimysium** (Fig. 2–1). These muscles are in turn partitioned into fasiculi (bundles of muscle fibers) by the **perimysium.** An

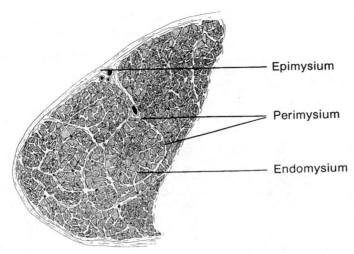

Figure 2-1. *Gross Appearance of Whole Skeletal Muscle.* This diagram of a small muscle in cross-section shows its connective tissue components and organization into bundles of muscle fibers. Epimysium encloses the entire muscle, perimysium surrounds each bundle of fibers, and endomysium lies between the individual fibers. (From Ham, AW and Cormack, DH: Histology, ed 8. JB Lippincott, Philadelphia, 1979, p 541, with permission.)

extension of the perimysium, the **endomysium**, extends into the interior of each bundle penetrating between all its fibers. These connective tissue elements are continuous with the connective tissue structures to which the muscle is attached, whether it is tendon, periosteum, or the dermis of the skin.

Each muscle fiber is a single muscle cell. As such, it has a cell membrane, the sarcolemma, and contains the usual cellular organelles distributed throughout the sarcoplasm. The cell membrane is covered by the protective basal lamina, which in turn is covered by a loosely woven network of collagen fibrils, referred to as the **reticular lamina.** In most muscles, the fibers extend the entire length of the whole muscle. Human fibers may thus be more than 30 cm long and range in diameter from 20 to 100 μm in adults. The muscle fibers are often arranged parallel with one another, but many other types of arrangement exist, each designed to efficiently carry out a particular type of movement.

When viewed microscopically, **the muscle fiber is seen to be nearly filled with closely packed, longitudinal myofibrils,** many of which run the entire length of the cell (Figs. 2-2 and 2-3). With a light microscope it can be seen that **the fibrils are distinctly banned or striated** with alternating light (I) and dark (A) bands. At the center of the A band is the dark transverse M line surrounded by a somewhat lighter region, the H zone. At the center of the I band runs the dense Z line. The region between two Z lines is termed a **sarcomere.** Beneath the cell membrane, as well as around and between the myofilaments, is an extensive, filamentous cytoskeleton that preserves the integrity of the muscle fiber during contraction and helps to transmit the force generated by contraction to the muscle membrane and its tendinous attachments. Large numbers of mitochondria are scattered throughout the muscle fiber interior. These are concentrated at sites where adenosine triphosphate (ATP) is most needed in energy-requiring processes such as contraction and ion transport. In addition, skeletal muscle cells are multinucleated with numerous nuclei distributed primarily near the cell membrane.

Electron microscopy or other forms of high-power visualization can show that the **myofibrils are in turn made up of thick and thin myofilaments** (Fig. 2-4). In fact, it is the elaborate three-dimensional arrangement of these filaments that gives rise to the characteristic striations of the myofibril. Specifically, the overlap of these two types of filaments creates a banded appearance when polarized light is passed through a thin section of muscle. **Fine cross-bridges between the thick and thin filaments can sometimes be observed in the**

Skeletal Muscle

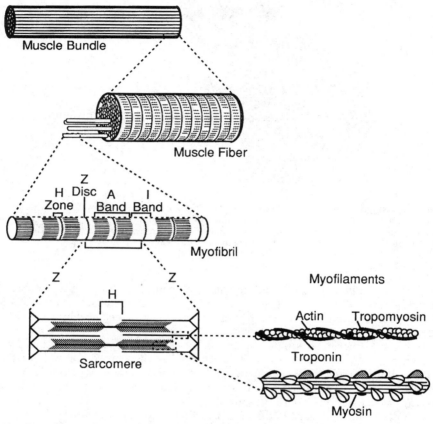

Figure 2–2. *Organization of Skeletal Muscle from the Gross to the Molecular Level.* Whole muscles are made up of bundles of individual fibers. Each fiber contains many closely packed striated myofibrils. The myofibrillar striations reflect the underlying arrangement of the thick and thin myofilaments.

areas of overlap. The thin filaments are linked together at one end by the dense meshwork of the Z line.

The myofilaments are in turn made up of at least four distinct proteins. A very large protein called *myosin* **forms the bulk of the thick filament.**[8] About 400 myosin molecules are aggregated to form each thick filament. The myosin molecule is composed of six polypeptide chains: two heavy chains (molecular weight: about 200,000 each), and two pairs of light chains (molecular weights: about 20,000 each). The two heavy chains are twisted around each other forming a long, rigid myosin "tail." One end of each one of these chains is formed into a globular protein mass, called the **myosin head.** Each myosin molecule thus has two heads attached to one end of the long tail. One polypeptide of each set of light chains is associated with each head of the molecule.

Myosin molecules aggregate in the cytoplasm to form thick filaments. The backbone of the filament is formed from aggregated tail segments, with the remainder of the molecule, including the globular heads, projecting laterally from the filament (Fig. 2–5). These projections form the cross-bridges sometimes seen between thick and thin filaments. Each cross-bridge is believed to be flexible at two points called *hinges*—one where the arm leaves the body of the myosin filament and the other where the two heads are attached to the arm.

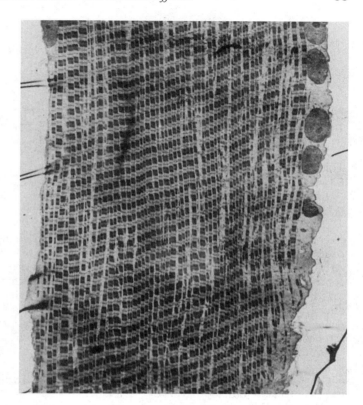

Figure 2–3. *Microscopic Appearance of a Single Human Skeletal Muscle Fiber.* The myofibrils and their characteristic banding pattern are clearly visible. At the edge of the fiber, several nuclei can be seen just below the surface membrane (×1600). (From Bourne, GH: The Structure and Function of Muscle, ed 2. Academic Press, New York, 1972, p 306, with permission.)

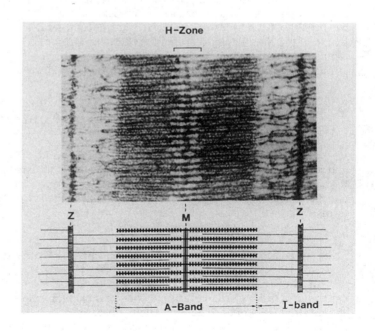

Figure 2–4. *Organization of a Skeletal Muscle Sarcomere.* This electron micrograph shows the distinct overlap of the thick and thin myofilaments that form the sarcomere and give rise to the characteristic striations of skeletal muscle. (From Squire, J: The Structural Basis of Muscular Contraction. Plenum Press, New York, 1981, p 9, with permission.)

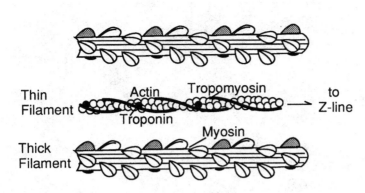

Figure 2–5. *Molecular Organization of Skeletal Muscle Myofilaments.* The thin filament is comprised of a double-stranded helix of G-actin molecules with strands of tropomyosin and globular troponin complexes lying along the grooves between the strands. The thick filament is an aggregate of myosin molecules, oriented so the myosin heads project from the filament surface toward adjacent thin filaments. (Adapted from Squire, JM: Molecular Mechanisms in Muscular Contraction. Trends Neurosci 6:409, 1983.)

These hinges allow the heads to move somewhat and are thought to participate in the actual contraction process. Since the myosin filament itself is twisted, the cross-bridges extend in all directions around the filament. The thick filaments are very uniform in length and contain an estimated 300 to 400 cross-bridges. Adjacent thick filaments seem to be linked together by fine structural filaments in the sarcomere, which contribute to their stability during contraction.

Contraction is dependent on the unique chemical properties of the myosin heads that form the cross-bridges. The myosin head, for example, has a strong affinity for binding to actin, the major protein constituent of the thin filament. It also possesses ATPase activity, particularly when bound to actin, which allows it to hydrolyze ATP and thereby provide energy for the contraction process. Two distinct forms of myosin have been identified, which have appreciably different levels of ATPase activity.

The **thin filament** is equally complex, and **is composed of three distinct proteins** (see Fig. 2–5).[8] The backbone of the thin filament is a long, twisted, two-stranded filament of **F-actin**. Each strand of F-actin is formed from globular G-actin molecules (molecular weight: 45,000) that polymerize under the conditions existing in the cytoplasm. Rod-shaped molecules of **tropomyosin** (molecular weight: 70,000) stretch along each F-actin strand. Attached near one end of each tropomyosin molecule is the protein, **troponin** (molecular weight: 80,000). As a result, troponin is located at intervals of approximately 400 Å along the length of the thin filament. Troponin is actually a complex of globular proteins with differing affinities for actin, tropomyosin, and Ca^{2+}. Specifically, one subunit (troponin T) has a strong affinity for tropomyosin, another (troponin I) for actin, and a third (troponin C) for Ca^{2+}.

Molecular Basis of Contraction

The function of skeletal muscle is to contract and thereby apply force to the skeleton and the other structures to which it is attached. To understand how muscle functions as a tissue, it is necessary to understand the process of contraction at the molecular level. In this context, skeletal muscle contraction can be described in both structural and biochemical terms.

Structural Basis of Contraction: The Sliding Filament Theory[5–7,9–15]

In the 1950s, HE Huxley and AF Huxley[9,10] and their colleagues proposed an explanation of how striated muscle contracts in the form of what has come to be known as the **Sliding Filament Theory.** Their observations have been reinforced by countless subsequent investigations, and the basic tenets of this theory continue to be universally

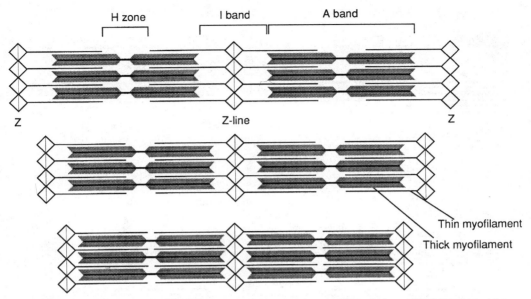

Figure 2–6. *The Sliding Filament Model of Contraction.* Shortening of the whole myofibril is achieved by an increase in the overlap of the thick and thin myofilaments in each sarcomere. During shortening, the I bands and H zones progressively narrow and may ultimately disappear. The A bands stay the same.

accepted today. According to this theory, the shortening of a skeletal muscle fiber reflects the aggregate shortening of the sarcomeres and hence the myofibrils of which the fiber is composed. This shortening is the result not of changes in the length of their component myofilaments, but of changes in their relative position (Fig. 2–6). Specifically, the thick and thin filaments slide past one another, increasing their overlap during contraction and decreasing their overlap during relaxation or stretch. In a relaxed muscle, about two thirds of the length of each thick filament and about half of that of each thin filament are overlapping. During contraction, cross-bridges form between the globular heads of the thick filaments and the G-actin units of the thin filaments, linking the overlapping portions of the filaments. These cross-bridges are rapidly formed and broken, each detaching itself from one site on the thin filament and reattaching itself to another site farther along, and so on, with the result that the thin filament slides along the thick filament. Relaxation occurs when cross-bridges cease to be formed, allowing the myofilaments to return to their resting level of interdigitation.

Biochemical Basis of Contraction: Binding of Actin and Myosin[5–7,11–16]

In the simplest terms, contraction is the consequence of a reversible binding between the proteins, actin and myosin, which is initiated by Ca^{2+} and results in the expenditure of ATP and energy. In actuality, **contraction is a complex cycle of biochemical reactions involving many steps.** The more important steps are illustrated in Figure 2–7.

Resting State

The relaxation of skeletal muscle occurs when actin and myosin are unable to bind to one another. Certain specific conditions have to be met to overcome the mutual affinity between these two proteins. Specifically, a high-energy nucleotide such as ATP must be bound to the myosin head. In addition, the ambient cytoplasmic concentration of Ca^{2+} must

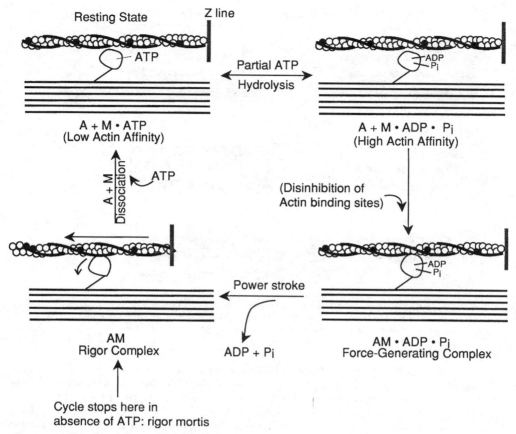

Figure 2–7. *Major Steps in the Crossbridge Cycle.* (*1*) In the relaxed state with ATP bound to the myosin head, actin and myosin have little affinity for one another. (*2*) With hydrolysis of the myosin-bound ATP to ADP and Pi, the myosin develops a high affinity for actin. (*3*) With increased ambient Ca^{2+}, the myosin binds tightly to actin; contraction follows. (*4*) With Ca^{2+} high and myosin shorn of its nucleotide, actin and myosin remain bound in the rigor complex. Replenishment of myosin-bound ATP and Ca^{2+} sequestration lead back to (*1*). (Adapted from Alberts, B, et al: Molecular Biology of the Cell, ed 2. Garland Publishing, Inc., New York, 1989, p 621.)

be low enough to maintain the inhibition of actin. At rest, the amount of free Ca^{2+} in the sarcoplasm is low (about 10^{-7} M), and the conformation of the troponin—tropomysin complex is such that the sites on the actin filaments to which the myosin heads might bind are blocked.

Force-generating Complex

After the dissociation of actin and myosin, the ATP bound to the myosin is split to ADP and inorganic phosphate. These hydrolysis products, however, are not released from the myosin but stay tightly bound to the myosin head. This new form of myosin has a higher affinity for actin. **If sarcoplasmic Ca^{2+} concentrations are increased and actin is consequently disinhibited, the myosin head will bind to actin, forming an unstable force-generating complex.** Through processes still poorly understood, this binding triggers the release of energy stored in the myosin. This somehow causes the head to bend and the bound actin to be moved. **Although the precise manner in which this interaction between the cross-bridges and actin causes contraction remains unknown, a reasonable explanation is termed the** *Ratchet Hypothesis.* As each myosin head attaches to an active site on actin, changes in intramolecular forces cause the head to tilt toward the arm, dragging the actin filament along with it. This is termed the **power stroke**. During cross-bridge movement myosin binds very firmly to actin. The binding of myosin to new ATP breaks this linkage and allows the cross-bridge to combine with a new site farther along the thin filament. In this way, the heads of the cross-bridges bend back and forth and step by step "walk" or "ratchet" along the thin filament, pulling it toward the middle of the sarcomere. Energy is somehow consumed in the movement of the myosin head and the resultant ratcheting of the myofilaments. Each cross-bridge is believed to operate independently of all the others, each attaching and pulling in a continuous but random cycle. Each thick filament has about 500 myosin heads, and each of these cycles about five times per second during contraction. Each cycle is estimated to shorten the muscle by about 1%.

Rigor Complex

After each power stroke, with the cytoplasmic Ca^{2+} concentration still high (about 10^{-5} M) and myosin shorn of its nucleotide, **actin and myosin remain strongly bound together in a rigor complex.** For relaxation to occur, the sarcoplasmic Ca^{2+} concentrations must be lowered, allowing the troponin-tropomyosin complex to reinhibit the cross-bridge binding sites on the actin filament. In addition, a fresh nucleotide (ATP) must be provided to bind to the myosin. In the absence of ATP, relaxation will be prevented. This explains the muscle tautness of contractures of fatigued muscle and of rigor mortis. In rigor mortis, for example, the muscles are stiff because ATP is depleted and the myosin heads cannot be released from the actin filament. They remain in rigor until the myofibrillar proteins themselves deteriorate.

Initiation of Contraction

In vivo initiation of the binding of actin and myosin, and hence skeletal muscle contraction, is dependent on three basic physiologic processes (Fig. 2–8). If any one of these processes is disturbed or disrupted, muscle weakness or paralysis may result.

Motor Impulse Generation and Propagation

Normal skeletal muscle is not spontaneously active, but depends on excitation by the somatic nervous system. This excitation comes in the form of action potentials arising in and propagated in somatic motor neurons. Impairment of impulse generation or conduction may result in difficulty in exciting skeletal muscle (i.e., weakness or paralysis) as discussed in Chapter 15. Many factors may impair motor neuron function, including local anesthetics and other drugs or chemicals, demyelination, trauma, ischemia, diabetes, and aging.

Neuromuscular Junction Transmission

The muscle cell membrane must be excited by the somatic motor neuron action potential. Since the motor neuron is not contiguous with the muscle cell but is separated from it by the neuromuscular junction, this excitation is accomplished indirectly by neurohumoral transmission. This is discussed at length in Chapter 3. Impairment of junctional activity can significantly impair muscle activity, as might be observed in poisoning by curare or other drugs, in botulism, and in myasthenia gravis.

Excitation-Contraction Coupling [5,12,13,17-22]

Once the muscle membrane is excited (i.e., an action potential has been initiated), this electrical activity must be coupled to the binding of actin and myosin. This coupling of electrical and mechanical processes is termed **excitation-contraction coupling**. This coupling is accomplished by release of intracellular Ca^{2+} stores and a resultant increase in intracellular Ca^{2+} levels to those required for actin and myosin binding.

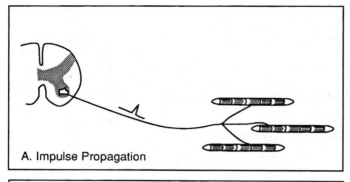

A. Impulse Propagation

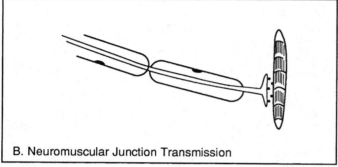

B. Neuromuscular Junction Transmission

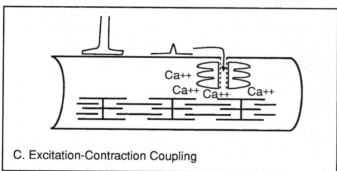

C. Excitation-Contraction Coupling

Figure 2–8. In Vivo Initiation of Contraction in Skeletal Muscle. The physiologic initiation of contraction is dependent upon three basic processes: (*A*) impulse propagation in motor neurons from the central nervous system to the nerve terminus, (*B*) neuromuscular junction transmission, and (*C*) linkage of a sarcolemmal action potential to intracellular Ca^{2+} release and actin/myosin binding.

About 5% of the total cell volume of skeletal muscle is occupied by an elaborate tubular system composed of transverse T tubules and longitudinal sarcoplasmic reticulum (Fig. 2–9). The T tubules are formed by invagination of the cell membrane and although they extend deep into the cell, they remain continuous with the extracellular space. The sarcoplasmic reticulum is an extensive vesicular network that surrounds each myofibril. Dilated portions of the sarcoplasmic reticulum called **terminal cisternae** (or lateral sacs) are located in close proximity to the T tubules and may actually be in contact with them via small structural bridges called **feet**. The terminal cisternae contain a calcium-binding protein, calsequestrin. The form that this tubular system takes varies somewhat among different types of skeletal muscle and is correlated with their performance characteristics. The more rapidly contracting muscles have the more extensive sarcoplasmic reticulum.

The **sarcoplasmic reticulum,** along with the mitochondria, **serves as an intracellular storehouse for Ca^{2+} and brings about excitation-contraction coupling by changing cytoplasmic Ca^{2+} levels.** Depolarization in the muscle cell membrane spreads through the

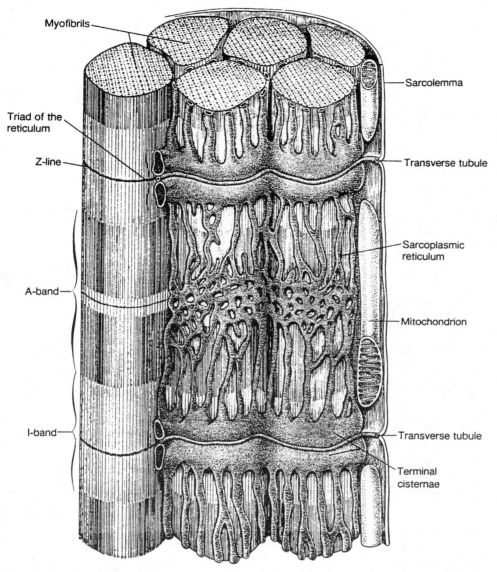

Myofibrils

Triad of the
reticulum

Z-line

A-band

I-band

Sarcolemma

Transverse tubule

Sarcoplasmic
reticulum

Mitochondrion

Transverse tubule

Terminal
cisternae

Figure 2–9. *Sarcoplasmic Reticulum.* Interspersed among the myofibrils is an elaborate tubular system comprised of the sarcoplasmic reticulum and transverse tubules. (From Fox, SI: Human Physiology, ed 2. Copyright © 1987 Wm C Brown Communications, Inc., Dubuque, Iowa. All rights reserved. Reprinted by permission.)

T-tubule system into the interior of the cell and leads to the release of Ca^{2+} from the sarcoplasmic reticulum that surrounds each myofibril (Fig. 2–10). The cytoplasmic Ca^{2+}, which is normally low, rapidly increases in the vicinity of the contractile apparatus, allowing actin and myosin binding and, hence, contraction to occur.

Although poorly understood, it is thought that the increased binding of Ca^{2+} to troponin C that accompanies the release of sarcoplasmic reticulum Ca^{2+} causes a conformational change in the troponin-tropomysin complex (Fig. 2–11). This change causes the complex to move, releasing the active sites on actin and thereby allowing myosin binding and contraction to occur. Relatively small changes in Ca^{2+} produce large changes in the

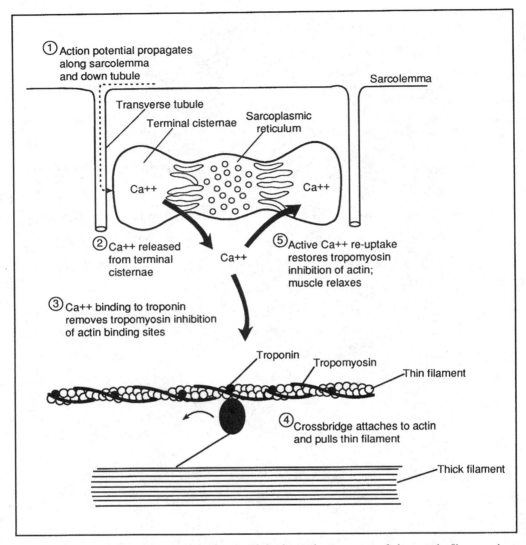

Figure 2–10. *Excitation Contraction Coupling in Skeletal Muscle.* Excitation of the muscle fiber membrane (sarcolemma) is linked to contraction by the release of intracellular stores of Ca^{2+} and its effects on the regulatory proteins, troponin and tropomyosin. (Adapted from Vander, AJ, Sherman, JH, and Luciano, DS: Human Physiology, ed 5. McGraw-Hill, New York, 1990, p. 295.)

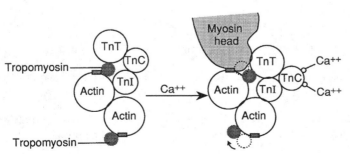

Figure 2–11. *Interaction Between Ca^{2+} and the Regulatory Proteins.* This is a cross-sectional view of actin, myosin, and the regulatory proteins, tropomyosin and troponin. When levels of cytoplasmic free Ca^{2+} are low, the actin binding sites are masked by tropomyosin, maintaining the relaxed muscle state. When free Ca^{2+} increases and binds to multiple sites on troponin, the regulatory complex moves, allowing myosin crossbridges to attach to the actin causing contraction.

number of cross-bridges formed and in the force developed. The fiber relaxes when Ca^{2+} is actively pumped back into the sarcoplasmic reticulum, and a low intracellular Ca^{2+} concentration is reestablished. It is notable that the resequestration of Ca^{2+} requires the expenditure of energy (derived from ATP hydrolysis), which may partly explain why relaxation may be delayed in fatigued muscle.

Although many of the pharmacologic agents used for the control of muscle spasticity act predominantly within the central nervous system, one agent, dantrolene, acts directly on skeletal muscle. Dantrolene reduces contractions of muscle by interfering with excitation-contraction coupling, apparently by reducing the amount of Ca^{2+} released by the sarcoplasmic reticulum.[22]

Muscle Performance

In addition to describing skeletal muscle in terms of the mechanisms by which contraction occurs, it can be viewed in terms of the characteristics of the tension it produces—in other words, in terms of what might be called "muscle performance." Skeletal muscle cells in all their morphologic and functional specialization are exquisitely flexible in their performance.

Types of Muscle Contractions

The force exerted by a contracting muscle on the system to which it is attached (whether it is a scientific measuring device or its natural bony attachments) is termed **muscle tension**. The external force applied to the muscle is known as **resistance** or **load**.[23] **Muscle contractions can be classified according to the relationship that exists between the muscle tension being produced and the concurrent resistance to contraction.** In characterizing this relationship, however, care must be taken to distinguish between the conditions existing in experimental settings in which skeletal muscles are detached from their bony attachments and the conditions that exist in the natural setting in which muscles are operating through the lever systems of the body.

Muscle physiologists using isolated muscle preparations have long divided muscle contractions into two types: isotonic and isometric. During an **isotonic contraction**, the muscle shortens, as might be observed while lifting a load vertically against gravity, so that the load on the muscle is constant throughout its shortening. Thus, there is movement of a force over a distance, and, by definition, external mechanical work is done. During an **isometric contraction**, the muscle is subjected to a resistance too great to overcome and thus the muscle does not shorten. Although no appreciable motion is accomplished and no external mechanical work is performed during an isometric contraction, cross-bridges are formed and broken and the sliding of myofilaments takes place. Muscle work is thus performed and energy expended.

In reality, the characterizations of muscle contraction that are derived from isolated muscle experiments do not necessarily apply to muscles operating under the conditions existing in the intact locomotor system. Truly isotonic contractions, for example, seldom, if ever, occur when muscles are acting through the natural lever systems of the body. Despite the fact that the term "isotonic" is often used to refer to a contraction that causes a joint bearing some load to move through a range of motion (e.g., flexing the elbow while holding an object in the hand), this is misleading because it does not take into account the leverage effects present at the joint. Although the weight being lifted remains the same throughout such a movement, the tension required to move the weight changes continuously throughout the movement in accordance with the changing leverage of the joint.

Muscle contractions in vivo do not always result directly in the production of joint movement, but may serve to hold a lever system in a fixed position. Since no change occurs in the length of the muscle under these circumstances, such a movement can be legitimately characterized as isometric. However, no shortening often occurs because the muscle is programmed to fixate some component of the musculoskeletal system (e.g., during the maintenance of upright posture), not because the muscle is subjected to some insurmountable load (e.g., an unmoving force-measuring device).

In the context of the intact locomotor system, two basic types of muscle contraction occur in which the length of muscle changes. When a muscle develops sufficient tension to overcome the resistance in the lever system to which it is attached, the muscle shortens and causes joint movement. This is a **concentric contraction.** When a muscle does not develop sufficient tension and is overcome by the external load, it will progressively lengthen rather than shorten. This is an **eccentric contraction.** Eccentric contractions often serve to decelerate the motion of a joint (e.g., when descending stairs the quadriceps works eccentrically to slow flexion of the knee).

All the various types of muscle contractions have a particular role to play in our motor behaviors. Isometric, concentric, and eccentric contractions seldom occur alone in normal human movement, but rather occur during different phases of a movement. Moreover, a specific muscle may contract both concentrically and eccentrically, depending on the direction of joint movement (e.g., flexor muscles of a joint contract concentrically during flexion and eccentrically during extension). It has been suggested that eccentric and isometric contractions occur more often in the proximal postural muscles, whereas concentric contractions occur more often in the muscles of the extremities in association with ambulation or the manipulation of objects in the environment.

The tension produced by a muscle varies with the type of contraction being performed. Isometric and eccentric contractions produce more tension than do concentric contractions of the same muscle. Less fibrillar shortening and slower contractions may permit more cross-bridges to be formed.

The Isometric Twitch

Although the characteristics of isotonic contraction are influenced by the nature of the load against which the muscle contracts, isometric contractions reflect strictly the force-generating properties of the muscle itself. For this reason, isometric systems are most often used in the study of muscle performance.

The simplest example of muscle performance is the muscle twitch (Fig. 2–12).[5,12] The twitch, by definition, is the response of muscle to a single, maximal stimulus. With each twitch, a brief but distinct delay occurs between the stimulus (action potential) and the appearance of external tension. This is called the **latency period.** This delay reflects the time necessary for excitation-contraction coupling to occur, in other words, for the release of sarcoplasmic reticulum Ca^{2+}, its diffusion to the vicinity of the myofilament binding sites, and the resultant binding of actin and myosin. Once begun, the twitch tension rapidly rises to a maximum in the **contraction time.** This interval varies markedly among skeletal muscle types. These differences in the speed with which tension develops reflect distinct differences in cell morphology and biochemistry. The interval from peak tension back to the resting baseline tension is the **relaxation time.** This interval also varies among skeletal muscle types and is typically proportional to the contraction time. Relaxation, with its own energy requirements, may be prolonged with fatigue and in the presence of certain metabolic diseases.

If one compares the internally generated tension of a twitch (in other words, the actual tension produced by the contractile apparatus) with that measured at external attachments to the muscle, they will be seen as being very different. The internal tension, known as **the active state**, develops more quickly and with greater magnitude but less duration than the **external tension.** This disparity exists because the tension produced by the contractile apparatus is transmitted only indirectly to the sarcolemma and the structures attached to it (e.g., tendons). The myofibrils are not directly connected to the muscle membrane. As they

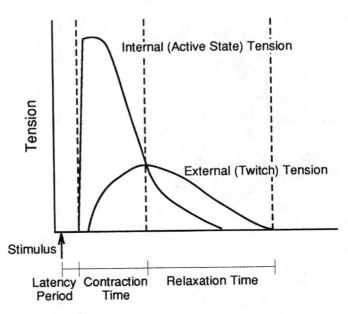

Figure 2–12. *Isometric Twitch of a Skeletal Muscle Fiber.* Note that the internally generated tension (active state) is appreciably different, in both duration and amplitude, from the externally expressed twitch tension. This reflects the presence of the "series elastic elements" interposed between the contractile apparatus and the cell surface.

shorten during contraction, tension is expressed only at the cell surface by the stretch that this shortening imparts to various elastic elements of the cell that surround the fibrils, such as filaments of the cytoskeleton and various cellular organelles. These may be described mathematically as the **series elastic elements**. This seemingly inefficient utilization of the internally generated tension provides a mechanism for somatic control over skeletal muscle performance by changes in the frequency of stimulation.

Types of Muscle Fibers[7,11,12,14,24–28]

It has long been known that **skeletal muscle is composed of different types of fibers.** Many different schemes have been used to classify skeletal muscle according to histochemical or physiologic criteria. In humans, because individual fibers are difficult to isolate and whole muscles tend to be more heterogeneous than those in other species, characterization of muscle fibers based on their physiologic properties has been difficult to achieve. In most studies of human muscle, a classification based on histochemical criteria has been used. Although many fiber types have been identified in human muscle using a variety of different histochemical techniques, **fiber typing is usually based on an assessment of myofibrillar ATPase activity.** This is done in thin muscle sections under conditions of varying acidity. For reasons not known, fast-twitch muscle myosin has a different pH sensitivity than slow-twitch muscle myosin, so that different types of muscle fibers will stain differently at different pHs (Fig. 2–13). This method can differentiate between fast-twitch fibers (type II) and slow-twitch fibers (type I). Moreover, type II fibers can be further classified into types IIA, IIB, and IIC. Numerous studies of the metabolic and physiologic properties of skeletal muscle conducted mainly in animals have suggested a functional classification of muscle into three basic types: slow contracting, fast contracting and resistant to fatigue, and fast contracting and rapidly fatiguing fibers (Table 2–1). These may correlate with human type I, IIA, and IIB fibers, respectively, as characterized by the ATPase-based histochemical scheme.

Type I fibers are relatively small, contract relatively slowly, and are difficult to fatigue. They have abundant mitochondria and lipid granules and make greater use of the Krebs cycle and oxidative metabolism. These muscles are reddish in appearance because of their

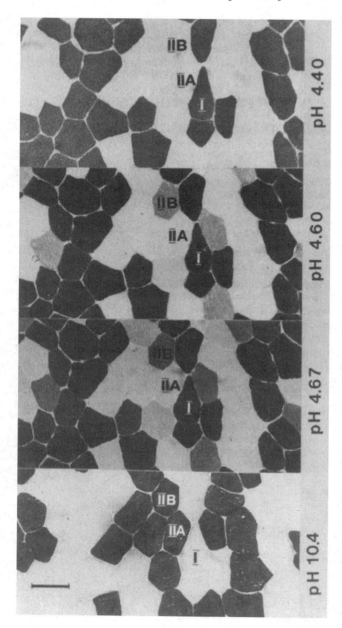

Figure 2–13. *Histochemically Typed Human Muscle Fibers.* Fiber typing in human muscle is usually based on an assessment of myofibrillar ATPase activity. The sensitivity of the ATPase staining reaction to pH varies among the different fiber types. These serial cross sections from vastus lateralis muscle display fiber types I, IIA, and IIB under different pH conditions. (From Baumann, et al,[46] p. 350, with permission.)

high myoglobin content and dense capillarization. Type I fibers are innervated by highly active motor neurons that fire at low frequencies and have slow conduction velocities. These fibers are best suited for long-lasting, low-level force production. **Type IIB fibers** are larger, more powerful, and contract more quickly, but are easily fatigued. They tend to have a higher glycogen content and fewer mitochondria, and they derive much of their energy from glycolysis. Type IIB fibers are best suited for intermittent, intense-force production. **Type IIA fibers** are intermediate to types I and IIB, with well-developed oxidative and glycolytic capabilities, and thus greater fatigue resistance. These fibers are capable of prolonged and relatively high-force production. Type II fibers are innervated by sporadically active motor neurons that fire at fast frequencies and have high conduction velocities.

Table 2–1. *Characteristics of Skeletal Muscle Fibers*

	Slow (Type I)	Fast, Fatigue-Resistant (Type IIA)	Fast, Rapidly Fatiguing (Type IIB)
Morphology			
Color	Red	Red	White
Fiber diameter	Small	Intermediate	Large
Motor neuron size	Small	Intermediate	Large
Metabolism			
Primary source of ATP	Oxidative phosphorylation	Oxidative phosphorylation	Anaerobic glycolysis
Glycolytic capacity	Low	Moderate to high	High
Oxidative capacity	High	High	Low
Glycogen content	Low	Intermediate	High
No. of mitochondria	Many	Many	Few
Capillaries	Abundant	Intermediate	Sparse
Myoglobin content	High	High	Low
Contraction			
Contraction velocity	Slow	Fast	Fast
Myosin ATPase	Slow	Fast	Fast
Rate of fatigue	Slow	Moderate	Fast

Type IIC fibers are rarely seen in normal adult muscle but are numerous in fetal muscle and occasionally present in disease. They may be significant in fiber-type transformation and may indicate a degree of undifferentiation such as might occur in regenerating muscle fibers.

Considerable evidence derived from animal experiments indicates that **fiber type is determined largely by its innervation.** For example, crossed reinnervation of a predominately fast-twitch muscle with a slow-twitch nerve will cause a conversion of both the physiologic and histochemical properties of the muscle fiber from fast to slow and vice versa.[33,34] In addition, all the muscle fibers innervated by the same motor neuron (i.e., a motor unit) are the same type.

Although motor units themselves are homogeneous, **fast-twitch and slow-twitch fibers are typically intermingled** in a random checkerboard pattern in most skeletal muscles (see Fig. 2–13). Their relative proportion, however, varies from one muscle to another. Fiber types are distributed in accordance with the type of function specific muscles are called on to perform. Accordingly, red slow-twitch fibers predominate in deep postural muscles (e.g., soleus), whereas white fast-twitch fibers predominate in the extraocular muscles, in flexors (e.g., tibialis anterior and flexor digitorum), and in superficial extensors (e.g., extensor digitorum longus and gastrocnemius). Within individual muscles, further stratification of fibers may be apparent. In the gastrocnemius, for example, type I and IIA fibers are situated in the deepest portions, whereas type IIB fibers predominate in the most superficial portions of the muscle.

Muscle fiber distribution also may vary markedly from one individual to another.[11,31] Although every person's muscles contain mixtures of the three fiber types, some people have relatively more of one variety. Top athletes in sports requiring either high speed or great endurance have very different fiber type compositions in their muscles (Fig. 2–14). For example, in marathon runners and professional cyclists, most fibers are type I slow-twitch fibers, whereas sprint runners or sprint swimmers have a high percentage (up to 90% or higher) of type II fast-twitch fibers. Weight lifters appear to have approximately equal proportions of fast-twitch and slow-twitch fibers. It remains a matter of debate as to what extent such extreme fiber type compositions are genetically predetermined or caused by the training these athletes perform. Both factors probably contribute.

Not only are muscle fiber types distributed in regular patterns within the motor system, but they are also recruited in predictable spatial patterns during motor activity.

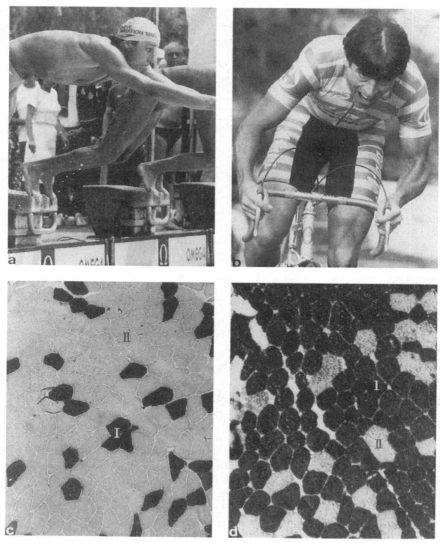

Figure 2–14. *Muscle Fiber Type Composition in Two Selected Top Athletes.* (A) A swimmer whose specialty is the 50-m crawl sprint. (B) A world class professional cyclist. In sections of vastus lateralis, type I fibers are stained dark, whereas type II fibers remain unstained. (C) The majority of the swimmer's fibers are type II (fast twitch). (D) The majority of the cyclist's fibers are type I (slow twitch). (From Komi, PV: Strength and Power in Sport. Blackwell Scientific Publications, Ltd., London, 1992, p 53, with permission.)

In Vivo Gradations of Contractile Force

Skeletal muscle is a tremendously adaptable effector tissue, which, together with the somatic nervous system, constitutes a motor system of immense flexibility. This system is capable of contractions ranging from those of extreme brevity and exquisite precision to those of great force and sustained duration. **This flexibility reflects both the functional characteristics of the muscle tissue itself, as well as the organizational powers of the somatic nervous system.** As a first step in developing an understanding of motor control, it is useful to consider the factors that influence force development at the level of the muscle tissue itself.

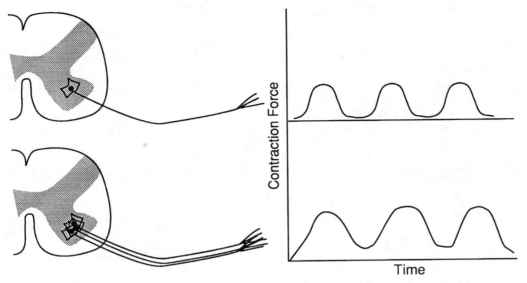

Figure 2–15. *Motor Unit Recruitment.* Activation of increasing numbers of motor neurons and hence more muscle fibers is one fundamental way of increasing the amount of force generated.

Number of Fibers Stimulated (Recruitment)[5,12,14,26–29]

Perhaps the most obvious influence on the amount of tension produced by skeletal muscle is the number of muscle fibers stimulated. Clearly, increasing the number of fibers activated will increase the force generated. This is a fundamental element of motor control. In this regard, it is important to recognize that the functional unit of muscle in vivo, the unit through which the somatic nervous system exerts its control, is not the whole muscle, the muscle bundle, or the muscle fiber; rather, it is the motor unit. A motor unit, by definition, is all the muscle fibers innervated by a single motor neuron. As somatic efferent neurons leave the central nervous system and travel to the periphery where skeletal muscle is located, they branch and thereby innervate multiple muscle fibers. The extent of this branching and hence the number of muscle fibers making up a motor unit vary markedly. In muscles controlling fine, precise movements, the motor units are made up of a small number of muscle fibers. Laryngeal, pharyngeal, and extraocular muscles, for example, have less than 10 muscle fibers per unit. Motor units of 10 to 125 fibers are attached to the bones of the middle ear. At the other extreme, large coarse-acting muscles may contain thousands of fibers per unit (e.g., 2000 per gastrocnemius unit). Motor units also differ from one another in the type of muscle fibers of which they are composed, although each individual motor unit necessarily contains only one type of fiber. The fibers of many motor units are scattered throughout a muscle bundle and intermingled with fibers of other units, including muscle fibers of different types.

Even the largest motor units are small, so that a strong contraction of skeletal muscle requires the participation of many motor units. **The somatic nervous system has the capacity to activate increasing numbers of motor units,** thereby increasing the force of contraction in accordance with the task at hand. This is termed *recruitment* (Fig. 2–15). Note that the **recruitment of motor units occurs in a specific, orderly sequence.**[12,14,26–29] In both voluntary and reflex muscle contractions, the smallest, weakest contractile units are usually recruited first, and the largest, most powerful units are recruited only during maximal efforts. In fact, some evidence exists that the largest motor units are so inexcitable that most persons cannot recruit them voluntarily. It has been proposed that this may account for the exceptional displays of strength exhibited under extraordinary circumstances. Changes in recruitment sequence or intensity may in part explain how individuals are able to train themselves to more readily perform tasks requiring great exertion (e.g., athletic tasks such as weight lifting or sprinting). Recruitment by muscle fiber size reflects the fact that the smaller fibers are innervated by smaller motor neurons, which are more readily excited in the central nervous system. In the spinal cord, for example, any given level of excitatory input produces more depolarization and hence a greater likelihood of excitation in the smallest neurons because of their smaller membrane areas. With increasing excitatory input, larger neurons will fire.

Recruitment by size (the "size principle") offers the advantage of recruiting highly oxidative fibers first. Hence the muscle fibers with the greatest endurance are those that are used most often and remain active for the longest periods of time. Large, glycolytic white fibers, on the other hand, which are the least fatigue-resistant (because of the rapid depletion of glycogen) are recruited last and for the briefest periods of time. In addition, with the recruitment of the smaller fibers first, movements begin with small gradations of tension, facilitating their control and direction. As a result of selective recruitment, not all parts of a muscle contribute an equal share of work. Small fractions of fibers (i.e., slow red fibers) do most of the work, whereas larger pale fibers may remain inactive for long periods and are used only on maximal exertion.

Because the large motor units are also the faster units, whole muscle contraction velocity can be increased by recruiting more motor units. Recruiting more units also contributes to an increase in speed by reducing the effective load on each cell, allowing faster cross-bridge cycling rates.

The duration and intensity of exercise strongly influence the types of muscle fibers recruited.[26–29] Type I slow-twitch fibers are preferentially recruited in submaximal endurance exercise, whereas type II fibers are selectively recruited for highly intense exercise, above aerobic threshold. In this way, recruitment is used not only to increase the force of contraction but also to match the metabolic characteristics of muscle fibers to the task underway. Beyond this, individuals can learn through proper training even more effective recruitment patterns. For example, one can learn to recruit large white fibers more rapidly and more extensively in support of motor tasks requiring extreme exertion (e.g., weight lifting).

Frequency of Stimulation (Summation/Tetanus)[5,12,14]

Up to a point, **increasing the frequency at which an individual fiber is stimulated will increase the force that it generates** (Fig. 2–16). If a muscle is stimulated repeatedly at intervals longer than the total twitch duration, a series of twitches of equal magnitude will

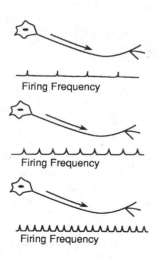

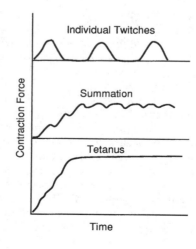

Figure 2–16. Skeletal Muscle Summation and Tetanus. As the frequency of stimulation increases, muscle tension development increases in the form of summation and ultimately tetanus.

result. If, however, the frequency of stimulation is increased so that each subsequent stimulus impinges on the muscle before relaxation is complete, an additive effect will be observed. If some relaxation is permitted to occur during the interstimulus intervals (i.e., stimulation occurs during the relaxation time of each twitch), **summation** will occur. If the frequency of stimulation is further increased so that no relaxation occurs between stimuli (i.e., stimulation occurs during the contraction time of each twitch), a sustained contraction will result, termed **tetanus**. In either case, the tension produced may be considerably greater than that of a single twitch, the maximum being achieved at tetanus. Tetanization may produce tension three to four times that of a single twitch. The particular frequency required to produce tetanus depends on the contraction time. Muscles that have long contraction times require slower stimulation to produce tetanus than do muscles with shorter contraction times.

Summation and tetanus can be explained by the series elastic elements and the manner in which they transmit active state tension to the muscle surface and its attachments. The actual binding of actin and myosin and the creation of tension at the level of the myofibrils constitute a brief phenomenon, which is quickly terminated by the pumping of Ca^{2+} back into the sarcoplasmic reticulum. By the time the series elastic elements are stretched, the tension-generating processes have already begun to dissipate. As a result, during a single twitch only a relatively small portion of the active state is actually expressed to the exterior of the muscle cell. As the frequency of stimulation is increased, less slack returns to the series elastic elements between stimuli, so that less time is required to stretch those elements with each subsequent contraction. Accordingly, more and more of the internally generated tension can be expressed to the muscle surface. This reaches its peak at the tetanizing frequency at which no relaxation occurs between stimuli; hence almost the entire active state can be used. In fact, if one compares the tension produced by tetanization with the active state, they are found to be essentially the same.

In providing a mechanism for responding to changes in the frequency of stimulation, the seemingly "inefficient" coupling of the contractile apparatus with the muscle surface provides another useful mechanism by which skeletal muscle output can be graded. Simultaneous recruitment of more motor units and increased firing rates of those motor units can markedly increase skeletal muscle force development.

Fiber Length at Stimulation[5,7,12,14,23,24,30]

A third factor that influences force development is the specific length at which a muscle fiber is positioned at the time of stimulation (Fig. 2–17). **When a skeletal muscle is stimulated at varying lengths, the force developed in response to each stimulus varies, reaching a peak at a specific optimal length.** This changing response to stimulation reflects changes occurring in the myofilament overlap as the muscle length is changed. Maximum tension will develop at the length (optimal length) at which myofilament overlap is ideal and maximal actin and myosin binding (cross-bridge formation) can occur. If this overlap is reduced by stretching the muscle, fewer cross-bridges can be formed. Similarly, if the muscle is overshortened, filaments from opposite ends of individual sarcomeres may interfere with one another and impede force development.

The optimal length in most muscles corresponds to what is termed the **resting length**, which is defined as the length that a given muscle assumes between its bony attachments in situ at rest. In fact, at the resting length most muscles are somewhat stretched and hence pre-positioned at a configuration at which tension production is highly effective. In this way, the peripheral locomotor system is held in a state of readiness, even at rest. When muscles are called on to operate at the extremes of overstretch or understretch (e.g., flexion of a limb against a significant resistance from a fully extended position), concomitant decreases in strength can be observed until those muscles can be returned to a position near the optimal length.

Pathologic alterations in muscle-bone relationships can also result in muscles operating at nonoptimal lengths. Length-tension factors, for example, must be considered in surgical

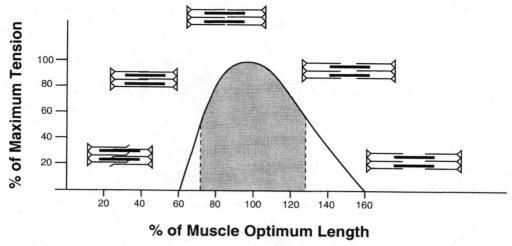

Figure 2–17. *Length-Tension Relationships in Skeletal Muscle.* Changes in muscle length are accompanied by changes in thick and thin filament overlap that affect cross-bridge formation and tension development. Maximum tension is generated at a muscle length (the optimal length) corresponding to the myofilament overlap permitting maximal cross-bridge formation.

procedures and in therapeutic programs. Outright releases, tenodeses, and transfers of muscles offer primary examples. Therapists, in lengthening muscle for the purpose of eliminating contractures, should avoid excessive lengthening that may remove the musculotendinous unit from the tension-generating range.

Maximal tension development in skeletal muscle thus occurs with convergence of optimal somatic recruitment and firing frequencies with optimal muscle positioning (i.e., length). This multifaceted control system provides the motor system with the tremendous flexibility and adaptability that will become more apparent in subsequent chapters on motor control.

Relationship Between Excitability and Force Development

As discussed in Chapter 1, **skeletal muscle is an excitable tissue,** with the same basic membrane properties shared by all muscle and nerve. The ability of muscle to contract is dependent on this excitability.

As you may recall, the muscle cell membrane is polarized, the inside being negative compared with the outside. This 90-mV resting membrane potential results from an unequal distribution of ions across the membrane and the selective permeability of the membrane to these ions. Both Na^+ and Cl^- have a greater concentration outside the cell and K^+, a higher concentration inside. The membrane is more permeable to Cl^- and K^+. Thus, the resting membrane potential is close to the equilibrium potential of these ions. For contraction to be initiated, an action potential must be generated and propagated throughout the muscle cell membrane. Ordinarily, this impulse is triggered by acetylcholine released from the somatic motor neuron but may also be initiated experimentally by electrical or chemical stimulation. Specifically, acetylcholine causes depolarization of the membrane by inducing an increased permeability to Na^+ (especially) and K^+. Depolarization beyond a threshold point leads to an action potential that will be propagated over the length of the fiber.

If the excitability of the muscle fiber is altered, the ability to contract may likewise be disturbed.[13] If, for example, excitability is diminished, muscle weakness or even paralysis may result. Hyperexcitability, on the other hand, may result in excessive muscle activity. **Although many factors may influence the excitability of muscle, it is most sensitive in this**

regard to changes in the concentrations of the electrolytes on which the membrane potential and action potential are based. Disturbances in potassium balance, for example, can cause marked changes in muscle excitability. Reduced extracellular K^+ (**hypokalemia**) causes excessive K^+ to leak out of the cell, the membrane to become hyperpolarized, and excitation to be more difficult. Muscle weakness is a characteristic sign of K^+ deficiency. **Hyperkalemia**, on the other hand, is associated with membrane depolarization and hyperexcitability. Calcium, although it does not contribute directly to the charge distribution across the muscle membrane, contributes to the stability of the membrane potential through its stabilizing effects on membrane ion channels. Reduced extracellular Ca^{2+} (**hypocalcemia**) may result in membrane instability, hyperexcitability, and excessive involuntary muscle activity, a condition termed **hypocalcemic tetany**. Increased extracellular Ca^{2+} (**hypercalcemia**), on the other hand, tends to overstabilize the membrane, making it less excitable and muscle contraction more difficult. Magnesium ion disturbances have similar effects. The direct effects of electrolyte disturbances on the muscle membrane may be exacerbated by concurrent effects on motor neuron and central nervous system activity.

A variety of pharmacologic agents exist, which can also impair muscle contraction by distorting the basic electrical processes in which these electrolytes are involved.[22] For example, a number of agents are used to purposely interfere with the effects of acetylcholine on ion fluxes and the membrane potential and thereby "block" muscle activation (see Chapter 3).

Muscle Metabolism (Provision of Energy)

Like all living cells, **the muscle fiber has an ongoing energy requirement arising merely from basal cellular activities**, such as maintaining ion gradients and synthesizing and degrading cellular constituents. **In addition, a much larger energy expenditure is required by the contraction cycle.** Each contraction reflects the cycling of tremendous numbers of cross-bridges, each one of which requires an ATP molecule. The rate at which this cycling occurs depends on both the load on the muscle and the speed of contraction. The activation of contraction requires an additional expenditure of energy in association with the action potential and sarcoplasmic reticulum Ca^{2+} release. Likewise, ATP is consumed during muscle relaxation, in the pumping of Ca^{2+} back into the sarcoplasmic reticulum and in the restoration of cellular energy stores such as creatine phosphate and glycogen.

The amount of ATP in muscle is sufficient to sustain maximal muscle activity for only a few seconds. It is therefore essential that new ATP be formed continuously. The metabolic machinery of the muscle cell provides a variety of pathways by which ATP can be supplied, each with its own particular role to play in support of contractile activity (Fig. 2–18).[5,11,12,30,31] First, **adenosine dephosphate (ADP) can be directly phosphorylated to ATP by creatine phosphate.** This is an extremely rapid process, but creatine phosphate stores are limited and sufficient to provide energy for only a few twitches. This reaction is important at the very beginning of contraction, while other systems for regenerating ATP are being turned on. Second, the glycogen stored in muscle can be split into glucose and the glucose then used in energy production. The initial stage of this process can occur entirely without the use of oxygen and is termed **anaerobic glycolysis.**[32] Although not as rapid as direct phosphorylation, anaerobic glycolysis can provide large amounts of ATP for short to moderate periods of time. The advantage of this system is that these reactions can be sustained even in the absence of oxygen. The disadvantage is that this pathway has a relatively low yield of ATP and is comparatively inefficient. It is also self-limiting to the extent that its main byproduct, lactic acid, accumulates rapidly and is highly detrimental to cell function. Moreover, glycogen stores can be rapidly depleted. Glycolysis alone can sustain maximal muscle contraction for only a minute or so. Finally, **oxidative metabolism (oxidative phosphorylation)** that takes place in mitochondria can produce large amounts of

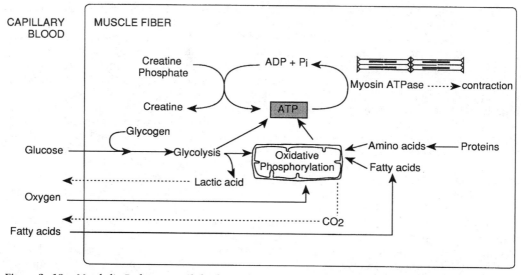

Figure 2–18. *Metabolic Pathways in Skeletal Muscle.* ATP is supplied via direct phosphorylation by creatine phosphate, glycolysis, and oxidative phosphorylation. (Adapted from Vander, AJ, Sherman, JH, and Luciano, DS: Human Physiology, ed 5. McGraw-Hill, New York, 1992, p 304.)

ATP from fatty acids, glucose, and amino acids. Although all are valuable substrates, by far the greatest proportion of energy comes from fatty acid metabolism. Oxidative phosphorylation is slower than either direct phosphorylation by creatine phosphate or anaerobic glycolysis, but it is more efficient (i.e., it produces more ATP/mole of substrate) and can be sustained for long periods of time. More than 95% of all energy used by the muscles for sustained, long-term contraction is derived from oxidative metabolism.

The specific pathways by which energy is provided to the muscle cell vary with the intensity and duration of the activity that it is performing and reflect the advantages offered by each system (Table 2–2; Fig. 2–19).[5,11,12,31,32] In a 100-m dash, for example, in which energy consumption is extremely rapid, about 85% of the energy consumed will be derived anaerobically. On the other hand, during a 60-minute long-distance run that requires the provision of energy at a relatively modest rate for a prolonged time, 95% of the energy will be provided oxidatively.

Table 2–2. *Basic Properties of Skeletal Muscle Energy Sources*

	Direct Phosphorylation	Anaerobic Glycolysis	Oxidative Phosphorylation
Maximum power generation (moles of ATP/min)	4	2.5	1
Endurance	8–10 s	1–2 min	Indefinitely
Advantages	Rapidity	Occurs in the absence of O_2	Efficient and sustainable
Disadvantages	Quickly depleted	Rapid depletion of glycogen; accumulation of lactic acid	Relatively lower power output
Muscle fiber type in which predominant	Fast twitch	Fast twitch	Slow twitch and fast twitch, fatigue-resistant (type IIA)
Activity in which this is primary energy source	Sprinting, jumping, weight lifting	400-m dash, 100-m swim, tennis, soccer	Marathon, cross-country skiing, jogging

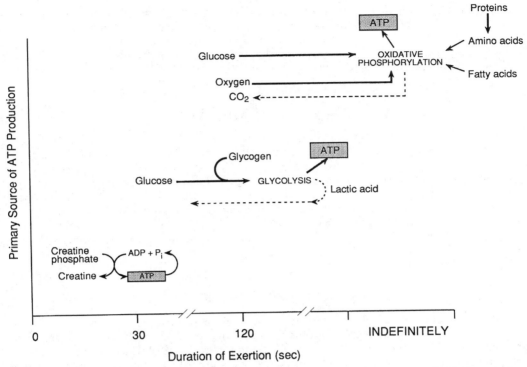

Figure 2–19. *Metabolism During Different Forms of Exertion.* Creatine phosphate may provide ATP for only the first few twitches. Anaerobic glycolysis may provide large amounts of ATP for several minutes of intense exertion. Long-term exertion of moderate intensity relies upon oxidative metabolism.

As discussed previously in this chapter (see Table 2–1), **considerable metabolic differences exist between the different types of skeletal muscle fibers.** Fast-twitch type II fibers have high glycolytic activity and relatively low oxidative activity and comparably few mitochondria. Slow-twitch type I fibers, have a more extensive oxidative capacity. In addition, fast-twitch fibers contain a form of myosin that is capable of high rates of ATP hydrolysis, expend energy rapidly, and thus have a much greater requirement for rapid ATP synthesis than do slow-twitch fibers. These basic metabolic differences underly the fatigue-resistance of type I fibers and the capacity of type II fibers for intense bursts of contractile activity and energy expenditure.

The **metabolic machinery of skeletal muscle is remarkably adaptable** and highly responsive to the functional demands placed on muscle. Those metabolic capabilities that best meet functional demands will be enhanced. Repeated activity requiring endurance results in improvement in the oxidative capacity (**conditioning**) of muscle, reflecting increased supplies of mitochondria and their oxidative enzyme systems. Conditioned athletes, for example, are capable of greater oxygen consumption by muscle and greater exertion without increased lactic acid production. These "training effects" are as evident in the patient undergoing rehabilitation as in the athlete and should be taken into consideration when designing rehabilitative exercise programs.

If skeletal muscle is not vigorously used, it quickly deconditions and the metabolic capacity to support vigorous contractile activity diminishes. This is particularly evident in the immobilized patient (see Chapter 23).

As capable and adaptable as the metabolic machinery of muscle is, it is wholly dependent on adequate supplies of substrate and oxygen. During exercise, the local changes that occur in blood flow, temperature, and pH all promote the delivery of substrate and oxygen to the muscle and the provision of energy to the contraction process. When circumstances occur that restrict the availability of these metabolic supplies, muscle performance is impaired. Insufficient blood flow (ischemia), hypoxia, anemia, diabetes, and malnutrition all can result in clinically significant impairment of muscle function. In addition, an assortment of genetic defects in specific enzyme pathways exist that result in deficient energy production and abnormal muscle activity (see Chapter 13).

Adaptive Response of Muscle to Exercise

The demands placed on the motor system are highly varied, and skeletal muscle is one of the most adaptable tissues in the body. Morphologic and functional changes in muscle can be stimulated by a variety of factors, including experimental manipulations such as crossed reinnervation or electrical stimulation, hormonal influences, and exercise.[33,34] With respect to exercise, it has become evident that **skeletal muscle is remodeled throughout life in response to the type of work that it performs.**[5,31,33–38] Muscle is affected not only by the frequency with which it is used but also by the duration and intensity of this activity (Table 2–3).

Strength Training

Skeletal muscle adapts to short-duration, high-resistance exercise, such as weight lifting or sprinting, **with increased muscle mass and strength.**[5,33–38,41] The increase in muscle size reflects an increase in the size of the individual fibers of which the whole muscle is composed. This is true hypertrophy and must be distinguished from the transient swelling

Table 2–3. *Adaptation of Skeletal Muscle to Specific Types of Exercise*

Strength Training*	Aerobic Training†
MORPHOLOGIC	
Significant overall muscle hypertrophy	No effect
Possible muscle fiber proliferation	No effect
Significant increase in muscle strength	No effect
↑ Cross-sectional area composed of fast-twitch fibers	↓ % of cross-sectional area composed of fast-twitch fibers
No consistent effect	↓ Number of type IIB fibers with a shift to either type I, IIA, or hybrid fibers
METABOLIC	
Enhanced creatine phosphate system	?
Enhanced glycolytic activity	Glycogen sparing effect
No effect	Enhanced oxidative capacity
	↑ Mitochondrial volume
	↑ Mitochondrial enzyme activity
	↑ FFA availability and utilization
↓ or no effect	↑ Capillary density

FFA = free fatty acids.
*Intermittent bouts of low-frequency repetitions (3–10 sets of 6–8 repetitions/set) with high loads (65–75% of maximum) and long recovery periods between training bouts (2–3 days).
†Involvement of large masses of muscle in rhythmic exercise of low resistance to an extent that whole body oxygen uptake's increased many times over the resting level.

of muscle that may be observed immediately after exercise as a result of increased local blood flow. Significant hypertrophy is most likely to occur in response to use of a muscle at or near its maximum force-generating capacity. In fact, brief periods of use at these levels of intensity will produce significant muscle growth within a period of weeks. This is an adaptive response in which muscle hypertrophies up to a level of size and strength that is consistent with a particular level of utilization. It remains at this level until the demands on it are changed. Additional growth occurs only with increased work intensity.

True **fiber hypertrophy reflects an actual net gain in the protein content of the muscle fiber**, which is brought about by increased protein synthesis and decreased protein degradation (catabolism).[39] Significant changes occur in the contractile apparatus itself. Increased numbers of both thick and thin myofilaments are produced, and the size and number of myofibrils increases. Sarcoplasmic reticulum and T-tubule volume increases in proportion to the change in myofibrils. The synthetic machinery itself is augmented, as manifested in increased RNA and DNA content and increased numbers of nuclei. In addition, cellular stores of energy-rich phosphates and glycogen are increased along with the activities of the enzymes necessary for their metabolism. The effects of forceful exercise are most evident in fast-twitch type II fibers which seem to be selectively hypertrophied. As a result, in any given muscle, type II fibers occupy an increasing proportion of the total cross-sectional area.

Although the bulk of work-induced muscle growth is due to fiber enlargement, **there is some evidence that the** *number* **of muscle fibers may also increase**. This is termed *hyperplasia*.[5,40,41] Under conditions of extremely forceful exercise (and under some conditions of reinnervation) new fibers have been shown to arise from the longitudinal splitting of enlarged fibers or even de novo synthesis from precursor cells. Hyperplasia, however, accounts for only a very small percentage of the overall increase in muscle size.

In addition to stimulating muscle cells, forceful exercise seems to stimulate fibroblasts to increase the synthesis of collagenous proteins in the supportive connective tissue structures of muscle. In this way, the size and strength of tendons and other muscular attachments increase as the strength of muscle increases.

Force development is determined not only by the size of the individual muscles but also by the ability of the nervous system to appropriately activate the muscles.[42] Early increases in strength, particularly in nontrained individuals, may occur without alterations in muscle size and are due to adaptive changes in the central nervous system that increase the capability to activate and recruit motor units. This is the neural component of strength training.

Aerobic Training

With exercise that is of low intensity but of long duration, such as long-distance running, swimming, or cycling, **the primary adaptation in skeletal muscle is an enhancement of fatigue resistance**.[5,33–38] Increased oxidative capacity is achieved by increasing the number of mitochondria and the specific activities of the mitochondrial enzymes of the fast-twitch and slow-twitch oxidative fibers that are recruited during this type of activity. Intracellular fat stores and the enzymes responsible for their metabolism are enhanced, enabling muscle cells to supply energy by using more fat and less glycogen. As a result of the increased activity of mitochondrial oxidative enzymes, the activities of extramitochondrial enzymes involved in anaerobic glycolysis are lower, and more power can be generated without producing lactate. Repeated long-term use also promotes expansion of the capillary network supplying muscle (i.e., increased capillary density) and increased blood flow. Although slow-twitch fibers may undergo some modest hypertrophy, simultaneous atrophy of some fast-twitch fibers leaves overall muscle size and power unaltered or even slightly diminished after endurance exercise. Concomitant changes in the respiratory and circulatory systems further improve fatigue resistance through improved delivery of oxygen and fuel to skeletal muscle.

Fiber Transformation

Theoretically, exercise might enhance the capabilities of a muscle for endurance or power activities by transforming the muscle fibers of which that muscle is composed into the most appropriate types.[33-38] Fiber type conversions have been shown to occur with crossed reinnervation and chronic electrical stimulation of human skeletal muscle and in young developing animals. It is unclear, however, whether exercise can induce actual transformation of one type of muscle fiber to another in adult animals, especially humans.[43-46]

In humans, at very intense exercise levels some fiber transformation probably does occur (Fig. 2–20).[37,43-46] However, this transformation makes a relatively small contribution to the overall adaptation of muscle to increased use. It is likely that intense endurance training over several months does induce conversion of type B fast-twitch fibers to type A and possibly conversion of a few type A fast-twitch fibers to slow-twitch type I fibers. Although heavy resistance training may induce meager conversion of fast-twitch subtypes, there is no evidence that strength training increases the proportion of fast-twitch fibers. Although fast-twitch fibers occupy an increased proportion of the cross-sectional area of strength-trained muscle, this is a reflection of their increased size, not an increase in their numbers either from hyperplasia or fiber transformation. The similar proportions of fast-twitch and slow-twitch fibers in trained and untrained muscles of elite athletes argues against any significant muscle fiber transformation even with prolonged training. The extremely high proportion of slow-twitch fibers in endurance athletes and fast-twitch fibers in power athletes is more likely inherited, than a result of the specific training undergone by these individuals.[31]

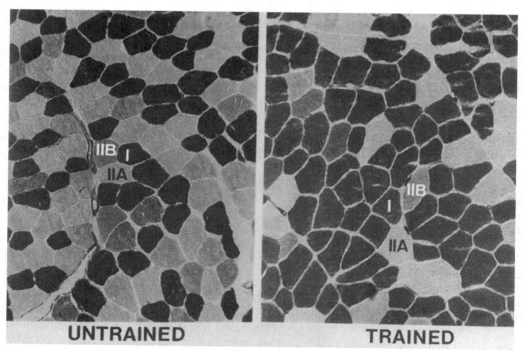

UNTRAINED   **TRAINED**

Figure 2–20. *Effect of Short-Term Endurance Training on Fiber Type Composition in the Vastus Lateralis Muscle.* Cross sections taken from biposies before and after the training period show an increase in type I fibers and a decrease in type IIA and IIB fibers. (From Baumann, et al,[46] p 351, with permission.)

Understanding the Mechanisms of Muscle Change

Even though the effects of increased use on skeletal muscle may be extensive, the mechanisms by which changes in mechanical activity elicit alterations in muscle cell morphology and function are poorly understood. Clearly, whatever the mechanisms may be, the fibers most actively recruited during exercise are affected the most. In general, during any muscular activity the slow-twitch oxidative fibers are recruited first. With any additional requirement for more rapid movement or for the generation of more force, increasing numbers of type IIA and type IIB fast-twitch fibers will be recruited. Accordingly, in rapid power movements or high-intensity isometric contractions (e.g., associated with athletic throwing events or weight lifting) all types of fibers are recruited, and the muscles involved become larger through hypertrophy of all fiber types. During repetitive low-intensity exercise (e.g., long-distance running or cycling) and postural activity, the slow-twitch fibers are predominantly activated, whereas fast-twitch fibers are hardly ever recruited. Although slow-twitch fibers may consequently undergo some hypertrophy, the simultaneous atrophy of some (seldom-used) fast-twitch fibers leave the muscle size and power unaltered or even slightly diminished.

Although recruitment order explains which fibers are most affected by different types of use, it does not explain how changes in mechanical activity affect basic cellular processes. **The final arbiter of cellular transformation must be the gene, which directs the synthesis of cellular proteins.** Muscle activity can influence genetic expression in terms of both the amounts and specific kinds of proteins synthesized.[43–46] Genetically determined alterations have been shown in myofibrillar proteins (myosin and the regulatory proteins), the Ca^{2+} regulatory system (T tubule and sarcoplasmic reticulum), and enzymatic activities. Myosin and many of the other proteins involved in contraction occur in different isoforms, and genes can be switched from one form to another, thus altering the basic contractile properties of fibers. Muscle is a tissue in which genetic expression is strongly influenced by mechanical signals, and, although not well understood, these signals seem to promote subtle changes at many sites of gene regulation. Increased overall nuclear synthetic activity is reflected in enhanced amino acid utilization and increased RNA translation and DNA transcription.

All the adaptations of skeletal muscle to exercise are reversible.[33,34,47,48] When exercise is stopped, the components of muscle that changed as a result of that exercise will slowly revert over a period of months to their state before exercise began. **This is termed** *deconditioning.* Even more severe deterioration of muscle occurs with immobilization or denervation. Physical therapy treatment strategies are designed to both prevent and reverse the disabling deconditioning of skeletal muscle. When muscle is allowed to deteriorate, functional loss is heightened and rehabilitation impeded. The deterioration and atrophy of muscle are further discussed in the context of locomotor dysfunction in Chapters 13 and 23.

Just as exercise choices are made in a program of athletic training with a view toward specific changes in muscle, these changes must be considered in planning patient care. If the goal of rehabilitation is stamina and endurance, exercises should specifically stress type I fibers. Where the aim is strength or power, exercise patterns should selectively promote type II fiber enhancement.

Hormone-Induced Effects on Muscle

A variety of hormones have significant effects on skeletal muscle function and performance. Although a detailed discussion of these substances and their interrelationships is beyond the scope of this chapter, several are briefly discussed here. All of these hormones are necessary for normal growth and development of muscle and its maintenance.[49,50]

Testosterone

Testosterone has powerful growth-promoting (anabolic) effects on skeletal muscle, which revolve around stimulation of protein synthesis and inhibition of protein catabolism.[50,51] Testosterone propels the rapid growth of muscle during puberty and accounts for the marked differences that exist between men and women in muscle size and strength. A man with little muscular activity, but adequate testosterone, will have appreciably more muscle growth, and hence strength, than his female counterpart. These growth-promoting properties of testosterone have prompted the development of a whole assortment of testosterone-related anabolic steroids,[50,51] designed to maximize anabolic while minimizing androgenic effects. Although there are legitimate medical indications for their use, these substances are most widely known for their illicit use in efforts to improve athletic performance. In men, when testosterone is deficient, because of aging or pathologic hypogonadism, muscle size and strength will decline.

Insulin

Insulin has important influences on muscle function through effects on both protein synthesis and glucose metabolism.[50] In the absence of insulin, the muscle cell membrane is only slightly permeable to glucose, which explains why most of the time muscle depends, not on glucose, but on fatty acids for its energy. In the presence of insulin, however, large quantities of glucose are transported into the muscle cell and either used for energy production or stored for future use in the form of glycogen. Insulin promotes protein synthesis and storage in muscle via stimulatory effects on amino acid uptake, ribosomal RNA translation, and gene DNA transcription, and inhibitory effects on protein catabolism. Insulin deficiency is associated with impaired muscle energetics, impaired performance, and atrophy.

Growth Hormone

Growth hormone has effects on muscle protein metabolism very similar to those of insulin, promoting protein synthesis, while inhibiting catabolism.[50,52] In fact, insulin and growth hormone exert synergistic effects on muscle.

Thyroid Hormone

Thyroid hormone has effects on nearly every organ system of the body. It exerts these effects by binding to nuclear receptors and thereby influencing the synthesis of many enzymatic, structural, and transport proteins, as well as other substances. **The net effect of thyroid hormone is a generalized increase in cellular activity throughout the body, including muscle.**[50] Slight increases in thyroid hormone usually enhance muscle contraction. In the presence of excessive amounts (hyperthyroidism) muscle atrophy, weakness, and fatiguability are common. Although the biochemical basis of these effects is uncertain, they may be related to increased protein catabolism and an inability of thyrotoxic muscle to phosphorylate creatine. In hypothyroidism, muscle cramps, but not muscle weakness, are common.

Glucocorticoids

Glucocorticoids, such as cortisol, mobilize amino acids from extrahepatic tissues, especially muscle, by producing a decrease in protein synthesis and an increase in protein catabolism.[50] The mobilized amino acids are then used in liver gluconeogenesis. In the normal state, glucocorticoids thus maintain blood sugar and the glycogen content of liver and muscle. In cases of excessive glucocorticoid levels, such as Cushing's syndrome or clinical treatment with steroids, excessive mobilization of amino acids from muscle (catabolism) may result in generalized muscle wasting and muscle weakness.[53,54] Moreover, excessive glucocorticoids may produce a diabeteslike state because of their ability to raise blood sugar and to decrease the sensitivity of muscle and other tissues to insulin.

Skeletal Muscle and Aging

Certain **characteristic changes occur in skeletal muscle as people age**.[48,55–63] It is difficult, however, to distinguish between alterations in muscle that result from aging per se and those due to factors that often accompany aging, such as reduced physical activity, poor nutrition, or disease. It is generally recognized that both **total muscle mass and the size of individual muscles decline throughout adult life**, a process that accelerates at about 60 years of age. This decline in muscle size is usually **accompanied by a loss of isometric and dynamic muscle strength**, although the age at which this decline occurs is variable and depends on the specific muscle in question. Variations in physical activity may explain some of the differences in the degree of atrophy and loss of strength among muscle groups. Muscles used continuously throughout life for the basic activities of daily living (e.g., gripping objects, ambulation, or breathing) tend to retain their strength the longest. Although aged muscles are smaller, their actual ability to generate force per unit of cross-sectional area remains relatively constant. Also, there appears to be little decline in the metabolic potential for either aerobic or anaerobic activity as the person ages, at least up to about age 70.

The primary cause of the age-dependent decline in muscle size and strength is not a decrease in the size of individual muscle fibers, but an actual loss of fibers.[58,59,62] **With age, a neurogenic loss of motor units occurs**. Deleterious changes in somatic nerves result in the denervation of motor units and their eventual disappearance. As somatic contacts are lost, a dynamic process of reorganization and reinnervation seems to occur among the surviving muscle fibers. Evidence of this is found in the fact that muscles contain motor units composed of more muscle fibers (i.e., they include some fibers from other denervated units) and more groupings of like fiber types.[60]

What happens to the size and relative numbers of specific fiber types during aging is much less clear. There is some evidence that fast-twitch fibers suffer the most, possibly reflecting a selective loss of the largest and fastest conducting motor neurons that innervate type II fibers.[57–59,61,62]

Most individuals significantly reduce their level of physical activity at a surprisingly early age; so it is likely that the changes occurring in aging muscle reflect both directly age-related factors as well as relative disuse. Even in old age, muscle function adapts to usage and many of these muscle alterations can be reversed by increased physical activity.[56–62] In men in their 70s, for example, strength training can significantly increase muscle size and strength and the relative area devoted to fast-twitch fibers. Although the age-dependent loss of motor units is inevitable, it is likely that much of the deterioration of the remaining muscle fibers can be forestalled or minimized by lifelong physical activity.

RECOMMENDED READINGS

Abernethy, PJ, Thayer, R, and Taylor, AW: Acute and Chronic Responses of Skeletal Muscle to Endurance and Sprint Exercise. Sports Med 10(6):365, 1990.

Astrand, P-O and Rodahl, K. Textbook of Work Physiology. Chapter 2. The Muscle and Its Contraction. McGraw-Hill, New York, 1986.

Binder-Macleod, S (ed): Special Series: Skeletal Muscle. Phys Ther 73(12):826, 1993.

Booth, FW and Thomason, DB: Molecular and Cellular Adaptation of Muscle in Response to Exercise: Perspectives of Various Models. Physiol Rev 71(2):541, 1991.

Carter, RJM: Age-Related Changes in Skeletal Muscle Function. Aging 2:27, 1990.

Eastwood, AB: Normal Structure of Skeletal Muscle. Chapter 1. In Adachi, M and Sher, JH (eds): Neuromuscular Disease. Igaku Shoin, New York, 1990.

Engel, AG and Franzini-Armstrong, C (eds): Myology. Part I, ed 2. McGraw-Hill, New York, 1994.

Florini, JR: Hormonal Control of Muscle Growth. Muscle Nerve 10:577, 1987.

Gordon, T and Pattullo, MC: Plasticity of Muscle Fiber and Motor Unit Types. Exerc Sport Sci Rev 21:331, 1993.

Guyton, AC: Textbook of Medical Physiology, ed 8. Chapter 6. Contraction of Skeletal Muscle. WB Saunders, Philadelphia, 1991.

Huxley, AF: Review Lecture: Muscular Contraction. J Physiol (Lond) 243:1, 1974.

Komi, PV (ed): Strength and Power in Sport. Blackwell Scientific Publications, London, 1992.

Lieber, RL: Skeletal Muscle Structure and Function. Chapters 1, 2, and 4. Williams & Wilkins, Baltimore, 1992.

Murphy, RA: Skeletal Muscle Physiology. Chapter 18. In Berne, RM and Levy, MN (eds). Physiology, ed 3. Mosby-Year Book, St. Louis, 1993.

Patton, HD, et al (eds): Textbook of Physiology, ed 2. Chapters 6–9. WB Saunders, Philadelphia, 1989.

Peachy, LD, Adrian, RH and Geiger, SR (eds): Handbook of Physiology. Section 10: Skeletal Muscle. American Physiological Society, Bethesda, MD, 1983.

Rogers, MA and Evans, WJ: Changes in Skeletal Muscle with Aging: Effects of Exercise Training. Exerc Sport Sci Rev 21:65, 1993.

Sugi, H and Pollack, GH (eds): Mechanism of Myofilament Sliding in Muscle Contraction. Plenum Press, New York, 1993.

REFERENCES

1. Eastwood, AB: Normal Structure of Skeletal Muscle. Chapter 1. In Adachi, M and Sher, JH (eds): Neuromuscular Disease. Igaku-Shoin, New York, 1990.

2. Landon, DN: Skeletal Muscle: Normal Morphology, Development, and Innervation. Chapter 1. In Mastaglia, FL and Walton, Lord Detchant (eds): Skeletal Muscle Pathology, ed 2. Churchill Livingstone, Edinburgh, 1992.

3. Fischbeck, KH: Structure and Function of Skeletal Muscle. Chapter 11. In Asbury, AK, McKhann, GM and McDonald, WI (eds): Diseases of the Nervous System: Clinical Neurobiology, ed 2. WB Saunders, Philadelphia, 1992.

4. Lieber, RL: Skeletal Muscle Structure and Functions. Chapter 1. Skeletal Muscle Anatomy. Williams & Wilkins, Baltimore, 1992.

5. Guyton, AC: Textbook of Medical Physiology, ed 8. Chapter 6. Contraction of Skeletal Muscle. WB Saunders, Philadelphia, 1991.

6. Murphy, RA: Contractile Mechanism of Muscle Cells. Chapter 17. In Berne, RM and Levy, MN (eds): Physiology, ed 3. Mosby-Year Book, St. Louis, 1993.

7. Astrand, P-O and Rodahl, K: Textbook of Work Physiology: Physiological Basis of Exercise, ed 3. Chapter 2. The Muscle and Its Contraction. McGraw-Hill, New York, 1986.

8. Craig, R: The Structure of the Contractile Filaments. Chapter 5. In Engel, AG and Franzini-Armstrong, C (eds): Myology, ed 2. McGraw-Hill, New York, 1994.

9. Huxley, AF: Muscle Structure and Theories of Contraction. Prog Biophys 7:255, 1957.

10. Huxley, HE and Hanson, J: Changes in the cross-striations of muscle during contraction and stretch and their structural interpretation. Nature 173:973, 1954.

11. Billeter, R and Hoppeler, H: Muscular Basis of Strength. Chapter 3. In Komi, PV (ed): Strength and Power in Sport. Blackwell Scientific Publications, Oxford, 1992.

12. Murphy, RA: Skeletal Muscle Physiology. Chapter 18. In Berne, RM and Levy, MN (eds): Physiology, ed 3. Mosby-Year Book, St. Louis, 1993.

13. Barchi, RL: The Muscle Fiber and Disorders of Muscle Excitability. Chapter 33. In Siegel, GJ, et al (eds): Basic Neurochemistry. Molecular, Cellular, and Medical Aspects, ed 4. Raven Press, New York, 1989.

14. Ghez, C: Muscles: Effectors of the Motor Systems. Chapter 36. In Kandel, ER, Schwartz, JH and Jessell, TM (eds): Principles of Neural Science, ed 3. Appleton & Lange, Norwalk, CT, 1991.

15. Gordon, AM: Molecular Basis of Contraction. Chapter 8. In Patton, HD, et al (eds): Textbook of Physiology, ed 21. WB Saunders, Philadelphia, 1989.

16. Homsher, E: The Cross-Bridge Cycle and the Energetics of Contraction. Chapter 13. In Engel, AG and Franzini-Armstrong, C (eds): Myology, ed 2. McGraw-Hill, New York, 1994.

17. Perry, SV: Activation of the Contractile Mechanism by Calcium. Chapter 20. In Engel, AG and Franzini-Armstrong, C (eds): Myology, ed 2. McGraw-Hill, New York, 1994.

18. Ruegg, JC: Calcium in Muscle Contraction: Cellular and Molecular Physiology, ed 2. Chapters 1–4. Springer-Verlag, Berlin, 1992.

19. Almers, W: Excitation-Contraction Coupling in Skeletal Muscle. Chapter 7. In Patton, HD, et al (eds): Textbook of Physiology, ed 21. WB Saunders, Philadelphia, 1989.

20. Catterall, WA: Excitation Contraction Coupling in Vertebrate Skeletal Muscle: A Tale of Two Calcium Channels. Cell 64:871, 1991.

21. Fleischer, S and Inui, M: Biochemistry and Biophysics of Excitation-Contraction Coupling. Ann Rev Biophys Biophys Chem 18:333, 1989.

22. Cedarbaum, JM and Schleifer, LS: Drugs for Parkinson's Disease, Spasticity, and Acute Muscle Spasms. Chapter 20. In Gilman, AG, et al (eds): Goodman and Gilman's The Pharmacologic Basis of Therapeutics, ed 8. McGraw-Hill, New York, 1993.

23. Lieber, RL and Bodine-Fowler, SC: Skeletal Muscle Mechanics: Implication for Rehabilitation. Phys Ther 73(12):844, 1993.

24. Lieber, RL: Skeletal Muscle Structure and Function. Chapter 2. Skeletal Muscle Physiology. Williams & Wilkins, Baltimore, 1992.

25. Kelly, AM and Rubenstein, NA: The Diversity of Muscle Fiber Types and Its Origin During Development. Chapter 4. In Engel, AG and Franzini-Armstrong, C (eds): Myology, ed 2. McGraw-Hill, New York, 1994.

26. Burke, D and Gandevia, SC: Peripheral Motor System. Chapter 6. In Paxinos, G (ed): The Human Nervous System. Academic Press, San Diego, 1990.

27. Burke, RE: The Physiology of Motor Units. Chapter 17. In Engel, AG and Franzini-Armstrong, C (eds): Myology, ed 2. McGraw-Hill, New York, 1994.

28. Peters, SE: Structure and Function in Vertebrate Skeletal Muscle. Am Zool, 29:221, 1989.

29. Clamann, HP: Motor Unit Recruitment and the Gradation of Muscle Force. Phys Ther 73(12):830, 1993.

30. Gordon, AM: Contraction of Skeletal Muscle. Chapter 9. In Patton, HD, et al (eds): Textbook of Physiology, ed 21. WB Saunders, Philadelphia, 1989.

31. Guyton, AC: Textbook of Medical Physiology, ed 8. Chapter 84. Sports Physiology. WB Saunders, Philadelphia, 1991.

32. Spriet, LL: Anaerobic Metabolism in Human Skeletal Muscle During Short-Term, Intense Activity. Can J Physiol Pharmacol 70(1):157, 1992.

33. Roy, RR, Baldwin, KM, and Edgerton, VR: The Plasticity of Skeletal Muscle: Effects of Neuromuscular Activity. Exerc Sport Sci Rev 19:269, 1991.

34. Gordon, T. and Pattullo, MC: Plasticity of Muscle Fiber and Motor Types. Exerc Sport Sci Rev 21:331, 1993.

35. Abernethy, PJ, Thayer, R, and Taylor, AW: Acute and Chronic Responses of Skeletal Muscle to Endurance and Sprint Exercise. Sports Med 10(6):365, 1990.

36. Booth, FW and Thomason, DB: Molecular and Cellular Adaptation of Muscle in Response to Exercise: Perspectives of Various Models. Physiol Rev 71(2):541, 1991.

37. Lieber, RL: Skeletal Muscle Structure and Function. Chapter 4. Skeletal Muscle Adaptation to Increased Use. Williams & Wilkins, Baltimore, 1992.

38. Goldspink, G: Cellular and Molecular Aspects of Adaptation in Skeletal Muscle. Chapter 8A. In Komi, PV (ed): Strength and Power in Sport. Blackwell Scientific Publications, Oxford, 1992.

39. Goldspink, DF: Exercise-Related Changes in Protein Turnover in Mammalian Striated Muscle. J Exp Biol 160:127, 1991.

40. McDougall, JD: Hypertrophy or Hyperplasia. Chapter 8B. In Komi, PV (ed): Strength and Power in Sport. Blackwell Scientific Publications, Oxford, 1992.

41. Tesch, PA: Skeletal Muscle Adaptations Consequent to Long-Term Heavy Resistance Exercise. Med Sci Sports Exerc 20(5):S132, 1988.

42. Sale, DG: Neural Adaptation to Strength Training. Chapter 9A. In Komi, PV (ed): Strength and Power in Sport. Blackwell Scientific Publications, Oxford, 1992.

43. Pette, D and Dusterhoft, S: Altered Gene Expression in Fast-Twitch Muscle Induced by Chronic Low-Frequency Stimulation. Am J Physiol 262:R333, 1992.

44. Goldspink, G, et al: Gene Expression in Skeletal Muscle in Response to Stretch and Force Generation. Am J Physiol 262:R356, 1992.

45. Booth, FW and Kirby, CR: Control of Gene Expression in Adult Skeletal Muscle by Changes in the Inherent Level of Contractile Activity. Biochem Soc Trans 19:374, 1991.

46. Baumann, H: Exercise Training Induces Transitions of Myosin Isoform Subunits with Histochemically Typed Muscle Fibres. Pfluger's Arch 409:349, 1987.

47. Lieber, RL: Skeletal Muscle Structure and Function. Chapter 5. Skeletal Muscle Adaptation to Decreased Use. Williams & Wilkins, Baltimore, 1992.

48. Jennekens, FGI: Disuse, Cachexia, and Aging. Chapter 23. In Mastaglia, FL and Walton, Lord Detchant (eds): Skeletal Muscle Pathology, ed 2. Churchill Livingstone, Edinburgh, 1992.

49. Florini, JR: Hormonal Control of Muscle Growth. Muscle Nerve 10:577, 1989.

50. Kraemer, WJ: Hormonal Mechanisms Related to the Expression of Muscular Strength and Power. Chapter 4. In Komi, PV (ed): Strength and Power in Sport. Blackwell Scientific Publications, Oxford, 1992.

51. Celotti, F and Negri Cesi, P. Anabolic Steroids: A Review of Their Effects on the Muscles, of Their Possible Mechanisms of Action, and of Their Use in Athletics. J Steroid Biochem Mol Biol 43(5):409, 1992.

52. Yarasheski, KE: Growth Hormone Effects on Metabolism, Body Composition, Muscle Mass, and Strength. Exerc Sport Sci Rev 22:285, 1994.

53. Hickson, RC and Marone, JR: Exercise and Inhibition of Glucocorticoid-Induced Muscle Atrophy. Exerc Sport Sci Rev 21:135, 1993.

54. Almon, RR and Dubois, DC: Fiber-Type Discrimination in Disuse and Glucocorticoid-Induced Atrophy. Med Sci Sports Exerc 22(3):304, 1993.

55. Wilmore, JH: The Aging of Bone and Muscle. Clin Sports Med 10(2):231, 1991.

56. Vandervoort, AA: Effects of Ageing on Human Neuromuscular Function: Implications for Exercise. Can J Sport Sci 17(3):178, 1992.

57. Klitgaard, H, et al: Function, Morphology, and Protein Expression of Ageing Skeletal Muscle: A Cross-Sectional Study of Elderly Men with Different Training Backgrounds. Acta Physiol Scand 140:41, 1990.

58. Rogers, MA and Evans, WJ: Changes in Skeletal Muscle with Aging: Effects of Exercise Training. Exerc Sport Sci Rev 21:65, 1993.

59. Doherty, TJ, Vandervoort, AA, and Brown, WF: Effects of Ageing on the Motor Unit: A Brief Review. Can J Appl Physiol 18(4):331, 1993.

60. Cartee, GD: Aging Skeletal Muscle Response to Exercise. Exerc Sport Sci Rev 22:91, 1994.

61. Thompson, LV: Effects of Age and Training on Skeletal Muscle Physiology and Performance. Phys Ther 74(1):71, 1994.

62. Hopp, JF: Effects of Age and Resistance Training on Skeletal Muscle: A Review. Phys Ther 73(6):361, 1993.

63. Seto, JL and Brewster, CE: Musculoskeletal Conditioning of the Older Athlete. Clin Sports Med 10(2):401, 1991.

CHAPTER 3

■

The Neuromuscular Junction: The Nerve/Muscle Interface

Christopher M. Fredericks, PhD

- *Structure*
- *Transmission of Excitation*
- *Pharmacologic Modification of Neuromuscular Transmission*
- *Trophic Interactions Between Motor Neurons and Muscle*

*I*n a healthy individual, skeletal muscles are not spontaneously active but are dependent on external stimulation for their excitation. This is normally provided by excitatory impulses (action potentials) occurring in the motor neurons with which the muscles are innervated. Although these neurons do not actually touch the muscle fibers, they are closely associated with them at the neuromuscular junction. The specialized structure and function of this junction permit their excitation to be transmitted to the muscle fiber. Disturbances of neuromuscular junction function can result in clinically significant, even life-threatening impairments of skeletal muscle activity.

Skeletal muscles are innervated by somatic motor neurons whose cell bodies are located in either the cranial nerve motor nuclei of the brainstem or the anterior horns of the spinal cord. These motor neurons have long, large-diameter, myelinated axons that travel without interruption from the central nervous system to skeletal muscle. Along its course, each axon branches. This branching allows a single axon to innervate many individual muscle fibers. Each axon, together with the muscle fibers that it innervates, forms the functional unit (the effector) of the somatic system called a **motor unit** (Fig. 3–1). The number of muscle fibers within a single motor unit varies tremendously, ranging from only a few fibers to thousands of fibers.

The neuromuscular junction is a chemical synapse that is specialized both anatomically and functionally to facilitate the transmission of a signal from the motor nerve terminal to the muscle fiber. In some respects, the neuromuscular junction resembles other chemical synapses; in other respects, it is unique.

Structure[1–3]

Both the motor neuron terminal and the adjacent muscle cell membrane are highly specialized anatomically to facilitate communication between these two excitable tissues.

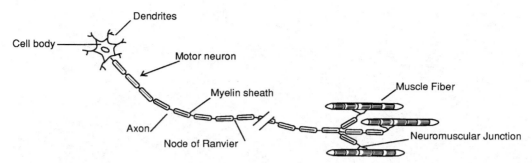

Figure 3–1. *A Motor Unit.* Each motor unit consists of a motor neuron and all of the muscle fibers that it innervates.

As the axon supplying a skeletal muscle fiber approaches its termination, it loses its myelin sheath and branches into an array of smaller terminal filaments. This array spreads in various directions over the surface of a specialized region of the sarcolemma called the **motor end plate** and may occupy several thousand square micrometers of the muscle fiber membrane (Fig. 3–2). The form and extent of this array depend on the specific muscle. Each unmyelinated filament lies embedded in a trough or indentation formed in the thickened membrane of the end plate, termed a **primary junctional cleft**. The surface of each primary cleft is in turn covered with many deep, closely spaced secondary clefts or junctional folds (Fig. 3–3). The branching of the terminal motor axon and the extensive convolutions of the adjacent motor end plate both serve to increase the surface area of the opposing excitable

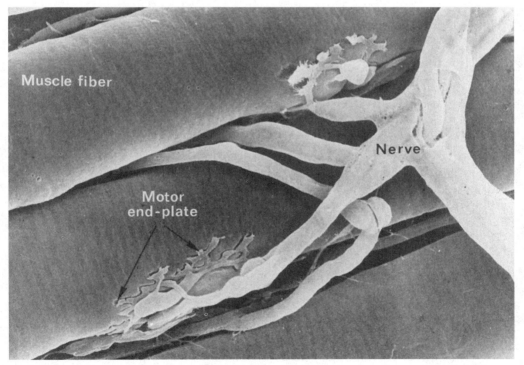

Figure 3–2. *Surface Appearance of the Neuromuscular Junction.* This is a scanning electron micrograph of a motor neuron and two motor endplates on adjacent skeletal muscle fibers. (Micrograph from Desaki, J and Uehara, Y: J Neurocytol 10:101, 1981 as published in Fawcett, DW: Textbook of Histology, ed. 11, p 291, with permission. Copyright © 1986 Chapman & Hall, New York.)

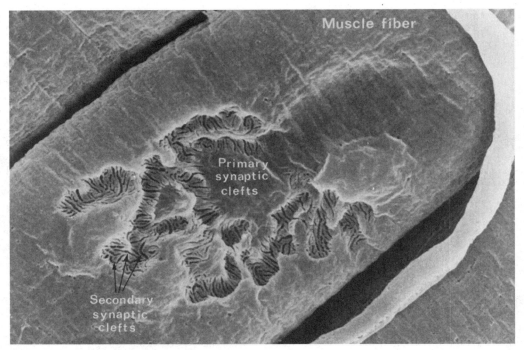

Figure 3–3. *Surface Appearance of the Motor Endplate.* This is a scanning electron micrograph of a skeletal muscle fiber from which the nerve terminal has been pulled away, revealing the underlying primary and secondary synaptic clefts of the motor endplate. (Micrograph from Uehara, Y, Desaki, J, and Fujiwara, T: Biomed Res 2: Suppl 139, 1981 as published in Fawcett, DW: Textbook of Histology, ed. 11, p 291, with permission. Copyright © 1986 Chapman & Hall, New York.)

tissues of the neuromuscular junction. Junctional folds are not found in other synapses. At synapses that lack junctional folds, the surface area of the presynaptic and postsynaptic membranes are essentially the same. The junctional folds of the neuromuscular junction, however, produce a five- to- sixfold increase in the postjunctional surface. The complexity and size of these folds vary according to species, type of innervation, and muscle fiber type. Fast-twitch (type IIB) muscle fibers, for example, generally have better developed and more complex junctional folds than slow-twitch (type I) muscle fibers.

The motor nerve terminal has many of the features observed in other chemical synapses (Figs. 3–4 and 3–5). Mitochondria and small, clear vesicles are abundant. In addition, electron-dense "active zones" may be demonstrated by electron microscopy on the axonal membrane opposite the openings to the secondary clefts, and they probably represent sites for transmitter release. The axonal vesicles seem to be congregated within the axoplasm just opposite the openings of the secondary clefts and are clustered around these active zones.

The synaptic space between the nerve terminal and the muscle membrane is continuous with the extracellular space around the junction. A layer of carbohydrate-rich material termed the **basement membrane** (or basal lamina) covers both the prejunctional and postjunctional membranes and follows the contour of both the primary and secondary clefts.[4] This basal lamina is rich in the enzyme, acetylcholinesterase, which extends all the way down to the bottom of the clefts. Although all chemical synapses have a cleft separating the presynaptic axon terminal from the postsynaptic cell, the gap in the neuromuscular junction is wider than in most other synapses.

The muscle membrane is also highly specialized. Tightly packed intramembraneous particles, which are believed to be acetylcholine receptors, are concentrated on top of the folds of the motor end plate. The sarcoplasm within the folds contains a complex

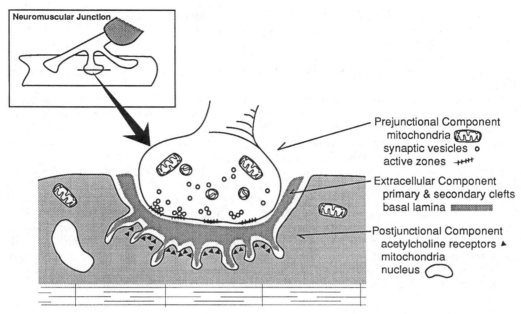

Figure 3-4. *Morphologic Features of a Typical Neuromuscular Junction.* The prejunctional axoplasm contains mitochondria and many small vesicles. The vesicles are clustered around active zones in the neural membrane, which may represent sites for their release. The postjunctional membrane is folded into primary and secondary clefts and contains the acetylcholine receptors. Nuclei, mitochondria, and other organelles abound within the muscle cell, along with the contractile apparatus. The synaptic cleft contains a central layer of basal lamina.

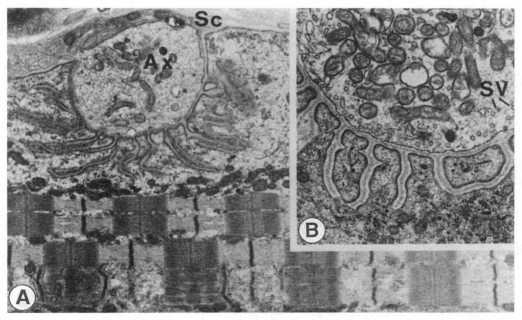

Figure 3-5. *Photomicrographs of Human Neuromuscular Junction.* (A) The axon terminal (Ax) lies in a groove or primary cleft in the muscle fiber. Secondary clefts radiate into the fiber from the primary cleft. A Schwann cell process (Sc) covers the axon (×10,000). (B) This portion of another neuromuscular junction shows synaptic vesicles (SV) and basal lamina in the junctional gap between the axon and muscle fibers (×25,000). (Micrograph from Adachi, M and Sher, SH: Neuromuscular Disease. Igaku-Shoin, New York, 1990, p 7, with permission.)

cytoskeleton of fine microtubules and filaments, which may be involved in the maintenance of the infolding or in anchoring the acetylcholine receptors. Mitochondria and nuclei are abundant within the adjacent sarcoplasm.

The outer surface of the terminal nerve filament is covered by a thin layer of Schwann cells. This layer forms a protective cap over the junction, insulating it from the surrounding fluids.

Only one motor neuron terminates at each motor end plate. There is no convergence of multiple neural inputs, such as usually observed in other synapses. In most synapses, the postsynaptic cells are excited only when the outputs of many presynaptic neurons are summated. At the neuromuscular junction, however, the depolarization of the motor end plate caused by a single motor neuron impulse is more than large enough under normal circumstances to trigger an action potential in the muscle fiber. In addition, a typical skeletal muscle fiber has only one neuromuscular junction. Exceptions do exist, however. In human extraocular muscles and certain laryngeal, esophageal, middle ear, and facial fibers, multiple junctions have been demonstrated. Although the multiple end plates observed on these multiply innervated muscle fibers appear to be innervated by the same neuron in most instances, in some there is probably polyneuronal innervation.[1] It is interesting that although muscle fibers in the fetus are multiply innervated, during postnatal development they undergo an orderly process of elimination of neuromuscular junctions whereby each loses all but one of the multiple inputs with which it is endowed at birth.[5]

Transmission of Excitation

One of the most basic functions of the neuromuscular junction is to mediate motor neuron excitation of skeletal muscle. This is accomplished by the release of an excitatory neurotransmitter, acetylcholine, from the nerve terminal, which diffuses across the neuromuscular junction to excite the muscle membrane. This whole process of chemical excitation is termed **neuromuscular transmission**. The neuromuscular junction may be the most thoroughly studied of all synapses, and the general mechanisms of neuromuscular transmission are well established (Fig. 3–6).[13]

Acetylcholine Synthesis[9,14,15]

Acetylcholine is synthesized from choline and acetylcoenzyme A in the axoplasm of the prejunctional neuron (Fig. 3–7). This reaction is catalyzed by the enzyme, choline acetyltransferase (formerly called choline acetylase). Choline acetyltransferase is synthesized in the motor neuron cell body and is transported to the axon terminal, where it is concentrated. Acetylcoenzyme A is synthesized in the mitochondria of the axon terminal from pyruvate. Only a small store of choline is in motor nerves; most of that needed for acetylcholine synthesis is derived from the extracellular fluid bathing the junction. The choline in the extracellular fluid bathing the neuromuscular junction comes not only from supplies in the plasma but also from the intrajunctional hydrolysis of acetylcholine that has previously been released from the nerve ending.[15] In this way, about 50% of the choline derived from released acetylcholine is conserved by re-uptake into the nerve terminal. Most of the plasma choline comes from the diet, but some is synthesized, principally in the liver. Acetylcholine synthesis in motor nerve endings is enhanced by nerve stimulation.

Acetylcholine Storage[14–16]

Acetylcholine is present throughout the motor neuron axoplasm, but it is most abundant in the axon terminals. Small agranular vesicles are present in large numbers in the terminals and contain about 80% of the total acetylcholine. Acetylcholine is in solution in

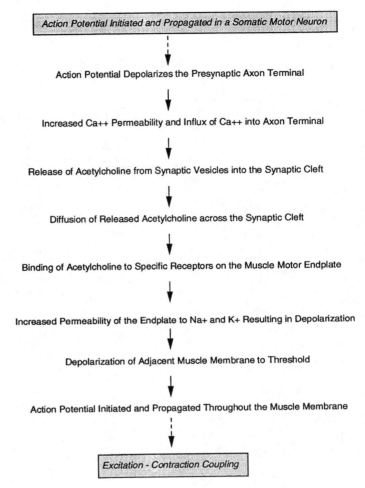

Figure 3–6. *Overview of Neuro-muscular Transmission.*

these vesicles at a concentration considerably higher than that in the surrounding axoplasm. Since acetylcholine is synthesized outside the vesicles, an active transport mechanism must exist to carry the transmitter and concentrate it inside the vesicles. Each nerve terminal contains thousands of vesicles. These vesicles are probably initially formed in the cell body of the neuron and then carried along the axons to the nerve terminals by fast axonal transport. The amount of acetylcholine contained in a single vesicle is termed a **quantum.**

Acetylcholine Release[9,10,13–18]

Considerable experimentation has been carried out in an effort to define how the nerve impulse is coupled to the actual release of acetylcholine. The best evidence suggests that local currents initiated by the action potential flow through the membrane of the nerve terminal and depolarize it, causing the opening of voltage-operated Ca^{2+} channels. The resultant influx of Ca^{2+} causes a Ca^{2+}-dependent temporary fusion of vesicular membranes to the membrane of the nerve terminal at the active sites (Fig. 3–8). This results in the vesicular contents being expelled by exocytosis. **As each neurotransmitter vesicle fuses, its outer surface ruptures through the neuronal cell membrane, causing exocytosis of acetylcholine into the synaptic cleft.** Usually about 200 to 300 vesicles rupture with each

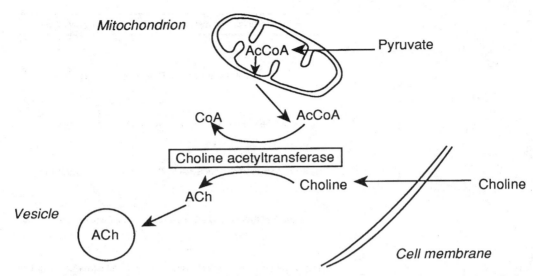

Figure 3–7. *Acetylcholine Synthesis.* Acetylcholine is synthesized in the motor neuron terminal through the choline acetyltranferase catalyzed coalescence of acetyl CoA and choline. The acetyl CoA is produced in axoplasmic mitochondria. The choline is acquired from the extracellular fluid, having originally been derived from dietary sources. The acetylcholine is concentrated and stored in numerous vesicles in the nerve terminal.

action potential. Specifically, the release of acetylcholine occurs from the vesicles nearest to the active sites. The rapidity with which acetylcholine is released upon the arrival of a nerve impulse at the nerve ending suggests that only those vesicles within about a vesicle diameter of the release sites can participate in the exocytosis. The actual mechanism underlying fusion of the vesicular membrane with the plasma membrane has not yet been fully elucidated.

Interestingly, the vesicles seem to be reformed, refilled, and reused repeatedly. The rapidity with which vesicles appear to be reformed may account for the fact that is it difficult to detect any reduction in the number of vesicles during even the most intense nerve stimulation. Objections have been raised to the vesicular hypothesis of quantal acetylcholine release, however, and other mechanisms of release have been proposed. A membrane gate hypothesis, for example, proposes that the acetylcholine held within vesicles represents a reserve store, and that transient opening of membrane gates allows the escape of the axoplasmic acetylcholine involved in neuromuscular transmission.[15]

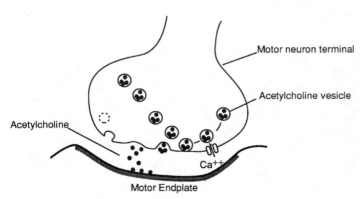

Figure 3–8. *Acetylcholine Release by Exocytosis.* Depolarization of the nerve terminal causes an influx of Ca^{2+}, which promotes fusion of transmitter vesicles to active sites in the neuronal membrane. This results in vesicle rupture and expulsion of the acetylcholine into the synaptic cleft.

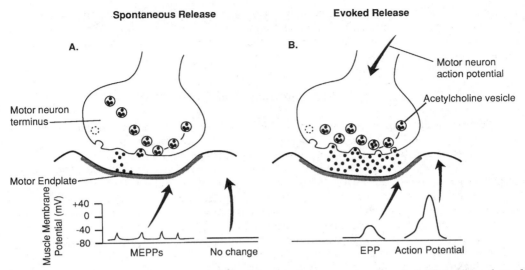

Figure 3–9. *Acetylcholine Release.* Acetylcholine release is both spontaneous and evoked. (*A*) Small numbers of vesicles are continually released spontaneously, giving rise to miniature end-plate potentials. These small depolarizations (0.5 to 1.0 mV) are not conducted beyond the end plate and do not excite the cell. (*B*) Large numbers of vesicles are evoked to release their contents by an action potential. This gives rise to an end-plate potential (15 to 40 mV), which normally elicits an action potential in the adjacent sarcolemma.

Acetylcholine release from the nerve terminal is both spontaneous and evoked by neuron impulse (Fig. 3–9).[13–18] In the absence of nerve impulses, a small amount of acetylcholine is released spontaneously causing miniature end-plate potentials of about 0.5 to 1 mV in amplitude to develop in the postjunctional membrane. Each miniature end-plate potential seems to arise from the spontaneous release of the acetylcholine contained within a single vesicle (i.e., a quantum) that occurs when a vesicle randomly collides in the appropriate way with a release site in an active zone of the terminal membrane. The release of the acetylcholine that causes the miniature end-plate potentials is Ca^{2+}-dependent. Generally, there is sufficient Ca^{2+} stored within the axoplasm to support this release. Spontaneous release of acetylcholine, and hence miniature end-plate potential frequency, is greatly increased by procedures that enhance axoplasmic Ca^{2+} concentration. Other types of spontaneous acetylcholine release also occur, including nonquantal molecular leakage that is not calcium dependent. Vesicle release giving rise to miniature end-plate potential is, however, the only form analogous to the transmitter release that is evoked by nerve impulses. The amplitude of a miniature end-plate potential is normally well below the minimum depolarization necessary to trigger a muscle fiber action potential and subsequent contraction.

A nerve impulse or any other means of depolarizing the nerve terminal, will cause the evoked release of acetylcholine, provided that there is adequate Ca^{2+} present in the extracellular fluid. This release seems to involve a consistent number of vesicles. The depolarization of the motor end plate evoked by a nerve impulse is called the *end-plate potential*. The end-plate potential represents the effect of only a small percentage (<1%) of the total amount of acetylcholine present in the nerve terminal. Nonetheless, the amount of acetylcholine released by a single isolated nerve impulse is considerably in excess of that required to evoke the degree of end-plate depolarization necessary to cause muscle contraction. This excess capacity represents a "safety factor" built into transmitter release, which has been estimated to be about fivefold.[12,13]

One of the most interesting features of junctional transmitter release is that the transmitter itself may serve to facilitate its own release through a form of positive feedback.[14,15] Released acetylcholine may act on receptors on the prejunctional membrane to enhance the availability of stored acetylcholine for release. In this way, when the traffic of nerve impulses is high, the availability of transmitter for release is increased to match the demand for it.

Postjunctional Binding of Acetylcholine[6–10,13,19–22]

When acetylcholine is released from the motor nerve terminal, it diffuses across the synaptic space and binds to acetylcholine receptors that are located on the upper portion of the junctional folds of the motor end plate (Fig. 3–10). This induces a conformational change in the membrane, which rapidly increases the permeability to Na^+ and to a lesser degree other cations, such as K^+, Ca^{2+}, and Mg^{2+}. These ions then flow through the membrane in accordance with their concentration and electrical gradients. The main result is an influx of Na^+. **This produces an end-plate current, which depolarizes the end-plate membrane to produce the end-plate potential.** The end-plate potential, in turn, creates local circuit currents that open Na^+ gates in the surrounding muscle fiber membrane initiating an action potential, which is propagated throughout the muscle fiber. Meanwhile, acetylcholine is inactivated and the end-plate conductance and membrane potential are restored to their resting values. Because this is accomplished before the end of the refractory period of the muscle fiber membrane, the acetylcholine released by a single nerve impulse causes only a single sarcolemmal action potential. This action potential passes throughout the sarcolemma to activate the contractile mechanisms of the muscle fiber (see Chapter 2).

An end-plate potential differs from an action potential in a number of significant ways. The end-plate potential is the result of a permeability increase caused by a chemical (acetylcholine), whereas the action potential is triggered by electric current flow; the end-plate potential is graded, whereas the action potential is all or nothing; unlike the action potential, the end-plate potential is not propagated; and the end-plate potential is without a refractory period, so successive nerve impulses can cause summating end-plate potentials.

As previously mentioned, the amplitude of the end-plate potential following a single nerve impulse is normally more than that necessary to trigger a muscle action potential (i.e., the safety factor). Any change that reduces the probability of successful acetylcholine-receptor interaction will impinge upon this safety margin and increase the risk of neuromuscular transmission failure. The importance of a loss of this margin is apparent in the muscle weakness or paralysis accompanying many disorders of the neuromuscular junction (see Chapter 14).

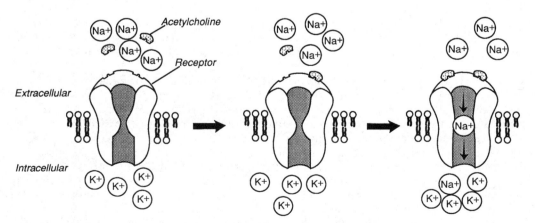

Figure 3–10. *Activation of the Endplate Acetylcholine Receptor.* Two acetylcholine molecules bind to the receptor and induce a conformational change in the receptor. This results in the opening of a cation channel, which allows Na^+ to diffuse into the muscle fiber. Binding of the first acetylcholine molecule to the receptor facilitates binding of the second.

The Acetylcholine Receptor[8,9,13,19–22]

The acetylcholine receptor is perhaps the most thoroughly studied of all biologic receptors. Knowledge of this receptor has been advanced by the availability of certain toxins that bind strongly and specifically to the active sites of the receptor and by the ready availability of analogous receptors in certain electric eels and rays. **The *acetylcholine receptor is a glycoprotein*** made up of five subunits **which is embedded in and spans the postjunctional membrane** (Fig. 3–11). Each receptor molecule contains an ion channel and two recognition or binding sites for acetylcholine. When acetylcholine binds to these receptor sites, a conformational change occurs, resulting in rapid opening of the ion channel. In normal, innervated muscle fibers these receptors are largely restricted to the crests of the junctional folds, where they are held in fixed clusters by filaments of the cytoskeleton.[1,2] The receptors are synthesized intracellularly and inserted into the membrane. In fetal muscle fibers before innervation, acetylcholine receptors are distributed over the entire surface of the cell membrane and relatively free to change their position. As these fibers become innervated, however, the receptors become clustered and anchored in the folds of the motor end plate.[5] Acetylcholine receptors undergo relatively slow turnover, their degradation involving active internalization into the muscle cell and proteolytic destruction in lysosomes. In denervated muscle, there is a marked increase in the synthesis of extrajunctional receptors, which turn over more than 10 times faster than the more stable junctional receptors.[5,19] Changes in receptor turnover rate may play a role in the pathogenesis of such junctional disorders as myasthenia gravis. Genes for fragments of human acetylcholine receptors have already been cloned, and the future availability of synthetic receptors may have important therapeutic applications.

Acetylcholine Inactivation[8,9,19,23]

The entire process of neuromuscular junction transmission is very rapid and is terminated by junctional mechanisms that quickly remove acetylcholine. Acetylcholine is hydrolyzed by the enzyme, **acetylcholinesterase,** which is found in high concentration on the postjunctional membrane and in the basal lamina. Enzyme inactivation is so rapid that each acetylcholine molecule has the chance to react with no more than one acetylcholine receptor and no accumulation of released acetylcholine occurs from one nerve impulse to the next, even at the highest frequencies of stimulation. Acetylcholinesterase is a glycoprotein enzyme, which exists in a number of different molecular forms. It is not yet clear

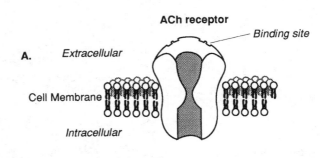

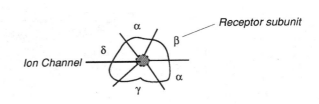

Figure 3–11. *Structure of the Acetylcholine Receptor.* This diagram depicts five subunits arranged around a central, funnel-shaped pore, the ion channel itself. Each subunit consists of a twisted amino acid chain that crosses back and forth across the membrane four or five times. (*A*) Side view. (*B*) Top view. (Adapted from Kistler, J, et al: Structure and Function of an Acetylcholine Receptor. Biophys J 37:371, 1982, p 377.)

whether this enzyme is synthesized in the nerve cell and released into the junctional cleft or whether the neuron somehow induces its synthesis in the basement membrane and sarcolemma. The hydrolysis of acetylcholine occurs in two stages. Choline is first split off, leaving an acetylated site on the enzyme. The latter then reacts with water to release the acetate and reactivate the enzyme. As mentioned previously, about 50% of the choline that is freed into the junctional cleft is taken back up by the motor neuron terminal to be used in the synthesis of new acetylcholine. In addition to enzymatic destruction, junctional acetylcholine is removed by diffusion away from the junction and nonspecific membrane binding.

Pharmacologic Modification of Neuromuscular Transmission

Virtually every step in the process of neuromuscular transmission can be altered by one or more chemical agents (Fig. 3–12). Although relatively few of these have proved to have much value as therapeutic agents, many have proved to be extremely useful in the study of junctional activity. One way to categorize these agents is in terms of whether their primary site of action is prejunctional or postjunctional.

Prejunctional Effects[14,24,25]

The motor neuron terminal is the site of acetylcholine synthesis, uptake and storage in vesicles, and release into the synaptic cleft. All these processes have been shown to be modified by a variety of chemical substances.

Theoretically, **acetylcholine synthesis could be inhibited by interfering with either choline acetyltransferase activity or with the availability of choline to that enzyme system.** Although a number of compounds have been developed that seem to inhibit this enzyme directly, none is very specific in this effect. Hemicholinium-3 is the best-known and most effective of a group of compounds that inhibit the transport of choline across the cell membrane, depriving choline acetyltransferase of one of its substrates and thereby inhibiting acetylcholine synthesis. The effect of hemicholinium-3 is most pronounced during continuous nerve stimulation, when rapid uptake of choline is needed to replenish the supply of acetylcholine in the nerve terminal. Junctional transmission could also be blocked if the

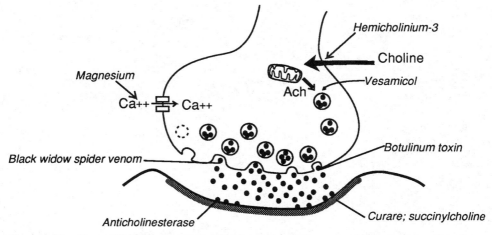

Figure 3–12. *Sites at Which Drugs or Toxins May Interfere with Neuromuscular Transmission.* Virtually every step in junctional transmission can be altered by one or more chemical agents.

vesicles from which acetylcholine is released were prevented from accumulating this transmitter. A substance called **vesamicol** is the most potent of a number of compounds that prevent vesicular uptake (loading) of acetylcholine and hence quantal release.[26]

A number of potent agents exist that disturb both the spontaneous and evoked release of acetylcholine. Interestingly, many of these are toxins of biologic origins.[14,24,25,27,28] Botulinum toxin, for example, which is produced by the anaerobic bacterium *Clostridium botulinum,* produces a powerful blockade of neuromuscular transmission by blocking acetylcholine release that results in a clinical syndrome of (often life-threatening) muscle paralysis (see Chapter 14).[29,30] Recently, botulinum toxin has been used therapeutically to treat a number of conditions characterized by pathologic muscle spasms. β-Bungarotoxin is a protein isolated from the venom of the Taiwan krait, which binds with the prejunctional membrane to irreversibly suppress acetylcholine release.[14,24,27] The active zones of the membrane where vesicle fusion and acetylcholine release occur seem to be irreversibly modified. The venom of the black widow spider (main protein, α-latrotoxin) greatly increases vesicle fusion with the nerve terminal membrane and inhibits vesicle recycling. This soon depletes the nerve terminal of releasable acetylcholine, so that transmission failure occurs. Both spontaneous and evoked vesicle release of acetylcholine is dependent on junctional calcium. The presence in the junction of other alkaline earth metals, such as magnesium or strontium, which are less effective in promoting transmitter release, will inhibit junctional activity.[24] Other metallic cations (e.g., manganese, cobalt, zinc, beryllium, nickle, lead, and cadmium) are also antagonistic to calcium binding and depress evoked transmitter release.

Postjunctional Effects

Most substances that modify prejunctional events are not used for this purpose in the clinic. Much more extensive use is made of those modifying postjunctional activity. These agents are of considerable clinical value, including their use in the treatment of certain neuromuscular disorders, and warrant consideration in more detail than other agents.

The most important of the pharmacologic agents that alter junctional activity are the neuromuscular blocking agents and anticholinesterases. **The term *neuromuscular blocking agent* usually refers to a group of drugs that block neuromuscular transmission through effects on the motor end-plate acetylcholine receptors** and are often used to produce muscle relaxation in association with anesthesia induced by other agents.[19,25,31–33] On the basis of distinct differences in their mechanism of action, these agents are described as either competitive blocking agents (of which curare is the classic example) or as depolarizing blocking agents (e.g., succinylcholine).

In brief, curare-type (curariform) drugs bind to the acetylcholine receptor sites at the postjunctional membrane and thereby competitively block access of acetylcholine to its receptor. The muscle cell becomes insensitive to motor neuron impulses and to directly applied acetylcholine. However, the muscle fiber still responds to direct electrical stimulation. The first agent of this type to be widely used clinically was D-tubocurare, which is still used as a neuromuscular blocking agent during surgical anesthesia. However, the difficulty and expense of obtaining adequate quantities of this naturally occurring alkaloid, combined with occasional undesirable side effects, have led to the development of numerous synthetic substitutes (e.g., alcurium, gallamine, pancuronium, vecuronium, atracurium), many of which have the advantage of greater potency and shorter duration.

The depolarizing agents act by a different mechanism. Their initial action is to depolarize the membrane by opening channels in the same manner as acetylcholine; however, since they persist at the junction, the depolarization is longer lasting. This results in a brief phase of repetitive excitation, which may be manifested by transient muscle fasciculations. This phase is followed by blockade of neuromuscular transmission and flaccid paralysis. Succinylcholine is the only blocking agent of the depolarizing type that is currently used in Europe and the United States.

As with the prejunctional membrane, a number of venoms that bind to postjunctional sites have been identified. The elapid snakes (kraits and cobras), for example, produce a group of toxins that bind to the acetylcholine receptor in a highly specific and long-lasting fashion.[19,29] One of these toxins, α-bungarotoxin, which binds irreversibly to the receptor, has been particularly useful in studying these receptors, as well as the effects of long-term junctional blockade. Cobra toxins from several species of cobra have also been isolated and shown to bind reversibly to the acetylcholine receptor.

As described previously in this chapter, acetylcholine released into the neuromuscular junction is rapidly metabolized by acetylcholinesterase present at the postjunctional membrane. **Several groups of compounds have been identified that slow or prevent hydrolysis of acetylcholine by acetylcholinesterase** at the neuromuscular junction, as well as at other sites of cholinergic transmission. **These compounds are termed** *anticholinesterases.*[15,19,34] As a result of the inhibition of the hydrolysis of acetylcholine, the transmitter accumulates and the action of acetylcholine that is liberated by nerve impulses, or that spontaneously leaks from the nerve ending, is enhanced. Motor end-plate potentials become prolonged because each molecule of acetylcholine can now move along the motor end plate and make multiple contacts with successive receptors before escaping by diffusion from the junctional cleft. As a result, repetitive muscle potentials may occur. Too much acetylcholinesterase inhibition can result in the accumulation of excessive amounts of acetylcholine in the neuromuscular junction, resulting in impairment of junctional transmission and a resultant muscle weakness or paralysis. Long-term acetylcholinesterase blockade may produce adverse effects on the neuromuscular junction, including decreased acetylcholine synthesis, decreased acetylcholine receptors, and damage to the postjunctional membrane.

Although anticholinesterase agents have received more extensive application as toxic agents in the form of agricultural insecticides and chemical agents (nerve gases) for warfare, several members of this class of compounds have proved to be clinically useful. These therapeutic agents are all **carbamyl esters**, which produce a relatively brief, reversible inhibition of acetylcholinesterase activity. The drugs of this group that are most commonly used for their actions at the neuromuscular junction are neostigmine, pyridostigmine, and edrophonium. They are used to reverse the neuromuscular junction blockade produced by curarelike agents and to improve junctional activity in myasthenia gravis and similar disorders (see Chapter 14). Organophosphates are a group of compounds that produce an **irreversible** inhibition of acetylcholinesterase and permanent junctional blockade, making them attractive for military and agricultural purposes.[35] The venom of the green mamba, a snake, has been shown to contain an irreversible anticholinesterase.[15]

Trophic Interactions Between Motor Neurons and Muscle

In addition to mediating cholinergic excitation of skeletal muscle per se, the neuromuscular junction mediates other important interactions between the nerve and muscle. Motor neurons and the muscles they innervate are strongly dependent on one another for their normal development and the maintenance of their normal function. This interdependence reflects a variety of "trophic" interactions, which depend on synaptic contact and become most apparent when this contact is interrupted.

Motor neurons exert powerful influences on the differentiation and development of both embryonic and mature skeletal muscle.[2,5,36–38] During embryogenesis, the differentiation of muscle fibers is strongly dependent on the parallel development of adjacent motor neurons. If embryonic muscles are deprived of innervation, the muscle cells atrophy and are replaced by fat and connective tissue. Contact with innervating motor neurons stimulates a number of aspects of muscle development, including synthesis and localization of acetylcholine receptors in the region of the neuromuscular junction[39]; thickening and folding of the motor end plate; secretion of the basal lamina and the synaptic acetylcholinesterase that it contains[23]; and definition of the speed of contraction and other basic contractile properties. Many of the basic properties of mature muscle also depend on synaptic contact. If, for example, the nerves to mature fast-twitch and slow-twitch fibers are experimentally switched (i.e., crossed reinnervation), the muscles will largely reverse their contractile properties and assume the characteristics of the opposite type of muscle. These changes are associated with the expression of new molecular forms of myosin, changes in muscle ultrastructure, and altered levels of protein synthesis and glycolytic and oxidative enzymes.[36,37] The profound effect each motor neuron has on the muscle it innervates is further evidenced by the observation that all the fibers within one motor unit are functionally and histochemically the same.

The importance of neural influences in sustaining the health of muscle is clearly revealed by the disastrous effects of denervation.[5,36-38] Although gross muscle atrophy is perhaps the most obvious consequence of denervation, other postsynaptic changes are quickly and consistently apparent. These include a fall in the resting membrane potential, dissemination of acetylcholine receptors to extrajunctional sites, increased acetylcholine sensitivity, loss of acetylcholinesterase, sharp declines in the rate of synthesis of muscle protein, increased protein degradation, changes in contraction kinetics, and fibrillations.

Although the exact nature of the neural influence is not known, several possible mechanisms for trophic regulation have been proposed.[36-38] The pattern and intensity of activity itself (electrical and mechanical) may influence the muscle fiber directly. Severely decreased muscle activity, for example, results in many (but not all) of the effects of denervation. The role of activity itself is also suggested by the effectiveness of direct stimulation in slowing or reversing the effects of denervation. How varying levels of activity actually affect the synthetic processes of the muscle cell is not known, although associated alterations in free intracellular calcium or various metabolites may be involved. Healthy motor neurons may also synthesize and release special trophic substances. The denervation-like changes in muscle that can be produced by blockade of axonal transport, nerve conduction block, and blockade of transmitter release, suggest the presence of such substances. Acetylcholine, through its own membrane effects, may exert trophic effects. The roles of the proteins, ATP, and prostaglandins that are released by nerve stimulation are not known. In addition, degeneration of the motor nerve may lead to the presence of breakdown products not normally present, which may lead to localized denervation-like changes in muscle. These effects may be greatly enhanced by muscle inactivity. Although poorly understood at present, it seems likely that all of these factors are important.

In much the same way that the motor neuron influences the muscle fiber, muscle exerts powerful regulatory influences on the nerves that innervate it.[36,37,40,41] Muscle influences nerve during both embryonic development and normal growth and maturation. The importance of these influences is illustrated by the effects of partial denervation on motor neurons and their central connections. During experimental denervation, for example, intact axons are stimulated to sprout new branches that innervate old end-plate sites on the denervated muscle fibers; metabolic and electrophysiologic changes occur in the motor neurons; and morphologic changes even occur in the central synapses on the motor neuron cell bodies.[36,37,40,41] Many of these changes can be stimulated by pharmacologic blockade[41] of the junction, indicating that the trophic effects of muscle on nerve depend on neuromuscular transmission.

Given the variety and importance of these trophic interactions, it is inevitable that some neuromuscular diseases must result from defective trophic regulation. Conversely, pathologic disorders of nerve and muscle are likely to disturb trophic interactions. Important clinical strides will ultimately be made when these processes are more fully understood and mechanisms are developed for minimizing the debilitating effects of denervation and for directly stimulating muscle or neuronal growth in disorders of both muscle or nerve.

RECOMMENDED READINGS

Aidley, DJ: The Physiology of Excitable Cells, ed 3. Chapter 7. Neuromuscular Transmission. Cambridge University Press, Cambridge, 1989.

Alberts, B, et al (eds): Molecular Biology of the Cell, ed 2. Chapter 19. The Nervous System. Garland Publishing, New York, 1989.

Aquilonius, SM and Gillberg, PG: Section IIA. Neuromuscular Transmission. In Cholinergic Neurotransmission: Functional and Clinical Aspects. Proceeding of Nobel Symposium 76. Prog Br Res 84:63, 1990.

Bowman, WC: Pharmacology of Neuromuscular Function, ed 2. Wright, London, 1990.

Chou, SM: Pathology of the Neuromuscular Junction. Chapter 17. In Mastaglia, FL and Detchant, Lord Walton (eds): Skeletal Muscle Pathology, ed 2. Churchill Livingstone, Edinburgh, 1992.

Engel, AG: Myasthenic Syndromes. Chapter 68. In Engel, AG and Franzini-Armstrong, C (eds): Myology: Basic and Clinical, ed 2. McGraw-Hill, New York, 1994.

Engel, AG: The Neuromuscular Junction. Chapter 9. In Engel, AG and Franzini-Armstrong, C (eds): Myology, ed 2. McGraw-Hill, New York, 1984.

Grinnel, AD: Trophic Interaction Between Nerve and Muscle. Chapter 10. In Engel, AG and Franzini-Armstrong, C (eds): Myology, ed 2. McGraw-Hill, New York, 1994.

Hall, ZW and Sanes, JR: Synaptic Structure and Development: The Neuromuscular Junction. Cell 72 (suppl): 99, 1993.

Hille, B: Neuromuscular Transmission. Chapter 6. In Patton, HD, et al (eds): Textbook of Physiology. WB Saunders, Philadelphia, 1989.

Magleby, KL: Neuromuscular Transmission. Chapter 16. In Engel, AG and Franzini-Armstrong, C (eds): Myology. McGraw-Hill, New York, 1994.

Nastuk, WL: Neuromuscular Transmission. Chapter 5. In Mountcastle, VB (ed): Medical Physiology. CV Mosby, St. Louis, 1980.

Newson-Davis, J: Diseases of the Neuromuscular Junction. Chapter 15. In Asbury, AK, McKhann, GM, and McDonald, WI (eds): Diseases of the Nervous System. Clinical Neurobiology, vol 1, ed 2. WB Saunders, Philadelphia, 1992.

Pascuzzi, RM (ed): Disorders of Neuromuscular Transmission. Semin Neurol 10(1):1, 1990.

Riederer, P, Kopp, N, and Pearson, J: An Introduction to Neurotransmission in Health and Disease. Oxford University Press, Oxford, 1990.

Salpeter, MM (ed): The Vertebrate Neuromuscular Junction. Alan R Liss, New York, 1987.

Senanayake, N and Roman, GC: Disorders of Neuromuscular Transmission Due to Natural Environmental Toxins. J Neurol Sci 107:1, 1992.

Taylor, P: Agents Acting at the Neuromuscular Junction and Autonomic Ganglia. Chapter 9. In Gilman, AG (ed): Goodman and Gilman's The Pharmacologic Basis of Therapeutics, ed 8. McGraw-Hill, New York, 1993.

Taylor, P and Brown, JH: Acetylcholine. Chapter 11. In Siegel, GJ, et al (eds): Basic Neurochemistry. Molecular, Cellular, and Medical Aspects, ed 5. Raven Press, New York, 1994.

REFERENCES

1. Salpeter, MM: Vertebrate Neuromuscular Junctions: General Morphology, Molecular Organization, and Functional Consequences. Chapter 1. In Salpeter, MM (ed): The Vertebrate Neuromuscular Junction. Alan R Liss, New York, 1987.

2. Engel, AG: The Neuromuscular Junction. Chapter 9. In Engel, AG and Franzini-Armstrong, C (eds): Myology, ed 2. McGraw-Hill, New York, 1994.

3. Ogata, T and Yamasaki, Y: The Three-Dimensional Structure of Motor Endplates in Different Fiber Types of Rat Intercostal Muscle: A Scanning Electron-Microscopic Study. Cell Tissue Res 241:465, 1985.

4. Slater, CR: The Basal Lamina and Stability of the Mammalian Neuromuscular Junction. Prog Br Res 84:73, 1990.

5. Salpeter, MM: Vertebrate Neuromuscular Junctions: General Morphology, Development, and Neural Control of the Neuromuscular Junction and of the Junctional Acetylcholine Receptor. Chapter 2. In Salpeter, MM (ed): The Vertebrate Neuromuscular Junction. Alan R Liss, New York, 1987.

6. Nastuk, WL: Neuromuscular Transmission. Chapter 5. In Mountcastle, VB (ed): Medical Physiology. CV Mosby, St. Louis, 1980.

7. Hille, B: Neuromuscular Transmission. Chapter 6. In Patton, HD, et al (eds): Textbook of Physiology. WB Saunders, Philadelphia, 1989.

8. Alberts, B, et al (eds): Molecular Biology of the Cell, ed 2. Chapter 19. The Nervous System. Garland Publishing, New York, 1989.

9. Taylor, P and Brown, JH: Acetylcholine. Chapter 11. In Siegel, GJ, et al (eds): Basic Neurochemistry. Molecular, Cellular, and Medical Aspects, ed 5. Raven Press, New York, 1994.

10. Aidley, DJ: The Physiology of Excitable Cells, ed 3. Chapter 7. Neuromuscular Transmission. Cambridge University Press, Cambridge, 1989.

11. Newsom-Davis, J: Diseases of the Neuromuscular Junction. Chapter 15. In Asbury, AK, McKhann, GM, and McDonald, WI (eds): Diseases of the Nervous System: Clinical Neurobiology, ed 2. WB Saunders, Philadelphia, 1992.

12. Guyton, AC: Textbook of Medical Physiology, ed 8. Chapter 7. Excitation of Skeletal Muscle Contraction, Neuromuscular Transmission, and Excitation-Contraction Coupling. WB Saunders, Philadelphia, 1991.

13. Magleby, KL: Neuromuscular Transmission. Chapter 16. In Engel, AG and Franzini-Armstrong, C

(eds): Myology, ed 2. McGraw-Hill, New York, 1994.

14. Jones, SW: Presynaptic Mechanisms at Vertebrate Neuromuscular Junctions. Chapter 5. In Salpeter, MM (ed): The Vertebrate Neuromuscular Junction. Alan R Liss, New York, 1987.

15. Bowman, WC: Pharmacology of Neuromuscular Function, ed 2. Chapter 3. Neuromuscular Transmission: Prejunctional Events. Wright, London, 1990.

16. Kelly, RB: Storage and Release of Neurotransmitters. Cell 72 (suppl):43, 1993.

17. Betz, WJ and Bewick, GS: Optical Monitoring of Transmitter Release and Synaptic Vesicle Recycling at the Frog Neuromuscular Junction. J Physiol (Lond) 287:4603, 1993.

18. Ceccarelli, B and Hurlbut, WP: Vesicle Hypothesis of the Release of Quanta of Acetylcholine. Physiol Rev 60:396, 1980.

19. Bowman, WC: Pharmacology of Neuromuscular Function, ed 2. Chapter 5. Neuromuscular Transmission: Post-Junctional Events. Wright, London, 1990.

20. Anderson, DJ: Molecular Biology of the Acetylcholine Receptor: Structure and Regulation of Biogenesis. Chapter 7. In Salpeter, MM (ed): The Vertebrate Neuromuscular Junction. Alan R Liss, New York, 1987.

21. Lindstrom, J: Acetylcholine Receptors: Structure, Function, Synthesis, Destruction, and Antigenicity. Chapter 27. In Engel, AG and Franzini-Armstrong, C (eds): Myology, ed 2. McGraw-Hill, New York, 1994.

22. Kandel, ER and Siegelbaum, BA: Directly Gated Transmission at the Nerve-Muscle Synapse. Chapter 10. In Kandel, ER, Schwartz, JH, and Jessell, TM (eds): Principles of Neural Science, ed 3. Appleton & Lange, Norwalk, CT, 1991.

23. Rotundo, RL: Biogenesis and Regulation of Acetylcholinesterase. Chapter 6. In Salpeter, MM (ed): The Vertebrate Neuromuscular Junction. Alan R Liss, New York, 1987.

24. Bowman, WC: Pharmacology of Neuromuscular Function, ed 2. Chapter 4. Pharmacological Manipulation of Prejunctional Events. Wright, London, 1990.

25. Taylor, P: Agents Acting at the Neuromuscular Junction and Autonomic Ganglia. Chapter 9. In Gilman, AG (ed): Goodman and Gilman's The Pharmacologic Basis of Therapeutics, ed 8. McGraw-Hill, New York, 1993.

26. Prior, C, Marshall, IG, and Parsons, SM: The Pharmacology of Vesamicol: An Inhibitor of the Vesicular Acetylcholine Transporter. Gen Pharmacol 23(6):1017, 1992.

27. Senanayake, N and Roman, GC: Disorders of Neuromuscular Transmission Due to Natural Environmental Toxins. J Neurol Sci 107(1):1, 1992.

28. Minton, SA: Neurotoxic Snake Envenoming. Semin Neurol 10(1):52, 1990.

29. Humbleton, R: *Clostridium botulinum* Toxins: A General Review of Involvement in Disease, Structure, Mode of Action, and Preparation for Clinical Use. J Neurol 239(1):16, 1992.

30. Gonnering, RS: Pharmacology of Botulinum Toxin. Int Ophthalmol Clin 33(4):203, 1992.

31. Larijani, GE, et al: Clinical Pharmacology of the Neuromuscular Blocking Agents. DICP 25(1):54, 1991.

32. Marakhur, RK: Newer Neuromuscular Blocking Drugs: An Overview of Their Clinical Pharmacology and Therapeutic Use. Drugs 44(2):182, 1992.

33. Bowman, WC: Pharmacology of Neuromuscular Function. Chapter 6. Neuromuscular-Blocking Agents, ed 2. Wright, London, 1990.

34. Tayor, P: Anticholinesterase Agents. Chapter 7. In Gilman, AG (ed): Goodman and Gilman's The Pharmacological Basis of Therapeutics, ed 8. McGraw-Hill, New York, 1993.

35. Gutmann, L and Besser, R: Organophosphate Intoxication: Pharmacologic, Neurophysiologic, Clinical, and Therapeutic Considerations. Semin Neurol 10(1):46, 1990.

36. Grinnel, AD: Trophic Interaction Between Nerve and Muscle. Chapter 10. In Engel, AG and Franzini-Armstrong, C (eds): Myology, ed 2. McGraw-Hill, New York, 1994.

37. Hall, ZW and Sanes, JR: Synaptic Structure and Development: The Neuromuscular Junction. Cell 72 (Suppl):99, 1993.

38. Salpeter, MM, et al: Regulation of Molecules at the Neuromuscular Junction. In Kelly, AM and Blau, HM (eds): Neuromuscular Development and Disease. Raven Press, New York, 1992.

39. Colman, H and Lichtman, JW: Interactions Between Nerve and Muscle: Synapse Elimination at the Developing Neuromuscular Junction. Dev Biol 156(1):1, 1993.

40. Crews, LL and Wigston, DJ: Dependence of Motor Neurons on Target Muscle During Postnatal Development of the Mouse. J Neurosci 10:1643, 1990.

41. Pinter, MJ, et al: Axotomy-like Changes in Cat Motor Neurons. Electrical Properties Elicited by Botulinum Toxin Depends on the Complete Elimination of Neuromuscular Transmission. J Neurosci 11:657, 1991.

CHAPTER 4

Basic Sensory Mechanisms and the Somatosensory System

Christopher M. Fredericks, PhD

- ■ *Basic Sensory Mechanisms*
- ■ *Classification of Senses*
- ■ *The Somatosensory System*
- ■ *Touch and Proprioception*
- ■ *Other Somatic Sensations*

When we think of motor activity, we tend to intuitively focus on the effector component of this system, that is, the action of skeletal muscle. It should be emphasized that the overall motor system has both afferent and efferent components and that sensory and motor mechanisms are intimately intertwined. Continuous, detailed sensory feedback is required for much of normal motor activity. Sensory information both triggers volitional and reflex motor behaviors and allows them to be carried to completion. Locomotor activity, ranging from the most basic postural adjustments to the most refined volitional tasks, is dependent on the integrity of sensory systems. Many locomotor disorders, in fact, have a significant sensory component. Disruption of sensory mechanisms may contribute directly to distortion or loss of locomotor capability. In this chapter, after basic sensory mechanisms and principles are introduced, attention will be focused on the somatosensory system. Of all the sensory systems, this is the one most closely linked to motor activity.

Basic Sensory Mechanisms[1-9]

Sensory Receptors

Information about the internal and external environment reaches the central nervous system in the form of afferent nerve impulses. These impulses arise from the stimulation of sensory receptors. These receptors function as energy transducers, converting the energy inherent in various stimuli into electrical activity, which culminates in the generation of action potentials (Fig. 4–1). Sensory receptors are strategically distributed over the body surface, as well as deep within the viscera and musculoskeletal system. Afferent nerve fibers from these receptors transmit information to many levels of the central nervous system

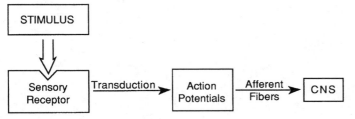

Figure 4-1 ***Sensory Transduction.*** Sensory receptors convert (transduce) energy inherent in the stimuli to which they are sensitive into graded electrical activity. With sufficient stimulation this culminates in afferent neuron action potentials.

including the spinal cord, brainstem, cerebellum, and cerebral cortex. Sensory information is received and used at both conscious and unconscious levels.

Although all sensory receptors are analogous to the extent that they respond to some form of external stimulation and in doing so excite afferent neurons, they differ markedly in their form, function, and complexity (Fig. 4–2). The simplest sensory receptors are merely the distal **free nerve endings** of relatively unspecialized afferent fibers. More common are receptor cells, which are specialized to be most readily stimulated by some particular kind of stimulus. Some receptor cells resemble ordinary neurons except for the specialization of their dendritic (receptive) terminals; their own axon serves as an afferent fiber, carrying

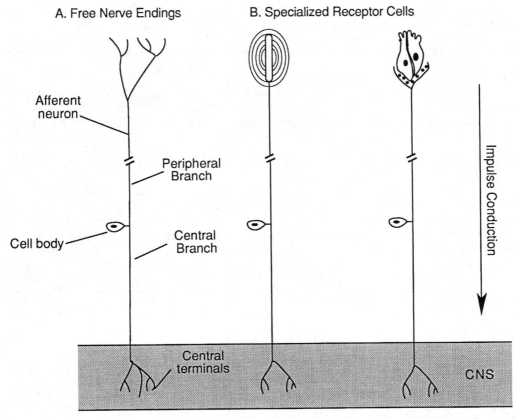

Figure 4-2 ***Types of Sensory Receptor Cells.*** Sensory receptors are cells that are highly sensitive to specific stimuli. There are two general types of receptors: (*A*) unspecialized afferent nerve endings and (*B*) specialized neural cells, which may or may not give rise to their own afferent axon.

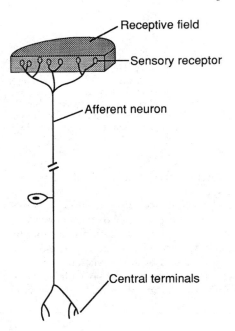

Figure 4–3   *A Sensory Unit and Its Receptive Field.* A sensory axon with all of its receptor endings is a sensory unit. The region of a sensory surface (i.e., the skin) innervated by these receptive endings is its receptive field.

information to the central nervous system. Other receptor cells have little or no axon and on stimulation release a chemical messenger that stimulates an adjacent afferent neuron. In some cases, **receptor cells** rely on specialized nonneural accessory structures with which they are organized into complex **sense organs.** These auxiliary structures assist the receptor cells in interacting efficiently and selectively with the most appropriate stimuli. In the eye, for example, accessory structures focus light on the retina. In the muscle spindle of skeletal muscle, accessory structures allow adjustment of its sensitivity.

Each receptor responds most readily to one particular form of energy, which is called its *adequate stimulus.* Receptors also respond to forms of energy other than the adequate stimulus, but the threshold for these nonspecific responses is much higher. The receptors of the eye, for example, normally respond to light, but they can be activated by an intense mechanical stimulus like a blow to the eye.

A single sensory axon with all of its receptor endings constitutes a sensory unit (Fig. 4–3). In a few cases, a sensory neuron may terminate in a single receptor, but most often the peripheral ending of a sensory nerve divides into many fine branches—each terminating at a receptor. For some units, the area of the body occupied by these receptors (the receptive field) may be very large; in others, it is very small and discrete. Usually, the areas supplied by one unit overlap with areas supplied by other units. Consequently, stimulation of any one region may activate several sensory units. All the receptors of a single unit are preferentially sensitive to the same type of stimulus. The central processes from a sensory unit terminate in the central nervous system.

Stimulus Transduction[1,4,6–8]

Regardless of the specific type of receptor cell or sense organ, the final outcome of sensory stimulation is the same: production of afferent nerve action potentials. These impulses provide information to the central nervous system. Although each type of sensory receptor customarily reacts to some specific type of stimulus, the general mechanisms of receptor stimulation and afferent neuron excitation are the same for all types of receptors (Fig. 4–4). **Each stimulus impinges on the receptor membrane in such a way that ion permeabilities are altered and a change in the membrane potential occurs. This potential**

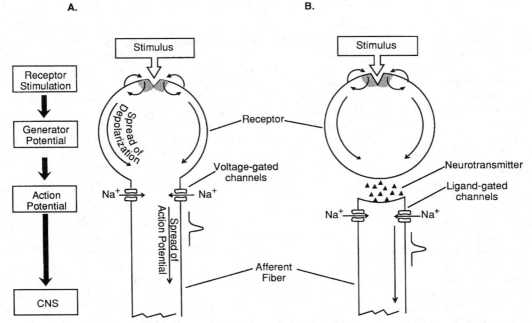

Figure 4–4 *Major Steps in Sensory Transduction.* During sensory transduction, each adequate stimulus impinges on a receptive membrane altering ion permeabilities and hence the membrane potential. Such a stimulus may affect ion channels directly or indirectly via receptors coupled to ion channels. (*A*) Depolarizing receptor potentials can spread by current flow to contiguous afferent fibers or (*B*) by the release of transmitter substance to nearby noncontiguous fibers. If great enough, these potentials will trigger afferent action potentials.

change is called the *receptor* or *generator potential.* Generator potentials are local, graded potentials that vary in magnitude and duration with the strength of the stimulus. Although not well understood, the ionic events underlying a typical generator potential appear to be similar to those of an excitatory postsynaptic potential induced by a neurotransmitter acting on a postsynaptic membrane. The sensory stimulus somehow causes membrane ion channels to open, the permeability to certain ions to increase, and these ions to redistribute according to the electrical and chemical gradients present across the cell membrane. As a consequence, there is usually a net movement of positive charges into the cell, producing a decrease in the membrane potential (depolarization). It should be noted that there are a few instances in which interaction with the adequate stimulus causes permeability changes that result in a hyperpolarizing receptor potential; such as in the visual system. **This transformation of stimulus energy into electrochemical events in the sensory receptor is termed** *sensory transduction.*

The stimulus may act on either simple nerve endings or on specialized receptor cells, depending on the type of sensory modality. In either case, the receptive region of the cell, much like a typical dendrite, can be depolarized but is not excitable. This depolarization, however, can spread by local current flow to a nearby area of the cell that is excitable (Fig. 4–4A). In myelinated afferent nerve fibers, this region is usually at the first node of the myelin sheath. In the case of receptor cells that have little or no axon, the generator potential induces the secretion of a chemical transmitter that acts on the dendrites of an adjacent afferent neuron in a manner similar to that of an excitatory synapse (Fig. 4–4B). In any case, **if the generator potential is great enough to bring the membrane of the afferent fiber to threshold, an action potential will be initiated.** As long as the excitable region of the afferent neuron remains depolarized to threshold, action potentials will continue to be generated and to propagate along the neuron. The more the receptor potential rises above the threshold, the greater becomes the action potential frequency.

Receptor Adaptation[1,2,4,6,7,9]

When a continuous stimulus is applied to a sensory receptor, the receptor typically responds at a high impulse rate initially, then at a progressively lower rate until firing may finally be completely extinguished (Fig. 4–5). This decline in afferent response is termed adaptation. **Adaptation is a characteristic shared by all sensory receptors, although the pattern of adaptation varies greatly.** Some receptors adapt to the point of extinction within fractions of seconds; others require hours or days to completely adapt. **The slowly adapting receptors continue to transmit impulses to the central nervous system as long as they are subjected to appropriate stimulation.** In this way, they provide a continual stream of sensory information to central processing areas. One good example is the muscle spindle of skeletal muscle that continues to fire as long as the muscle is under stretch, providing ongoing information about skeletal muscle length. Because the slowly adapting receptors can continue to transmit information for many hours, **they are called** *tonic receptors.* Many of these receptors ultimately adapt to extinction if the stimulus intensity remains constant for several hours or days. This, however, seldom occurs with normal levels of physical activity, and these receptors seldom reach a state of complete adaptation. **Rapidly adapting receptors, on the other hand, are characterized by a rapid decline in action potential frequency in the face of sustained stimulation.** Because these receptors respond primarily to changes in stimulus intensity rather than to continual stimulation, **they are termed** *phasic receptors.* These receptors provide information about the onset and termination of stimulation, as well as about the rate at which stimulation takes place, with the number of afferent impulses directly related to the rate at which change in the stimulus occurs. For example, some sensory receptors in and around joints are excited by acceleration or deceleration of joint movement, but adapt quickly when the movement ceases. Sensing the rate at which some change in the body is taking place allows prediction of the state of the body a few

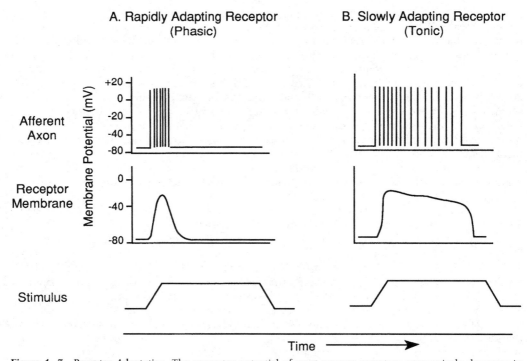

Figure 4–5 *Receptor Adaptation.* The generator potential of most sensory receptors progressively decreases in response to a continuous stimulus. This is adaptation. (*A*) Rapidly adapting (phasic) receptors respond only at the beginning of the stimulus, whereas (*B*) slowly adapting (tonic) receptors continue responding to prolonged stimulation.

seconds or even a few minutes later. For example, when one is running, information from receptors detecting the rates of movement of the joints and hence the movement of different parts of the body will allow anticipatory corrections in limb position to be continually made. Without this predictive ability, it would be impossible for the person to run.

Classes of Afferent Fibers[1–3,8,9]

The speed at which an afferent fiber conducts an action potential is related to the diameter of the fiber and whether the fiber is myelinated. The conduction velocity is less in smaller myelinated fibers than in larger ones, and still less in small unmyelinated fibers. **A number of different schemes have been used to categorize the various types of sensory fibers according to their diameters and conduction velocities** (Table 4–1). Sensory fibers are commonly divided into groups I, II, III, and IV. The speed of conduction in sensory fibers is important, because the faster that action potentials are conducted, the more quickly the central nervous system receives the information. Some signals need to be transmitted to the central nervous system extremely rapidly; otherwise the information would be useless. An example of this is the sensory signals that apprise the brain of the momentary positions of the limbs at each fraction of a second during locomotor activity. At the other extreme, some types of sensory information, such as that depicting prolonged, aching pain or mild temperature changes do not need to be transmitted rapidly at all, and small, unmyelinated (slow) fibers will suffice.

Coding of Sensory Information[1–5]

Regardless of the type of sensory receptor or the nature of the afferent nerve fiber, sensory stimulation is manifested as action potentials conducted to the central nervous system. These action potentials are identical. How is it then that the specific quality, location, and intensity of stimulation are communicated centrally?

MODALITY **The quality or type of a sensation is its modality.** Examples of sensory modalities include touch, warmth, cold, sound, vision, and so forth. Each sensory modality has a discrete pathway to the brain, and the sensation perceived (as well as the part of the body to which it is localized) is determined by the particular part of the brain activated. As a result, **any time a given pathway is stimulated, the sensation (i.e., the modality) will be the same** (Fig. 4–6). This is termed the **labeled line principle.** Stimulation of a specific nervous pathway at any point along its course gives rise to the sensation quality that would have occurred if the receptor at the beginning of the pathway had been stimulated by its natural stimulus. If, for example, the optic nerve or even specific sites in the brain are electrically stimulated, a sensation of light is produced.

Table 4–1. *Classes of Afferent Fibers*

Fiber Group Classification	I	II	III	IV
Axon diameter*	12–20 μm	5–12 μm	2–5 μm	0.1–1.5 μm
Conduction velocity	70–120 m/s	30–70 m/s	5–30 m/s	0.5–2 m/s
Myelination	Yes	Yes	Yes	No
Receptor types	Primary muscle spindle (Ia) Golgi tendon organ (Ib)	Secondary muscle spindle Rapidly adapting touch receptors (fine) Pressure receptors	Touch receptors (coarse) Nociceptors (fast) Thermoceptors (cold)	Nociceptors (slow) Thermoceptors (cold, warm) Itch; tickle
Fiber type classification	A alpha	A beta	A delta	C

*Includes myelin sheath, where present.

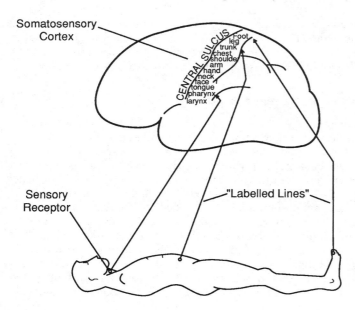

Somatosensory Cortex

CENTRAL SULCUS

Foot
leg
trunk
chest
shoulder
arm
hand
neck
face
tongue
pharynx
larynx

Sensory Receptor

"Labelled Lines"

Figure 4-6 *The Labeled-Line Principle.* Both stimulus location and modality are coded in the specific sensory pathway activated and the cortical areas in which it terminates.

LOCATION Most sensations convey a sense of the location from which the stimulus originates, whether it is on the body surface, within the body, or in the external environment. No matter where a particular sensory pathway is stimulated, whether it is in the periphery or at the cortex itself, the conscious sensation will usually be referred to the location of the receptor (the law of projection). One dramatic example of the law of projection is seen in amputees. These patients may complain of pain and proprioceptive sensations in an absent limb (i.e., phantom limb pain). These sensations are due in part to pressure on the stump of the amputated limb stimulating the firing of impulses in the sensory fibers that previously came from the sensory receptors in that limb. These impulses travel to the sensory cortex as if the entire pathway were intact, and the sensations evoked are perceived as if they emanate from where the receptors were originally located. Another interesting example of the dependence of sensory localization on the stimulation of a specific pathway to the brain is a phenomenon called referred pain. Referred pain is pain that arises at one site, but is perceived as arising from another. Referred pain often has visceral origins. This central misinterpretation of stimulus location is due to the convergence of visceral and somatosensory nociceptive fibers on the same ascending fibers in the spinal cord. The higher centers incorrectly attribute the source of the visceral pain to the site of origin of the somatosensory fibers. Additional information about stimulus location is provided by the relative intensity of excitation of the overlapping sensory units present in the area being stimulated. Since the receptor density is usually greatest at the center of a given sensory unit, stimulation in the center of the receptive field will activate more receptors and generate more action potentials in the afferent neuron. Because multiple sensory units are usually stimulated, the pattern of firing frequencies among these units helps to localize the stimuli (i.e., the greatest frequency arises from the sensory unit within which the stimulus is most centrally located).

INTENSITY There are two ways in which information about the intensity of stimulation is conveyed to the brain: by variation in the frequency of the action potentials generated by the activity in a given sensory unit and by variation in the number of receptors—hence sensory units—activated (Fig. 4-7). As we have seen, generator potentials vary in magnitude with the strength of stimulation. As stimulus intensity increases, the amplitude of the generator potential increases. Up to a point, the greater the generator potential, the greater will be the frequency of afferent action potentials (frequency coding). In this way, the intensity of stimulation is encoded in the frequency of afferent firing

A. Frequency Coding

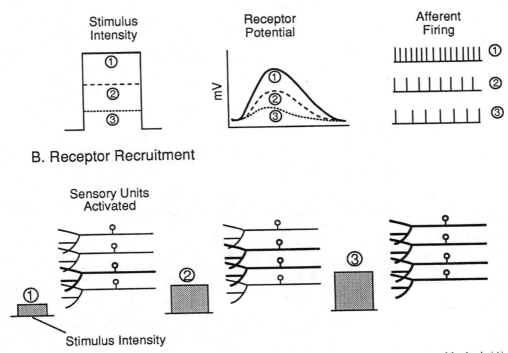

Figure 4–7 *Coding of Stimulus Intensity.* The intensity of sensory stimulation is communicated by both (A) the frequency of afferent neuronal firing and (B) the number of afferent neurons activated (recruited).

in individual afferent fibers. In addition, as the strength of a stimulus increases, it tends to spread over a larger area and to activate (recruit) more sensory receptors (population coding). Some of the increased number of receptors activated are part of the same sensory unit, and impulse frequency in the unit therefore increases. Other receptors are in overlapping units, and so more units fire. In this way, more afferent pathways are activated, with greater frequencies of firing, and this is interpreted in the brain as an increase in the intensity of the sensation.

Classification of Senses[1–4,7–9]

Many different schemes have been proposed in an effort to classify sensory receptors and the "senses" that they mediate (Table 4–2). Sensory receptors have been classified according to the specific form of energy to which they are most responsive (chemical, mechanical, thermal, or electromagnetic energy). They may also be characterized in terms of the sensation (modality) that they arouse (sound, sight, touch, hot, cold, or pain). Traditionally, the senses have been divided into the special senses (smell, vision, hearing, taste, and balance), the cutaneous senses of the skin, and the visceral senses monitoring the internal environment. A similar scheme divides afferent impulses into general somatic afferents (information from skin, skeletal muscle, and joints), general visceral afferents (information from visceral and smooth muscle), special somatic afferents (information related to vision, audition, and equilibrium), and special visceral afferents (information related to taste and smell).

Table 4–2. *Classification of Sensory Receptors and Senses*

RECEPTOR ACCORDING TO TYPE OF STIMULUS DETECTED	
Mechanoreceptors	Respond to mechanical forces such as touch, pressure, vibration, and stretch
Chemoreceptors	Respond to chemicals in solution
Thermoreceptors	Respond to changes in temperature
Photoreceptors	Respond to light
Nociceptors	Respond to potentially damaging stimuli; virtually all receptor types may function as nociceptors
RECEPTOR ACCORDING TO LOCATION OF STIMULUS	
Exteroceptors	Respond to stimuli arising within the external environment
Interoceptors	Respond to stimuli arising within the internal environment
Proprioceptors	Respond to deformation of tissues within the musculoskeletal system to signal body position or movement
COMMON CLINICAL CLASSIFICATION OF SENSES	
Cutaneous (superficial) sensations	Arise from receptors present in skin; include touch, pain, temperature, and 2-point discrimination
Deep sensations	Arise from receptors present in skeletal muscles, tendons, joints, and bone; include proprioception, vibration sense, and deep muscle pain
Visceral sensations	Arise from receptors present in viscera and relayed by autonomic afferent fibers; include hunger, nausea, and visceral pain
Special sensations	Arise from receptors of distinct embryologic origins; found within complex sense organs of the head and mediated by cranial nerves; include smell, vision, hearing, taste, and equilibrium
FUNCTIONAL CLASSIFICATION OF AFFERENT FIBERS	
General somatic afferents	Arise from skin, skeletal muscle, and joints
General visceral afferents	Arise from viscera and smooth muscle, largely unconscious in nature
Special somatic afferents	Related to vision, audition, and equilibrium
Special visceral afferents	Related to taste and smell

One functional approach is to divide the sensory systems into three categories: exteroceptive, proprioceptive, and interoceptive. Exteroceptive systems are sensitive to external stimuli; these include vision, hearing, skin sensation, and some chemical senses. Proprioceptive systems provide information about the position of body segments relative to one another and about the position of the body in space. Interoceptive systems are concerned with stimuli arising from the internal environment, such as blood pressure or osmolarity. Unlike exteroceptive and proprioceptive stimuli, which usually produce conscious sensations, interoceptive signals usually do not reach consciousness. All these systems of classification are somewhat arbitrary. **In reality, human perceptions and responses (especially motor responses) are usually determined by a combination of sensory modalities and are not easily explained in terms of these classification schemes.**

The Somatosensory System

The somatosensory system, with which this chapter is primarily concerned, transmits and processes information from sensory receptors on both the body surface and in the muscles, tendons, joints, and connective tissue of the musculoskeletal system. This system

Table 4-3. Characteristics of the Somatosensory System

- Somatosensory endings are less complex than those of the special sense organs.
- Somatosensory endings are distributed throughout the body, both on its surface and deep within its tissues.
- Somatosensory endings are diverse and highly specialized morphologically and functionally.
- Somatic sensibility is conveyed to the CNS by a variety of peripheral axons, ranging from large myelinated fibers (group I) to small unmyelinated fibers (group IV).
- Somatosensory pathways are composed of three major neurons: primary, secondary, and tertiary neurons.
- Primary somatic afferent fibers enter the CNS via either spinal nerve roots or cranial nerves; their cell bodies are usually located outside the CNS in sensory ganglia.

CNS = central nervous system.

has certain general characteristics (Table 4-3). As we shall see, the somatosensory system encompasses elements of our overall sensory capacity most closely linked to locomotor activity.

The Receptors[9-12]

The somatosensory receptors are numerous and highly varied, but **can be classified into three general types:** (1) mechanoreceptors, which are stimulated by mechanical displacement of some tissue of the body and mediate both tactile and proprioceptive senses; (2) thermoreceptors, which detect heat and cold; and (3) nociceptors, which are activated by damaging stimuli and serve to arouse pain (Table 4-4).

The mechanoreceptors are the most numerous and are highly specialized in their morphology, distribution, and function. They are found throughout both the surface of the body and the musculoskeletal system. These receptors give rise to our sense of the position of body parts (proprioception) and of body movement (kinesthesia). In this regard, they are intimately involved in all locomotor activity. These receptors will be emphasized in the following discussion of somatosensation.

Table 4-4. Principal Somatosensory Receptors

Receptor Type	Adequate Stimulus	Adaptation	Associated Sensation
Mechanoreceptors			
Cutaneous			
Merkel's cell	Skin distortion	Slow	Touch-pressure
Meissner's corpuscle	Vibration	Rapid	Flutter, contact
Ruffini's ending	Skin distortion	Slow	Touch
Pacinian corpuscle	Vibration	Very rapid	High-frequency vibration
Hair follicle	Hair movement	Rapid	Contact, touch
Free ending	Distortion	Rapid	Contact (coarse)
Musculoskeletal			
Muscle spindle—1° endings	Spindle stretch	Slow	Proprioception
Muscle spindle—2° endings	Spindle stretch	Slow	Proprioception
Golgi tendon organ	Tendon tension	Slow	Proprioception
Joint receptor	Joint movement and pressure	Slow	Proprioception
Thermoreceptors			
Free ending	15–30°C	Intermediate	Cold
Free ending	30–42°C	Intermediate	Warm
Nociceptors			
Free ending	Noxious	Slow	Pricking pain
Free ending	Noxious	Slow	Burning pain

From Patton, HD, et al: Textbook of Physiology, vol 1, ed 21. WB Saunders, Philadelphia, 1989, p 301.

The Ascending Pathways[9,10,13–19]

The somatosensory systems are designed to not only transduce sensory stimuli and to receive sensory information but also to relay this information from the periphery to higher neural areas. This occurs in several parallel sensory pathways that convey information to various regions of the nervous system (Fig. 4–8). These **somatosensory pathways have a characteristic configuration.** Receptor cells begin each pathway by transducing stimulus energy into action potentials in afferent nerve fibers. Thus, the first neuron in each pathway is the receptor neuron. The cell bodies of these **first-order neurons** are outside the central nervous system in a dorsal root or cranial nerve ganglion. The distal axon of each of these cell bodies receives information from the sensory receptor, whereas the proximal axon enters the spinal cord or brainstem by a dorsal root or cranial nerve. Each receptor neuron encodes and transmits information from a restricted locality, that neuron's receptive field. These first-order neurons then converge onto **second-order neurons** within the central nervous

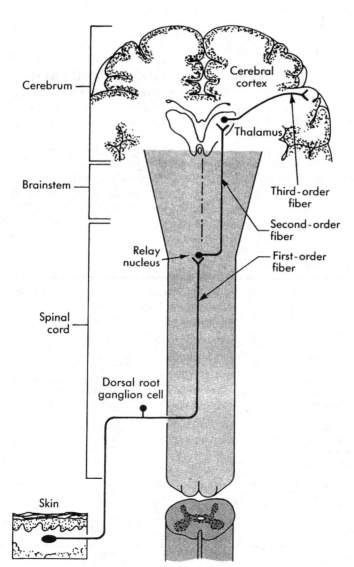

Figure 4–8   General Arrangement of Sensory Pathways. The typical ascending sensory pathway consists of three major neurons. It is notable that in each pathway the axon of the second-order neuron crosses the midline, so that sensory information from one side of the body is transmitted to the opposite side of the brain. (From Berne, RM and Levy, MN: Physiology, ed 3. Mosby–Year Book, St. Louis, 1993, p 122, with permission.)

system. The cell bodies of the second-order neurons lie within the dorsal gray matter of the spinal cord or in analogous areas of the brainstem. The axons of the second-order fibers cross to the opposite side of the neural axis (decussate) at some level of their ascent. First- and second-order neurons as they ascend in the spinal tract, are grouped into tracts (fasciculi) that are located primarily in the white matter of the cord. The second-order neurons, which may be located in the spinal cord or medulla, project to **third-order neurons** in the thalamus. Third-order neurons, their cell bodies in the thalamus, then project to the somatosensory areas of the cerebral cortex. This area of the cerebral cortex is concerned with the reception and conscious appreciation of somatosensory impulses.

In addition to joining ascending pathways, some sensory information is conveyed directly or via interneurons to spinal motor neurons, forming a basis for certain motor reflexes (see Chapter 5). Afferent projections also go to supraspinal structures other than the cerebral cortex, such as the cerebellum or reticular formation, which also participate in motor control.

In each of the ascending somatosensory pathways, there are several levels at which synapses occur. These junctures constitute sites at which ascending sensation can be influenced by activity in other parts of the central nervous system. Important sources of descending influences are the cerebral cortex and reticular formation. Descending fibers modify data transmission and processing within the ascending pathways and serve to control the intensity and character of sensory input to the cerebral cortex.

The Dorsal Column–Medial Lemniscal and the Anterolateral Systems

Most somatosensory information is carried along the neural axis in two major parallel ascending systems: the dorsal column–medial lemniscal system and the anterolateral system (Fig. 4–9). The first-order sensory neurons of **the dorsal column system** begin as peripheral sensory receptors and project central axonal branches into the spinal cord by way of the dorsal horn.[13–18] These fibers ascend in the dorsal columns of the ipsilateral spinal cord and ultimately synapse on second-order neurons in the dorsal column nuclei of the medulla. Above the midthoracic spinal level, the dorsal columns are divided into two bundles (fascicles) of axons: the medial gracile fascicle and the cuneate fascicle. The gracile fascicle contains the ascending branches of afferent fibers from levels caudal to the midthoracic region, whereas the cuneate fascicle contains afferent fibers from midthoracic to upper cervical levels. These two bundles terminate in different dorsal column nuclei (the gracile nucleus and cuneate nucleus, respectively). From there, the fibers decussate and project in a compact bundle called the **medial lemniscus** to the ventral posterior nucleus of the thalamus. Neurons in this nucleus then project through the internal capsule to the primary somatosensory cortex.

The central axonal branches of the first-order neurons of **the anterolateral system** do not themselves ascend in the spinal cord, but on entering the cord, synapse with second-order neurons within the nucleus proprius of the dorsal horn.[13–16,19] These neurons cross immediately to the contralateral side of the spinal cord and ascend in the anterolateral portion of the lateral column. Unlike the medial lemniscal fibers, which terminate almost exclusively in the thalamus, the anterolateral pathways terminate in various regions of the brainstem and hypothalamus, as well as in the thalamus. The three major pathways of the anterolateral system, as defined by the location of their terminations, are the spinothalamic, spinoreticular, and spinomesencephalic (spinotectal) tracts. The fibers of the spinothalamic tracts synapse on neurons in the thalamus but in more varied nuclei than the medial lemniscus. As a result, neurons from these nuclei then project to more diverse cortical areas than do the medial lemniscal. Fibers in the spinoreticular tracts terminate on neurons in the reticular formation of the medulla and pons, which in turn relay information to the thalamus and other structures in the diencephalon. The spinomesencephalic (or spinotectal) tracts terminate primarily in the superior colliculus of the midbrain but also project to the region around the cerebral aqueduct.

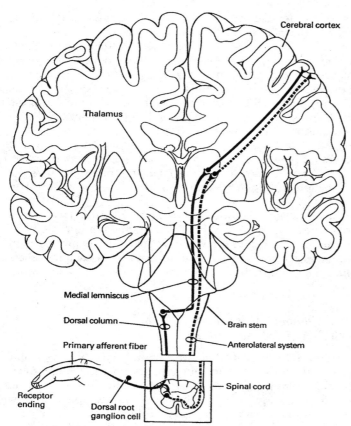

Figure 4–9   *Primary Somatosensory Spinal Cord Tracts.* The main pathway for tactile sensations (discriminative touch, proprioception, and vibration) is termed the dorsal column-medial lemniscal system (*Solid Line*). Pain, temperature and, to a much lesser extent, tactile sensations travel to the brain via the anterolateral system (*Broken Line*). (From Kandel, ER, Schwartz, JH, and Jessell, TM (eds): Principles of Neural Science, ed 3. Appleton & Lange, Norwalk, CT, 1991, p 333, with permission.)

These somatosensory systems are used to conduct information regarding pain, temperature, touch, and proprioception from the extremities and trunk. Somatosensory information from the face, mouth, and head is supplied primarily by the trigeminal nerve and its central connections.

Although the dorsal column–medial lemniscal system and the anterolateral system are analogous in some respects, they differ significantly in the types of information that they convey and in their basic transmission characteristics (Table 4–5). The dorsal

Table 4–5. *Differences Between the Dorsal Column–Medial Lemniscal and Anterolateral Systems*

- Anterolateral has large contingent of uncrossed ascending fibers.
- Anterolateral crossing occurs in the spinal cord; lemniscal occurs in the medulla.
- Most axons in the lemniscal terminate in the thalamus; anterolateral fibers terminate throughout the brainstem as well as in the thalamus.
- Lemniscal system contains larger, more rapidly conducting nerve fibers.
- Lemniscal system transmits sensory information with greater specificity and more precise localization.
- Lemniscal system conveys sensations of fine touch, vibration, and joint position; anterolateral system conveys sensations of pain, temperature, and crude touch.
- Lemniscal system may be assessed by vibration, two-point discrimination, and stereognosis; anterolateral by pinprick, heat, and cold testing.

column system is concerned primarily with highly discriminative aspects of sensation. This system conveys information regarding fine touch (e.g., the tactile recognition of shapes and textures), awareness of the position and movement of the body (i.e., proprioception), and vibration. This system is capable of great spatial and temporal discrimination. The tracts and nuclei of this system have a high degree of spatial orientation (somatotopy), which reflects with great precision the specific origins of sensory information. In addition, this system is composed of large myelinated nerve fibers that transmit this information rapidly through the central nervous system to the cerebral cortex. The anterolateral system, on the other hand, is concerned with the conveyance of a broad spectrum of more diffuse information, including pain and temperature. It is also the main pathway for the less discriminative form of touch, usually referred to as **light touch**. This system has inherently less ability to discriminate spatially and is slower conducting.

Because there is a degree of functional overlap or redundancy between these two parallel systems, if one system is damaged some residual sensory capability may be provided by the other.[9,13,16] Patients with lesions of the dorsal columns, for example, may retain some crude tactile sensibility. Moreover, because these two systems are physically separated, pathology may disrupt the sensations mediated by one system without affecting the other. A good example is the distinctive pattern of mixed sensory loss that occurs with certain kinds of spinal cord injury (e.g., the Brown-Séquard syndrome; see Chapter 17).

Although tactile and proprioceptive information from most of the body is conveyed by the dorsal column–medial lemniscal system, a few fibers carrying position and movement signals from the lower extremities take a different route. These ascend with the dorsal spinocerebellar tract. Specifically, most of the afferent fibers from lower extremity proprioceptors synapse on the spinal cord nucleus dorsalis. Fibers from this nucleus then ascend with the dorsal spinocerebellar tract to the medulla, where they exit and synapse in the cerebellum. This provides input for use in the cerebellar modulation of gait and posture (see Chapter 8). Some collateral spinocerebellar fibers do project by routes poorly understood (possibly by rejoining the medial lemniscus) to the cerebral cortex, contributing to conscious perception of gait and posture.[13–18]

The Trigeminal System[13,14,20]

The back of the head and much of the external ear are supplied by branches of the second and third cervical nerves, whose central connections are via the medial lemniscus and anterolateral systems. The rest of **the head, face, and mouth are innervated almost entirely by branches of the trigeminal nerve.** The arrangement of the first-order (primary afferent) fibers of the trigeminal system is analogous to that of the spinal somatosensory systems. As with spinal nerves, the primary afferent fibers of the trigeminal nerve are the peripheral axons of pseudounipolar neurons whose cell bodies are located in a ganglion outside of the central nervous system (Fig. 4–10). The central axons of these **first-order cells** enter the pons and divide into ascending and descending tracts that terminate in the pontine or spinal trigeminal nuclei, respectively. The pontine trigeminal nucleus is also called the **principal sensory nucleus.** Information from these nuclei then reaches the thalamus via the **second-order neurons** of the trigeminal lemniscus, which travels with the medial lemniscus. These projections are primarily (not exclusively) contralateral, and most terminate in the same regions of the thalamus (the ventral posterior nucleus) that receive spinal somatosensory information. Like the spinal system, the trigeminal information in the thalamus is somatotopically organized. Information from the thalamus is then relayed in **third-order neurons** to the somatosensory cortex. The representation of the face, and especially the mouth and tongue, is greatly exaggerated in the cortex, reflecting the extremely high-innervation density of these regions. Small areas of the skin and some areas of the mucous membrane are supplied by components of other cranial nerves (i.e., facial, glossopharyngeal, and vagus nerves). The central connections of the somatosensory components of these nerves, however, are essentially the same as for the trigeminal nerve.

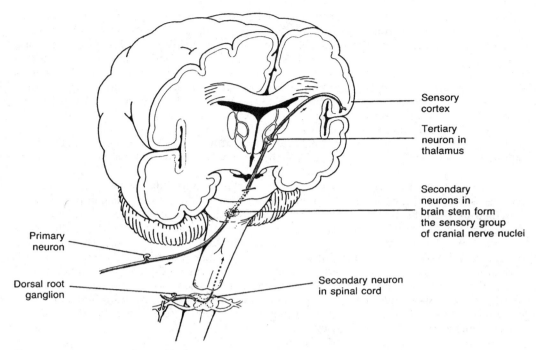

Figure 4–10 *Sensory Pathways from the Head.* Pathways carrying somatosensory information from the head are also composed of three major neurons. The first-order neurons form the trigeminal cranial nerve and synapse with second-order neurons in brainstem cranial nerve nuclei. Afferent fibers then generally cross the midline to project to third-order neurons in the thalamus. (From Wilson-Pauwels, L, Akesson, EJ, and Stewart, PD: Cranial Nerves: Anatomy and Clinical Comments. BC Decker, Inc., Toronto, 1988, p XI, with permission.)

The Somatosensory Cortex[9,10,12–15]

Extending horizontally across each hemisphere of the cortex is a deep central fissure (the central sulcus), which provides a superficial landmark for delineating the cortical sensory and motor areas. In general, sensory signals terminate in the cerebral cortex posterior to this fissure. The portion of the cortex anterior to the central fissure is devoted to motor control and to some aspects of analytical thought. **Somatosensory information is projected to the somatosensory cortex, which lies immediately behind the central fissure in the postcentral gyrus of the parietal lobe** (Fig. 4–11). The somatosensory cortex is composed of two components—somatosensory areas I and II. **Somatosensory area I is the most important and best understood.** The somatosensory fibers projecting from the thalamus to somatosensory area I have a specific spatial arrangement, giving rise to a distinct spatial orientation in the sensory information reaching the cortex. Various parts of the body are represented sequentially along the postcentral gyrus, with the legs on top and the head at the foot of the gyrus. **The sensory information is not only distributed over somatosensory area I in accordance with body location, but also the size of the cortical representation for impulses from that particular part of the body is roughly proportional to the number of receptors in that locality.** The relative size and distribution of cortical receptor areas may be diagrammatically represented as the sensory homunculus (Fig. 4–12). Some evidence suggests that it may be too simplistic to think in terms of one sensory homunculus; rather, each subsection of somatosensory area I may have its own complete homunculus of the contralateral body. The cortical areas for sensation from the trunk and back are small, implying relatively indiscriminate perception, whereas very large areas are concerned with impulses from the hand and parts of the face (especially the lips). Remember that each

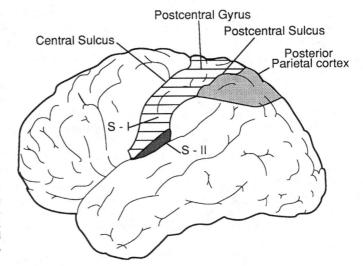

Figure 4–11 *The Somatosensory Cortex.* This lateral view of a cerebral hemisphere illustrates the somatic sensory receiving areas: somatosensory areas I and II and the posterior somatic association areas. (Adapted from Kandel, ER, Schwartz, JH, and Jessell, TM (eds): Principles of Neural Science, ed 3. Appleton & Lange, Norwalk, CT, 1991, p 364.)

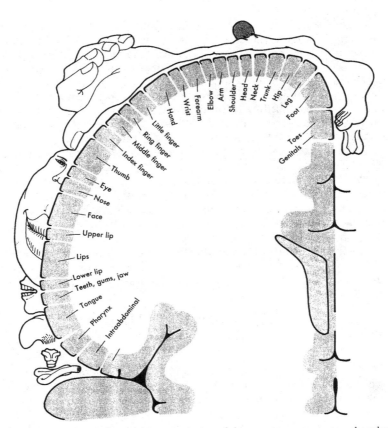

Figure 4–12 *The Sensory Homunculus.* In this coronal view of the somatosensory cortex, the relative amount of cortical tissue devoted to each area of the body surface is indicated by the size of the adjacent diagrammatic body part. This type of representation of the somatotopic organization of the sensory cortex is termed the sensory homunculus. (From Berne, RM, and Levy, MN: Physiology, ed 3. Mosby–Year Book, St. Louis, 1993, p 136, with permission.)

hemisphere of the cortex receives sensory information from the opposite (contralateral) side of the body, with the exception of a small amount of sensory information from the same (ipsilateral) side of the face. Direct stimulation of the sensory cortex dramatically demonstrates the specificity with which stimulus location and sensory modality are represented in the cortex.

The cerebral cortex is a complex structure composed of many layers of different types of cells. The layers of cells in the postcentral gyrus appear to be organized into vertical columns extending through all of the separate neuronal layers of which it is composed. Each of these columns is activated by afferents from a particular part of the body, mediating the same specific sensory modality.

Somatosensory area II is much smaller and lies posterior and inferior to the lateral end of somatosensory area I. The degree of localization of sensory information from different parts of the body is very poor compared with that of area I. Although this area seems to further process information received from area I, relatively little is known about its overall function. It is interesting that removal of an entire cerebral hemisphere causes contralateral difficulty in sensory localization but not complete anesthesia. Bilateral input received by area II from the remaining hemisphere may be responsible for this residual sensory capability.[9]

Cortical lesions do not affect the various somatic sensations to the same extent.[9,16] Proprioception and fine touch, the most refined and discrete sensibilities, are most affected. Temperature sensibility is less affected, and pain sensibility is only slightly affected. Upon recovery, pain sensibility returns first, followed by temperature sense and finally proprioception and fine touch.

As complex as the cortical sensory areas are, a significant degree of adaptability or plasticity seems to be present. It is likely that cortical maps are subject to constant modification on the basis of their use. If, for example, an area of the cortex is no longer activated because a digit is lost or the nervous connections to that digit are disrupted, that area will become activated by other parts of the body. By the same token, increased use and hence increased sensory feedback from some part of the body may increase its cortical representation.[22,23]

Deciphering of sensory information does not end in the primary sensory cortex, but **continues on in somatic association areas.**[9,10,12,24] These seem to be areas where signals denoting several aspects of a stimulus are integrated into a meaningful, complete pattern. For example, electrical stimulation in the somatic association areas can cause an individual to experience a complex somatic sensation, even to the extent of "feeling" an intact object such as a ball. With damage to these areas of the brain, a person is aware of sensation but is unable to put the data to use. Such a patient may suffer abnormalities in body image and an inability to recognize complete objects through otherwise normally functioning sensory channels (agnosia).[24] Clearly these areas are important for deciphering and further integrating information that enters the somatosensory areas. Functions that the association areas may subserve include integration of simultaneous inputs from many different modalities, attachment of emotional significance to sensory perceptions, exploration of the environment, and participation in such functions as arousal, learning, and memory.

Information Processing in the Ascending Pathways[10,12,17,19,21]

As we have seen, **sensory information arising in the periphery ascends the neural axis in specialized pathways terminating in the sensory cortex.** It is important to realize that this sensory information is not only transmitted in a headward direction by these pathways but also is processed and integrated along the way. Each of these pathways is composed of at least three orders of afferent neurons, each of which communicates synaptically with the next higher order. At these synapses, the processing of sensory input takes place.

The flow of sensory information through the ascending pathways is subject to extensive control, and much of it is reduced or even abolished by inhibition from other

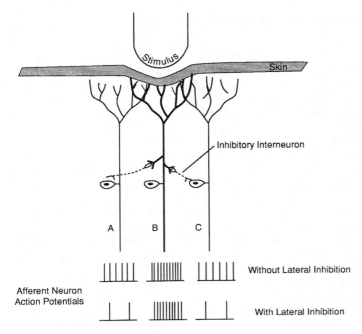

Figure 4–13 *Lateral Inhibition.* Although the sensory neuron at the center of the stimulus is activated to the greatest extent, adjacent receptors are also stimulated. In the absence of lateral inhibition, neurons A, B, and C would all discharge in accordance with this stimulation. With lateral inhibition, the lateral pathways are inhibited, emphasizing the activity in the central pathway. Localization of the stimulus is thus accentuated.

neurons. Inhibitory influences arise from many sources, including collateral fibers of the afferent neurons themselves, local interneurons, and descending pathways from higher areas such as the reticular formation and cerebral cortex. Inhibitory mechanisms at each level are complex and involve both presynaptic and postsynaptic inhibitory influences.

Descending inhibitory pathways transmit signals to relay centers in the thalamus, medulla, and spinal cord, imposing a degree of control over the overall flow of information and over the sensitivity of sensory input. When sensory input becomes too great, these inhibitory signals may automatically decrease transmission in relay nuclei. In this way, the sensory system can be kept operating at a sensitivity that is not so low as to be ineffective, nor so high that the system is overwhelmed. This type of inhibition is especially evident in the anterolateral pathways mediating pain. Pain-carrying pathways are tonically inhibited, which provides the flexibility of either reducing the inhibition to increase signal transmission or of increasing the inhibition to block the signals more completely.

In pathways carrying the most precise and discriminant information (dorsal column–medial lemniscal pathways), more discrete inhibitory influences are used to refine sensory input. A process called **lateral inhibition** enhances the ability to distinguish between adjacent stimuli.[2,12,21] As each sensory pathway gives rise to excitatory signals, it also gives rise to concurrent inhibitory signals that spread laterally. This inhibits the peripheral spread of the signal, further delineating the central excitatory message (Fig. 4–13). Dorsal column neurons, for example, exert this effect through short collateral fibers transmitting inhibitory signals to surrounding neurons. These inhibitory signals occur at each synaptic level of the ascending pathway. The net result is to increase the degree of contrast or sharpness in the cerebral cortex. Although lateral inhibition occurs to some extent in the pathways of most sensory modalities, it is most extensively used in the pathways providing the most discrete localization of stimuli. For example, a pointed object lightly touching the skin or slight deflection of skin hairs can be highly localized, whereas stimuli activating temperature receptors whose pathways lack such lateral inhibition are localized poorly. Two-point discrimination, the ability to distinguish between two needles pressed lightly against the skin, is strongly dependent on lateral inhibition and is a method frequently used clinically to test tactile capability.

Touch and Proprioception

The tactile senses involve a complex interplay between different types of tactile receptors and sensations. There are two basic tactile capabilities: (1) simple touch, which consists of relatively crude touch and pressure sensations and is only poorly localized on the surface of the body, and (2) tactile discrimination, which consists of touch, pressure, and position senses, the intensity and locality of which are perceived in great detail. **All tactile sensation is mediated by mechanoreceptors** (see Table 4–4). These receptors can be classified into two major categories.[2,6,26] About 50% of the receptors are **slowly adapting mechanoreceptors**, which respond with a sustained discharge to an enduring stimulus. The other receptors are **rapidly adapting mechanoreceptors**, which respond primarily to changes in stimulus intensity. These characteristically respond with a burst of action potentials at the onset and termination of stimulation. Within each of these two categories, some receptors have small, well-defined receptive fields and are able to provide precise information about the location and contour of objects touching or pressing against the body. As might be expected, these receptors are concentrated at the fingertips, which are used for the exploration of objects by touch. In contrast, other receptors have larger receptive fields, with obscure boundaries; these cells are not involved in detailed touch discrimination, but signal information about crude touch, pressure, and vibration. Each receptor has its own particular morphology, functional characteristics, and distribution. In general, the receptors that communicate the most precise information transmit via the more rapidly conducting myelinated afferent fibers, whereas those that signal crude pressure, poorly localized touch, and the sensations of itch and tickle communicate via much slower nerve fibers (see Table 4–1).

Although each specific receptor mediates a particular type of tactile sensation, the natural stimuli that we encounter in our actual daily experiences usually activate a combination of mechanoreceptors producing somewhat different "hybrid" sensations.

Simple touch consists of relatively indistinct sensations of touch and pressure, as well as the sensations of itch and tickle. This system provides only a crude representation of stimulus location. Although some simple touch fibers may ascend in the dorsal column–medial lemniscal pathways, most travel upward in the anterolateral pathways following a course similar to that of pain and thermal sensation. The first-order neurons of this system do not synapse with cells in the spinal cord until a considerable amount of longitudinal dispersion has taken place and the axons have spread out over several spinal cord segments. The clinical manifestation of disturbances involving this pathway is primarily an inability to perceive light touch. However, because touch information is also transmitted in the dorsal pathways, complete loss of touch usually occurs only with extensive lesions involving all ascending tracts.

Tactile discrimination consists of sensations of touch and pressure with a high degree of localization, phasic sensations such as vibration or movement against the skin, and a sense of body position. This system mediates discriminatory tasks such as the ability to discern two separate points applied to the skin simultaneously (two-point discrimination), recognition of the size, shape, and texture of objects in the hand (stereognosis), and identification of letters or figures drawn on the skin (graphesthesia). This system also mediates proprioception and our vibratory sense (as might be tested clinically with a tuning fork). First-order neurons conveying tactile discrimination and proprioceptive information enter the spinal cord through the dorsal roots and immediately ascend in the dorsal column pathways to the lower medulla.

The term *proprioception* **is used to describe an awareness of the position or movement of the body.** This encompasses a sense of both the position of the body with respect to gravity and the relative position of any of its parts. **Of all the sensory modalities, proprioception is perhaps the one most closely linked to locomotor activity.** For motor function to proceed normally, the nervous system must be continually apprised of the position of the body and limbs. This is true whether motor activity is directed at maintaining a posture or producing movement. Proprioception is a complex sensory function, which uses information gathered from a variety of sources.

Proprioceptive information is processed at both conscious and unconscious levels. Conscious proprioception travels along with tactile discrimination information in the dorsal column–medial lemniscal pathways ultimately to be represented in the somesthetic areas of the cerebral cortex. In addition, first-order neurons conveying proprioceptor information may pass through the dorsal centers into the ventral horn and synapse directly on motor neurons (anterior horn cells) of the same segment. As will be discussed in Chapter 5, this direct link between first-order sensory fibers and motor fibers mediates the simplest of all motor reflexes, the skeletal muscle stretch reflex. Other receptor neurons may synapse with second-order neurons, which ascend in the spinocerebellar pathways and transmit information about the activity of muscles and limbs to the cerebellum, where it is integrated and processed (see Chapter 8). The cerebellum can use this feedback to ensure that movements are performed smoothly and accurately.

Proprioceptors in Muscle, Joint, and Skin

The sensors involved in proprioception provide information to the central nervous system about the relative position of the body parts and their movement. Central to a knowledge of body position is information regarding the degree of angulation of all joints in all planes and their rates of movement. **Many different types of mechanoreceptors are used to develop this information.** The receptors involved lie in the muscles, the tendons, the joints, and the skin (Fig. 4–14).[9,11,25–28]

Muscle Receptors [6,8,9,25–34]

Skeletal muscle contains a variety of specialized sensory receptors, which convey information to the central nervous system about muscle length, muscle tension, and velocity of stretch. Predominant among these receptors are the muscle spindle and Golgi tendon organ.

Muscle spindles are distributed throughout the fleshy part of skeletal muscle and are found in greatest abundance in muscles capable of delicate, phasic contractile activity.[28–33] Notable exceptions, however, are the tongue and ocular muscles, in which they are scarce.

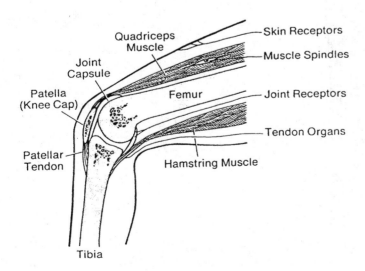

Figure 4–14 *Proprioceptors.* Many different types of mechanoreceptors contribute to proprioception. As illustrated by the knee joint, these receptors lie in the muscles, the tendons, the joints, and the skin. (From Shepherd, GM: Neurobiology, ed 2. Oxford University Press, New York, 1988, p 271, with permission.)

Each muscle spindle consists of 2 to 10 muscle fibers enclosed in a connective tissue capsule (Fig. 4–15). The small muscle fibers within the spindle are called **intrafusal fibers** and are morphologically and functionally distinct from the **extrafusal fibers** of the muscle itself. Although capable of contracting, the intrafusal fibers do not contribute to the overall tension-generating capability of the muscle; rather, they play a role in adjusting the sensitivity of the muscle spindle itself. The intrafusal fibers are arranged parallel with the rest of the muscle fibers, with the ends of the spindle capsule attached to either the tendon at either end of the muscle or to the side of an extrafusal fiber.

Each spindle contains two types of intrafusal fibers, which differ principally in the overall arrangement of their nuclei. The first type contains many nuclei clustered in a dilated central area and is called a **nuclear bag fiber**. The second type, which is thinner, shorter, and lacking a nuclear bag, has its nuclei arranged in single file. This is the **nuclear chain fiber**. The nuclear-bag–type and nuclear-chain–type intrafusal fibers also differ in the kind of contractile activity that they exhibit. Bag fibers contract more slowly than chain fibers.

Two kinds of sensory endings are associated with the muscle spindle. The **primary endings** are small group Ia afferent fibers that wrap around both the nuclear bag and nuclear chain fibers. The **secondary endings** are terminations of group II sensory fibers that are located near the ends of only the nuclear chain fibers. These sensory endings have also been called the **annulospiral** and **flowerspray endings**, respectively, because of their characteristic appearance. The primary afferents seem to have a lower threshold to stretch than do the secondary.

In general, when muscle spindles are stretched the primary and secondary endings are stimulated, resulting in increased firing in the group Ia and II afferent fibers. The primary and secondary endings of the muscle spindle, however, seem to respond differently to specific phases of stretch. Both types respond to tonic (steady-state) stretch, although the

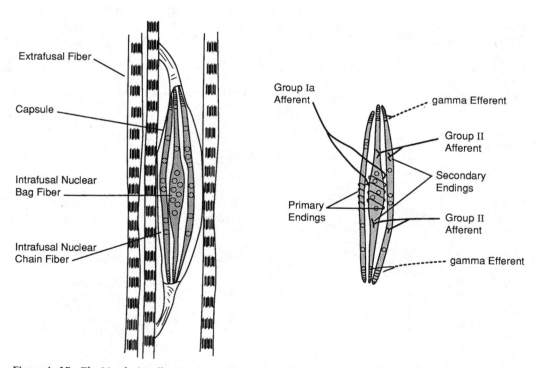

Figure 4–15 *The Muscle Spindle.* Muscle spindles consist of a thin capsule containing 2 to 10 intrafusal fibers. Group Ia sensory fibers have stretch-sensitive endings on both nuclear-bag–type and nuclear-chain–type intrafusal fibers. Group II sensory fibers have stretch-sensitive endings on the nuclear chain fibers. Gamma motor axons innervate the contractile portions of both types of intrafusal fibers.

secondary endings are a bit more sensitive. During the dynamic phase of stretch, however, when the muscle is actually changing length, it is the primary endings that are discharging most rapidly. Thus, the secondary endings are mainly sensitive to the length of the muscle, whereas the primary endings are sensitive to both changes in the length of the muscle and to changes in the rate of stretch. The responsiveness of the primary endings to the phasic as well as the tonic events in muscle is important because the sensitivity of the spindle to the velocity of stretch helps to minimize oscillations that would otherwise occur during changes in muscle length. Without this damping effect, tremor would develop.[12]

Muscle spindles, in addition to their sensory connections, have their own motor supply. **Both types of intrafusal fibers are innervated by small motor fibers from the ventral horn called** *gamma motor neurons.* The extrafusal fibers, on the other hand, are innervated by large alpha motor neurons. The gamma motor neurons innervate the intrafusal fibers at their polar regions, where the contractile elements of the fibers are located. The central region of the fibers is almost devoid of contractile apparatus. **Gamma activation has the effect of contracting and shortening the intrafusal fiber at its ends, thereby stretching the central nuclear region.**

There are two types of gamma motor neurons: gamma dynamic, which innervate nuclear bag fibers, and gamma static, which innervate nuclear chain fibers. These inputs seem to specifically regulate the sensitivity of the spindles either to dynamic or to static phases of stretch. As will be discussed in Chapter 5, gamma motor input, by shortening the intrafusal fibers, increases tension in the spindle and hence its sensitivity to stretch. In this way, the level of gamma efferent discharge may influence alpha motor activity and muscle tone. Abnormal gamma activity can significantly distort motor function.

Golgi tendon organs are located among the tendon fasicles near the transition between muscle and tendon.[29,30,34,35] These sense organs are less numerous than muscle spindles in any given muscle and are most abundant in more slowly contracting muscles. A single tendon organ is composed of a network of small unmyelinated fibers enclosed in a fine capsule (Fig. 4–16). Each tendon organ is in series with 15 to 20 extrafusal fibers; when the muscle fibers actively contract or are stretched, the nerve endings are distorted, causing them to fire. Afferent connections are type Ib myelinated fibers. They have no motor innervation.

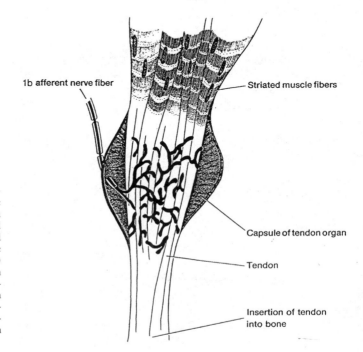

Figure 4–16 The Golgi Tendon Organ. Golgi tendon organs, which are located at the transition between muscle and tendon, consist of small bundles of tendon fibers enclosed within a thin capsule. Several large myelinated afferent fibers (Group Ib) penetrate the capsule to terminate in numerous unmyelinated branches interspersed among the tendon bundles. (From Ham, AW and Cormack, DH: Histology, ed 8. JB Lippincott, Philadelphia, 1979, p 584, with permission.)

1b afferent nerve fiber

Striated muscle fibers

Capsule of tendon organ

Tendon

Insertion of tendon into bone

The Golgi tendon organs have traditionally been described as high-threshold stretch receptors with a function limited to signaling dangerously high muscle tensions.[9,25-27,34,35] More recently, however, it has become evident that tendon organs are very sensitive muscle receptors, particularly sensitive to actively generated muscle force, and that they have a more widespread role in movement control. Although the tendon organs are much less sensitive to passive stretch than the muscle spindles, they are highly sensitive to the stretch imposed on them by contraction of the muscle fibers with which they are attached in series. Some tendon organs are probably activated even in the weakest of contractions. The function of the tendon organ is to monitor muscle contraction. It is a misnomer to call it a stretch receptor.

Muscle spindles are thus arranged parallel with extrafusal fibers, whereas Golgi tendon organs are situated in series with muscle fibers. These anatomic arrangements explain in large part the differing responses of spindles and tendon organs to muscle stretch and contraction (Fig. 4-17).[27,29,30] Passive stretching of muscle distorts and thereby activates both the tendon organ and the muscle spindle receptors; thus, the afferent output of both increases. Active muscle contraction, on the other hand, affects these two sensors very differently. Because the tendon organs are in series with extrafusal fibers, they are stretched and activated by muscle contraction. The parallel muscle spindles, on the other hand, are unstretched by muscle contraction and deactivated. The discharge of tendon organs is thus increased and the discharge of muscle spindles is decreased during muscle contraction. In this way, the **tendon organs sense more directly active muscle tension, whereas the spindle organs sense increasing muscle length.**

Differences in the response of spindles and tendon organs are well illustrated by afferent findings during mechanically or electrically induced muscle contraction. In response to a tendon tap, for instance, tendon organs fire during the active phase of contraction, whereas spindles fire in response to the stretch produced by the tap itself. During electrically induced muscle twitches, the tendon organs respond during the twitch, the period in which the spindles are silent.

Two additional types of sensory nerve endings are found in muscle: paciniform corpuscles and free nerve endings.[8,25-28] Although little is known about the physiologic

A. Passive Muscle Stretch

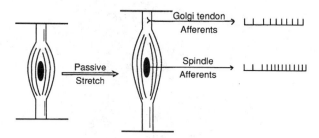

B. Active Muscle Contraction

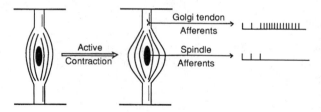

Figure 4-17 Responses of Muscle Spindles and Golgi Tendon Organs to Muscle Stretch and Muscle Contraction. (A) During passive stretch of the muscle, both afferents discharge; the Golgi tendon organ discharges less than the spindle. (B) However, when the muscle is made to actively contract by stimulation of its motor neuron, the spindle is unloaded and therefore becomes silent; the tendon organ output is further increased.

function of either type of ending, they constitute a significant proportion of the total sensory innervation of the muscle. There are more free nerve endings in muscle than any other type of sensory receptor, and the number of paciniform corpuscles may reach 30% of the total number of muscle spindles.

The **paciniform corpuscles**, although smaller, are similar to those found in the skin. They are most frequently observed at the musculotendinous junction in the vicinity of tendon organs and are supplied by a large-diameter (group II) myelinated fiber, which may innervate several separate corpuscles. They are probably rapidly-adapting end organs sensitive to high frequency vibration like true pacinian corpuscles in the skin.

Free nerve endings are found in close association with almost every structure in muscle (spindles, tendon organs, muscle fibers, fascia, fat, and blood vessels, excluding capillaries). All nonmyelinated fibers and most small group III myelinated axons terminate as free nerve endings. These endings are rarely excited by classic proprioceptive stimuli such as muscle stretch or contraction or muscle vibration. Instead, they are primarily activated by high-threshold mechanical stimulation of muscle, such as pinching or pricking, and have been termed "pressure-pain" receptors. They also respond to other nociceptive stimuli. Some of these endings may play a role in mediating local vascular reflexes.

Joint Receptors[8,9,25–27,36]

Three main types of endings are associated with the synovial joints of the body. Free nerve endings, which are the most numerous type of joint receptor, are found throughout the connective tissue. These are innervated by group III or nonmyelinated fibers. **Golgi's endings** similar to tendon organs are found in the joint ligaments and are innervated by large diameter group I myelinated fibers. **Ruffini's endings** similar to those found in the skin are found in the joint capsule. These are innervated by group II fibers. There are no nerve endings on the cartilaginous surfaces of the joint or in the synovial membranes.

The physiologic function of these afferents is not very well understood. During passive movement of the joint, most of the joint afferents fire only at the extremes of joint rotation. It seems likely that the joint receptors with group I and II afferent fibers (i.e., Golgi's and Ruffini's endings) are responsive only to deformation of the joint capsule or ligaments. At joint positions where no stress is placed on the capsule, the receptors remain silent. These receptors, as well as free nerve endings, may mediate some protective function when potentially harmful stress is placed on the joint. Active movement of the joint may create stresses very different from those arising from passive movement and may well involve these receptors in physiologic functions yet to be defined. Moreover, the receptors that signal joint position may differ for different joints.

Cutaneous Receptors[8,9,25–27,37,38]

Three types of receptors are found in the skin: thermoreceptors, nociceptors, and mechanoreceptors.[37] **The mechanoreceptors, however, convey proprioceptive information and play an important role in the control of movement.** This is particularly true of the densely innervated regions of the hand and foot. Signals from pressure sensors in the soles of the feet are used in balance.[27,39] Peripheral neuropathies, which cause loss of sensation in the extremities, may result in patients' being unable to stand unassisted with their feet together when they close their eyes. Although the neuropathy may involve muscle receptor input from the intrinsic muscles of the foot, the major contribution to pressure sensation is believed to come from cutaneous receptors. Without information regarding the differential distribution of pressure on the soles of the feet, the reflexes from the vestibular system of these patients are unable to maintain balance alone. In the same way, any complex manipulation of objects in the hand is grossly impaired by cutaneous anesthesia; writing with a pen or picking up small objects becomes much more difficult, even when vision of the hand and object is allowed. Cutaneous mechanoreceptors include Merkel's disks, Meissner's corpuscles, Ruffini's endings, and pacinian corpuscles.

Summary of Proprioceptors

Normal movement is accompanied by active and passive changes in the length and tension of all muscles acting on the moving joint, by distortion of the joint capsule and ligaments, and by deformation of skin. The afferent activity generated by movement comes from all these sources. **The particular contribution made by specific receptors to proprioception varies,** however, from one part of the body to another.[9,25–27,36] In the finger, for example, where skin receptors are particularly abundant, as much as half of position recognition is probably determined via skin receptors. On the other hand, in most of the larger joints of the body, deep tissue receptors are more important. It is interesting that joint afferents themselves may not be that important in sensing either limb position at rest or during movement. [9,25–27,36] Patients with total hip replacement and thus no innervation to their joints are still able to detect the direction of passive limb movement. By the same token, cutaneous receptors are not necessary. Anesthetizing the skin around the knee joint has no effect on estimation of knee joint angle. **The most important receptors are probably the muscle spindles.** When the angle of a joint is changing, some of the associated muscles become loosened, whereas others are stretched; this information can be used to monitor the movement of this joint. At the extremes of joint angulation joint afferents and stretch receptors in the ligaments and deep tissues surrounding the joints provide important additional information. The importance of specific proprioceptive inputs also seems to vary from one kind of motor task to another. Our overall proprioceptive sense requires input regarding both body movement and absolute body position. Although these two senses are interrelated, they are each derived from information arising from somewhat different combinations of somatic receptors.

Relatively little is known about the *conscious* component of our sense of limb position or joint movement. Although muscle has for many years been described as insensient, experiments suggest that inputs from both muscle spindles and tendon organs contribute to our conscious sense of limb position.[25,27] The contribution from joint receptors themselves is less sure. These receptors respond predominantly to extremes of rotation, with many of them not distinguishing in the process between extreme flexion and extension. Such characteristics do not seem very useful for sensing joint position. Their role is further obscured by the observation that the conscious position sense of patients with total hip joint replacement is nearly as good as normals with intact joint receptors. The contribution of cutaneous receptors remains equally ill defined.

Importance of Input from Other Sensory Systems

It is important to remember that our overall proprioceptive capability relies on sensory information in addition to that provided by the proprioceptive sensors described previously. **Essential contributions to the coordination of body movements and the maintenance of upright posture are made by both the vestibular and visual systems.**

The Vestibular System

The vestibular system revolves around a complex sensory apparatus containing specialized receptors, which is located in the inner ear on either side of the head.[40] Like the proprioceptors scattered throughout the body, these receptors are mechanoreceptors. In this case, they are stimulated by mechanical stresses generated by the force of gravity and movement of the head. Specifically, the vestibular apparatus includes the semicircular canals, which are stimulated by angular acceleration, and the utricles and saccules, which are stimulated by linear acceleration and by changes in the orientation of the head in relation to gravity. **Information from the vestibular apparatus, which senses the position and motion of only the head, is integrated with information from proprioceptors in the neck, as well**

as in other parts of the body. This information is conveyed directly into the vestibular and reticular nuclei of the brainstem and indirectly by way of the cerebellum (see Chapters 6 and 8). The whole apparatus functions to keep the body balanced, to coordinate head and body movements, and to enable the eyes to remain fixed on a point in space in spite of changes in the position of the head. Its normal operation is essential for the performance of most motor behaviors.

The Visual System

Vision provides the motor system with information about the horizon and about the location of objects and the body in space. Visual cues are important in balance, gait, and many skilled motor activities.[41] The importance of this information is well illustrated by the contribution of vision to equilibrium. After destruction of the vestibular apparatus, and even after loss of most proprioceptive information from the body, a person can still use the visual mechanisms for maintaining equilibrium. Even slight linear or rotational movement of the body shifts the visual images on the retina, and this information is relayed to the equilibrium centers. Many persons with complete destruction of the vestibular apparatus have almost normal equilibrium as long as their eyes are open and as long as they perform motions slowly. Although visual and proprioceptive input complement one another, each type of information may be better suited for different types of motor tasks. Visual input, for example, is much better suited for limb movements to targets in extrapersonal space, since these targets usually cannot be located with proprioceptive input. Proprioceptive input, on the other hand, is better adapted for finely controlled movements, such as handwriting.[41]

The control of movement and posture requires that the motor systems be provided with a continuous flow of information about both the context in which motor activity is occurring and the status of the motor system itself. The vestibular apparatus and vision convey information about our position with respect to gravity and to objects in our environment. Proprioceptors simultaneously provide information about the position of the body in space, the angles of the joints, and the length and tension of muscles.

Other Somatic Sensations

Pain

The receptors that respond selectively to damaging or potentially damaging stimuli are nociceptors, and the sensation that they arouse is pain.[2,8,9,26,37,42–47] Nociceptors are found in the skin, and the muscles, joints, and viscera. There are four basic types of nociceptors: (1) mechanical nociceptors, which are activated most readily by strong mechanical stimulation, especially by sharp objects; (2) heat and cold nociceptors, which respond when the receptive field is heated to greater than 45°C or cooled to less than about 18°C, respectively; (3) chemical nociceptors, which respond to specific chemicals in the tissues, such as bradykinin, histamine, acids, and proteolytic enzymes; and (4) polymodal nociceptors, which respond to many types of noxious stimuli. The main types of cutaneous nociceptors are mechanical nociceptors and polymodal nociceptors, which respond well to noxious mechanical, thermal, and chemical stimuli. Morphologically **all nociceptors are free nerve endings and are found in almost every tissue of the body.** It is not known whether nociceptors respond directly to the noxious stimuli or indirectly by means of one or more chemical intermediaries released from the traumatized tissue. In contrast to most other sensory receptors, pain receptors adapt very little or not at all. The intensity of the pain is proportional to the number of nerve impulses stimulated, at least for brief stimuli. However, central mechanisms may be involved in pain produced by prolonged stimuli, since the pain may increase despite a reduction in afferent discharge.

Even though all pain endings are free nerve endings, these endings use two separate pathways for transmitting pain signals into the central nervous system, both within the anterolateral system.[42-47] Fast-twitch pain fibers transmit mainly mechanical and thermal pain, whereas slow-twitch chronic pain fibers convey more dull, chronic pain. **Fast sharp pain** apprises the person very rapidly of a damaging influence and plays an important role in stimulating immediate, protective withdrawal from the stimulus. **Slow pain** tends to increase over time, giving rise to the suffering of chronic pain. The fast sharp type of pain can be localized much more exactly than slow chronic pain, which is consistent with its role in prompting specific protective movements. Patients often have great difficulty in localizing the source of some chronic types of pain.

Although not directly involved in the normal control of motor activity, painful stimuli can strongly influence motor activity. Fast sharp pain can forcefully stimulate reflexive and volitional withdrawal and avoidance behaviors, which may involve extensive activation of motor systems. Slow, enduring pain, does not trigger these types of activities but has strong arousal effects on all types of nervous activity. In addition, the overall reaction to pain includes autonomic reflexes, endocrine changes, and emotional responses.

Pain is perhaps the most common reason why people seek medical attention, and it is a component of many somatic and visceral disorders. It is beyond the scope of this discussion to consider the clinical implications of pain in any detail. Suffice it to say that pain often accompanies locomotor dysfunction, and its thorough clinical assessment can provide insight into both the neurogenic and myogenic causes of motor problems. Muscle spasm, for example, is a common cause of pain and is the basis of many clinical pain syndromes. Pain itself can cause involuntary muscle contractions, protective reactions ("guarding"), and abnormal motor patterns that interfere with normal movement.

Temperature[8-11,26,37,45]

There are two distinct thermal sensations: warmth and cold. When the skin is kept at 32°C to 34°C, no thermal sensation is noted. However, when the temperature of the skin is altered in either direction from this level, a sense of warmth or cold results. Thermal gradations are sensed by separate warmth and cold receptors. These receptors are located immediately under the skin at discrete but separate points having a stimulatory diameter of about 1 mm. In most areas of the body, there are many more cold receptors than warmth receptors; the numbers and proportions of these receptors vary in different areas of the body. Although free nerve endings probably function as warmth receptors and some as cold receptors, a distinct cold receptor has been histologically identified. Once the stimulus temperature exceeds about 45°C or drops below about 18°C, pain fibers begin to be stimulated. The thermal senses respond markedly to changes in temperature, as well as to thermal steady states. One way in which this is manifested is the extreme degree of heat or cold that one feels on first entering a tub of hot or cold water. Although not well understood, cold and warmth receptors are believed to be stimulated by changes in their metabolic rates induced by changes in the ambient temperature. Thermoreceptors are insensitive to mechanical stimulation, but they are stimulated by certain chemical agents evoking sensations of warmth or cold. Menthol, for example, produces a sensation of cold when applied topically.

In general, thermal signals are transmitted in parallel with pain signals. The primary neurons terminate in the same areas of the dorsal horns as do pain fibers. After a small amount of processing by one or more cord neurons, the signals enter long, ascending thermal fibers that cross to the opposite anterolateral sensory tract and terminate in the reticular areas of the brainstem and thalamus. A few thermal signals are relayed from the thalamus to the somatosensory cortex. Removal of the postcentral gyrus in humans reduces the ability to distinguish gradations of temperature.

RECOMMENDED READINGS

Barr, ML and Kiernan, JA: The Human Nervous System, ed 6. Chapter 19. General Sensory Systems. JB Lippincott, Philadelphia, 1993.

Berne, RM, and Levy, MN (eds): Physiology, ed 3. Chapters 7 and 8. Mosby-Year Book, St. Louis, 1993.

Brookhart, JM and Mountcastle, VB (eds): Handbook of Physiology, Section 1. The Nervous System, vol III. Sensory Processes. Parts 1 and 2. American Physiological Society, Bethesda, MD, 1984.

Carpenter, MB: Core Text of Neuroanatomy, ed 4. Williams & Wilkins, Baltimore, 1991.

Guyton, AC: Textbook of Medical Physiology, ed 8. Chapters 46–48. WB Saunders, Philadelphia, 1991.

Hall, JL: Anatomy of Pain. Chapter 3. In Tollison, CD (ed): Handbook of Chronic Pain Management, ed 2. Williams & Wilkins, Baltimore, 1994.

Kandel, ER, Schwartz, JH, and Jessell, TM (eds): Principles of Neural Science, ed 3. Chapters 23–27. Appleton & Lange, Norwalk, CT, 1991.

Martin, JH: Neuroanatomy: Text and Atlas. Chapter 5. The Somatic Sensory System. Appleton & Lange, Norwalk, CT, 1989.

Mountcastle, VB (ed): Medical Physiology, ed 14. Chapters 9 and 10. CV Mosby, St. Louis, 1980.

Patton, HD, et al (eds): Textbook of Physiology, ed 21. Chapters 13–16, WB Saunders, Philadelphia, 1989.

Rothwell, JC: Control of Human Voluntary Movement. Chapter 4. Proprioceptors in Muscle, Joint, and Skin. Aspen Publishers, Rockville, MD, 1987.

Stern, EB: The Somatosensory Systems. Chapter 3. In Cohen, H (ed): Neuroscience for Rehabilitation. JB Lippincott, Philadelphia, 1993.

Willis, WD, Jr and Coggeshall, RE: Sensory Mechanisms of the Spinal Cord, ed 2. Plenum Press, New York, 1991.

Yaksh, TL (ed): Spinal Afferent Processing. Plenum Press, New York, 1986.

Zimmermann, M: Neurophysiology of Sensory Systems. Chapter 2. In Schmidt, RF (ed): Fundamentals of Sensory Physiology. Springer-Verlag, New York, 1978.

REFERENCES

1. Guyton, AC: Textbook of Medical Physiology, ed 8. Chapter 46. Sensory Receptors: Neuronal Circuits for Processing Information. WB Saunders, Philadelphia, 1991.

2. Brown, AC: Introduction to Sensory Mechanisms. Chapter 13. In Patton, HD, et al (eds): Textbook of Physiology, ed 21. WB Saunders, Philadelphia, 1989.

3. Martin, JH and Jessell, TM: Modality Coding in the Somatic Sensory System. Chapter 24. In Kandel, ER, Schwartz, JH, and Jessell, TM (eds): Principles of Neural Science, ed 3. Appleton & Lange, Norwalk, CT, 1991.

4. Willis, WD, Jr: The Peripheral Nervous System. Chapter 7. In Berne, RM and Levy, MN (eds): Physiology, ed 3. Mosby-Year Book, St. Louis, 1993.

5. Martin, JH: Coding and Processing of Sensory Information. Chapter 23. In Kandel, ER, Schwartz, JH, and Jessell, TM (eds): Principles of Neural Science, ed 3. Appleton & Lange, Norwalk, CT, 1991.

6. Nicholls, JG, Martin, AR, and Wallace, BG: From Neuron to Brain. Chapter 14. Transduction and Processing of Sensory Signals. Sinauer Associates, Sunderland, MA, 1992.

7. Detwiler, PB: Sensory Transduction. Chapter 5. In Patton, HD, et al (eds): Textbook of Physiology, ed 21. WB Saunders, Philadelphia, 1989.

8. Willis, WD, Jr and Coggeshall, RE: Sensory Mechanisms of the Spinal Cord, ed 2. Chapter 2. Peripheral Nerves and Sensory Receptors. Plenum Press, New York, 1991.

9. Stern, EB: The Somatosensory Systems. Chapter 3. In Cohen, H (ed): Neuroscience for Rehabilitation. JB Lippincott, Philadelphia, 1993.

10. Willis, WD, Jr: The Somatosensory System. Chapter 8. In Berne, RM and Levy, MN (eds): Physiology, ed 3. Mosby-Year Book, St. Louis, 1993.

11. Brown, AC: Somatic Sensation: Peripheral Aspects. Chapter 14. In Patton, HD, et al (eds): Textbook of Physiology, ed 21. WB Saunders, Philadelphia, 1989.

12. Guyton, AC: Textbook of Medical Physiology, ed 8. Chapter 47. Somatic Sensations: I. General Organization: The Tactile and Position Senses. WB Saunders, Philadelphia, 1991.

13. Barr, ML and Kiernan, JA: The Human Nervous System: An Anatomical Viewpoint, ed 6. Chapter 19. General Sensory Systems. JB Lippincott, Philadelphia, 1993.

14. Phillips, JO and Fuchs, AF: Somatic Sensation: Central Processing. Chapter 15. In Patton, HD, et al (eds): Textbook of Physiology, ed 21. WB Saunders, Philadelphia, 1989.

15. Martin, JH and Jessell, TM: Anatomy of the Somatic Sensory System. Chapter 25. In Kandel, ER, Schwartz, JH, and Jessell, TM (eds): Principles of Neural Science, ed 3. Appleton & Lange, Norwalk, CT, 1991.

16. Willis, WD, Jr and Coggeshall, RE: Sensory Mechanisms of the Spinal Cord, ed 2. Chapter 6. Ascending Sensory Pathways in the Cord White Matter. Plenum Press, New York, 1991.

17. Willis, WD, Jr and Coggeshall, RE: Sensory Mechanisms of the Spinal Cord, ed 2. Chapter 7. Sensory Pathways in the Dorsal Funiculus. Plenum Press, New York, 1991.

18. Davidoff, RA: The Dorsal Columns. Neurology 39:1377, 1989.

19. Willis, WD, Jr and Coggeshall, RE: Sensory Mechanisms of the Spinal Cord, ed 2. Chapter 9. Sensory Pathways in the Ventral Quadrant. Plenum Press, New York, 1991.

20. Dodd, J and Kelly, JP: Trigeminal System. Chapter 45. In Kandel, ER, Schwartz, JH, and Jessell, TM (eds): Principles of Neural Science, ed 3. Appleton & Lange, Norwalk, CT, 1991.

21. Kandel, ER and Jessell, TM: Touch. Chapter 26. In Kandel, ER, Schwartz, JH, and Jessell, TM (eds): Principles of Neural Science, ed 3. Appleton & Lange, Norwalk, CT, 1991.

22. Kandel, ER: Cellular Mechanisms of Learning and the Biological Basis of Individuality. Chapter 65. In Kandel, ER, Schwartz, JH, and Jessell, TM (eds): Principles of Neural Science, ed 3. Appleton & Lange, Norwalk, CT, 1991.

23. Merzenich, MM, et al: Cortical Representational Plasticity. In Rakic, P and Singer, W (eds): Neurobiology of Neocortex. John Wiley & Sons, New York, 1988.

24. Kupfermann, I: Localization of Higher Cognitive and Affective Functions: The Association Cortices. Chapter 53. In Kandel, ER, Schwartz, JH, and Jessell, TM (eds): Principles of Neural Science, ed 3. Appleton & Lange, Norwalk, CT, 1991.

25. Matthews, PBC: Proprioceptors and Their Contribution to Somatosensory Mapping: Complex Messages Require Complex Processing. Can J Physiol Pharmacol 66:430, 1988.

26. Willis, WD, Jr and Coggeshall, RE: Sensory Mechanisms of the Spinal Cord. Chapter 10. The Sensory Channels, ed 2. Plenum Press, New York, 1991.

27. Rothwell, JC: Control of Human Voluntary Movement. Chapter 4. Proprioceptors in Muscle. Aspen Publishers, Rockville, MD, 1987.

28. Burke, D and Gandevia, SC: Peripheral Motor System. Chapter 6. In Paxinos, G (ed): The Human Nervous System. Academic Press, San Diego, 1990.

29. Willis, WD, Jr: Spinal Organization of Motor Function. Chapter 12. In Berne, RM and Levy, MN (eds): Physiology, ed 3. Mosby-Year Book, St. Louis, 1993.

30. Gordon, J and Ghez, C: Muscle Receptors and the Spinal Reflexes: The Stretch Reflex. Chapter 37. In Kandel, ER, Schwartz, JH, and Jessell, TM (eds): Principles of Neural Science, ed 3. Appleton & Lange, Norwalk, CT, 1991.

31. Poppele, RE: The Muscle Spindle. Chapter 6. In Dyck, PJ and Thomas, PK (eds): Peripheral Neuropathy, ed 3. WB Saunders, Philadelphia, 1993.

32. Barker, D and Banks, RW: The Muscle Spindle. Chapter 11. In Engel, AG and Franzini-Armstrong, C (eds): Myology, ed 2. McGraw-Hill, New York, 1994.

33. Hunt, CC: Mammalian Muscle Spindle: Peripheral Mechanisms. Physiol Rev 70:643, 1990.

34. Proske, V: The Golgi Tendon Organ. Chapter 7. In Dyck, PJ and Thomas, PK (eds): Peripheral Neuropathy, ed 3. WB Saunders, Philadelphia, 1993.

35. Jami, L: Golgi Tendon Organs in Mammalian Skeletal Muscle: Functional Properties and Central Actions. Physiol Rev 72(3):623, 1992.

36. Edin, BB: Finger Joint Movement Sensitivity of Non-Cutaneous Mechanoreceptor Afferents in the Human Radial Nerve. Exp Brain Res 82:417, 1990.

37. Light, AR and Perl, ER: Peripheral Sensory Systems. Chapter 8. In Dyck, PJ and Thomas, PK (eds): Peripheral Neuropathy, ed 3. WB Saunders, Philadelphia, 1993.

38. Valbo, AB and Johansson, RS: Properties of Cutaneous Mechanoreceptors in the Human Hand Related to Touch Sensation. Hum Neurobiol 3:3, 1984.

39. Do, MC, Bussel, B, and Breniere, Y: Influence of Plantar Cutaneous Afferents on Early Compensatory Reactions to Forward Fall. Exp Brain Res 79:319, 1990.

40. Kelly, JP: The Sense of Balance. Chapter 33. In Kandel, ER, Schwartz, JH, and Jessell, TM (eds): Principles of Neural Science, ed 3. Appleton & Lange, Norwalk, CT, 1991.

41. Cordo, PJ and Flanders, M: Sensory Control of Target Acquisition. Trends Neurosci 12:110, 1989.

42. Hall, JL: Anatomy of Pain. Chapter 3. In Tollison, CD (ed): Handbook of Chronic Pain Management, ed 2. Williams & Wilkins, Baltimore, 1994.

43. Balter, K: A Review of Pain Anatomy and Physiology. Pain Dig 2:306, 1992.

44. Melzack, R: Pain: Past, Present, and Future. Can J Exp Psychol 47(4):615, 1993.

45. Guyton, AC: Textbook of Medical Physiology, ed 8. Chapter 48. Somatic Sensations: II. Pain, Headache, and Thermal Sensations. WB Saunders, Philadelphia, 1991.

46. Jessell, JM and Kelly, DD: Pain and Analgesia. Chapter 27. In Kandel, ER, Schwartz, JH, and Jessell, TM (eds): Principles of Neural Science, ed 3. Appleton & Lange, Norwalk, CT, 1991.

47. Henry, JL: Concepts of Pain Sensation and its Modulation. J Rheumatol 16 (suppl 19):104, 1989.

SECTION

II

CONTROL OF MOTOR ACTIVITY

Systems That Regulate and Coordinate Movement

Overview

The human motor repertoire is remarkably adaptable and diverse. Human motor responses vary from the simplest reflexive reactions to noxious stimuli to the complex movements of volition. Whatever the form of motor behavior, it is ultimately determined by the pattern of excitatory impulses generated in the central nervous system and transmitted via motor neurons to the pertinent muscle groups in the periphery. In Section I of this text, the fundamental properties of the cells and tissues of the motor effector unit were described, with an emphasis on the nature of their response to excitation. The purpose of the section to follow is to describe the control of this excitation. This is **motor control**. This discipline pursues an understanding of how motor activities are planned, initiated, and carried efficiently and accurately to completion. Considerable interest is also focused on the adaptability of the motor system, both in the context of normal goal-directed behavior and in the context of motor rehabilitation.

In Chapters 6 through 9, an emphasis is placed on the anatomy of the major structures of the motor system, the principal pathways that interconnect them, and what is known of their physiologic properties. An understanding of overall motor function, however, requires more than a familiarity with the function of the individual anatomic components of the nervous system. In this regard, Chapters 10 and 11 take a broader look at the integrated output of the motor system.

In Chapter 10, various theories of motor control are discussed. Classic neuroanatomic and neurophysiologic approaches have reinforced the view that motor activity is largely under hierarchial control. According to this model, higher central nervous system centers plan and direct movement, delegating the requisite motor programs to lower centers for their execution. As it has become evident, however, that traditional hierarchial models cannot account for much of what is known about motor behavior, newer theories have been developed. Systems models, for example, suggest that instead of being directed by a single command center, movements emerge as a result of interactions among many systems, with each contributing to different aspects of control. Action or dynamical models shift emphasis further away from anatomic and physiologic explanations to more behavioral perspectives. Accordingly, movements are viewed as strategies that emerge in varying contexts, to accomplish specific tasks. Motor behaviors are considered highly adaptable, with specific outcomes attainable by a number of different movement patterns. Although many traditional assumptions remain useful in some aspects of neurologic rehabilitation, the assumptions inherent in newer models of motor control are leading therapists to novel, more effective therapeutic approaches.

One of the primary goals of rehabilitation is to assist the patient to learn or relearn the motor skills required to obtain optimal function. For example, patients who have experienced a stroke with resultant paralysis may need to relearn the motor skills required to achieve safe independent ambulation. Therefore, it is important for rehabilitation professionals to understand not only the principles involved in motor control but also the factors that influence a person's ability to acquire motor skills. These factors include practice variables such as frequency of feedback and blocked versus random practice schedules. In Chapter 11, the critical terms associated with motor learning, the variables that influence motor learning, and information regarding the application of motor learning principles to clinical situations are discussed.

CHAPTER 5

■

Motor Control at the Spinal Cord Level

Christopher M. Fredericks, PhD

- ■ *Review of Spinal Cord Anatomy and Physiology*
- ■ *Information Processing: General Principles*
- ■ *Neuronal Interconnections and the Integration of Information*
- ■ *Spinal Contributions to Motor Control*
- ■ *Influences Descending from Supraspinal Areas*
- ■ *Integration of the Spinal Cord into Overall Motor Control*

*T*he spinal cord is more than just a conduit that transmits impulses from one part of the central nervous system to another. In reality, the spinal cord is a complex neuronal system capable of extensive processing of both sensory and motor information. The cord contains dozens of different types of cells, neuronal circuits, and neurochemicals and has a tremendous inherent capacity for directing, sorting, collating, and integrating information. On its own, the spinal cord can generate and coordinate a variety of simple and complex motor behaviors. Without the special capabilities of the cord, even the most powerful control systems of the brain would be unable to cause any purposeful muscle activity.

The purpose of this chapter is to discuss the basic contributions that the spinal cord makes to overall motor control. An emphasis is placed on the underlying neuroanatomic substrates and physiologic mechanisms that make these contributions possible. A more detailed exploration of the location of specific sensory and motor tracts within the cord is undertaken in Chapter 17 in the context of explaining the functional deficits that accompany spinal cord disease or injury.

Review of Spinal Cord Anatomy and Physiology[1-3]

The spinal cord is an elongated cylindrical mass of nervous tissue that occupies the spinal canal of the vertebral column and extends from the foramen magnum to the lower border of the first lumbar vertebra (Fig. 5–1). The spinal cord is noticeably enlarged in the cervical and lumbar regions, where the increased numbers of neurons responsible for the

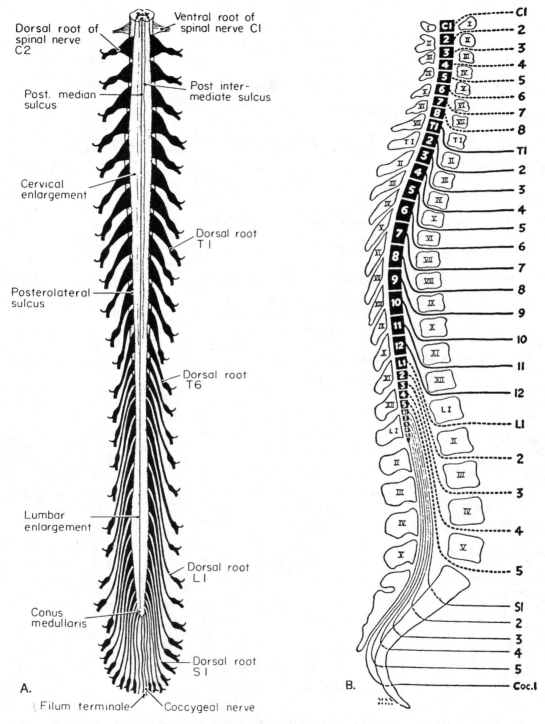

Figure 5–1. *Gross Anatomy of the Spinal Cord and Vertebral Column.* (*A*) Posterior view of the spinal cord showing attached dorsal roots and spinal ganglia. (*B*) Position of the spinal cord segments with reference to the bodies and spinous processes of the vertebrae. (Adapted from Carpenter, MB and Sutin, J: Human Neuroanatomy, ed 8. Copyright © Williams & Wilkins, Baltimore, 1983, pp 233, 235, with permission.)

control of the upper and lower extremities (respectively) are congregated. Examination of a transverse section of the cord reveals a deep anterior (ventral) median fissure and a shallower posterior (dorsal) median sulcus, which divide the cord into symmetric right and left halves joined together centrally. **Nerve fibers enter and exit along the length of the cord via spinal nerve roots** (Fig. 5–2). The dorsal nerve roots are attached to the spinal cord along a shallow longitudinal groove, the posterolateral sulcus, whereas the ventral nerve roots exit by way of the anterolateral sulcus. **The dorsal and ventral roots join laterally to form the spinal nerves.** Thirty-one pairs of spinal nerves are thus formed and divide the cord into 8 cervical, 12 thoracic, 5 lumbar, 5 sacral, and 1 coccygeal segment.

The names of the spinal nerves correspond to the names of the segment from which they arise. Within the cord itself, however, there are no distinct boundaries between these segments. Each of the first cervical nerves leaves the vertebral canal *above* the corresponding vertebra.[3] Because there are only seven cervical vertebrae, the eighth cervical nerve leaves between the seventh cervical and first thoracic vertebrae, whereas each of the subsequent nerves leaves *below* the corresponding vertebra (See Fig. 5–1).

Each spinal segment, except the first and last, has both a dorsal and ventral root emerging from each side of the cord. In the dorsal root of a typical spinal nerve, a dorsal root ganglion containing the cell bodies of the root's neurons lies close to the junction with the ventral root. Most dorsal root ganglia are located immediately outside the points where the nerve roots pass through the dura mater. The cell bodies of the nerve fibers of the ventral root lie within the cord. The ventral roots are composed primarily of myelinated fibers, including the large-diameter alpha motor neurons to skeletal muscle fibers, the smaller gamma motor neurons to the intrafusal fibers of the muscle spindles, and the preganglionic fibers of autonomic nerves to the viscera. The dorsal roots contain both myelinated and unmyelinated afferent (sensory) fibers arising in somatic (skin, joint, and muscle) and visceral structures. **A spinal nerve is thus composed of a mixture of motor, sensory, and autonomic fibers** united in a single structure. Each spinal nerve exits the spinal canal through a bony channel between adjacent vertebrae called the **intervertebral foramen** (see Fig. 15–2). Because the nerve is surrounded by rigid bony tissue, it is particularly vulnerable at this site to injury (e.g., by compression due to a tumor or herniated disk).[4]

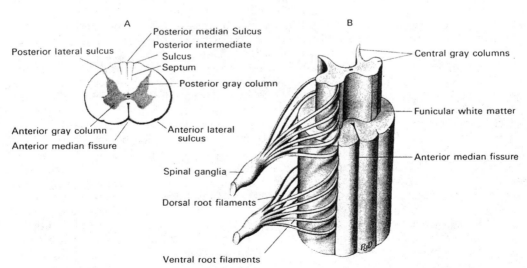

Figure 5–2. Spinal Cord. (A) Diagram showing the internal arrangement of the gray and white matter. (B) External and internal topography of cervical spinal cord. Dorsal and ventral root filaments coalesce to form spinal nerves. (From Carpenter, MB and Sutin, J: Human Neuroanatomy, ed 8. Copyright © Williams & Wilkins, Baltimore, 1983, p 238, with permission.)

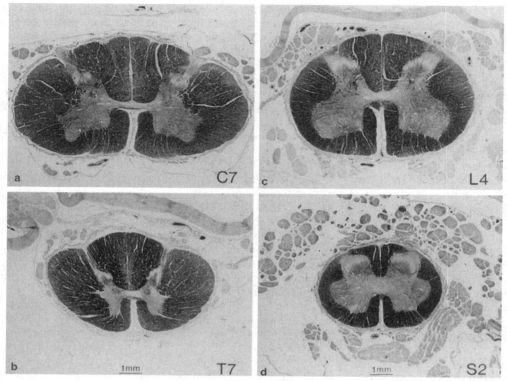

Figure 5–3. *Configuration of the Spinal White and Gray Matter at Levels C7, T7, L4, and S2, Respectively.* Note the changing shape and proportions of white and gray matter. (From Schoenen and Faull,[7] 1990, p 48, with permission.)

The tissue of the spinal cord is heterogeneous and is composed of many different types of cells in a very specific arrangement. **If we look at a cross section of the cord** (Fig. 5–3), **two basic types of tissue are readily apparent:** an H-shaped central region of gray matter and an area of white matter surrounding it (see Fig. 5–2).

The gray matter is a longitudinally continuous mass of nerve cell bodies, dendrites, myelinated and unmyelinated axons, and glial cells. Gray matter is considered to be made up of three horns. The anterior (ventral) horn contains the cell bodies of the large motor neurons that innervate skeletal muscle. The posterior (dorsal) horn consists mainly of interneurons and tract cells that transmit various types of somatic and visceral sensory information. Intermediate gray matter contains the cell bodies of preganglionic sympathetic fibers, as well as various tract cells and interneurons synapsing on both sensory and motor fibers. In addition, the intermediate gray matter includes at some levels (especially the lower thoracic) a distinct region called **Clark's nucleus** (column), which seems to play an important role in relaying sensory information to the cerebellum and thalamus. Because of its role in sensory processing, Clark's nucleus is sometimes considered part of the dorsal horn.

Although a detailed discussion of the cytoarchitecture of gray matter is beyond the scope of this chapter,[5–7] it is notable that gray matter is divided into clusters of nerve cell bodies that extend along the spinal cord for various distances as cell columns. Furthermore, gray matter may be subdivided histologically into distinct layers of like neurons called **laminae**[5] (see Chapter 17). Different functions predominate in each lamina, reflecting the prominence of specific types of nerve fibers.[5–7] Laminae I and II, for example, contain terminations of primarily pain and temperature afferents, whereas lamina IX contains many motor neurons.

Table 5–1. *Major Tracts of the Spinal Cord White Matter*

Descending Tracts	
Corticospinal	Arise in either hemisphere of the cerebral cortex; fibers descend in the lateral and ventral columns; terminate mainly on alpha motor neurons and interneurons of the ventral gray horn; also on neurons of the dorsal gray column.
Reticulospinal	Arise in the brainstem reticular formation; fibers descend in the ventral and lateral columns; terminate mainly on gamma motor neurons and interneurons of the ventral gray horn; also on neurons of the dorsal gray column.
Vestibulospinal	Arise in the lateral vestibular nucleus; fibers descend in the ventrolateral columns; terminate on both alpha and gamma motor neurons of the ventral gray horn.
Rubrospinal	Arise in the red nucleus; fibers descend in the lateral column; terminate on motor neurons and interneurons of the ventral gray horn.
Tectospinal	Arise in the superior colliculus; fibers descend in the cervical ventral column; terminate on interneurons of the ventral gray horn.
Ascending Tracts	
Dorsal column (medial lemniscal)	Arise in mechanoreceptors of skin, joints, and tendons; fibers ascend in dorsal column; terminate in medullary nuclei.
Spinothalamic (anterolateral or ventrolateral)	Arise in pain and thermoreceptors of skin (lateral), as well as touch and pressure receptors (ventral); synapse in the dorsal gray horn, then ascend in the ventral portion of the lateral column; terminate in the thalamus; collateral to reticular formation.
Dorsal and ventral spinocerebellar	Arise in mechanoreceptors of skin, muscle, deep tendons, and joints; synapse in the dorsal gray horn, then ascend in the lateral column; terminate in the cerebellum.

Three general types of neurons predominate in the gray matter. Efferent (motor) fibers arise in the anterior and lateral horns and send axonal projections out of the cord through the ventral roots to terminate on extrafusal and intrafusal muscle fibers or on the cell bodies of postganglionic autonomic nerve fibers. Afferent (sensory) fibers—their cell bodies in the dorsal root ganglia—enter the cord and send branches into specific areas of both the white and gray matter. The most abundant cells are the interneurons, which are distributed throughout the gray matter but do not project beyond it. Although many interneurons terminate only within the segment in which they originate, others may project along the cord in either direction before terminating. Descending pathways from the brain (e.g., corticospinal and reticulospinal tracts) also send projections that terminate in localized areas of the gray matter.

Gray matter is surrounded by white matter, which is organized into analogous posterior, lateral, and anterior funiculi (also called *columns*). The posterior funiculus is the largest column and is composed almost exclusively of long ascending and short descending fibers that arise from cells in the spinal ganglia.[1] Tracts composing the lateral and anterior funiculi are both ascending and descending. Ascending tracts in these funiculi arise from cells within the spinal gray matter; long descending tracts arise from nuclei in the brainstem and the cerebral cortex. The white matter is composed of both myelinated and unmyelinated fibers, with the abundance of myelin giving it its white appearance. Fast-conducting, myelinated fibers having similar courses and connections travel up and down the cord in bundles known as tracts or fasciculi.[8,9] The location and function of the major ascending and descending tracts of the white matter are summarized in Table 5–1 and will be considered in more detail in subsequent discussions of supraspinal motor control (see Chapter 17).

Nerve fibers within the white matter are of three general types.[3] (1) Long ascending fibers convey sensory information to the thalamus, cerebellum, and various brainstem nuclei (see Chapter 4). (2) Long descending fibers project from the cerebral cortex and various brainstem nuclei to both the motor neurons and the interneurons of the spinal gray matter. (3) Shorter propriospinal fibers interconnect various spinal cord levels. The propriospinal fibers are largely concentrated in a thin layer surrounding the gray matter called the **propriospinal tract** or **fasciculus proprius**. As we shall see, the lateral and ventral white columns contain tracts that are not as well delineated as those of the dorsal columns.

The relative amounts of gray and white matter and their configuration vary appreciably among the different levels of the spinal cord (see Fig. 5–3). Cervical spinal segments contain the greatest number of fibers in the white matter, whereas the lumbosacral segments contain the largest amount of gray matter, both in relation to the size of the cord segments and to the amount of white matter.[1]

Information Processing: General Principles

The spinal cord is composed of countless neurons of different shapes and sizes. One of the fundamental properties of these neurons is their ability to rapidly conduct impulses along the length of their axons. In doing so, they provide an efficient mechanism for transmitting information from one point of the nervous system to another. The spinal cord, however, is more than just a conduit that carries impulses from the periphery of the body to the brain and back again or from sensory fibers to local motor neurons. In reality, **the spinal cord is a complex neuronal system capable of extensive processing of both sensory and motor information**. The capacity of the spinal cord for information processing resides in its synapses, in the physical arrangement of the diverse cells of which it is made up, and in the functional circuitry arising from these interconnections.

Synapses[10–12]

The overall activity of the spinal cord, whether it is the transmission of impulses along the neural axis or the programming of local patterns of movement, depends on the same basic neuronal interactions that occur throughout the nervous system. The excitable cells of the spinal cord, regardless of their specific morphology, have the same basic properties of all excitable cells, as described in Chapter 1.

Throughout the spinal cord, neurons communicate with one another at synapses. Synaptic transmission within the cord is chemical, with each presynaptic neuron influencing each postsynaptic cell via the release of a neurotransmitter. Each neurotransmitter interacts with specialized reactive sites (receptors) on the postsynaptic membrane to induce characteristic conformational changes in that membrane, which result in changes in ion permeabilities and conductances, and hence in the membrane potential. Excitatory neurotransmitters induce graded depolarizations of the postsynaptic membrane (excitatory postsynaptic potentials [EPSPs]), which may ultimately trigger the firing of an action potential (Fig. 5–4). Inhibitory neurotransmitters, on the other hand, induce graded *hyper*polarizations of the postsynaptic membrane (inhibitory postsynaptic potentials [IPSPs]), which, by shifting the membrane potential away from the action potential threshold, make impulse generation less likely.

Although not fully understood, **spinal synaptic transmission is thought to be mediated by a variety of neurotransmitters.** Substances that have been implicated in central nervous system transmission in general, and in spinal function in particular, include various amino acids, biogenic amines (e.g., catecholamines, histamine, and serotonin), neuropeptides (e.g., endorphins and substance P), prostaglandins, and nucleotides. Perhaps the best understood among these are the neurally active amino acids. One of the primary neurotransmitters mediating spinal excitatory transmission (EPSPs) is glutamate.[11,12] IPSPs, on the other hand, are mediated primarily by the inhibitory neurotransmitters, glycine and γ-aminobutyric acid (GABA).

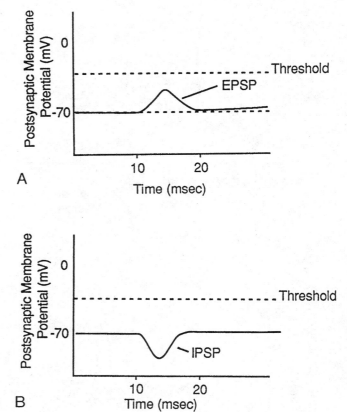

Figure 5–4. *Postsynaptic Membrane Potentials.* (A) An excitatory postsynaptic potential (EPSP) involves depolarization *toward* the excitation threshold (B). An inhibitory postsynaptic potential (IPSP) involves hyperpolarization *away* from the excitation threshold.

Most spinal cord neurons receive inputs from many presynaptic cells. Moreover, these presynaptic neurons may themselves be influenced by other neurons impinging on their axon terminals (e.g., presynaptic inhibition). **The overall electrical status of the postsynaptic cell (i.e., the likelihood of action potential firing) is the net consequence of the influences exerted by all of these participating cells.** In other words, the excitatory and inhibitory influences impinging on each postsynaptic cell membrane are "summated" or integrated to yield a net inclination or disinclination to fire (Fig. 5–5). This summation may occur temporally, spatially, or both ways. The firing pattern of each spinal motor neuron, for example, is the result of thousands of complementary and conflicting influences converging on each anterior horn cell body.

Synapses provide a convenient site for the control of information transmission. They may serve to route information by determining the direction that nervous signals spread in the cord, often channeling signals in many different directions, rather than simply in one direction. Signals from other areas in the nervous system can control synaptic activity, sometimes facilitating transmission and at other times inhibiting transmission through a specific synapse. Synapses may also perform a selective action, often blocking weak signals, while allowing the stronger signals to pass. Alternately, they may select and amplify certain weaker signals.

Neuronal Circuitry[13-16]

The extensive interconnections among the diverse cells of the spinal cord create a neuronal circuitry, which, although extremely complex, functions according to certain basic organizational principles. In general, **neurons within the spinal cord,** as well as throughout

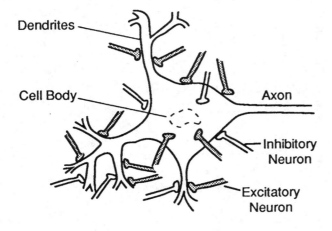

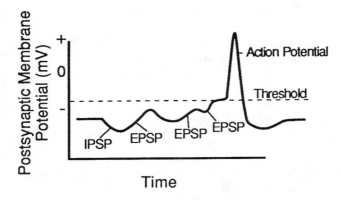

Figure 5–5. Summating Synaptic Inputs. Complementary and conflicting influences (i.e., EPSPs, IPSPs) are summated or "integrated" by the neuron cell body to yield a net increase or decrease in the likelihood of generating an action potential.

the rest of the central nervous system, **are organized into neuronal pools.** Some of these functional pools contain only a few neurons, whereas others contain vast numbers of cells. **Although each pool has its own particular organization that allows it to process information in a particular way, they all embody certain basic types of neuronal organization.**

By definition, any given pool of neurons has a number of input neurons connected to a number of output neurons. Typically, each input fiber subdivides many times, giving rise to a large number of terminal filaments that spread over a large area of the pool to synapse with the dendrites or cell bodies of numerous neurons within the pool. The neuronal area stimulated by each incoming neuron is called its **stimulatory field.** The terminal filaments of each input fiber are concentrated in the center of this field, with progressively fewer terminals located toward the periphery of the field (Fig. 5–6). In this way, output fibers in the central portion of the field receive more terminal filaments and are thus more likely to be sufficiently excited by the incoming fibers to fire. The area encompassed by these fibers is termed the **discharge** or **excited zone.** Away from this central zone, neurons are facilitated but not excited. This is defined as the facilitated, subthreshold, or subliminal zone (or fringe). A discharge zone and a facilitated zone can thus be defined for the group of neurons contacted by any given input fiber.

Interactions between these zones and the analogous zones of other interconnected sets of neurons provide a mechanism by which incoming signals may be amplified or suppressed.

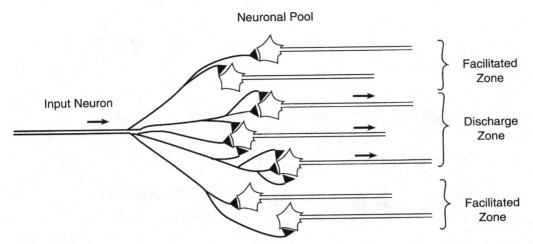

Figure 5–6. *A Neuronal Pool.* Input neuron terminals are concentrated in the center of the neuronal pool creating a region more likely to be excited (the discharge zone). Away from this central zone, neurons are facilitated but not excited (the facilitated zone).

Suppose, for example, that a second input fiber branches and projects onto a number of neurons in the same neuronal pool as the first input fiber. Although the population of neurons contacted by the second neuron may not be identical with that contacted by the first, some of these cells are likely to be located in the subliminal fringe and some in the discharge zone of the original neuron. Where overlap occurs in their subliminal fringes, an additive effect will occur through spatial summation. The effect of stimulating the two fibers simultaneously will then be greater than the sum of the effects of stimulating each individually, a form of signal amplification called **facilitation**. In contrast, within the overlap of the discharge zones, the effect of stimulating the fibers simultaneously may be less than the sum of the effects of stimulating them individually, a phenomenon called **occlusion**. In a pool such as this, an additional dimension is added to the signal processing by the possibility that some of the incoming fibers may be inhibitory rather than excitatory neurons. Each of these then creates its own inhibitory zone, the center of which contains the most inhibitory terminals and thus exerts the strongest inhibitory effect. Sometimes an input to a neuron pool (e.g., of motor neurons) can produce both excitatory and inhibitory outputs. An input fiber might, for example, directly excite an excitatory output pathway while concurrently stimulating an inhibitory interneuron, which would then inhibit a second output pathway from the pool. A use of this type of arrangement is in controlling antagonistic pairs of muscle, as might occur in the coordination of flexors and extensors in limb movement. This phenomenon is termed **reciprocal innervation** or **inhibition**.

In any neuronal pool, two basic types of signal transmission may occur—signal divergence and signal convergence. **Divergence** refers to the process by which a single neuron, by branching into multiple terminal filaments, may synapse on (and thus influence) multiple target neurons (Fig. 5–7). Divergence often results in the amplification of a signal whereby a single input can influence large numbers of neurons. A command signal in a single descending corticospinal fiber, for instance, may excite literally thousands of spinal cord motor neurons. Divergence also provides a means of directing a signal to multiple destinations, thereby promoting its dispersion to many different areas. Many afferent fibers, upon entering the cord, branch out and synapse with many different types of neurons, including interneurons, motor neurons, and ascending second-order fibers. A single afferent fiber (Ia) from a muscle spindle may give rise to 500 or more branches within the spinal cord.

Divergent Circuits

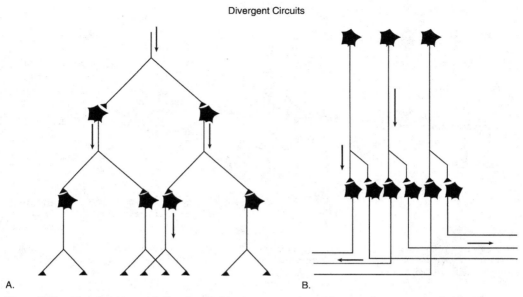

A.   B.

Figure 5–7. *Divergent Neuronal Circuits.* (A) Divergence causes amplification of an input signal. (B) Divergence causes direction of input signals to multiple areas. (Adapted from Guyton, AC: Basic Neuroscience. Anatomy and Physiology, ed 2. WB Saunders, Philadelphia, 1991, p 109.)

Convergence refers to the coming together of axon terminals from many neurons onto a single neuron (Fig. 5–8). In this way, multiple inputs, none of which alone is capable of discharging a neuron, may summate to reach the threshold of excitation for a given neuron. The firing rate of spinal motor neurons, for example, is the result of thousands of converging (summating) signals. The converging inputs may arise from a single type of source (e.g., many group Ia sensory fibers converging on a single motor neuron) or more often may arise from many different sources (e.g., convergence of afferent fibers, interneurons, and descending pathways on a single motor neuron).

Referred pain is an interesting example of one clinical consequence of the convergence of different types of input. In referred pain, nociceptive stimulation of one site is perceived as arising in another. This is thought to be due to the convergence of disparate pain fibers on the same ascending pathways in the spinal cord.

Convergent Circuits

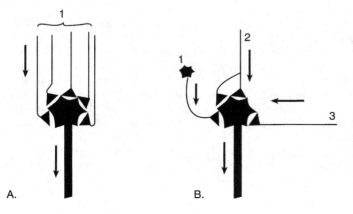

A.   B.

Figure 5–8. *Convergent Neuronal Circuits.* Multiple inputs may converge on an output neuron having arisen from (A) a single neuron or (B) multiple neurons.

Feedback Circuits

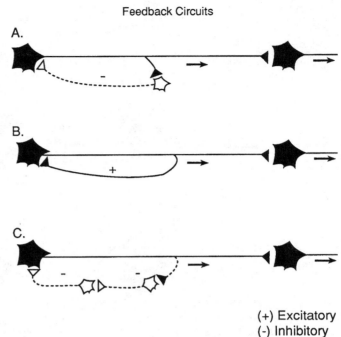

Figure 5–9. *Feedback Neuronal Circuits.* Neurons may feed back upon themselves in such a way that their (*A*) output is diminished (negative feedback) or (*B,C*) their output is enhanced (positive feedback).

(+) Excitatory
(-) Inhibitory

Although the circuits discussed so far have involved signals constantly moving forward along a series of neurons, in many instances signals may also be directed back on a neuronal chain to further modify signal transmission. These are termed **feedback circuits** (Fig. 5–9). One example of such feedback is that exerted by the spinal cord Renshaw cell. The Renshaw cell is an interneuron found in the ventral horn of the spinal cord, which is inhibitory to motor neurons. Motor neurons often give rise to collateral branches that terminate on Renshaw cells. These cells in turn project back onto the motor neurons that innervate them. This creates a **negative feedback circuit** that serves to limit the discharge of the motor neurons. These types of circuits can also create positive feedback, which serves to facilitate neuronal discharge. One type of circuit that is dependent on this type of feedback is the **reverberating or oscillating circuit** (Fig. 5–10). Here, the output of a neuronal circuit feeds

Reverberating Circuit

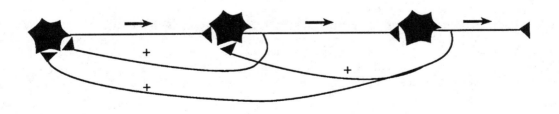

(+) Excitatory

Figure 5–10. *Reverberating Neuronal Circuit.* The output of this circuit feeds back upon itself to re-excite the circuit. This arrangement permits a prolonged signal to be generated with a minimal amount of new input. If both excitatory and inhibitory neurons are involved, a prolonged, oscillating output signal may be automatically generated.

Gating Circuits

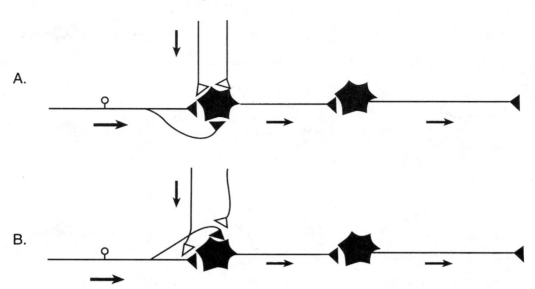

Figure 5–11. *Gating Neuronal Circuits.* The flow of information through these circuits is modulated (i.e., gated) by either (A) postsynaptic or (B) presynaptic influences. These influences are often inhibitory, resulting in a suppression of information (e.g., sensory) transmittal.

back on itself to re-excite the circuit. Consequently, once stimulated, the circuit tends to discharge repetitively for a long period of time. Such circuitry permits a prolonged signal to be generated with a minimal amount of new input. If both excitatory and inhibitory neurons are incorporated into the circuit, a protracted, oscillating signal may be automatically generated. These kinds of circuits are particularly useful in the activation of motor neurons during rhythmic muscular activities such as locomotion. A reverberating circuit can greatly simplify the work of higher centers, since all that is required to command fairly complex motor behavior is a command sequence that initiates the oscillation of that circuit.

Groups of neurons can also act to **gate information**, giving priority to certain signals, while suppressing others (Fig. 5–11). In this way, certain signals can be selected and given preeminence. Traffic in nociceptive fibers in the dorsal horn, for example, may be overridden by activity in other sensory pathways. Activity in large somatosensory afferent fibers may discharge on interneurons, which in turn cause presynaptic inhibition of smaller nociceptive afferent fibers, effectively closing off or "gating" the nociceptive signal. Signals may also be selectively gated by activity in descending pathways terminating on interneurons or through presynaptic effects directly on the terminals of afferent fibers. In this way, higher centers can control at the local level of the cord the impact that peripheral sensory input has on motor activity.

In reality, the histology, neurochemistry, and circuitry of the spinal cord is much more complex than that described above. Dozens of different cell types, neurotransmitters, and neuromodulators have been identified. The cord plays a major role in the ongoing processing of sensory and motor information that is necessary for both reflex and volitional activity.

Neuronal Interconnections and the Integration of Information[17-22]

The spinal cord is composed of millions of cells of many different types. These cells vary considerably in their function and morphology. This cellular heterogeneity and the diversity of the interconnections among these cells endow the spinal cord with a tremendous capacity for directing and processing impulse traffic and hence information. As discussed, the spinal cord can be grossly differentiated into white matter and gray matter. **Most of the processing of information takes place within the gray matter.**[17-22] Among the various components of gray matter, **the elaborate interconnections formed by the interneurons provide the anatomic basis for most of the information processing.**

Interneurons

Interneurons are present in all areas of the gray matter and are the most common of the spinal neurons. They are 30 times more numerous than motor neurons. Interneurons are small and highly excitable cells, often spontaneously active, and capable of extremely high firing rates. **Interneurons have extensive interconnections with each other, as well as with afferent fibers, motor neurons, and descending motor control pathways.**[17-22] They accomplish this by means of elongated, extensively branched dendrites and axons, which may cross from one side of the cord to the other as well as ascend or descend to other spinal cord segments. Some interneurons may extend into the brainstem as well. Intersegmental projections may travel in the white matter of the cord for varying numbers of segments before re-entering the gray matter to terminate. Such fibers may extend over only a few segments or may actually extend over much of the length of the spinal cord. These wide ranging interneurons are known as **propriospinal neurons** and form the fasciculus propius that surrounds the gray matter. The distinction between interneurons and proprioneurons is arbitrary however, since most interneurons are involved in coordinating the activity of neurons in several segments.

Spinal interneurons are organized into networks that constitute much of the actual circuitry mediating the reflex behaviors and more complex motor patterns that arise from the cord. Extensive interconnections among interneurons within these circuits coordinate the activity of separate muscle groups (e.g., between limbs), ensure the synergy of agonists and antagonists, and establish the rhythmicity of muscle contractions specific for different gaits.[17-20] These networks are influenced by afferent impulses from the periphery, motor signals descending from supraspinal centers, and even by the output of the lower motor neurons themselves (Fig. 5–12). In this way, the output of these neuronal pools and ultimately the spinal output funneled through the alpha motor neurons to skeletal muscle is continually modified. Spinal output is highly adaptable and continually responsive to the needs of the organism.

A distinction is usually made between the afferent and efferent neurons of the spinal cord and the so-called interneurons that are interposed between them. It should be

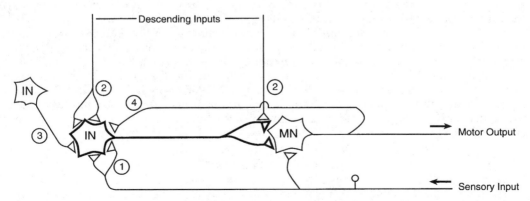

Figure 5–12. *Potential Sources of Input to a Spinal Interneuron.* This spinal interneuron (IN) is influenced by (*1*) segmental afferent fibers (*2*) descending control fibers (*3*) other spinal interneurons, and (*4*) recurrent motor neuron (MN) axon collaterals.

recognized, however, that this distinction is not entirely justified.[19,20] The alpha motor neurons, for example, not only function as output neurons but also serve via their intraspinal axon collaterals as segmental interneurons that coordinate the activity of other neurons and interneurons. Similarly, a number of ascending (sensory) tract cells can act as interneurons via their own axon collaterals. **All spinal fiber types may** thus **function to some degree as interneurons.**

By virtue of the diversity of their own interconnections with other neurons, the afferent and efferent cells of the spinal cord also contribute to the coordination of motor activity at the spinal level. The motor neurons themselves have unusually extensive dendrites and receive large numbers of axon terminals from afferent fibers, interneurons, and descending motor pathways. The only comparable dendritic outreach is found in large cells of the reticular formation that receive signals from throughout the nervous system. Afferent fibers give rise to multiple axonal branches, which may terminate on many other neurons, including local motor neurons, interneurons, and second-order ascending fibers.

It will become evident in the following discussions of the role of higher centers in motor control that the entire local spinal circuitry is subject to the influence of axons that descend from supraspinal areas. These axons modulate the flow of sensory input, control receptor sensitivities (as in the fusimotor control of muscle spindle receptor sensitivity), influence the interneurons of reflex and pattern generating circuits, and terminate directly on motor neurons themselves.

Spinal Contributions to Motor Control

Different theories of motor control imply different contributions by the spinal cord to motor control (see Chapter 10).[23] According to the *Reflex Model* of motor control, movement reflects a compounding of chains of reflexes arising at spinal, brainstem, and cortical levels. These reflexes arise from rigid neuroanatomic substrates and are characterized as stereotypical and relatively immutable. They are elicited and controlled by sensory stimuli. In this context, the contribution of the spinal cord to motor control would be limited to the various spinal reflexes. A related model, the *Hierarchial Model,* proposes that movement is created by motor programs available at various levels of the neural axis. These motor programs are controlled by an ascending, hierarchial control system. This model presumes a somewhat more flexible (albeit more abstract) capability in the spinal cord for creating specific programs specifying particular muscle activation patterns. The output of the central pattern generators underlying the rhythmicity of locomotion and scratching might represent one example of such a motor program. Finally, the *Systems Model* of motor control presumes that normal movements arise, not from muscle activation patterns prescribed by sensory pathways (reflexes) or from central motor programs, but from movement strategies shaped by specific tasks. Implicit in this thinking is the notion that many different muscle strategies may be capable of accomplishing the same goal. Most of the theorizing related to this model remains at a fairly abstract level and is difficult to relate to what is known objectively about the neuroanatomy and physiology of the spinal cord.

Much of the discussion to follow focuses on the traditional notion of spinal reflexes. The reflex concept espoused early on by Sherrington[24] (1906) is by far the best understood in terms of actual neuroanatomic and physiologic mechanisms. We will see, however, that within this most concrete of motor domains many of the fundamental assumptions are being questioned.

Reflexes in General[24]

The most basic example of integrated neural activity is the reflex. A reflex may be defined in general terms as a subconscious, unlearned, automatic response to a stimulus. **Each reflex is usually elicited by a particular type of stimulus and involves the generation**

Segmental Reflex Arc

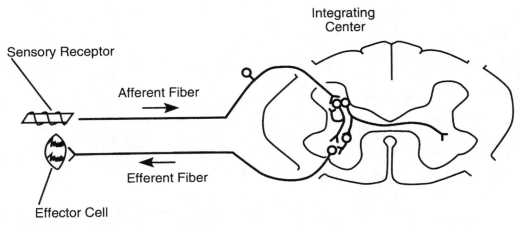

Figure 5–13.   Prototypical segmental reflex arc.

of a limited repertoire of responses. Reflexes are organized at practically all levels of the nervous system and participate in many different types of physiologic activity. Reflexes play a fundamental role in the control of somatic activity, as well as in the regulation of a variety of visceral functions.

The anatomic pathway mediating a reflex is termed the *reflex arc* (Fig. 5–13). This arc consists of a sense organ whose stimulation initiates an impulse; an afferent neuron that transmits this impulse to the central nervous system; one or more synapses in a central integrating station; an efferent neuron that transmits the resultant impulses from the central nervous system to an effector; and the effector (usually a muscle or gland) that actually produces the reflex response. Interruption of the reflex arc at any point abolishes the entire response.

There are many different types of reflexes, and they can be classified according to many different criteria (Table 5–2). Reflexes have been classified, for example, according to the type of sensory input by which they are elicited, the level of the nervous system at which the reflex is integrated (spinal, brainstem, cerebellum), and the functional significance of the effector response itself. In any case, the following discussion focuses primarily on the reflexes of the spinal cord that control somatic (skeletal muscle) activity.

Spinal Cord Reflexes[14,15,24–28]

The simplest type of motor control is at the level of the spinal reflex, in which a specific sensory input induces a specific motor response. In lower animals in which instinctive, stereotypical motor activities predominate, spinal reflexes mediate the bulk of motor function. In humans, despite the fact that higher brain centers are more developed and the spinal cord is subject to considerably more regulation by these centers, the spinal reflexes remain an indispensable component of motor control.

The spinal reflex arc is analogous to that based in any region of the central nervous system, with afferent, integrative, and efferent components (see Fig. 5–13). In the case of the spinal reflex, the afferent neurons enter by way of the dorsal roots, whereas the efferent fibers arise in the ventral horn and leave by way of the ventral roots. The principle that in the spinal cord the dorsal roots are sensory and the ventral roots are motor is known as the **Bell-Magendie law.** In actuality, this distinction is not entirely accurate.

Table 5–2. *Approaches to Classifying Spinal Reflexes*

Afferent Connections
Somatosensory
   Tactile (touch pressure)
   Thermal (warmth/cold)
   Nociceptive (pain)
   Proprioceptive (position/rate of movement)
Visceral

Level of Central Integration
Spinal
Supraspinal
  Bulbar
  Midbrain
  Cerebellar

Complexity of Reflex Arc
Monosynaptic, polysynaptic
Segmental, multisegmental (intersegmental)
Interlimb

Functional Significance of the Motor Response
Postural
Locomotor
Defensive

The simplest conceivable reflex involves only two neural elements—an afferent neuron, which is in direct contact with an efferent (motor) neuron. This is termed a **monosynaptic reflex.** In most spinal reflex arcs, however, one or more interneurons are interposed between the sensory neurons and the motor neurons. This constitutes a **polysynaptic** or **pleurisynaptic reflex.** With the addition of multiple interneurons and the variety of interconnections that these may form, reflex pathways can become complex.

Spinal reflexes share certain basic characteristics. They are all very stimulus-specific. Each reflex is characteristically stimulated most readily by a specific type of stimulation. Moreover, the location of the stimulus dictates which particular muscles contract. The dependence of the exact response on the location of the stimulus is known as **local sign.** For example, the exact flexor pattern of the withdrawal reflex in a limb varies precisely with the part of the limb that is stimulated. Reflexes are also usually **graded**, so that the intensity of the stimulation governs the intensity of the response. Inherent in every spinal reflex is some degree of **delay** between the stimulus and the response. The more complex the reflex pathway (the number of interneurons), the slower the spread of excitation through the pathway and the greater the delay. Most spinal reflexes are highly consistent in their response pattern and are usually described as producing stereotypical or **stereotyped motor activity.**

Traditionally, the spinal reflexes have been considered highly rigid, inflexible responses elicited by specific sensory stimuli. In fact, this is how they are usually described in physiology and neuroscience textbooks. **It has become apparent, however, that the reflexive motor behaviors arising in the spinal cord are much more complex and adaptable than previously thought.**[16–18] It has long been assumed that spinal reflexes function as parallel, separate systems, each of which serves as an exclusive pathway for a single muscle or small group of muscles. It is now thought that activity in one class of reflex is likely to exert a variety of influences on other segmental pathways and may actually have neurons in common with other pathways.[16–18] Specific interneurons are probably influenced by numerous classes of afferent fibers and participate in a variety of motor behaviors. Moreover, a specific motor outcome can probably be accomplished by differing cohorts of neurons, depending on the circumstances. In addition, spinal reflexes are strongly influenced (both inhibited and excited) by axons that descend from many areas in the brain.

Many different somatic reflexes are mediated by the spinal cord. One convenient way to discuss these reflexes is to organize them in terms of their basic anatomic complexity and then to consider them from the simplest to the most complex.

The Stretch Reflex[13–15,25–30]

Perhaps the simplest of all the spinal cord reflexes is the so-called stretch reflex. Although this reflex is often described in terms of the least complicated of all conceivable reflex arcs, the monosynaptic pathway, it is actually much more complex. It is extremely important for both the maintenance of posture and for locomotion.

It was pointed out in Chapter 4 that an assortment of sensory receptors continuously provide the central nervous system with information regarding body position. This sensory capability is called **proprioception.** Many different types of mechanoreceptors are used to develop this sense, including a variety of receptors found in skeletal muscle itself. These sensory receptors convey information to the central nervous system regarding muscle length, muscle tension, and the velocity of stretch. Predominant among these are the muscle spindles and the Golgi tendon organs. **The contractile response initiated by afferent discharge from the muscle spindles is the stretch reflex.**

The stretch reflex actually has two separate components: the phasic stretch reflex and the tonic stretch reflex.[13,14,29,30] **The phasic (or dynamic) stretch reflex** is elicited by rapid muscle stretch and functions to oppose sudden changes in muscle length. Rapid stretch discharges the primary endings of the muscle spindle and the group Ia afferent nerve fibers. These large myelinated fibers project to the dorsal horn and give rise to branches that ascend in the dorsal columns to higher centers and to segmental branches that terminate largely within the segment of entry. The ascending fibers provide information on muscle length to various supraspinal structures, such as the cerebellum and cerebral cortex. Most of the segmental branches project directly onto alpha motor neurons innervating muscle from which the afferent fibers originated (homonymous muscle) (Fig. 5–14). Some group Ia afferent fibers also terminate directly on motor neurons that innervate the synergists of these muscles. The reflex pathways mediating the activation of both the primary homonymous muscle and its synergists thus involve direct afferent-to-efferent fiber contact. For this reason, the stretch reflex is often characterized as a monosynaptic reflex. The complete reflex, however, is not this simple.[16–18,30–32] In addition to making monosynaptic contact with alpha motor neurons, group Ia fibers send collateral projections to spinal interneurons, which in turn inhibit the motor neurons of muscles antagonistic to the homonymous muscle. In this way, when a muscle is stretched, the alpha motor neurons innervating that muscle and its synergists are excited, whereas those innervating antagonistic muscles are inhibited. This is a good example of reciprocal innervation. It is a prominent feature in spinal organization and serves in this case to integrate the actions of agonists and antagonists.

A second component of the response to muscle stretch is the **static** or **tonic stretch reflex.** This results from a slower stretch of the muscle, as might occur during passive movement of a joint. The reflex pathways for the tonic reflex involve essentially the same connections as the phasic reflex, but group II afferent fibers from the secondary endings of the muscle spindle are also involved. These fibers make monosynaptic excitatory connections with the alpha motor neurons projecting to the homonymous muscle. When a muscle is slowly, passively stretched, continuous tonic receptor signals evoked at both primary and secondary endings stimulate motor units within the muscle and create a resistance to that movement. This resistance to movement is termed **muscle tone.** The tonic stretch reflex is slowly adapting and continues to cause muscle contraction as long as the muscle is maintained at excessive length. This is in contrast to the dynamic stretch reflex, which ceases within a fraction of a second after the muscle has been stretched to its new length. Although this reflexive activity is a major contributor to muscle tone, other factors also contribute, including the inherent, viscoelastic properties of the muscle itself.

The muscle spindle is an unusual sensory organ in that it has its own motor input in addition to its sensory connections (see Chapter 4). The nerves mediating this input are

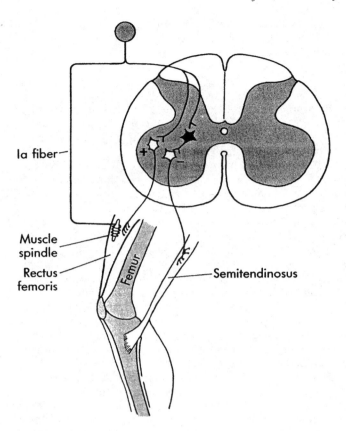

la fiber

Muscle
spindle

Rectus
femoris

Femur

Semitendinosus

Figure 5–14. *Reflex Arc of the Stretch Reflex.* The interneuron shown in black is a group Ia inhibitory interneuron. (From Berne and Levy, [15] p 204, with permission.)

small myelinated gamma fibers, which constitute about 30% of the motor fibers of the ventral root. **Changes in the gamma motor input to the intrafusal fibers of the spindle (fusimotor control) alter the sensitivity of this sense organ and hence the overall activity of the stretch reflex.** The ability of the central nervous system to control the sensitivity of the stretch reflex has many physiologic implications and is fundamental to motor control. As we shall see in later chapters, when gamma control is pathologically disturbed, motor activity may be grossly distorted.

Because the intrafusal fibers of muscle spindles are arranged parallel with the extrafusal fibers of the whole muscle, contraction of the muscle causes the length of the spindles to shorten (Fig. 5–15). Unless a mechanism were available for simultaneously adjusting the length of the muscle spindle, this would result in an "unloading" of the spindle and a decrease in afferent firing. A mechanism to prevent this is provided by the gamma motor neurons.[13–15,29,30] The gamma efferent fibers stimulate contraction of the intrafusal fibers on either side of their noncontractile central regions. This contraction stretches the central regions, activating their receptors and increasing afferent nerve discharge. When the gamma motor neurons are active during muscle contraction, the resultant intrafusal fiber contractions are sufficient to prevent the "slack" that would develop in the spindle. This allows the spindle to maintain a high degree of sensitivity over a wide range of different lengths, during both reflex and voluntary contraction. **It is likely that movements are normally initiated by coactivation of both alpha and gamma motor neurons.**[13–15,29,30] This parallel activation of both extrafusal and intrafusal fibers prevents unloading of the muscle spindles. The fact that group Ia fibers continue to discharge after voluntary contraction of skeletal muscle attests to the effectiveness of this mechanism. Recordings made from muscle spindle afferents in human subjects during voluntary contraction of extensor muscles indicate that gamma motor neurons are recruited in an orderly manner along with alpha motor neurons.[30]

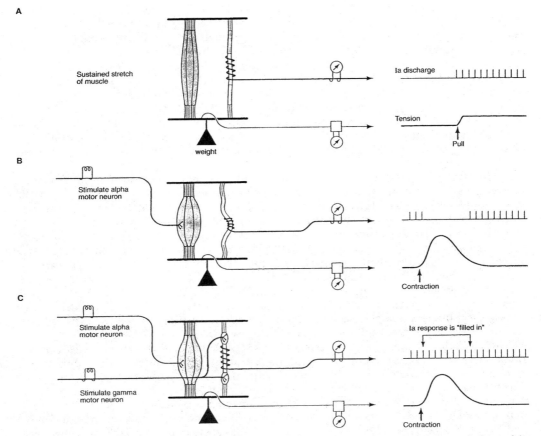

Figure 5–15. *Effect of Gamma Activation on Muscle Spindle Activity.* (A) Sustained tension elicits steady firing of the Ia afferent. (B) A characteristic pause occurs in ongoing Ia discharge when the muscle is caused to contract by stimulation of its alpha motor neuron alone. The Ia fiber stops firing because the spindle is unloaded by the contraction. (C) If during a comparable contraction a gamma motor neuron to the spindle is also stimulated, the spindle is not unloaded during the contraction and the pause in Ia discharge is "filled in." (From Kandel, ER, Schwartz, JH, and Jessell, TM: Principles of Neural Science, ed 3. [adapted from Hunt, CC and Kuffler, SW: Stretch receptor discharge during muscle contraction. J Physiol 113:298-315, 1951] Appleton & Lange, Norwalk, CT, 1991, p 572, with permission.)

Individual spindle endings thus respond promptly to changes in load and are active at specific contraction strengths.

The gamma motor neurons innervating a muscle are activated in much the same way as alpha motor neurons, being influenced by both local, segmental activity and descending influences from higher centers. The motor neurons of the gamma system are regulated to a large degree by descending tracts from a number of supraspinal areas, especially in the brainstem (see Chapter 6). Through these pathways, the sensitivity of the muscle spindles and hence the threshold of the stretch reflexes in various parts of the body can be adjusted to meet the needs of motor control. Gamma efferent discharge is also influenced by sensory input. Stimulation of the skin, for example, especially by noxious agents, increases gamma discharge to ipsilateral flexor muscles, while decreasing gamma input to extensors.

Modulation of the stretch reflex is also possible on the output side of the reflex through the inhibitory actions of the Renshaw cell.[17,22,30-32] This interneuron receives monosynaptic excitation from alpha motor neuron collateral branches and feeds back onto the homonymous and synergistic alpha (and gamma) motor neurons to produce recurrent inhibition. The Renshaw cells also suppress activity in the group Ia inhibitory interneurons directed to the antagonistic pool, thereby decreasing the reciprocal inhibition of these muscles. The excitability of the Renshaw cell is subject to supraspinal control. The fact that Renshaw cells are subject to facilitory and inhibitory control from both segmental reflex pathways and descending tracts suggests that the feedback regulation provided by this recurrent pathway can be used in a versatile way during different types of movements. During voluntary contraction, for example, Renshaw cell activity may be suppressed, disinhibiting the active motor neuron pool and promoting reciprocal inhibition of the antagonists.[30,31] This facilitates the movement and helps to prevent undesirable activation of the stretch reflex in antagonists stretched during the movement. Renshaw cell inhibition may also serve to enhance "contrast" within the active motor neuron pool by inhibition of the subliminal fringes. In patients presenting with spasticity, the level of recurrent inhibition produced by Renshaw cells seems to be normal or increased, but the ability to modulate the inhibition is lost.

The stretch reflex and the systems that modulate it play a number of important roles in overall motor control. Basically, this reflex serves to maintain a constant muscle length. When muscle is stretched, activation of this reflex serves to resist that stretch. This inherent resistance to muscle lengthening is fundamental to many aspects of motor activity.

The stretch reflex is a primary (but not sole) source of muscle tone.[30,33] This resistance is created by the activation of muscle fibers by means of the stretch reflex. In the absence of this reflex, there is little resistance to movement and little tone, and the muscle is flaccid. Clinically significant alterations in muscle tone are common and accompany lesions at many levels of the central nervous system.[30] Disruption of the reflex pathway at the local, segmental level, such as by disruption of the dorsal roots, results in a dramatic decrease in muscle tone. Interruption of descending influences that are facilitatory to the gamma system, such as by spinal cord disruption or cerebellar disease, also results in hypotonia.

At the other extreme, certain lesions may interfere with inhibitory influences on the gamma motor neurons, thereby increasing the sensitivity of the stretch reflex and causing abnormalities in muscle movement. Another finding characteristic of hyperactive stretch reflexes is a phenomenon called **clonus.** Clonus is a rapid, involuntary alternation of muscle contraction and relaxation, which may often be induced in spastic or hyperreflexive limbs by muscle stretch. Ankle clonus, for example, is elicited by brisk, maintained dorsiflexion of the foot, and the response is rhythmic plantar flexion (gastrocnemius contraction) at the ankle.

The stretch reflex, particularly its static component, is also necessary for the maintenance of upright posture.[15] This reflex continuously activates proximal extensor and axial muscles, stabilizing the trunk and limbs and counteracting the force of gravity. When a person is standing upright, for example, gravity tends to flex the knees, stretching the quadriceps muscles. This stretching force elicits a sustained reflex contraction of the quadriceps. This assists in the maintenance of extension at the knee joint and hence upright posture. Because this component of the reflex shows little adaptation, the stretch reflex contraction can be sustained as long as the stretch is imposed.

The muscle spindle and gamma efferent system also play a more subtle role in the "smoothing" of voluntary movements.[13] If alpha motor neurons were the only fibers activated by descending motor commands then, with every muscle contraction, spindles would be unloaded and the stimulatory effect of their discharge on the alpha motor neurons would diminish. This would result in involuntary fluctuations or oscillations in contraction force and a jerkiness of movement. However, the smoothness of normal movement is due to coactivation of gamma fibers along with alpha fibers, which prevents this oscillation from occurring.

The dynamic stretch reflex may be evoked clinically by tapping a tendon to produce a sudden stretch of muscle. This may be readily accomplished at a variety of joints, such as the knee or ankle, at which tapping the tendon produces contraction of the extensor muscles and relaxation of the antagonistic flexor muscles. Perhaps **the stretch reflex most commonly observed clinically is the contraction of the quadriceps elicited by tapping the patellar tendon, the so-called knee jerk reflex** (Fig. 5–16).[13–15] A number of analogous monosynaptic reflexes are also routinely tested as part of the neurologic examination. Similar reflexes can be obtained from almost any muscle of the body either by striking the tendon of the

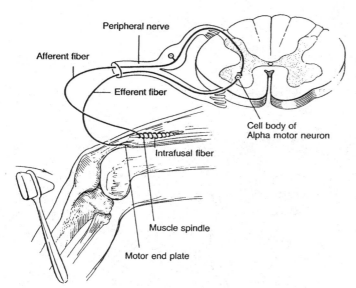

Peripheral nerve

Afferent fiber

Efferent fiber

Cell body of
Alpha motor neuron

Intrafusal fiber

Muscle spindle

Motor end plate

Figure 5–16. Schematic Diagram of the Knee Jerk Reflex. This stretch reflex is elicited by tapping the patellar tendon, which induces a rapid stretch of the gastrocnemius. (From Geneser, F: Textbook of Histology. Copyright © Lea & Febiger, Philadelphia, 1986, p 322, with permission.)

muscle or by striking the belly of the muscle itself. Such reflexes are variously termed myotatic reflexes, stretch reflexes, tendon-jerk reflexes, or deep tendon reflexes. This last term is used extensively in the clinic but is somewhat misleading in implying that the receptors for the reflex reside within the tendon. In fact, they reside in the spindles of the muscle itself. Nonetheless, examination of the phasic stretch reflex provides valuable information regarding both supraspinal and segmental motor control mechanisms. For example, diminished reflex activity may accompany reduced supraspinal facilitation (e.g., spinal shock), disruption of muscle afferent fibers (e.g., destruction of dorsal roots), or motor neuron damage (e.g., peripheral neuropathy). Excessive reflex activity, on the other hand, may result from a loss of supraspinal inhibition (e.g., upper motor neuron lesion), excessive supraspinal activation (e.g., basal ganglia disorders), excessive spinal activation (e.g., segmental spinal pathology), or enhanced motor neuron excitability (e.g., hypocalcemia).

The Inverse Stretch Reflex[13–15,25–30]

Up to a point, the harder a muscle is stretched, the stronger the reflex contraction will be in the muscle. **A tension will be reached, however, at which contraction will suddenly cease and the muscle will relax. This relaxation occurs as a result of the inverse stretch reflex. The receptors for this reflex reside in the Golgi tendon organs of the muscle,** and project to the spinal cord as group Ib myelinated nerve fibers. Like the group Ia afferent fibers from the primary endings of the muscle spindles, the group Ib fibers transmit signals into both local areas of the spinal cord and through long pathways to the brain. The group Ib fibers terminate in the cord primarily on inhibitory interneurons, which in turn terminate on alpha motor neurons supplying the muscle in which the tendon organs are located (Fig. 5–17). As a result, stimulation of the group Ib fibers causes inhibition of the muscle being stretched. Similar inhibitory connections are made with the synergists of the homonymous muscle. Like the stretch reflex, the inverse stretch reflex includes reciprocal innervation of antagonistic muscles, resulting in this case in their activation.

The inverse stretch reflex also includes a crossed component. For example, if the reflex action is to relax the quadriceps muscle of one limb, the crossed component will excite the motor neurons of the contralateral quadriceps muscle. In this way, relaxation of the antigravity muscles in one limb will be offset by their contraction in the other limb, thus maintaining some postural support. With the imposition of the inhibitory neuron between the group Ib afferent fibers and the homonymous alpha motor neurons, a bisynaptic pathway

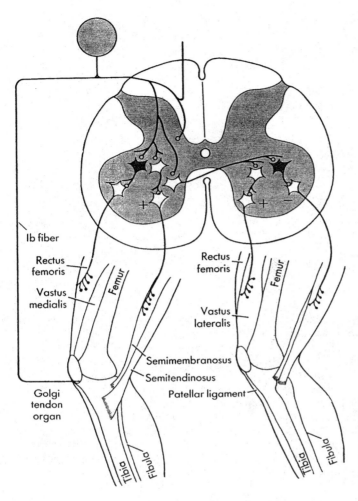

Ib fiber

Rectus femoris

Vastus medialis

Rectus femoris

Vastus lateralis

Femur

Femur

Semimembranosus

Semitendinosus

Patellar ligament

Golgi tendon organ

Tibia

Fibula

Tibia

Fibula

Figure 5–17. *Reflex Arc for the Inverse Stretch (Myotatic) Reflex.* The interneurons include both excitatory (*Clear*) and inhibitory (*Black*) interneurons. (From Berne, RM and Levy MN: Physiology, ed 2. Mosby–Year Book, St. Louis, 1988, p 209, with permission.)

is created. Because of this, the inverse reflex is often described as a bi(di) synaptic reflex. As is the case in designating the stretch reflex as a monosynaptic reflex, this is something of an oversimplification when the reflex response is viewed in its entirety.

The stretch and inverse stretch reflexes clearly differ in that one contracts the primary muscle and the other relaxes it. These two reflexes also differ fundamentally in the manner in which they are stimulated. As described in Chapter 4, the muscle spindles are arranged parallel with the extrafusal fibers, whereas the Golgi tendon organs are situated in series with the muscle fibers. Because of these differing anatomic arrangements, the spindles and tendon organs respond differently to muscle stretch and contraction (Fig. 5–18). Passive stretching of muscle distorts and thereby activates both the tendon organ and muscle spindle receptors. Active muscle contraction activates only the tendon organs.

The sensitivity of the Golgi tendon organ to *passive stretch* is relatively low, in part because elastic fibers within the muscle take up much of the stretch. This is why it takes a strong stretch to produce relaxation. **However, tendon organ discharge is readily produced by *active contraction* of the muscle.**[13,15,34] Some tendon organs are probably activated even in the weakest of contractions. The Golgi tendon organs have often been described as high-threshold stretch receptors with a function limited to protecting muscle from dangerously high tension levels. It is now evident that tendon organs are very sensitive muscle receptors, particularly to actively generated muscle force, and they have an important role in proprioception and motor control.

A. Passive Muscle Stretch

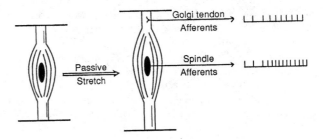

B. Active Muscle Contraction

Figure 5–18. Response of Muscle Receptors to Passive Stretch and Active Contraction. Because the muscle spindles are arranged in parallel with the muscle fibers, whereas the Golgi tendon organs are situated in series with these same muscle fibers, these two sensors respond very differently to (*A*) passive muscle stretch and (*B*) active muscle contraction.

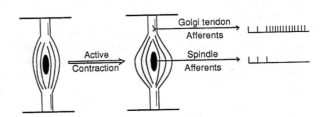

The inverse stretch reflex has been implicated in a variety of spinally organized motor patterns. For example, it may be involved in the rotational recruitment of motor units during sustained contraction and the rapid switching between flexion and extension required for behaviors such as running.[13] This reflex may also play a role in spreading a contractile load over many fibers of a whole muscle, so that no particular small group of fibers is subject to excessive, potentially damaging force.

Although the stretch reflexes depend on the activity of the muscle spindle and Golgi tendon organ, afferent fibers from these sensors constitute only a small fraction of the total afferents coming from muscle. Natural movement is accompanied by active and passive changes in the length of all muscles acting on the moving joint, by distortion of the joint capsule, and by deformation of the skin. The afferent activity generated by movement comes from all of these sources and strongly influences the stretch reflexes. In pathologic states such as spasticity, a normally innocuous afferent volley from these receptors can produce excessive reflex activity such as flexor spasms.

Unlike the stretch reflex that can be easily evoked clinically, the inverse stretch reflex cannot be demonstrated in a normal limb. It can be elicited in hypertonic muscle.[15,30] if, for example, one begins to flex a spastic lower limb at the knee, increasing resistance to the stretch of the extensor muscles is encountered. This resistance continues to increase as more force is applied until a point is reached at which the inverse stretch reflex is actuated. This inhibits the extensor contraction, allowing the limb to passively flex. A similar sequence would be elicited by passive flexon of the elbow. This sequence of resistance followed by release when a limb is moved passively is known clinically as the **clasp-knife reaction**. It is also termed **the lengthening reaction** because it refers to the response of a spastic muscle to lengthening. Although the Golgi tendon organs (group Ib afferents) are involved in this response, they cannot by themselves produce the complete suppression of reflex contraction that occurs; therefore, other inhibitory inputs must be involved as well.[30] The most likely sources of this inhibition are certain non–spindle muscle mechanoreceptors.

Forceful muscle stretching is often effective in relieving certain types of muscle hyperactivity (e.g., cramps). This may be due in part to activation of the inverse stretch reflex.

The Withdrawal (Flexor) Reflex[13-15,25-30]

If an individual were walking in bare feet and suddenly stepped on a sharp object, his or her walking would be immediately and automatically interrupted and the injured foot drawn away from the offending stimulus (Fig. 5–19). **This is an example of the withdrawal reflex.** The withdrawal reflex is a polysynaptic reflex that is evoked by stimulation of a diverse group of somatosensory receptors. This response is particularly marked in response to stimulation of nociceptors signaling pain and tissue injury but may also be elicited by stimulation of a variety of other receptors in the skin, muscle, and joints.[26,30] This group of afferents includes secondary muscle spindle endings, joint receptors, pacinian corpuscles, and free nerve endings. The collective term "flexor reflex afferents" is sometimes used to lump these sensors into a group, since they all seem to be able to elicit the same actions.[30]

Afferent discharge arising from stimulation of these receptors travels to the spinal cord in small myelinated group II and III nerve fibers and unmyelinated group IV nerve fibers. Upon entering the cord, these fibers diverge widely, traveling along the cord in both directions and terminating extensively among the interneurons of many segments. Through complex, multisynaptic pathways, these fibers ultimately excite motor neurons that innervate flexor muscles in the offended body part, causing it to be withdrawn from the stimulus. When a strong noxious stimulus is applied to a limb, the response is heightened and may spread to include extension of the opposite limb. This is the *crossed-extensor response.*

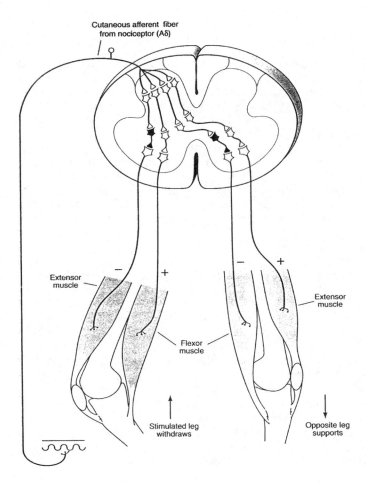

Cutaneous afferent fiber
from nociceptor (Aδ)

Extensor
muscle

Extensor
muscle

Flexor
muscle

Stimulated leg
withdraws

Opposite leg
supports

Figure 5–19. Reflex Arc for the Flexion (Withdrawal) Reflex. The flexion withdrawal reflex produces flexion of the stimulated limb and extension of the opposite limb. Stimulation of cutaneous afferents, such as an A delta fiber from a nociceptor, produces excitation of ipsilateral flexor muscles and inhibition of ipsilateral extensor muscles, while producing the opposite response in the contralateral limb (the crossed extensor reflex). The cutaneous input is distributed over many spinal segments, so that the full reflex involves contraction of muscles at all joints of both limbs. The pathways are schematically illustrated here for one spinal segment only. (From Kandel, ER, Schwartz, JH, and Jessell, TM (eds): Principles of Neural Science, ed 3. [adapted from Schmidt, RF and Thews, G (eds): Human Physiology. Springer Verlag, New York, 1993, p 90] Appleton & Lange, Norwalk, CT, 1991, p 588, with permission.)

Although the flexion of the ipsilateral limb serves to protect the body from possible harm, the contralateral crossed-extensor response serves as a postural adjustment made in compensation for the loss of antigravity support provided by the limb that is flexed. Like the stretch and inverse stretch reflexes, reciprocal innervation functions in each component of the withdrawal response to inhibit the appropriate antagonists.

Despite the extensive divergence of nerve fibers involved in the withdrawal response, the actual motor response is highly specific and succinctly defined by the nature and location of the stimulus. Slight variations in the location of the stimulation of a limb cause corresponding changes in the form of the motor response. The specific muscles that are activated result in a final limb position that is closely linked to the exact site of stimulation and hence is most effective in moving the limb away from the stimulus. If the medial part of a limb is stimulated, for example, the response will include some abduction, whereas stimulation of the lateral surface will produce some adduction. This principle, which is called **local sign,** applies to any part of the body but is especially evident in the limbs where the flexor reflexes are most highly developed.

An interesting characteristic of the withdrawal reflexes, especially those occurring in response to strong, painful stimuli, is that they may override reflex activity occurring in other pathways. Nociceptive afferent discharge seems to be able to preempt pathways mediating less pressing responses.

Because of their particular organization, some of the basic properties of the withdrawal response are different from those of the simpler stretch reflexes.[13,15] Since more slowly conducting afferent fibers (e.g., smaller, less myelinated) are involved and more extensive intraspinal circuitry must be activated, the delay or **latency** inherent in the withdrawal response is greater. As with other spinal reflexes, this latency diminishes somewhat with increased stimulus intensity and the resultant increase in spatial and temporal facilitation occurring at synapses along the reflex pathway. The withdrawal response also tends to last longer. Although the stretch reflex ceases abruptly with stimulus termination, the flexor response persists even after the body part is removed from the stimulus. This results from recurrent pathways and reverberating circuits that excite persistent neuronal activity within the spinal circuitry mediating this reflex. These circuits may continue to transmit impulses to motor neurons for several seconds after the incoming sensory signal is completely gone. This prolonged, repeated firing of the motor neurons is termed **afterdischarge.** The physiologic significance of this persistence is that it serves to maintain withdrawal for a sufficient time to allow other reflexes and behaviors to prevent recontact with the offending stimulus (e.g., move the entire body away from the threat). The crossed-extensor component continues for an even longer period than the flexor response.

A more subtle difference in the reflexes is apparent in the relationship between the stimulus and response intensities. In the stretch response, a close, nearly linear relationship exists between the intensity of stretch and the reflex contraction, a relationship that holds over a wide range of stimulus intensities. At low-stimulus intensities the withdrawal response is also weak, and a rather restricted flexor pattern results. However, with stronger stimulation such as when nociceptive fibers are activated, a full response develops quickly that is augmented a little by further increasing the stimulus.

Although this discussion has focused on the obvious protective function of the withdrawal reflex, it is also probably involved in other aspects of motor control. For example, it is likely that lower threshold, non-nociceptive receptors help modulate limb movement in locomotion.

A number of other cutaneous or superficial reflexes are mediated by polysynaptic spinal pathways similar to those of the withdrawal reflex. Some of these may be readily elicited as part of a neurologic examination and may be diagnostic of certain central nervous system lesions. Plantar flexion of the toes in response to painful stimulation of the sole of the foot is a good example. In the presence of corticospinal tract disease, this response is disturbed and a more primitive form of the flexion reflex occurs called **Babinski's sign** (see Fig. 12–20). In this case, the big toe responds to plantar stimulation with dorsiflexion. The abdominal contraction normally induced by cutaneous stimulation of the abdomen and the cremasteric contraction (elevating the testicles) normally induced by stimulation along the inner aspect of the thigh are both forms of the withdrawal reflex and may be disrupted by corticospinal lesions.

Intersegmental Reflexes[27–30,32,35,36]

Complex spinal reflexes may involve integration of activity at many levels (segments) of the spinal cord. These are termed *intersegmental reflexes.* Links between segments may be provided by divergence of afferent fibers (such as in the withdrawal response) or by propriospinal or other interneurons. These intersegmental connections allow coordination of motor activity among the limbs and allow axial muscles, which tend to be innervated from many segments, to be activated in concert. Complex intersegmental reflexes include limb-supporting reactions, righting responses, and rhythmic stepping reflexes, all of which are fundamental to posture and locomotion. These reflexes can be demonstrated in spinal animals in which the intact spinal cord is operating without connection to supraspinal centers.

Supraspinal Reflexes[35,36]

Complex motor reflexes are also mediated by centers in the brainstem, cerebellum, basal ganglia, and other areas of the brain. Notable among these supraspinal reflexes are the tonic neck reflexes and labyrinthine reflexes, which respond to changes in head position and assist in the maintenance of overall posture (see Chapter 6). Abnormalities in these reflexes are responsible for many clinically evident abnormalities in body righting, balance, posture, and locomotion.

Visceral (Autonomic) Reflexes

It is important to remember that in addition to the many somatic reflexes controlling skeletal muscle, **numerous reflexes exist in the spinal cord that regulate primarily visceral activity.** These autonomic reflexes control such phenomena as thermoregulatory adjustments in vascular tone and sweating, gastrointestinal tract motility, urine storage and bladder emptying, and sexual function. Spinal cord damage may lead to profound disturbances in these reflexes and clinically significant visceral disturbances often accompany the somatic disturbances of cord dysfunction (see Chapters 17 and 24).

Central Pattern Generators[14,18,37–43]

It has long been known that "spinal" animals whose spinal cords are surgically disconnected from the brain can perform the rhythmic, coordinated limb movements associated with locomotion. A spinal dog or cat can emit coordinated stepping movements as long as its weight is supported and the ground (a treadmill) is moving beneath its feet. **Considerable evidence suggests that this "spinal locomotion" is generated by neuronal networks located within the spinal cord itself. These systems have been termed *central pattern generators* (CPGs).** Stepping activity continues in spinal animals even after dorsal root transections, indicating that these spinal circuits are capable of generating a sustained motor output without rhythmic input from either supraspinal structures or peripheral sensory fibers.[14,41]

The precise nature of these pattern generators is still uncertain because the exact connections of so few interneurons are known.[18,37–41] Theoretically, all that would be required to generate alternating extension and flexion of a limb would be two CPGs linked together, each tending to be rhythmically active and each inhibiting the other so that only one was active at a time (Fig. 5–20).[14,18,37–41] It is likely that complex, multijoint

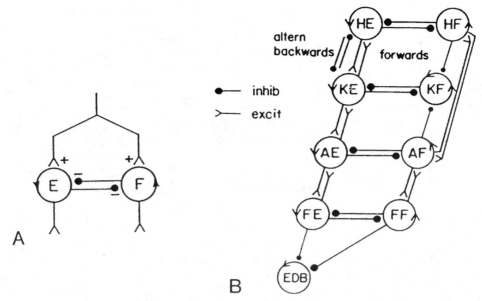

Figure 5–20. *Locomotor Central Pattern Generators (CPGs).* (*A*) A simple scheme to generate alternating extensions and flexions of a limb. Two "unit" CPGs, each rhythmically active, are linked to one another by reciprocal inhibition. Both are driven by tonic excitatory input. (*B*) Multiple interconnected CPGs establish the coordinated movement of an entire limb. E-extensor; F-flexor; H-hip; K-knee; A-ankle; F-foot; EDB-extensor digitorum brevis (short toe flexor). (Adapted from Brooks, VB: The Neural Basis of Motor Control. Oxford University Press, New York, 1986, pp 187, 188.)

movements of entire limbs require the linking together of many local control centers ("unit" CPGs) in extended flexible networks. Each of the unit CPGs might govern specific, individual muscle synergies (e.g., knee flexion or ankle extension) but might be coordinated with the activities of CPGs throughout the network. Flexibility would be gained by the interconnection of individual unit CPGs because individual synergies could be uncoupled from the group as circumstances dictated.

Like the spinal reflexes, **the pattern-generating circuits of the cord do not operate in a vacuum but are subject to a variety of influences that ensure ongoing adaptation of these behaviors to the changing environment of the animal.**[14,18,37–41] Controlling signals arrive from higher centers, peripheral sensors, and other CPGs. Peripheral feedback from muscle, joint, and cutaneous receptors and from spinal reflex circuits (e.g., stretch reflexes) exert important control over CPGs. This control regulates the specific duration and amplitude of the different phases of the step cycle. Although this sensory feedback is not necessary for the generation of a rhythmic locomotor pattern, the locomotion will be slowed and less well coordinated without this input. The reliance of the CPGs on higher centers increases with the extent to which locomotion is purposeful. Goal-directed or purposeful locomotion requires more involvement of tonic signals from midbrain and brainstem, both for the maintenance of posture and balance in a moving body and for the adaptation of the locomotor pattern to the changing environment and to the achievement of behavioral goals.

Like the spinal reflexes, the CPGs are an innate part of the spinal circuitry. They are present in cats, for example, whose spinal cords have been transected only 1 or 2 weeks after birth.[14] The movement patterns they produce, however, seem less stereotyped and more adaptable. In the limb of the spinal cat, the pattern of muscle activation is not simply stereotyped flexion and extension, but it consists of the true muscle synergies seen in normal cats.[14] The CPGs may interact with the spinal reflexes and may actually share some of the neuronal elements of the reflex pathways. Group Ia inhibitory interneurons, for example, are driven by CPGs in the absence of any excitation from group Ia afferent fibers.

Although almost all of what we know about these CPGs has been derived from animal experiments, there is reason to believe that analogous systems function in humans.[14] Even though humans with complete transection of the spinal cord are incapable of rhythmic stepping movements, developmental studies indicate that human infants are born with innate reflex circuitry capable of rhythmic pattern generation. Newborn infants exhibit rhythmic stepping when placed on a moving treadmill. It is also likely that the bipedal locomotion of humans places greater demands on the descending systems that control posture and balance during locomotion than is required in quadripedal animals.[14]

Influences Descending from Supraspinal Areas[14,16-22,29,32,39-41]

As self-contained as the spinal reflex and pattern generating networks are, they are constantly influenced (both facilitated and inhibited) by descending pathways from supraspinal regions. Several areas of the brain can directly influence the activity of the spinal cord via their descending fiber connections. The main fiber tracts are the corticospinal, rubrospinal, tectospinal, reticulospinal, and vestibulospinal tracts. Although each fiber tract is usually considered separately, it should be noted that under normal physiologic conditions they seldom act alone. This is because each region of origin is influenced by input from many other areas of the brain (as well as afferent input from sensory systems) and in turn asserts its effects via other supraspinal areas. For example, the cerebral cortex does not influence the spinal cord solely by way of the corticospinal tracts, but also via its interconnections with structures such as the red nucleus, reticular formation, and tectum. There may also be significant collateral connections between these descending pathways.

At one time, it was believed that the descending tracts were involved only with efferent motor commands. It is now evident that these tracts have important actions on afferent systems as well. Afferent fiber systems usually exert their influences on motor neurons by means of polysynaptic pathways, so there are many sites at which descending pathways might exert their effects. These systems may regulate transmission of sensory information from the spinal cord to the brain, influence the excitability of spinal interneurons, or terminate directly on motor neurons. In this way, supraspinal regions can facilitate or suppress reflex responses to afferent stimulation as well as evoke preprogrammed motor sequences.

Integration of the Spinal Cord into Overall Motor Control

The spinal cord acting in concert with higher centers makes many significant contributions to motor control. The spinal cord both mediates stereotypical unconscious responses to afferent stimulation and constitutes a reservoir of preprogrammed motor sequences available to higher centers for activation in conscious, voluntary activity.

It may be difficult to imagine the contribution that these relatively simple activity patterns make to the seemingly limitless repertoire of motor responses at our disposal until we consider all of the possible combinations that might be derived from portions or all of these synergies. Moreover, the motor programs described in detail in this chapter are only the most simple and best understood. Many more complex and flexible systems of motor programming undoubtedly exist at the spinal level of the motor control.

RECOMMENDED READINGS

Anderson, ME and Binder, MD: Spinal and Supraspinal Control of Movement and Posture. Chapter 26. In Patton, HD, et al (eds): Textbook of Physiology, vol 1, ed 21. WB Saunders, Philadelphia, 1989.

Berne, RM and Levy, MN: Physiology, ed. 3. Chapter 12. Spinal Organization of Motor Function. Mosby-Year Book, St. Louis, 1993.

Binder, MD: Peripheral Motor Control: Spinal Reflex Actions of Muscles, Joint, and Cutaneous Receptors. Chapter 24. In Patton, HD, et al (eds): Textbook of Physiology, vol 1, ed 21. WB Saunders, Philadelphia, 1989.

Brooks, VB (ed): Handbook of Physiology. Section 1. The Nervous System, vol II. Motor Control. The American Physiological Society, Bethesda, MD, 1981.

Burke, D and Lance, JW: The Myotatic Unit and Its Disorders. Chapter 20. In Asbury, AK, McKhann, GM, and McDonald, WI (eds): ed 2. WB Saunders, Philadelphia, 1992.

Carpenter, MB: Neuroanatomy, ed 4. Chapter 3. Spinal Cord: Gross Anatomy and Internal Structure. Williams & Wilkins, Baltimore, 1991.

Carpenter, MB: Neuroanatomy, ed 4. Chapter 4. Tracts of the Spinal Cord. Williams & Wilkins, Baltimore, 1991.

Davidoff, RA and Hackman, JC: Aspects of Spinal Cord Structure and Reflex Function. Neurol Clin 9(3):533, 1991.

Gordon, J and Ghez, C: Muscle Receptors and Spinal Reflexes: The Stretch Reflex. Chapter 37. In Kandel, ER, Schwartz, JH, and Jessell, TM (eds): Principles of Neural Science, ed 3. Appleton & Lange, Norwalk, CT, 1991.

Gordon, J: Spinal Mechanisms of Motor Coordination. Chapter 38. In Kandel, ER, Schwartz, JH, and Jessell, TM (eds): Principles of Neural Science, ed 3. Appleton & Lange, Norwalk, CT, 1991.

Guyton, AC: Basic Neuroscience, Anatomy and Physiology, ed 2. Chapter 8. Sensory Receptors: Neuronal Circuits for Processing Information. WB Saunders, Philadelphia, 1991.

Guyton, AC: Textbook of Medical Physiology, ed 8. Chapter 54. Motor Functions of the Spinal Cord: The Cord Reflexes. WB Saunders, Philadelphia, 1991.

Jankowska, E: Interneuronal Relay in Spinal Pathways from Proprioceptors. Prog Neurobiol 38(4):335, 1992.

Kottke, FJ: The Neurophysiology of Motor Function. Chapter 11. In Kottke, FJ and Lehmann, JF: Krusen's Handbook of Physical Medicine and Rehabilitation, ed 4. WB Saunders, Philadelphia, 1990.

Martin, JH: Neuroanatomy: Text and Atlas. Chapter 9. Descending Projection Systems and the Motor Function of the Spinal Cord. Appleton & Lange, Norwalk, CT, 1989.

Noback, CR, Strominger, NL, and Demarest, RJ: The Human Nervous System: Introduction and Review, ed 4. Chapter 8. Reflexes and Muscle Tone. Lea & Febiger, Philadelphia, 1991.

Nolte, J: The Human Brain, ed 3. Chapter 7. The Spinal Cord. Mosby-Year Book, St. Louis, 1993.

Shepherd, GM and Koch, C: Introduction to Synaptic Circuits. Chapter 1. In Shepherd; GM (ed): The Synaptic Organization of the Brain, ed 3. Oxford University Press, New York, 1990.

REFERENCES

1. Carpenter, MB: Neuroanatomy, ed 4. Chapter 3. Spinal Cord: Gross Anatomy and Internal Structure. Williams & Wilkins, Baltimore, 1991.

2. deGroot, J and Chusid, J: Correlative Neuroanatomy. Chapter 4. The Spinal Cord, ed 21. Appleton & Lange, Norwalk, CT, 1991.

3. Nolte, J: The Human Brain, ed 3. Chapter 7. The Spinal Cord. Mosby-Year Book, St. Louis, 1993.

4. Dorwart, RH and Genant, HK: Anatomy of Lumbosacral Spine. Radiol Clin North Am 21:201, 1983.

5. Rexed, B: The Cytoarchitectonic Organization of the Spinal Cord in the Cat. J Comp Neurol 96:415, 1952.

6. Brown, AG: Organization in the Spinal Cord. Springer-Verlag, Berlin, 1981.

7. Schoenen, J and Faull, RLM: Spinal Cord: Cytoarchitectural, Dendroarchitectural, and Myeloarchitectural Organization. Chapter 2. In Paxinos, G (ed): The Human Nervous System. Academic Press, San Diego, 1990.

8. Martin, JH: Neuroanatomy: Text and Atlas. Chapter 9. Descending Projection Systems and the Motor Function of the Spinal Cord. Appleton & Lange, Norwalk, CT, 1989.

9. Carpenter, MB: Neuroanatomy, ed 4. Chapter 4. Tracts of the Spinal Cord. Williams & Wilkins, Baltimore, 1991.

10. Shepherd, GM and Koch, C: Introduction to Synaptic Circuits. Chapter 1. In Shepherd, GM (ed): The Synaptic Organization of the Brain, ed 3. Oxford University Press, New York, 1990.

11. Speckmann, EJ and Lucke, A: Interneuronal Information Transfer: Recent Advances in Synaptology. Int J Clin Pharmacol 30(11):425, 1992.

12. Alberts, B, et al: Molecular Biology of the Cell. Chapter 19. The Nervous System. Garland Publishing, New York, 1989.

13. Guyton, AC: Basic Neuroscience, Anatomy and Physiology, ed 2. Chapter 8. Sensory Receptors: Neuronal Circuits for Processing Information. WB Saunders, Philadelphia, 1991.

14. Gordon, J: Spinal Mechanisms of Motor Coordination. Chapter 38. In Kandel, ER, Schwartz, JH, and Jessell, TM (eds): Principles of Neural Science, ed 3. Appleton & Lange, Norwalk, CT, 1991.

15. Berne, RM and Levy, MN: Physiology, ed. 3. Chapter 12. Spinal Organization of Motor Function. Mosby-Year Book, St. Louis, 1993.

16. McCrea, DA: Spinal Cord Circuitry and Motor Reflexes. Exerc Sport Sci 14:105, 1986.

17. Baldissera, F, Hultborn, H, and Ilert, M: Integration in Spinal Neuronal Systems. In Brooks, VB (ed): Handbook of Physiology, Section 1, vol II. American Physiological Society, Bethesda, MD, 1981.

18. Davidoff, RA and Hackman, JC: Aspects of Spinal Cord Structure and Reflex Function. Neurol Clin 9(3):533, 1991.

19. Jankowska, E and Edgley, S: Interactions Between Pathways Controlling Posture and Gait at the Level of Spinal Interneurons in the Cat. Prog Brain Res 97:161, 1993.

20. Jankowska, E: Interneuronal Relay in Spinal Pathways from Proprioceptors. Prog Neurobiol 38(4):335, 1992.

21. Schomburg, ED: Spinal Functions in Sensorimotor Control of Movements. Neurosurg Rev 13(3):179, 1990.

22. Anderson, ME and Binder, MD: Spinal and Supraspinal Control of Movement and Posture. Chapter 26. In Patton, HD, et al (eds): Textbook of Physiology, vol 1, ed 21. WB Saunders, Philadelphia, 1989.

23. Horak, FB: Assumptions Underlying Motor Control for Neurological Rehabilitation. Chapter 4. In Contemporary Management of Motor Control Problems. Proceedings of the II Step Conference Foundation for Physical Therapy, 1991.

24. Sherrington, CS: The Integrative Action of the Nervous System. Yale University Press, New Haven, CT, 1906.

25. Burke, RE: Spinal Cord: Ventral Horn. Chapter 4. In Shepherd, GM (ed): The Synaptic Organization of the Brain, ed 3. Oxford University Press, New York, 1990.

26. Binder, MD: Peripheral Motor Control: Spinal Reflex Actions of Muscle, Joint, and Cutaneous Receptors. Chapter 24. In Patton, HD, et al (eds): Textbook of Physiology, vol 1, ed 21. WB Saunders, Philadelphia, 1989.

27. Guyton, AC: Textbook of Medical Physiology, ed 8. Chapter 54. Motor Functions of the Spinal Cord: The Cord Reflexes. WB Saunders, Philadelphia, 1991.

28. Ganong, WF: Review of Medical Physiology, ed 16. Chapter 6. Reflexes. Appleton & Lange, Norwalk, CT, 1993.

29. Gordon, J and Ghez, C: Muscle Receptors and Spinal Reflexes: The Stretch Reflex. Chapter 37. In Kandel, ER, Schwartz, JH, and Jessell, TM (eds): Principles of Neural Science, ed 3. Appleton & Lange, Norwalk, CT, 1991.

30. Rothwell, JC: Control of Human Voluntary Movement. Chapter 5. Reflex Pathways in the Spinal Cord. Aspen Publishers, Rockville, MD, 1987.

31. Windhorst, V: Activation of Renshaw Cells. Prog Neurobiol 35:135, 1990.

32. Stein, RB and Capaday, C: The Modulation of Human Reflexes During Functional Motor Tasks. Trends Neurosci 11:328, 1988.

33. Davidoff, RA: Skeletal Muscle Tone and the Misunderstood Stretch Reflex. Neurology 42(5):951, 1992.

34. Proske, U: The Golgi Tendon Organ. Chapter 7. In Dyck, PJ and Thomas, PK (eds): Peripheral Neuropathy, ed 3. WB Saunders, Philadelphia, 1993.

35. Kottke, FJ: The Neurophysiology of Motor Function. Chapter 11. In Kottke, FJ and Lehmann, JF: Krusen's Handbook of Physical Medicine and Rehabilitation, ed 4. WB Saunders, Philadelphia, 1990.

36. Gowitzke, BA and Milner, M: Scientific Bases of Human Movement, ed 3. Chapter 10. Proprioceptors and Allied Reflexes. Williams & Wilkins, Baltimore, 1988.

37. Grillner, S and Wallen, P: Central Pattern Generators for Locomotion, with Special Reference to Vertebrates. Ann Rev Neurosci 8:233, 1985.

38. Grillner, S, Wallen, P, and Viana di Prisco, G: Cellular Network Underlying Locomotion as Revealed in a Lower Vertebrate Model: Transmitters, Membrane Properties, Circuitry and Simulation. Cold Spring Harbor Symp Quant Biol 55:779, 1990.

39. Grillner, S: Control of Locomotion in Bipeds, Tetrapods and Fish. Chapter 26. In Brooks, VB (ed): Handbook of Physiology. Section 1, vol 2. Motor Control. American Physiological Society, Bethesda, MD, 1981.

40. Grillner, S: Interactions Between Control and Peripheral Mechanisms in the Control of Locomotion. Prog Brain Res 50:227, 1978.

41. Brooks, VB: The Neural Basis of Motor Control. Chapter 10. Locomotion. Oxford University Press, New York, 1986.

42. Lydic, R: Central Pattern-Generating Neurons and the Search for General Principles. FASEB 3:2457, 1989.

43. Sqalli-Houssaini, Y, Cazalets, JR, and Clarac, F: Oscillatory Properties of the Central Pattern Generator for Locomotion in Neonatal Rats. J Neurophysiol 70(2): 803, 1993.

CHAPTER 6

■

The Brainstem and Motor Control

Christopher M. Fredericks, PhD

- *Superficial Anatomy of the Brainstem*
- *Descending Motor Control Tracts to the Spinal Cord*
- *Cranial Nerves*
- *Clinical Implications of Brainstem Damage*

*T*he brainstem begins immediately rostral to the spinal cord and extends to the level of the diencephalon. **Although the brainstem represents only a small portion of the overall brain, it is crowded with elements of many neural systems and is the site of a surprising variety of vital neurologic functions.** The brainstem is extensively involved in numerous aspects of motor control. Some of its contributions to somatic activity are reminiscent of those occurring in the spinal cord (see Chapter 5), whereas other contributions are peculiar to the brainstem itself.[1-4]

Because of its unique location in the neural axis, interposed between higher integrative centers and the spinal cord, **the brainstem serves as a critical conduit through which the principal motor and sensory tracts of the central nervous system must pass** (Fig. 6–1). Sensory pathways include tracts that arise in the spinal cord, as well as tracts that arise from cranial nerve nuclei within the brainstem itself. The principal ascending spinal tracts are the medial lemniscal pathways (conscious proprioception and fine touch), the anterolateral pathways (pain and temperature), and the spinocerebellar pathways (unconscious proprioception). Important cranial nerve tracts are trigeminal pathways mediating touch and proprioception from the face and mouth and lateral lemniscal pathways (auditory). Major motor pathways include all the descending cortical projections (corticospinal and cortico-bulbar tracts), as well as projections to the spine from the brainstem (reticulospinal, rubrospinal, and vestibulospinal tracts).

The brainstem also contains the nuclei and nerve fibers of 10 of the 12 cranial nerves, which, with one exception (the trochlear nerve), emerge bilaterally from the ventrolateral aspects of the brainstem (Fig. 6–2). The trochlear nerve exits from the dorsal side. The most rostral of these nerves is the oculomotor nerve (III), and the most caudal is the spinal accessory nerve (XI). Although much of the function of the cranial nerves is related to the control of skeletal muscle, some are involved in nonsomatic sensory function and visceral control. In general, the medulla contains the motor neurons for swallowing, tongue movements, talking, and certain visceral-motor functions; the pons contains the motor

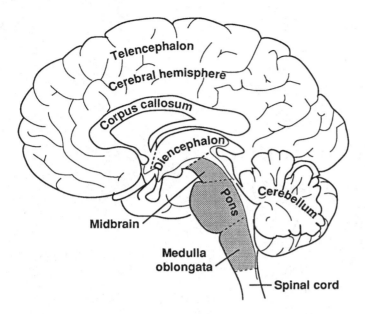

Figure 6–1. *The Major Subdivisions of the Central Nervous System.* The shaded areas constitute the brainstem. (From Noback, CR, Strominger, NL, and Demarest, RJ: The Human Nervous System. Introduction and Review, ed. 4. Copyright © Lea & Febiger, Philadelphia, 1991, p. 6, with permission.)

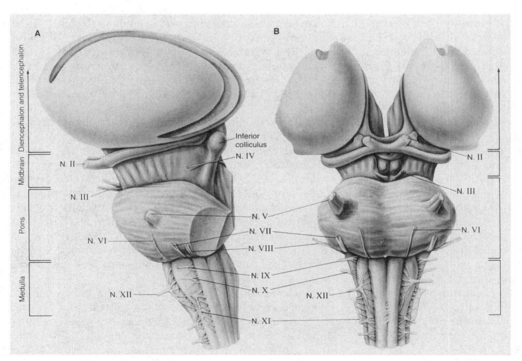

Figure 6–2. *Origins of the Brainstem Cranial Nerves.* (*A*) Lateral view. (*B*) Ventral view. (From Kandel, ER, Schwartz, JH, and Jessell, TM (eds): Principles of Neural Science, ed 3. Appleton & Lange, Norwalk, CT, 1991, p. 720, with permission.)

nuclei associated with facial expression, chewing, and abduction of the eye; and the midbrain contains the nuclei that govern eye movements (excluding abduction), blinking, and pupillary constriction and accommodation.

Dispersed throughout the core of the brainstem are the cells and fibers of the reticular formation. This elaborate neuronal network is entwined with the major tracts and nuclei of the brainstem throughout the medulla, pons, and midbrain. For many years, the reticular formation was thought to be a diffuse system involved primarily in controlling consciousness and modulating the sleep-wakefulness cycle. It is now known to be a highly organized neuronal system with discrete morphologically and biochemically distinct components. It is also known that in addition to its role in arousal, the reticular formation has important physiologic roles in many aspects of motor, sensory, and visceral activity.

Finally, it is important to remember that **the brainstem contains essential elements of the cerebrospinal fluid system, including the cerebral aqueduct (aqueduct of Sylvius) and the fourth ventricle** (Fig. 6–3).[5,6] Cerebrospinal fluid flows into this area through the narrow cerebral aqueduct, which connects the third and fourth ventricles. The fourth ventricle is located at the level of the medulla and pons. These structures form the floor of this ventricle, whereas the ventral cerebellum forms its roof. The fourth ventricle is in turn continuous with the central canal of the spinal cord. Cerebrospinal fluid leaves the ventricular system through three small openings in the roof of the fourth ventricle and then circulates around the brain and spinal cord within the subarachnoid space.

Since an in-depth consideration of all of the various functions of the brainstem is beyond the scope of this chapter, attention here is focused on those aspects of brainstem activity that most directly affect somatic motor control.

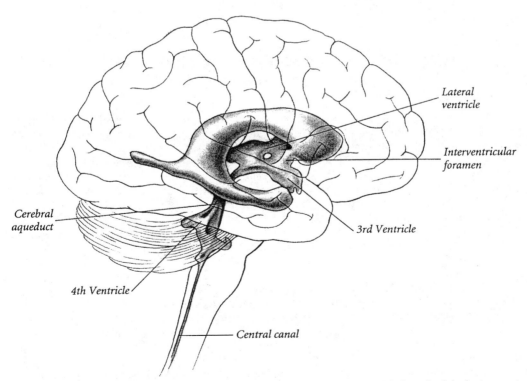

Figure 6–3. *The Ventricles of the Brain.* The fourth ventricle, which forms the roof of much of the brainstem, is connected with the third ventricle by the narrow cerebral aqueduct and is continuous with the central canal of the spinal cord. (From Cohen, H. ed: Neuroscience for Rehabilitation. JB Lippincott, Philadelphia, 1993, p. 18.)

Superficial Anatomy of the Brainstem[1,2,7-9]

The brainstem is not actually a specific anatomic entity, but is a group of neurologic structures that lie beneath the cerebral hemispheres. The definition of what specifically constitutes the brainstem varies somewhat among the scientists and clinicians using this term. According to the most common usage of this designation, the brainstem consists of those portions of the brain that remain after removal of the cerebral and cerebellar hemispheres (see Figs. 6–1 and 6–2). Accordingly, **the brainstem includes the medulla (derived from the myelencephalon), the pons (derived from the metencephalon), and the midbrain (derived from the mesencephalon).** The midbrain is the most rostral component of the brainstem and is continuous with the diencephalon. The midbrain is dominated by the paired superior and inferior colliculi on its posterior surface and by the paired cerebral peduncles on its anterior surface. The pons lies below the midbrain and consists of a large, protruding ventral portion (basis pontis) and the overlying pontine tegmentum, which forms part of the floor of the fourth ventricle. Finally, the medulla consists of a caudal or "closed" portion containing a central canal, which is continuous with the central canal of the spinal cord, and a rostral or "open" portion, in which the central canal expands as the fourth ventricle. Conspicuous in any cursory examination of the brainstem are the numerous pairs of cranial nerves that emerge (with one exception) from the ventrolateral aspects of this structure.

One of the problems with defining the exact boundaries of the brainstem is that certain structures, such as the red nucleus and substantia nigra, extend from the upper midbrain into the diencephalon, blurring the distinction between the two.[15] Other semantic problems arise because some authors include within the brainstem the cerebellum, which is also derived from mesencephalon, as well as part of the diencephalon.[1,7]

Descending Motor Control Tracts to the Spinal Cord

The brainstem contains several groups of neurons or nuclei that give rise to direct projections to the spinal cord.[1,2,10-12] These projections terminate on both spinal interneurons and motor neurons and thereby influence or control motor activity. Descending pathways from the midbrain include rubrospinal, tectospinal, and interstitiospinal tracts; those from the pons and medulla include vestibulospinal and reticulospinal tracts. **The primary pathways in humans are the rubrospinal, reticulospinal, and vestibulospinal tracts.** These pathways are known to be important in the maintenance of posture and muscle tone and in the modulation of spinal cord reflexes.

Descending pathways from the brainstem can be divided into two subgroups on the basis of their terminal distribution and functional properties (Fig. 6–4).[10,12,13] The **medial** (ventromedial) pathways end in the medial ventral horn of the spinal cord and primarily influence interneurons and motor neurons that control the axial musculature bilaterally. Functionally, this system is concerned with balance, control of posture, synergistic whole-limb movements, and coordination of movements of the head and body. Medial pathways include ventral corticospinal tracts, as well as the vestibulospinal, reticulospinal, and tectospinal tracts originating in the brainstem. The **lateral** (dorsolateral) pathways end on the neurons of the lateral spinal gray matter that innervate the more distal muscles of the limbs. Functionally, this system is primarily concerned with control of fine movements of the distal extremities (especially the elbow and hand). The lateral pathways include the large lateral corticospinal tracts, as well as the rubrospinal tracts originating in the brainstem.

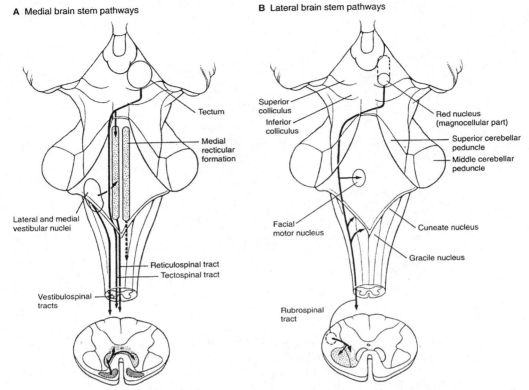

A Medial brain stem pathways

B Lateral brain stem pathways

Figure 6–4. Medial and Lateral Descending Brainstem Pathways. (A) The main medial pathways are the reticulospinal, vestibulospinal, and tectospinal tracts; these control primarily proximal muscles. (B) The main lateral pathway is the rubrospinal tract; this controls primarily distal muscles. (From Kandel, ER, Schwartz, JH, and Jessell, TM (eds): Principles of Neural Science, ed 3. Appleton & Lange, Norwalk, CT, 1991, p. 542, with permission.)

Rubrospinal Tract[10,11,15–18]

The main lateral descending pathway from the brainstem is the rubrospinal tract. Fibers of this tract arise from the red nucleus, an oval cell mass in the rostral part of the midbrain (Fig. 6–5). The red nucleus consists of a rostral component, the parvocellular (small-celled) division, and a caudal component, the magnocellular (large-celled) division.[10,11,15] These components vary markedly in size in different animals. In humans (and apes), the relatively sparse rubrospinal fibers originate in the large-celled component, which is extremely small. In cats, whose rubrospinal pathway is highly developed, tract fibers originate in both the large and small cells of the red nucleus. Rubrospinal fibers cross completely near their origins and descend in the contralateral brainstem giving off collaterals to many areas, including cerebellar and vestibular nuclei.[10–12,15–18] In the spinal cord, the fibers descend ventral and slightly lateral to the lateral corticospinal tracts. The fibers of these two tracts are intermingled and may share some interneurons. Fibers of the rubrospinal tract are somatotopically organized. **Fibers projecting to cervical spinal segments arise from dorsal and dorsomedial parts of the red nucleus, whereas fibers projecting to lumbosacral spinal segments arise from ventral and ventrolateral parts of the nucleus. Thoracic spinal segments receive fibers that arise from an intermediate region of the nucleus.** The sites of termination of the rubrospinal fibers in the spinal cord are about the same as the lateral corticospinal fibers (see Chapter 7). Few rubrospinal fibers reach the lower spinal cord; therefore, the main rubrospinal influence is on muscles of the upper extremities.

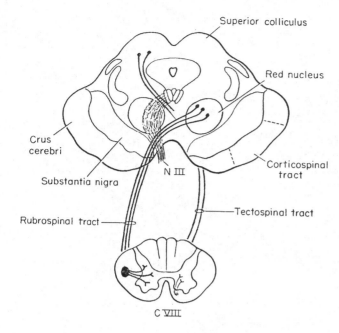

Superior colliculus

Red nucleus

Crus cerebri

Corticospinal tract

Substantia nigra

N III

Tectospinal tract

Rubrospinal tract

C VIII

Figure 6–5. The Rubrospinal and Tectospinal Tracts. The rubrospinal tract arises somatotopically from the magnocellar part of the red nucleus and decussates to descend in the contralateral spinal cord. (From Carpenter,[11] p. 100, with permission.)

The red nucleus receives extensive, somatotopically organized input from the motor cortex and the cerebellum. The synaptic linkage of corticorubral and rubrospinal fibers constitutes a nonpyramidal pathway between the motor cortex and the spinal cord. Fibers from the interposed nuclei of the cerebellum connect portions of the cerebellar cortex somatotopically with the magnocellular part of the red nucleus. Although fibers from the dentate nuclei of the cerebellum pass through or around the red nucleus, few actually terminate in this structure.

Considerable difference of opinion exists over the functional significance of the rubrospinal tract in humans.[10–12,15–18] In other animals such as the cat, this tract is highly developed and plays an important role in motor control. In humans, this tract is small and its cells of origin are few. **It is likely that in humans and apes much of the function of this system has been taken over by the lateral corticospinal tract.** The most important function of the rubrospinal tract may be to influence tone in flexor muscle groups, particularly in the upper extremities. Stimulation of cells in the red nucleus excites contralateral flexor alpha motor neurons, while inhibiting extensor motor neurons. These effects are most evident in distal muscles. The greatest clinical significance of the rubrospinal tract may be that it can mediate some residual motor function after damage to the lateral corticospinal pathways.

Reticulospinal Tracts

The reticular formation is an extensive network of cell clusters, loosely defined nuclei, and nerve fibers that extends throughout the core of the brainstem.[1–3,19–21] At most levels of the brainstem, the reticular formation can be roughly divided into three longitudinal zones. Arranged in a medial to lateral sequence, these regions are the midline raphe nuclei, the medial zone, and the lateral zone.[1–3] The medial zone contains a mixture of large and small neurons and is the source of most of the long ascending and descending projections from the reticular formation. The lateral zone is primarily concerned with cranial nerve reflexes and visceral functions. Specific nuclei or clusters of cells can be further delineated within these general zones using histochemical techniques.

Many of the neurons of the reticular formation are multipolar, with extensive branching of both their dendrites and axons.[2] This branching allows a single reticular neuron to synapse with many other cells and thereby to receive many inputs and exert influence over many other neurons. **Reticular cells project to multiple levels of the spinal cord, as well as to other centers in the brain, including the thalamus and hypothalamus.** Inputs to the reticular formation are innumerable and include collateral branches from primary ascending sensory pathways (anterolateral and lemniscal pathways), fibers from the cerebral cortex and collateral branches from the corticospinal and corticobulbar tracts, projections from other central nervous system structures (cerebellum, basal ganglia, hypothalamus, cranial nerve nuclei, and colliculi), and visceral afferents from the spinal cord and cranial nerves.[2,10,11]

Of particular relevance to motor control is the fact that the reticular formation is a source of several groups of fibers that descend to influence both the motor neurons and the interneurons of the spinal cord (Fig. 6–6).[4,10–12,22] Although the reticular formation extends throughout the brainstem, the reticulospinal fibers originate primarily in the pons and medulla. **The pontine reticulospinal fibers originate in cells in the pontine tegmentum** and descend uncrossed in the medial part of the ventral (anterior) funiculus of the spinal cord (see Chapter 17). **Medullary reticulospinal fibers originate in the medial two thirds of the medullary formation** and project bilaterally (crossed and uncrossed) in the anterior part of the lateral funiculus. Fibers crossing to the opposite side do so in the medulla and are less numerous than the uncrossed fibers. The pontine reticulospinal fibers are more numerous than the medullary fibers and more often descend the entire length of the spinal cord. Pontine fibers terminate primarily in ventromedial parts of the ventral horn (where vestibulospinal tracts also terminate), whereas medullary fibers terminate chiefly in dorsolateral parts of the ventral horn (where corticospinal and rubrospinal fibers also tend to terminate). Accordingly, pontine fibers primarily influence proximal muscle groups, whereas medullary fibers primarily influence more distal muscles. The regions of the reticular formation that give rise to the descending tracts receive input from many sources, but direct projections from widespread areas of the sensorimotor cortex are particularly abundant.

Both pontine and medullary reticulospinal fibers terminate primarily on interneurons of the spinal cord, although some medullary projections probably end directly on alpha motor neurons. Most influences of the reticular formation on **gamma** motor neurons are probably mediated at the segmental level by interneurons. Although neither group of reticulospinal fibers is somatotopically organized, specific regions of the reticular formation may exert their primary influence at particular levels of the spinal cord.

Although the role of the reticular formation in motor control is not entirely understood, it is evident that this system strongly influences segmental somatic reflex activity and hence muscle tone.[1,3,10–12,21–23] **Activity in the pontine reticulospinal fibers generally enhances extensor muscle tone, whereas activity in medullary fibers inhibits this tone. This inherent antagonism between the pontine and medullary influences is important in the support of the body against gravity and in motor behaviors such as locomotion.** During locomotion, for example, phasic activity is apparent in the reticulospinal tracts. These two competing reticulospinal systems receive different inputs. The pontine reticular formation receives important input from the major vestibular nuclei. The vestibulospinal tracts also excite extensor muscle activity in concert with the pontine reticular formation. Together they counteract the force of gravity. The medullary reticular formation, on the other hand, counteracts this antigravity activity in response to inputs from other structures, particularly the cerebral cortex.

Presumably, the cerebral cortex uses the medullary reticular system to diminish antigravity activity (i.e., muscle extension) during volitional movements requiring muscle flexion. The excessive activation of extensor motor neurons in decerebrate rigidity may in part reflect a gross imbalance in these opposing influences (see Chapter 12). With destruction of all descending pathways from above the pons (decerebration), descending cortical excitation of the medullary reticular system is lost. This results in a loss of the medullary inhibition of muscle tone and excessive pontine facilitation of extensor activity.

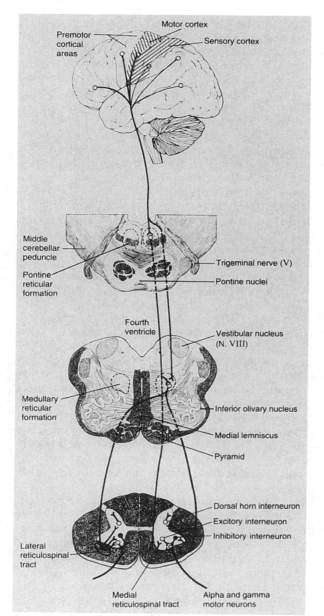

Premotor cortical areas
Motor cortex
Sensory cortex

Middle cerebellar peduncle
Pontine reticular formation
Trigeminal nerve (V)
Pontine nuclei

Fourth ventricle
Vestibular nucleus (N. VIII)

Medullary reticular formation
Inferior olivary nucleus
Medial lemniscus
Pyramid

Dorsal horn interneuron
Excitory interneuron
Inhibitory interneuron

Lateral reticulospinal tract

Medial reticulospinal tract
Alpha and gamma motor neurons

Figure 6–6.   The Reticulospinal and Corticoreticular Tracts. Pontine reticulospinal fibers originate in the pontine tegmentum and descend uncrossed in the medial part of the ventral funiculus of the spinal cord. Medullary reticulospinal fibers project bilaterally in the ventral part of the lateral funiculus of the spinal cord. (From Kandel, ER, Schwartz, JH, and Jessell, TM(eds): Principles of Neural Science, ed 3. Appleton & Lange, Norwalk, CT, 1991, p 601, with permission.)

The reticulospinal tracts mediate influences arising in both the reticular formation itself and other regions of the brain. For example, the regions of the reticular formation that give rise to these descending tracts receive extensive input from widespread areas of the motor cortex. These corticoreticulospinal connections may represent a significant nonpyramidal route by which the motor cortex can influence spinal segmental activity. This "alternate" pathway may become particularly important when the primary control pathways (corticospinal) are damaged. By the same token, the reticular formation has extensive connections with subcortical structures, such as the cerebellum, basal ganglia, and red nucleus, and undoubtedly participates in their involvement in motor control. The reticulospinal tracts may also carry motor commands generated within the reticular formation itself.[1] Much like the spinal cord (see Chapter 5), the reticular formation probably contains the neuronal circuitry necessary for generating relatively complex patterns of movement. A cat, for example, whose brainstem has been surgically separated from its diencephalon can, after a recovery period, walk and run spontaneously, right itself, and assume a variety of complex postures. Although a human with such a lesion would have so much rigidity that he or she could not demonstrate such motor behaviors, these types of experiments do suggest that some motor programming may arise in the reticular formation.

An additional group of medullary reticulospinal neurons descends in the dorsolateral column of the spinal cord and terminates in the dorsal horn. These pathways have a more significant influence on transmission in sensory systems than on motor pathways. They have been specifically implicated in the inhibition of pain transmission in the spinal cord.

Vestibulospinal Tracts

Maintenance of equilibrium requires both the ability to support the head and body against gravity and the ability to keep the body aligned and balanced over its base of support (the feet). This capability is necessary for all locomotor activity. To maintain balance and equilibrium, continuous information must be provided about the position and motion of all body parts. Three sources provide this information: the eyes, the proprioceptors throughout the body, and the vestibular apparatus of the inner ear.

The principal sensory organ of equilibrium is the vestibular apparatus. This elaborate sense organ is housed within a system of bony tubes and chambers located in the temporal skull, called the **bony labyrinth.**[4,24-27] The sensory apparatus contained within this bony housing is composed of a system of delicate membranous tubes and sacs, called the **membranous labyrinth.** The labyrinth is specifically composed of the cochlea, three semicircular ducts, and two large chambers, known as the utricle and saccule. The cochlea is the major sense organ for hearing and is not discussed here. The utricle, saccule, and semicircular ducts are involved in equilibrium. The utricle and saccule detect the orientation of the head with respect to gravity, especially during linear acceleration. The semicircular ducts detect rotary (angular) movement of the head, especially when accompanied by acceleration or deceleration.

The labyrinths are innervated by the vestibular portion of the eighth cranial nerve, and much of their output is transmitted to the vestibular nuclei located in the brainstem. A significant portion of the output of the labyrinths also goes directly to the vestibular parts of the cerebellum, particularly to the nodulus and ventral uvula (see Chapter 8). From the vestibulocerebellum, secondary afferents then go to the vestibular nuclei.

Inputs to the vestibular nuclei thus come primarily from the vestibular labyrinth and cerebellum.[4,10,11,25-27] Cerebellar projections are extensive, with both the cerebellar cortex and fastigial nuclei projecting to all four nuclei. Fibers also arrive from the reticular formation. The nuclei receive additional information from other sensory systems, the most important of which are the visual system and proprioceptors in various parts of the body, especially the neck and bottoms of the feet. Visual information is important in the maintenance of equilibrium. After complete destruction of the vestibular apparatus and even after loss of most proprioceptive information from the body, a person can maintain almost normal equilibrium as long as their eyes are open and they move slowly. Pressure sensations from the feet provide information regarding the distribution of weight between the two feet and the extent to which the weight is forward or backward. Because the vestibular apparatus detects the orientation and movement of only the head, it is essential that information be provided depicting the orientation of the head with respect to the body. This information is provided by proprioceptors of the neck and other parts of the body. This feedback flows directly to the vestibular and reticular nuclei of the brainstem, as well as indirectly to these nuclei by way of the cerebellum.

The vestibular nuclear complex contains four main structures (superior, medial, lateral, and inferior nuclei) and some smaller cell groups[10,11,16,24-27] (Fig. 6-7). The nuclei are

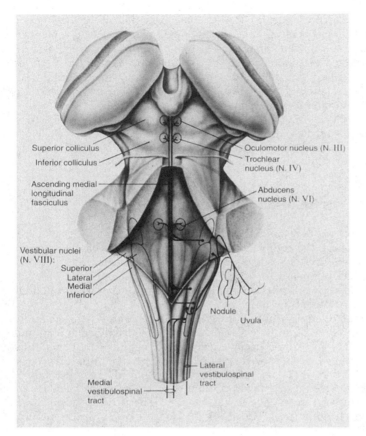

Figure 6–7. The Vestibular Nuclei and Their Connections. (From Kandel ER, Schwartz, JH, and Jessell, TM (eds): Principles of Neural Science, ed 3. Appleton & Lange, Norwalk, CT, 1991, p 509, with permission.)

located in the floor of the fourth ventricle, extending from the medulla a short distance into the pons. **The vestibular nuclei give rise to two descending vestibulospinal tracts. The main tract is the** *lateral* **vestibulospinal tract, which originates in the lateral vestibular nucleus, and is activated primarily by inputs from the utricle and saccule.** The fibers of this tract descend uncrossed (ipsilaterally) the length of the spinal cord in the anterior part of the lateral funiculus. Fiber terminations are most abundant in cervical and lower lumbar segments, where synaptic connections are made with the interneurons and alpha and gamma motor neurons of extensor muscles. **The** *medial* **vestibulospinal pathways arise primarily (but probably not exclusively) from the medial vestibular nuclei** and descend through the brainstem to the medial part of the ventral funiculus of the spinal cord. These fibers descend bilaterally to cervical and upper thoracic levels of the spinal cord and synapse both directly and through interneurons on motor neurons that innervate neck and back muscles. **These pathways are influenced chiefly by inputs from the semicircular ducts. Both tracts facilitate extensor motor neurons and inhibit flexor motor neurons in predominantly proximal muscles.**

Information generated by the vestibular labyrinth is used by the vestibular nuclei in the context of the so-called *vestibular reflexes.*[4,13,22,27–31] This group of reflexes causes actions on muscles of both the limbs (vestibulospinal reflexes) and neck (vestibulocollic reflexes) that are essential for the maintenance of proper posture and equilibrium. **Impulses in the lateral vestibulospinal tracts activate extensor limb muscles that support posture and resist falling.** For example, when the head is rotated to the left, extensor activity (postural support) increases on the left side. This increased support resists the tendency for the subject to fall to the left as head rotation continues. A disease process that eliminates labyrinthine function in the left ear causes the person to fall to the left. Conversely, a disease that irritates the right labyrinth causes the person to fall to the right. **Impulses in the medial vestibulospinal tracts cause contraction of neck muscles that tend to keep the head stable by opposing head movement.** For example, when the head is tilted forward without bending the neck, these reflexes return the head to the vertical position by contracting the dorsal neck muscles.

The vestibular reflexes function in concert with a group of *neck reflexes*, which are triggered by bending or turning the head relative to the body.[4,13,22,27-31] These reflexes are mediated by spindles in the neck muscles and receptors in the joints of the upper cervical vertebrae rather than input from the vestibular apparatus and evoke reflexive responses in both neck muscles (cervicocollic reflexes) and limb muscles (cervicospinal reflexes). Cervicocollic reflexes contract neck muscles that are stretched when the neck is bent and act in synergy with the vestibulocollic reflexes to realign the head. In contrast, the actions of the cervicospinal reflexes on limb muscles generally oppose those of the vestibulospinal reflexes.

The vestibular and neck reflexes are readily elicited in newborns and in patients with major cerebral lesions by tilting the head or bending the neck.[22] In normal adults, however, these effects are minimal. Passive bending or turning of the head produces only small changes in muscle activity, which are detectable only by electromyographic recordings. If the vestibular apparatus is damaged, however, the neck reflexes may become more prominent.

Activity in both the vestibulospinal tracts and the pontine reticulospinal tract enhance extensor muscle tone. In humans and many other animals, transection of the brainstem above the level of the vestibular nuclei but below the red nucleus produces a condition called **decerebrate rigidity.**[22,27] In quadrupeds, this condition is characterized by tonic extension of all four limbs in what looks like an exaggerated reaction against gravity. When decerebration is produced in primates or when it occurs in patients, a much less pronounced exaggeration of extensor tone occurs. In either case, it is likely that without the inhibitory influences of higher centers, the vestibulospinal and reticulospinal pathways are producing a heightened (disinhibited) facilitation of extensor tone. When transection of the brainstem occurs above the level of the red nucleus and other midbrain nuclei, decerebrate rigidity no longer occurs, presumably because the red nucleus and other midbrain nuclei serve to suppress or oppose the activity of the vestibulospinal and reticulospinal systems of the lower brainstem.

Humans with extensive lesions of the cerebral hemispheres, but whose brainstem is still intact, exhibit a postural state known as **decorticate rigidity.** In this condition, the extensors of the legs and flexors of the arms contract steadily. One possible explanation for this is that the rubrospinal tract in humans projects only as far as the cervical cord and may therefore be able to counteract vestibulospinal facilitation of arm, but not leg, extension.

Tectospinal and Interstitiospinal Tracts

Two additional tracts descend from the midbrain to the spinal cord. Both of these tracts are small, and little is known about their function in humans. The tectospinal tract originates in the superior colliculus of the rostral midbrain, crosses to the opposite side of the brainstem, and projects only as far as the cervical spinal segments.[10,14] This tract is believed to influence (via effects on interneurons) motor neurons to neck and possibly shoulder and upper trunk muscles. The principal input to the superior colliculus is from the visual cortex, and so the tract may take part in head- and neck-orienting reactions to visual stimuli. The other small descending tract is the interstitiospinal tract, which arises from cells in the interstitial nucleus of Cajal in the rostral midbrain and projects ipsilaterally along the entire length of the spinal cord.[10] Although inputs to this nucleus are known to originate in vestibular nuclei and cerebral cortex, the significance of this tract in humans is unknown. It may be involved in visual-motor coordination.

Table 6–1. *Brainstem Cranial Nerves*

Cranial Nerve	Functions
Medulla	
XII Hypoglossal	Motor to muscles of tongue
XI Spinal accessory	Motor to sternocleidomastoid and trapezius muscles
X Vagus	Motor to muscles of soft palate, pharynx, and larynx; parasympathetic fibers to thoracic and abdominal viscera; sensory fibers from pharynx and external auditory meatus; visceral sensory fibers from chest and abdominal cavity
IX Glossopharyngeal	Motor to pharyngeal muscles; sensory from pharynx, middle ear, and tongue; taste from posterior tongue; parasympathetic to salivary glands
Pons	
VIII Vestibulocochlear	Hearing and equilibrium
VII Facial	Motor to muscles of facial expression and stapedius of middle ear; parasympathetic to salivary and lacrimal glands; taste sensation from anterior tongue
VI Abducens	Motor to lateral rectus muscle of eye
V Trigeminal	Sensory from face; motor to muscles of mastication
Midbrain	
IV Trochlear	Motor to superior oblique muscle of eye
III Oculomotor	Motor to medial, superior, and inferior recti; inferior oblique muscles of eye and levator palpebrae of eyelid; parasympathetic to constrictors of pupil

Cranial Nerves[3,15,32–34]

The brainstem is also the site of origin of the majority of the cranial nerves. **Ten of the twelve pairs of cranial nerves enter and exit from various locations along the brainstem** (Table 6–1; see Fig. 6–2). In many respects, these nerves are analogous to the spinal nerves. Most emerge from the brainstem as cranial roots and pass through narrow bony foramina to reach the periphery. As in the spinal cord, the cell bodies of motor and sensory neurons are found in separate locations. The cell bodies of cranial motor neurons are located in motor nuclei within the brainstem and are analogous to the anterior horn cells congregated in the ventral horn of the spinal cord. The cell bodies of sensory fibers are found outside the brainstem, either in ganglia analogous to the dorsal root ganglia or within specialized end organs such as the eye. The peripheral cranial nerves are composed of a variable mixture of motor and sensory fibers and are structurally similar to the peripheral nerves originating in the spinal cord (see Chapter 15). Because of the presence of special sense organs, widespread connections with the body viscera, and the mixed embryologic origins of the muscles of the head, the cranial nerves contain several more classes of motor and sensory fibers than do the spinal nerves (Table 6–2).

The cranial nerves subserve many different physiologic functions. They are involved in various types of sensory perception, in autonomic regulation of many viscera, and in somatic motor activity. The senses of olfaction, sight, hearing, equilibrium, and taste all are centered in the head and are mediated by cranial nerves. Specifically, the olfactory and optic nerves project directly to the telencephalon and diencephalon, respectively; the others project to the brainstem. Preganglionic parasympathetic autonomic fibers arise from the brainstem to synapse with parasympathetic postganglionic fibers that regulate the lacrimal (tear), salivary, and sweat glands, blood vessels, smooth muscle of the pupil, and the activity of various body cavity viscera. In the vagus, the effector terminations are widespread, distributed throughout the viscera of the body cavities. Of most direct relevance to somatic function are the group of cranial nerves arising in the brainstem, which innervate the striated muscle of the head and neck.

Eight of the ten pairs of cranial nerves that emerge from the brainstem contain motor fibers controlling skeletal muscle (see Table 6–1).[3,15,32–34] As distinct from the

Table 6-2. Functional Classes of Cranial Nerves

Classification	Functions	Structures Innervated	Cranial Nerves
Sensory Fibers			
General somatic	Touch, pain, temperature, and proprioception	Skin, skeletal muscles of head and neck, mucous membrane of mouth, and teeth	V, VII, IX, X
Special somatic	Hearing, vision, balance	Cochlea, vestibular apparatus, retina	II, VIII
General visceral	Mechanical, pain, temperature, and proprioception	Pharynx, larynx, gut	V, VII, IX, X
Special visceral	Olfaction, taste	Taste buds, olfactory epithelium	I, VII, IX, X
Motor Fibers			
General somatic	Skeletal muscle control (somites)	Extraocular and tongue muscles	III, IV, VI, XII
General visceral	Autonomic control	Tear glands, sweat glands, gut	III, VII, IX, X
Special visceral	Skeletal muscle control (branchiomeric)	Muscles of facial expression, jaw, neck, larynx, and pharynx	V, VII, IX, X, XI

From Role and Kelly,[3] with permission.

rest of the body, however, the "bulbar" striated muscles have two different embryologic origins and are thus innervated by two distinct classes of neurons.[3,32-34] *Somatic* motor neurons innervate the extraocular muscles and the intrinsic muscles of the tongue (via nerves III, IV, VI, and XII). These muscles develop from the myotomes of the embryo in a manner similar to that of other striated muscles throughout the body. The somatic motor neurons resemble the large alpha motor neurons of the spinal cord. The *special visceral* (branchiomeric) motor neurons innervate the striated muscles of facial expression, the jaw (chewing), neck, larynx, and pharynx (via nerves V, VII, IX, X, and XI). These muscles develop from the branchial arches of the embryo.

The cranial nerve nuclei are arranged in six longitudinal columns within the brainstem (Fig. 6-8).[3,32,33] In general, columns containing nuclei that mediate cranial motor function are located medially, whereas sensory columns are located laterally. On the floor of the fourth ventricle, the sulcus limitans forms a boundary between the sensory and motor columns. The motor neurons that innervate the somatic muscles of the head arise from the nuclei of the somatic motor column, the most medial of the columns. This column is adjacent to the midline, immediately ventral to the floor of the fourth ventricle. The motor neurons that control the branchiomeric muscles arise from the nuclei of the special visceral column. They are lateral to the somatic motor column, but remain medial to the sulcus limitans.

The somatic motor column contains three nuclei which contain motor neurons that innervate extraocular muscles (the oculomotor, trochlear, and abducens nuclei) and the hypoglossal nucleus which controls the muscles of the tongue. Unlike other skeletal muscles, the extraocular muscles are not controlled by descending pathways from the primary motor cortex. The extraocular motor nuclei are controlled by projections from the frontal eye field and parieto-occipital eye field. The hypoglossal nucleus receives a predominantly contralateral projection from the motor cortex.

The special visceral column contains four cranial nerve nuclei (trigeminal, facial, and accessory nuclei and the nucleus ambiguous). The trigeminal motor nucleus, the most rostral of this column, innervates the muscles of mastication via the trigeminal nerve (V). This nucleus receives bilateral projections from the motor cortex. The facial nucleus

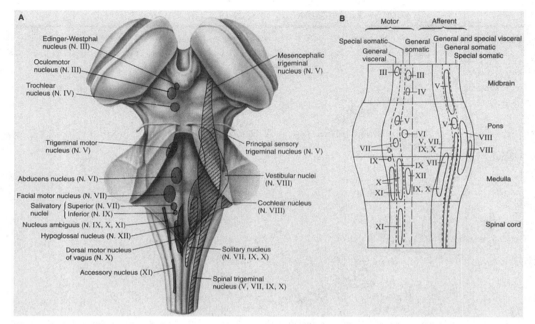

Figure 6–8. *Organization of the Cranial Nerve Nuclei into Discontinuous Columns.* (A) Dorsal view of the brainstem illustrates the location of the motor (*Left*) and sensory (*Right*) nuclei. (B) Schematic dorsal view of the columnar organization of the nuclei. (From Kandel, ER, Schwartz, JH, and Jessell, TM (eds): Principles of Neural Science, ed 3. Appleton & Lange, Norwalk, CT, 1991, p 688, with permission.)

innervates the muscles of facial expression via the facial nerve (VII). Note that motor neurons that innervate muscles of the upper face receive bilateral input from the motor cortex, whereas those innervating muscles of the lower face are controlled unilaterally by the contralateral motor cortex. Unlike the other cranial nerve nuclei, the nucleus ambiguus contains motor neurons whose axons contribute to multiple cranial nerves. This nucleus innervates the muscles of the palate, pharynx, and larynx via the glossopharyngeal nerve (IX), the vagus nerve (X), and the cranial root of the spinal accessory nerve (XI). The motor cortex exerts bilateral control over these muscles. The accessory nucleus is located at the caudal extreme of the brainstem at the junction of the medulla and spinal cord. This nucleus begins at the pyramidal decussation and may extend into the cord as far as the fifth cervical segment. Motor neurons arising in the accessory nucleus innervate the sternocleidomastoid and trapezius muscles. These fibers travel in the spinal root of the spinal accessory nerve, whereas the nucleus ambiguous motor neurons travel in the cranial root of this nerve.

As with spinal cord lesions, **an understanding of the functional consequences of lesions within the brainstem cranial nerve system may be derived from a knowledge of the organization of the cranial nerves and their nuclei.** For example, knowledge of the specific location of the motor and sensory columns within the brainstem explains the functional deficits created by discrete lesions within the brainstem. In the skeletal muscle motor columns, midline damage would have its greatest impact on somatic muscle control, whereas more lateral damage would have a greater impact on the branchiomeric muscles. By the same token, lesions at different levels of the brainstem affect different cranial nerve nuclei and hence specific muscles. Careful testing of the function of these muscle groups in a neurologic examination can define precisely the location of a specific lesion.

Even though the nuclei of motor, sensory, and autonomic cranial nerves lie in distinct regions within the brainstem, considerable mixing of different fiber types occurs in the periphery. Not only is there intermingling of fiber types within individual cranial nerves but also branches of different cranial nerves may be closely associated in their course through the periphery. This implies that a relatively small peripheral lesion may adversely affect a variety of functions simultaneously. For example, a lesion of the facial nerve as it exits from the brainstem may disturb the secretion of tears, alter hearing, and produce paralysis of the muscles of facial expression.[3]

Like the motor neurons of the spinal cord, the motor nuclei of the brainstem may receive either unilateral (contralateral) or bilateral projections from the motor cortex. Muscles innervated by motor neurons that receive bilateral input are little affected by a unilateral lesion of the motor cortex or its descending pathways.[3,33,35] Intact projections from the nonaffected side maintain normal or near normal muscle control. Muscles subject to only contralateral cortical control, however, are severely affected by disruption of this control. A classic example of this dichotomy is apparent in the effects of a contralateral lesion on the activity of the upper and lower facial muscles.[2,3,33] After a unilateral lesion of the descending corticobulbar fibers, the *bilaterally innervated* upper facial muscles retain the intact input from the side opposite the lesion and are thus relatively unaffected. The unilaterally innervated lower facial muscles are severely affected on the side contralateral to the lesion because their sole cortical input has been interrupted. Most cranial motor nerves receive bilateral cortical input; the major exceptions are the hypoglossal and lower facial nerves.

Clinical Implications of Brainstem Damage[35-38]

So many neuronal pathways and nuclei are crowded into the brainstem that with any brainstem damage, the potential exists for the pathologic disruption of many physiologic functions (Table 6–3). Even small lesions can have significant consequences. The consequences of widespread damage or suppression of brainstem function may be catastrophic, leading to the depression of vital functions such as consciousness, respiration, and cardiovascular control, and often to death.

One of the vital components of the brainstem is the reticular activating system.[19-21,39] This portion of the reticular formation is the primary mechanism responsible for maintaining consciousness. Brainstem reticular activating system neurons project

Table 6–3. *Potential Clinical Manifestations of Brainstem Damage*

Functional Deficits	Structures Damaged
Spinal muscle weakness	Corticospinal tracts
Cranial muscle weakness (larynx, pharynx, tongue, palate, jaw, face, neck, and extraocular)	Corticobulbar tracts or cranial nerves
Impaired touch, position, and vibratory sense	Medial lemniscus
Impaired cutaneous sensation in face and proprioception in jaw	Trigeminal tracts or nuclei
Impaired sense of pain and temperature	Anterolateral (spinothalamic) tracts
Limb ataxia and nystagmus	Cerebellar connections
Involuntary movements (tremor, chorea, athetosis)	Red nucleus
Deafness, tinnitus	Vestibulocochlear nerve or cochlear nucleus
Loss of taste	Solitary nucleus and associated tracts
Autonomic disturbances (miosis, ptosis, impaired sweating, abnormal respiration, cardiovascular abnormalities)	Autonomic tracts or nuclei
Vertigo, nausea, and vomiting	Vestibular nucleus and its connections
Nystagmus, diplopia, and oscillopsia	Vestibular nucleus and its connections
Decreased consciousness, stupor, or coma	Reticular formation
Hiccups	Uncertain (medullary respiratory centers?)

diffusely to the cerebral cortex, primarily via "nonspecific" thalamic nuclei. These projections exert powerful influences on broad areas of the cerebral hemispheres, evoking changes in the electroencephalographic pattern (EEG) that are associated with alertness and wakefulness. A healthy cerebral cortex cannot by itself maintain a conscious state (no matter what the sensory input), but depends on this activation by the reticular activating system.

The cerebral hemispheres, the reticular activating system, and the connections among them all participate in maintaining normal consciousness.[20,39] Accordingly, the principal causes of loss of consciousness (i.e., coma) are bilateral hemispheral damage or suppression by drugs or toxins and brainstem lesions that damage or suppress the reticular activating system. Large lesions in one or both hemispheres may also compress the brainstem, indirectly causing coma by damaging the reticular activating system.

In humans, lesions of the brainstem often produce disturbances of consciousness, which range from fleeting unconsciousness to sustained coma. With lesions of the lower brainstem, unconsciousness is often accompanied by respiratory and cardiovascular disturbances.[20] The loss of consciousness is frequently sudden and accompanied by life-threatening depression of vital functions. Lesions of the upper brainstem most frequently produce hypersomnia, characterized by muscle relaxation, slow respiration, and an EEG pattern characteristic of sleep.[20] If the patient develops decerebrate rigidity, coma has usually developed. At all levels of the brainstem, the likelihood of unconsciousness is related to the rapidity with which lesions develop. Lesions associated with hemorrhage usually produce sudden coma. On the other hand, slowly developing lesions (e.g., tumors) may not disturb consciousness for a considerable period of time.

Also located within the brainstem are several groups of cells or "centers," which are responsible for regulating specific visceral activities, particularly in the respiratory and cardiovascular systems.[40] Destruction of some areas of the medulla produces changes in heart rate, blood pressure, and peripheral circulation. Destructive lesions in the medulla and pons may result in abnormal patterns of respiration, hiccups, or total loss of breathing. Extensive interruption of brainstem activity is likely to produce both loss of consciousness and catastrophic disruption of vital visceral function.

More to the point of this chapter, **the brainstem is also the site of many important fiber tracts and nuclei involved in somatosensation and motor control.** As discussed in previous sections, important sensory (e.g., medial lemniscal and spinothalamic) and motor (e.g., corticospinal and corticobulbar) tracts traverse the brainstem, having arisen elsewhere in the central nervous system or having originated within the brainstem itself (e.g., cranial nerves and their nuclei). Destructive lesions within the brainstem may involve either sensory or motor tracts or both.

Although the potential always exists for disastrous outcomes, brainstem lesions vary markedly in severity. For example, small lesions just outside the brainstem, may interfere with individual cranial nerves. Small, isolated lesions in the corticospinal tracts of the medullary pyramids or basis pontis may produce a pure contralateral motor hemiplegia without cranial nerve or sensory tract involvement. Bilateral pontine lesions, on the other hand, may create such extensive impairment that a "locked-in" syndrome is produced in which a patient exists essentially as an alert consciousness unable to move or communicate.[35-38,41] As a result of interruption of the corticospinal and corticobulbar tracts on both sides, the patient with bilateral pontine lesions is quadriplegic, unable to speak, and incapable of facial movements. Although this state may resemble coma, the reticular formation is actually not injured and the patient is fully awake. Because the supranuclear ocular pathways lie dorsally, they are spared. Thus, vertical eye movements and blinking are intact and provide the only means of communication. In the most extensive and severe lesions of the brainstem, motor and sensory dysfunction is combined with coma and respiratory failure, progressing to death.

Because the cranial nerve nuclei and long-tract fibers are highly regimented within the brainstem, assessment of the functional status of the systems dependent on these pathways or nuclei can provide invaluable information regarding the precise location and extent of brainstem damage. At levels below the midbrain, lesions in long ascending and descending tracts lead to signs that indicate the extent to which damage is medial or lateral. Cranial nerve signs provide information about the level of the lesion. Modern imaging techniques confirm these impressions.

Vascular Lesions

Vascular lesions are among the most common and severe of the various pathologic conditions affecting the brainstem.[35-38] The typical clinical presentation of brainstem stroke is a "crossed" involvement of long tracts passing through the brainstem with deficits of cranial nerve nuclei (see Chapter 21). In these patients, the cranial nerve palsy (weakness) is ipsilateral to the lesion, whereas the long-tract signs are contralateral—hence, the term, "crossed." A good example of this dichotomy is the so-called medial medullary syndrome, which results from occlusion of the anterior spinal artery or its parent vertebral artery.[35-38] The anterior spinal artery supplies the ipsilateral pyramid, medial lemniscus, and hypoglossal nerve and nucleus. Its occlusion thus results in the following signs:

1. **Ipsilateral** paresis, atrophy, and fibrillation of the tongue (due to cranial nerve XII involvement). The protruded tongue deviates toward the lesion and away from the hemiplegia.
2. **Contralateral** hemiplegia (due to involvement of the pyramid) with sparing of the face.
3. **Contralateral** loss of position and vibratory sensation (due to involvement of the medial lemniscus).

The more dorsolateral spinothalamic tract is usually unaffected, so pain and temperature sensation are spared. Because the hypoglossal fibers run somewhat laterally to the medial lemniscus and pyramid, they are also occasionally spared. In some instances, only the pyramid is damaged, resulting in a **pure motor hemiplegia**, which spares the face.[37]

Many other specific ischemic brainstem syndromes have been described, each presenting with its own constellation of clinical features that reflect the level and extent of the lesion involved (see Chapter 21).[35-38]

Other Lesions of the Brainstem

Not all lesions in the brainstem are vascular in origin. Damage may also be produced directly by primary brainstem tumor, demyelination, or abscess, traumatic contusion and hemorrhage, encephalitis, and the effects of drugs or other toxins. Large lesions or other conditions displacing the cerebral hemispheres may compress or twist the tissue of the brainstem, indirectly damaging it.

RECOMMENDED READINGS

Brazis, PW: The Localization of Lesions Affecting in Brainstem. Chapter 14. In Brazis, PW, Masdeu, JC, and Biller, J (eds): Localization in Clinical Neurology, ed 2. Little, Brown & Company, Boston, 1990.

Daube, JR, et al (eds): Medical Neurosciences: An Approach to Anatomy, Pathology, and Physiology by Systems and Levels, ed 2. Chapter 14. The Posterior Fossa Level. Little, Brown & Company, Boston, 1986.

Fox, CR and Cohen, H: The Visual and Vestibular Systems. Chapter 5. In Cohen, H: Neuroscience for Rehabilitation. JB Lippincott, Philadelphia, 1993.

Guyton, AC: Textbook of Medical Physiology, ed 8. Chapter 55. Cortical and Brainstem Control of Motor Function. WB Saunders, Philadelphia, 1991.

Kelly, JP: The Sense of Balance. Chapter 33. In Kandel, ER, Schwartz, JH, and Jessell, TM (eds): Principles of Neural Science, ed 3. Appleton & Lange, Norwalk, CT, 1991.

Martin, JH: Neuroanatomy: Text and Atlas. Chapter 9. Descending Projection Systems and the Motor Function of the Spinal Cord. Appleton & Lange, Norwalk, CT, 1989.

Martin, JH: Neuroanatomy: Text and Atlas. Chapter 12. General Organization of the Cranial Nerve Nuclei and the Trigeminal System. Appleton & Lange, Norwalk, CT, 1989.

Martin, JH: Neuroanatomy: Text and Atlas. Chapter 13. The Somatic and Visceral Motor Functions of the Cranial Nerves. Appleton & Lange, Norwalk, CT, 1989.

Mitz, AR and Winstein, C: The Motor System I: Lower Centers. Chapter 7. In Cohen, H (ed): Neuroscience for Rehabilitation. JB Lippincott, Philadelphia, 1993.

Nolte, J: The Human Brain: An Introduction to Its Function, ed 3. Chapter 8. The Brainstem. Mosby-Year Book, St. Louis, 1993.

Role, LW and Kelly, JP: The Brainstem: Cranial Nerve Nuclei and the Monoaminergic Systems. Chapter 44. In Kandel, ER, Schwartz, JH, and Jessell, TM (eds): Principles of Neural Science, ed 3. Appleton & Lange, Norwalk, CT, 1991.

Ropper, AH and Martin, JB: Coma and Other Disorders of Consciousness. Chapter 26. In Isselbacher, KJ, et al (eds): Harrison's Principles of Internal Medicine, ed 13. McGraw-Hill, New York, 1994.

Rothwell, JC: Control of Human Voluntary Movement. Chapter 7. Ascending and Descending Pathways of the Spinal Cord. Aspen Publishers, Rockville, MD, 1987.

Rowland, LP: Clinical Syndromes of the Spinal Cord and Brainstem. Chapter 46. In Kandel, ER, Schwartz, JH, and Jessell, TM (eds): Principles of Neural Science, ed 3. Appleton & Lange, Norwalk, CT, 1991.

Stern, BJ, Wityk, RJ, and Lewis, RF: Disorders of the Cranial Nerves and Brainstem. Chapter 40. In Joynt, RJ (ed): Clinical Neurology, vol 3. JB Lippincott, Philadelphia, 1993.

Wall, M: Brainstem Syndromes. Chapter 30. In Bradley, WG, et al (eds): Neurology in Clinical Practice, vol II. Butterworth-Heinemann, Boston, 1990.

REFERENCES

1. Nolte, J: The Human Brain: An Introduction to Its Function, ed 3. Chapter 8. The Brainstem. Mosby-Year Book, St. Louis, 1993.

2. Daube, JR, et al (eds): Medical Neurosciences: An Approach to Anatomy, Pathology, and Physiology by Systems and Levels, ed 2. Chapter 14. The Posterior Fossa Level. Little, Brown & Company, Boston, 1986.

3. Role, LW and Kelly, JP: The Brainstem: Cranial Nerve Nuclei and the Monoaminergic Systems. Chapter 44. In Kandel, ER, Schwartz, JH, and Jessell, TM (eds): Principles of Neural Science, ed 3. Appleton & Lange, Norwalk, CT, 1991.

4. Guyton, AC: Textbook of Medical Physiology, ed 8. Chapter 55. Cortical and Brainstem Control of Motor Function. WB Saunders, Philadelphia, 1991.

5. Daube, JR, et al (eds): Medical Neurosciences: An Approach to Anatomy, Pathology, and Physiology by Systems and Levels, ed 2. Chapter 6. The Cerebrospinal Fluid System. Little, Brown & Company, Boston, 1986.

6. Nolte, J: The Human Brain: An Introduction to Its Functional Anatomy, ed 3. Chapter 4. Ventricles and Cerebrospinal Fluid. Mosby-Year Book, St. Louis, 1993.

7. Martin, JH: Neuroanatomy: Text and Atlas. Chapter 3. Internal Organization of the Central Nervous System. Appleton & Lange, Norwalk, CT, 1989.

8. Carpenter, MB: Core Text of Neuroanatomy, ed 4. Chapter 2. Gross Anatomy of the Brain. Williams & Wilkins, Baltimore, 1991.

9. Barr, ML and Kiernan, JA: The Human Nervous System, ed 6. Chapter 6. Brainstem: External Anatomy. JB Lippincott, Philadelphia, 1993.

10. Rothwell, JC: Control of Human Voluntary Movement. Chapter 7. Ascending and Descending Pathways of the Spinal Cord. Aspen Publishers, Rockville, MD, 1987.

11. Carpenter, MB: Neuroanatomy, ed 4. Williams & Wilkins, Baltimore, 1991.

12. Mitz, AR and Winstein, C: The Motor System I: Lower Centers. Chapter 7. In Cohen, H (ed): Neuroscience for Rehabilitation. JB Lippincott, Philadelphia, 1993.

13. Willis, WD, Jr: Descending Pathways Involved in Motor Control. Chapter 13. In Berne, RM and Levy, MN (eds): Physiology, ed 3. Mosby-Year Book, St. Louis, 1993.

14. Martin, JH: Neuroanatomy: Text and Atlas. Chapter 9. Descending Projection Systems and the Motor Function of the Spinal Cord. Appleton & Lange, Norwalk, CT, 1989.

15. Barr, ML and Kiernan, JA: The Human Nervous System, ed 6. Chapter 7. Brainstem: Nuclei and Tracts. JB Lippincott, Philadelphia. 1993.

16. Nathan, PW and Smith, MC: The Rubrospinal and Central Tegmental Tracts in Man. Brain 105:223, 1982.

17. Cheney, PD, Fetz, EE, and Mewes, K: Neural Mechanisms Underlying Corticospinal and Rubrospinal Control of Limb Movements. Prog Brain Res 87:213, 1991.

18. Houk, JC: Red Nucleus: Role in Motor Control. Curr Opin Neurobiol 1(4):610, 1991.

19. Barr, ML and Kiernan, JA: The Human Nervous System, ed 6. Chapter 9. Reticular Formation. JB Lippincott, Philadelphia, 1993.

20. Carpenter, MB: Core Text of Neuroanatomy, ed 4. Chapter 7. The Mesencephalon. Williams & Wilkins, Baltimore, 1991.

21. Daube, JE, et al (eds): Medical Neurosciences: An Approach to Anatomy, Pathology, and Physiology by Systems and Levels. Chapter 8. The Consciousness System. Little, Brown & Company, Boston, 1986.

22. Ghez, C: Posture. Chapter 39. In Kandel, ER, Schwartz, JH, and Jessell, TM (eds): Principles of Neural Science, ed 3. Appleton & Lange, Norwalk, CT, 1991.

23. Wilson, VJ and Peterson, BW: Vestibulospinal and Reticulospinal Systems. Chapter 14. In Brooks, VB (ed): Handbook of Physiology. Section 1. The Nervous System, vol II. Motor Control. American Physiological Society, Bethesda, MD, 1981.

24. Carpenter, MB: Neuroanatomy, ed 4. Chapter 6. The Pons. Williams & Wilkins, Baltimore, 1991.

25. Kelly, JP: The Sense of Balance. Chapter 33. In Kandel, ER, Schwartz, JH, and Jessell, TM (eds): Principles of Neural Science, ed 3. Appleton & Lange, Norwalk, CT, 1991.

26. Barr, ML and Kiernan, JA: The Human Nervous System, ed 6. Chapter 22. Vestibular System. JB Lippincott, Philadelphia, 1993.

27. Fox, CR and Cohen, H: The Visual and Vestibular Systems. Chapter 5. In Cohen, H: Neuroscience for Rehabilitation. JB Lippincott, Philadelphia, 1993.

28. Baloh, RW and Honrubia, V: Clinical Neurophysiology of the Vestibular System, ed 2. FA Davis, Philadelphia, 1990.

29. Cohen, B, Guedry, F, and Tomko, D (eds): Sensing and Controlling Motion: Vestibular and Sensorimotor Function. Ann NY Acad Sci 656:1, 1992.

30. Highstein, SM: The Central Nervous System Efferent Control of Organs of Balance and Equilibrium. Neurosci Res 12:13, 1991.

31. Keshner, EA and Cohen, H: Current Concepts of the Vestibular System Reviewed. 1. The Role of the Vestibulospinal System in Postural Control. Am J Occup Ther 43:320, 1989.

32. Martin, JH: Neuroanatomy: Text and Atlas. Chapter 12. General Organization of the Cranial Nerve Nuclei and the Trigeminal System. Appleton & Lange, Norwalk, CT, 1989.

33. Martin, JH: Neuroanatomy: Text and Atlas. Chapter 13. The Somatic and Visceral Motor Functions of the Cranial Nerves. Appleton & Lange, Norwalk, CT, 1989.

34. Barr, ML and Kiernan, JA: The Human Nervous System, ed 6. Chapter 8. Cranial Nerves. JB Lippincott, Philadelphia, 1993.

35. Rowland, LP: Clinical Syndromes of the Spinal Cord and Brainstem. Chapter 46. In Kandel, ER, Schwartz, JH, and Jessell, TM (eds): Principles of Neural Science, ed 3. Appleton & Lange, Norwalk, CT, 1991.

36. Wall, M: Brainstem Syndromes. Chapter 30. In Bradley, WG, et al (eds): Neurology in Clinical Practice, vol II. Butterworth-Heinemann, Boston, 1990.

37. Brazis, PW: The Localization of Lesions Affecting in Brainstem. Chapter 14. In Brazis, PW, Masdeu, JC, and Biller, J (eds): Localization in Clinical Neurology, ed 2. Little, Brown & Company, Boston, 1990.

38. Stern, BJ, Wityk, RJ, and Lewis, RF: Disorders of the Cranial Nerves and Brainstem. Chapter 40. In Joynt, RJ (ed): Clinical Neurology, vol 3. JB Lippincott, Philadelphia, 1993.

39. Ropper, AH and Martin, JB: Coma and Other Disorders of Consciousness. Chapter 26. In Isselbacher, KJ, et al (eds): Harrison's Principles of Internal Medicine, ed 13. McGraw-Hill, New York, 1994.

40. Daube, JR, et al (eds): Medical Neurosciences: An Approach to Anatomy, Pathology, and Physiology by Systems and Levels, ed 2. Chapter 10. The Visceral System. Little, Brown & Company, Boston, 1986.

41. Reznik, M. Neuropathology in Seven Cases of Locked-in Syndrome. J Neurol Sci 60:67, 1983.

CHAPTER 7

■

Cortical Motor Systems

Robert J. Morecraft, PhD
and
Gary W. Van Hoesen, PhD

- ■ *Principles of Cortical Organization*
- ■ *Basic Frontal Lobe Anatomy*
- ■ *Specific Connections and Functions of the Motor Cortices*
- ■ *Prefrontal Influence on the Motor Cortices*
- ■ *Limbic Influence on the Motor Cortices*
- ■ *Language and the Frontal Lobe*
- ■ *Synthesis*

*H*ughlings Jackson (1864) is regarded as one of the first to have advocated a role for the cerebral cortex in motor control.[1,2] He suggested that the highest motor centers of the nervous system are located at the cortical level and speculated further that the frontal lobe regulated the most "voluntary" and "complex combinations" of motor behavior.[3] Jackson's thinking developed from deductive observations of motor behavior produced by seizures, which he called "the experiment made on the brain by disease." Experimental studies in animals by Ferrier[4,5] and by Fritsch and Hitzig[6] lent support by demonstrating that electrical stimulation of the cerebral cortex produced discrete patterns of movement in the head and extremities.

The execution of voluntary movement requires an ongoing awareness of the internal and external environment, a motor plan or strategy, and axonal connections through which cerebral cortex can exert its influence on the musculoskeletal apparatus. To accomplish this, the cerebral cortex is equipped anatomically with (1) cortical areas that receive sensory information then relay it to the frontal lobe, (2) a mechanism by which the prefrontal and premotor cortices can forward information to the primary motor cortex, and (3) a host of descending projections that arise from the premotor and primary motor cortices and target, through direct or indirect pathways, motor neurons that give rise to peripheral motor nerves. The goal of this chapter is to condense an extensive body of literature, focusing on principles underlying the frontal lobe contribution to movement.

Supported by a USDSM Alumni Faculty Development Award (to RJM) and a NIH Javits Neuroscience Investigator Award (NS-14944)(to GWVH). We would like to thank Drs. Joyce Kiefer and Jo Moore for their helpful suggestions.

Principles of Cortical Organization

Fundamental Organization of the Cerebral Cortex

The cerebral cortex can be divided into five major lobes: the frontal, parietal, temporal, occipital, and limbic lobes (Fig. 7–1). Each contains a subdivision or area dedicated to subserving either one primary sensory modality or motor control. These areas are called *primary* or *unimodal areas*. The **primary motor cortex** is located in the frontal lobe, the **primary somatosensory cortex** in the parietal lobe, the **primary visual cortex** in the occipital lobe, the **primary auditory cortex** in the temporal lobe, and the **primary olfactory cortex** in the limbic lobe (Fig. 7–2). The **primary motor cortex is a major cortical output system for facilitating somatic movement.** The primary sensory cortices are major targets of sensory input arising from specialized receptors that monitor activity in the external and internal environments.

Although this chapter focuses on the frontal lobe, we will find that it is influenced directly or indirectly by all of the other cortical lobes. Therefore, recognizing the cortical location and functional specialization of each modality will foster an appreciation for the potential influence that each lobe has on frontal motor behavior.

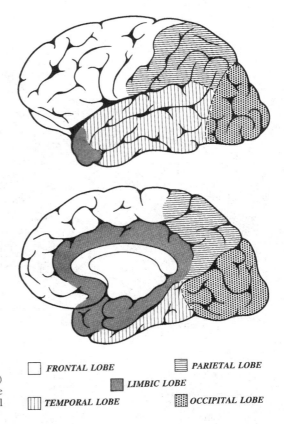

☐ *FRONTAL LOBE*	▤ *PARIETAL LOBE*
	▦ *LIMBIC LOBE*
▥ *TEMPORAL LOBE*	▩ *OCCIPITAL LOBE*

Figure 7–1. Lateral (*Top*) and medial (*Bottom*) views of the human cerebral cortex depicting the topography of the various lobes that form the cerebral hemisphere.

Functional Organization of the Cerebral Cortex

Within each lobe and associated with each primary area are primary association or multimodal association areas or both (see Fig. 7–2). Functionally, these areas operate at a more integrative level than the primary areas. Multimodal association cortex can be considered as being involved with the analysis of highly synthesized information relating to multiple modalities. Therefore, multimodal association cortex can be regarded as a site for shaping or processing a variety of higher-order behaviors.

The functional differences between primary and association cortices can be illustrated by examining the roles of the primary motor cortex compared with that of its related multimodal association cortex, the prefrontal cortex. Based on physiologic experiments, **stimulation of the primary motor cortex evokes movement on the opposite side of the body.** Such movements commonly affect a single joint or involve the digits.[7,8] Thus, the primary motor cortex relates to motor behavior in terms of simple, isolated movements. **In contrast, the prefrontal cortex does not produce movement when stimulated.** Behavioral and physiologic experiments demonstrate that it is associated with generating and mediating the programming component of voluntary motor activity.[9–12]

Situated between the primary motor cortex and prefrontal cortex is the **premotor cortex**. Stimulation in the premotor region elicits synergistic movement involving multiple joints, which is accompanied occasionally by postural movement.[19,48] Therefore, the premotor cortex is committed to influencing peripheral movement, but it relates to motor behavior at a more integrative level than does the primary motor cortex.

A somewhat analogous organization exists for sensory perception[13] (see Fig. 7–2). In the parietal lobe, the primary somatosensory cortex lies just posterior to the central sulcus; the multimodal association cortex is located caudally; and the **primary association cortex**

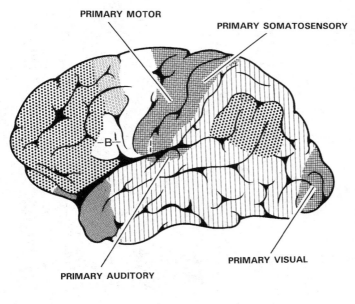

PRIMARY MOTOR

PRIMARY SOMATOSENSORY

–B–

PRIMARY VISUAL

PRIMARY AUDITORY

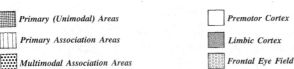

Primary (Unimodal) Areas

Primary Association Areas

Multimodal Association Areas

Premotor Cortex

Limbic Cortex

Frontal Eye Field

Figure 7–2. *Lateral View of the Human Cerebral Cortex Illustrating the Functional Organization of the Cerebral Cortex.* "B" indicates the approximate location of Broca's area.

can be located at midparietal levels. In the sensory cortices, the general flow of information by feedforward connections can be conceptualized as proceeding from the primary sensory cortex to the primary association cortex, and finally to the multimodal association cortex.[14] Therefore, at the level of multimodal association cortex, information is markedly transformed and has a great deal more meaning than the original sensory signal. For example, the primary area receives elementary information concerned with pain, temperature, discriminative touch, and conscious proprioception. Although this area may signal that an object has been touched, the association cortices are involved in the processing that would lead to recognition of an object by touch or stereognosis.

Connectional Organization of the Cerebral Cortex

To understand the processing of information that ultimately produces somatic movement, it is important to understand the flow of information within the cortex. For example, **adjacent cortices are usually interconnected.** The prefrontal cortex is interconnected with the premotor cortex which in turn is interconnected with the primary motor cortex (Fig. 7–3). In the parietal, occipital, and temporal lobes, the primary sensory cortex is interconnected with adjacent primary association cortex, which is in turn interconnected with more distal multimodal association cortex.

As a general rule, primary cortex does not connect directly with multimodal association cortex. Instead, the link between primary and multimodal association cortex is established by a series of connections passing through the intermediately situated premotor cortex (in the frontal lobe) or primary association cortices (in the parietal, occipital, and temporal lobes). Therefore, the primary areas and multimodal association areas lie at opposite ends of a sequential series of corticocortical connections.[15,16]

With one exception, it can also be stated that primary areas are not directly interconnected. This exception involves the primary motor and somatosensory cortices that are adjacent and directly interconnected. This relationship allows output from the primary motor cortex to be strongly and rapidly affected by peripheral feedback that has been subjected to little cortical transformation. A synergy between motor behavior and

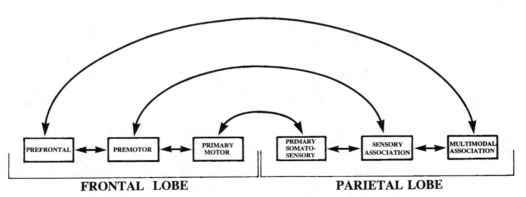

FRONTAL LOBE **PARIETAL LOBE**

Figure 7–3. A Simplified Diagram of Corticocortical Connections Between Frontal and Parietal Lobes. Several basic principles are illustrated. First, adjacent cortices are interconnected. Although the primary motor and primary somatosensory areas are interconnected (since they are adjacent to one another), this is the only circumstance in which primary areas are directly interconnected. Second, multimodal association areas are strongly interconnected. Third, cortex located between primary and multimodal areas are strongly interconnected. Note that primary and multimodal areas are not directly interconnected. Instead, the relationship between primary and multimodal association cortices is established through an intermediate series of connections. It is important to stress that this diagram does not take into account all connectional features, and in particular more minor ones. Also, it does not necessarily reflect the structural relation between all lobes.

somatosensory feedback is essential. For example, information regarding painful stimuli must be transmitted rapidly to the motor cortex to provide an adequate and timely response.

In each lobe, cortex located progressively away from the primary area can be characterized as having connections that are distributed to more widespread cortical sources. The cortical connections of the primary motor cortex involve primarily adjacent cortical regions that include parts of the frontal and parietal lobes. On the other hand, the cortical connections of the prefrontal cortex involve adjacent as well as distant cortical regions, which include parts of the parietal, occipital, temporal, and limbic lobes. For example, the prefrontal cortex is connected with the posterior parietal cortex (see Fig. 7–3). This general pattern of connectivity provides a basis for intracortical convergence and integration of higher-order information.[15,16]

Basic Frontal Lobe Anatomy

Motor Cortices of the Frontal Lobe

As our knowledge and insight regarding cortical motor systems have evolved, so has our understanding of frontal lobe organization. Although there are a number of views of motor cortex organization, there is good agreement that **the motor cortices include the primary motor cortex (M1), several premotor cortices, and the frontal eye field (FEF) (Fig. 7–4). The premotor cortices include the lateral premotor cortex (LPMC), supplementary motor cortex (M2), and cingulate motor cortex (M3).** Premotor cortex can be defined as parts of the frontal lobe that are directly interconnected with the primary motor cortex.[17] **Although influence of the prefrontal cortex on motor control will be discussed, it is not considered a motor cortical area.**

All the motor cortices are electrically excitable and thus produce peripheral movements when stimulated with electrical current. **Movement threshold is defined as the minimal current level needed to evoke a somatic response.** The primary motor cortex is characterized physiologically as having the lowest movement thresholds, whereas the premotor cortices and FEF have generally higher movement thresholds. Therefore, it is easier to evoke movement from the primary motor cortex than it is from the premotor cortices and FEF.

Somatotopic Organization of the Frontal Lobe

A fundamental feature of the frontal lobe is that its motor cortices are organized somatotopically. **Somatotopic organization refers in part to the view that regions of the body can be activated by stimulating discrete parts of the motor cortex.**[18,19] For instance, the primary, supplementary, and cingulate motor cortices have a head, upper extremity, and lower extremity representation (Fig. 7–5). Head representations project to brainstem motor nuclei involved in movements of the head and face, upper extremity representations project primarily to the cervical enlargement of the spinal cord and produce upper extremity actions, and lower extremity representations project to the lumbosacral enlargement of the spinal cord for lower extremity activation.[20,21] Between the motor cortices, similar body representations are interconnected. For example, the head representation of the primary, supplementary, and cingulate motor cortices are all interconnected.[17,28] Although this organization assists clinicians in localizing functional deficits following a lesion, **it is important to realize that maps depicting somatotopy are oversimplified,** since overlap of body parts and multiple representation of movement patterns are not reflected. **Multiple representation refers to the fact that identical *movement patterns* can be evoked from several noncontiguous cortical sites.**[7]

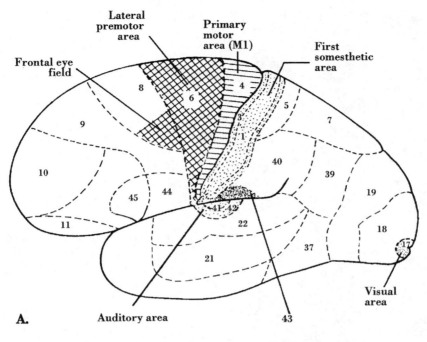

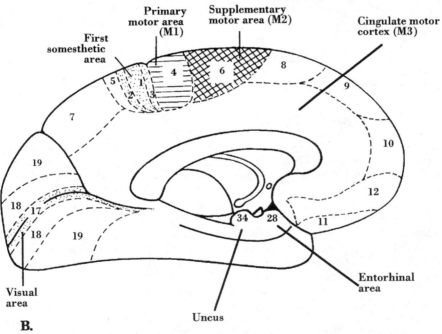

Figure 7–4. *The Topographic Organization of the Motor Cortices.* (A) Motor areas located on the lateral surface of the cortex. (B) Motor areas located on the medial side of the cortex. (Adapted from Barr, ML and Kiernan, JA. The Human Nervous System: An Anatomical Viewpoint, ed 6. JB Lippincott, Philadelphia, 1993, pp 240, 241, with permission.)

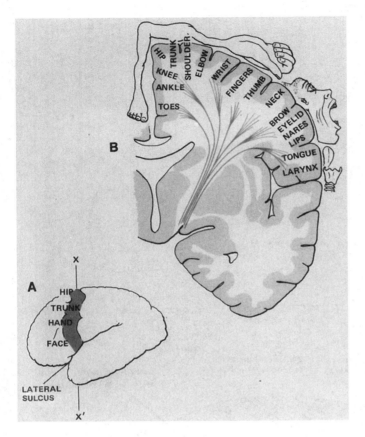

Figure 7–5. *Somatotopic Organization of the Motor Cortex.* The cortex is cut in a coronal section and a somatotopic map of the body and face is shown as a motor homunculus. Note that the cortical representation of the lower extremity is on the medial aspect of the hemisphere, while the trunk, hand, and face representations extend down the lateral surface. The size of different body parts indicates the amount of motor cortex devoted to the control of that part. (From Gilman, S and Newman, SW: Manter and Gatz's Essentials of Clinical Neuroanatomy and Neurophysiology, ed 8. FA Davis, Philadelphia, 1992, p 235, with permission.)

Cytoarchitecture of the Frontal Lobe

The study of the morphology of individual cells and the spatial arrangement of groups of cell bodies in the central nervous system is called *cytoarchitectonics,* which forms an important basis for brain organization. For example, when stained sections of the cerebral cortex are viewed microscopically, a laminar pattern distinct to each cortical region is apparent. The classical cortical pattern is a six-layered sheet of gray matter, with each layer numbered consecutively from the pia mater (externally) to the subcortical white matter (internally) (Fig. 7–6). From external to internal, the cortical layers are identified as I, the molecular layer; II, the external granular layer; III, the external pyramidal layer; IV, the internal granular layer; V, the internal pyramidal layer; and VI, the multiform layer. Layer I contains scattered neurons but is occupied primarily by axons and dendrites. Layers II and IV are formed by small cells and layers III and V are formed by larger cells called *pyramidal cells.* These pyramidal cells are the main projection neurons, whose axons leave the local environment and terminate in distal cortical and subcortical parts of the central nervous system. Layer VI contains cells of variable sizes and shapes. The small cells have short axons connecting layers of cortex.

At the turn of the century, Brodmann[22] systematically studied the cytoarchitectural organization of the primate cerebral cortex. Based on cytoarchitectural features, he partitioned the primate cerebral cortex into various areas and assigned each a specific number (Fig. 7–7). Over time, Brodmann's cytoarchitectural areas have been subdivided into more elaborate subsections, and many areas are now associated with unique functional properties. In the frontal lobe, the primary motor cortex is designated as **area 4.** In the premotor region, the lateral premotor cortex coincides with **area 6,** the supplementary motor cortex with

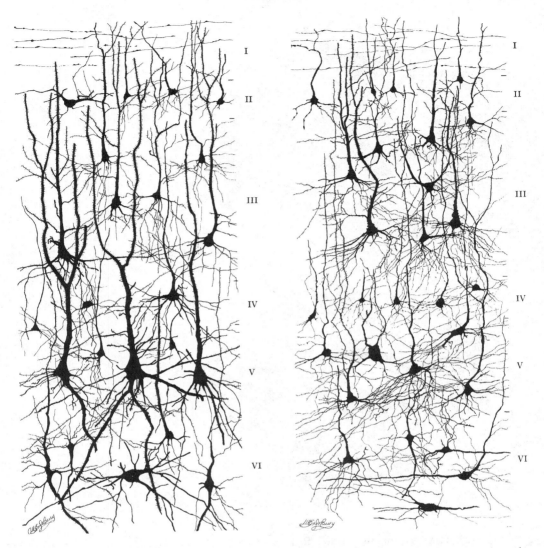

Figure 7–6. *Two Major Types of Cortex Found in the Frontal Lobe Are Shown in Golgi Reconstructions. Agranular cortex* (area 4 or primary motor cortex) is shown on the left and *granular cortex* (area 46 of the prefrontal cortex) is shown on the right. Note the granule (small) cells in layer 4 in the latter and their absence in the former. (From Conel, JL: The Postnatal Development of the Human Cerebral Cortex, Volume VIII: The Cortex of the Six Year Old Child. Harvard University Press, Cambridge, Plate 6, Figure 8 and Plate 30, Figure 56, Copyright © 1967. Reprinted by permission.)

area 6m, and the cingulate motor cortex with **area 24c.** The FEF corresponds to **area 8.** The prefrontal cortex is composed of several Brodmann's areas that include **areas 9, 46,** and **10** laterally and areas **9** and **10** medially.

Basic Patterns of Frontal Lobe Connections

When describing the neural circuitry of the central nervous system, the terms *efferent* and *afferent* are used to describe the anatomic relation of a set of projection neurons in a chain of neural connections. In general, **efferent projections** categorize neurons providing the output of a neural structure. **Afferent projections** categorize neurons providing the input to a neural structure.

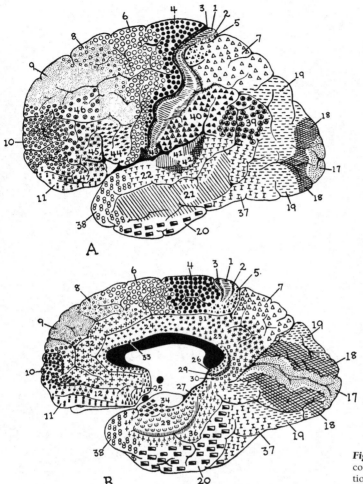

Figure 7-7. Brodmann's map of cortical cytoarchitectural organization in the human brain.

Corticocortical connections refer to projections that arise from and terminate within the cerebral cortex. **Corticobulbar connections** refer to projections that link the cerebral cortex directly with the brainstem motor nuclei of cranial nerves. **Corticofugal connections,** a general term, refers to all projections directed away from the cortex to subcortical targets. **Corticopetal connections** refers to projections directed toward the cortex from subcortical areas.

Corticocortical Connections

INTRINSIC CONNECTIONS. In the frontal lobe, information passes from the prefrontal cortex to the premotor cortex and finally to the primary motor cortex.[9] However, it is important to realize that reciprocal connections occur in this chain, so that the primary motor cortex projects to the premotor cortex, which projects to the prefrontal cortex (see Fig. 7-3). The reciprocal nature of these connections allows the prefrontal cortex to receive information from the motor cortices.

Another characteristic of intrinsic frontal lobe connections is that all the motor cortices (excluding the FEF) are reciprocally interconnected[16,23-28] (Fig. 7-8). For example, the LPMC projects to the primary, supplementary, and cingulate motor cortices,

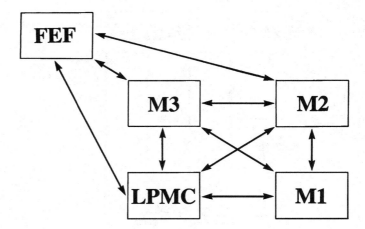

Figure 7–8. Schematic Diagram Showing the Basic Interconnections of the Motor Cortices. FEF = frontal eye fields; M1 = primary motor cortex; M2 = supplementary motor cortex; M3 = cingulate motor cortex; and LPMC = lateral premotor cortex.

and the primary, supplementary, and cingulate motor cortices project back to the lateral premotor cortex. These reciprocal lines of communication allow different parts of the motor cortex to directly exchange information. **This information not only informs adjacent motor cortex but also may mediate its input as well as regulate its output.** The FEF is an exception, since it is reciprocally connected with the lateral premotor, supplementary, and cingulate motor cortices, but not with the primary motor cortex[29,30] (see Fig. 7–8).

EXTRINSIC CONNECTIONS. The primary motor, premotor, and prefrontal cortices each can be characterized by their overall distribution of corticocortical connections. **The primary motor cortex has limited corticocortical connections,** which involve primarily, a small set of adjacent cortical areas.[27] This restricted pattern of corticocortical connections and the fact that somatotopic representations within the primary motor cortex are not interconnected may relate to physiologic observations showing that simple movements, confined to an isolated body region, are commonly evoked following stimulation of the primary motor cortex.

In contrast, **the prefrontal cortex is characterized by widespread corticocortical connections.**[10,15,16,31–33] These connections involve adjacent as well as distant sites in many regions of the cerebral cortex. The widespread nature of this projection pattern, and the fact that prefrontal connections involve parts of the other lobes that assimilate information from more than one modality (multimodal association cortices), establish a structural basis for the prefrontal cortex in regulating complex motor behavior.

In general, **the cortical connections of the premotor cortices vary with respect to each premotor region.** For instance, the cortical connections of the LPMC involve adjacent areas, as well as a few distant sites.[23,25,26] Furthermore, the LPMC has a limited number of connections with multimodal association cortex.[23,26,31] On the other hand, the cortical connections of cingulate motor cortex involve adjacent and many widespread parts of the cortical mantle.[34] In particular, the connections involve a variety of multimodal association cortices, and what is established with the prefrontal cortex is relatively dense. This widespread pattern of connections may relate to the complex movements elicited by stimulation of the anterior cingulate gyrus.

Descending Motor Pathways

A fundamental anatomic feature of motor cortex is that more than any other area, it sends projections to subcortical structures that influence somatic motor activity. **This link occurs through a variety of descending pathways.**[35] Major subcortical structures that subserve motor function include the spinal cord, reticular formation, pontine nuclei, red

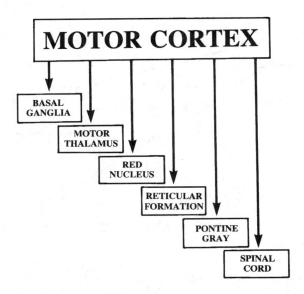

Figure 7–9. Schematic diagram illustrating characteristic descending corticofugal projections from motor cortices.

nucleus, motor thalamus, basal ganglia, and cranial nerve motor nuclei (Fig. 7–9). It is important to stress that many of these structures contribute uniquely to the motor act; thus, they are supportive to the whole plan and its ideal execution, but not essential for motor behavior per se. **Direct** cortical motor pathways arise from cell bodies in the motor cortices, which give rise to axons that terminate in subcortical targets containing motor neurons whose axons leave the central nervous system to form peripheral nerves. In the simplest sense, direct pathways constitute a two-stage neuronal relay from cerebral cortex to skeletal muscle. **Indirect** cortical pathways arise in the motor cortex and terminate in subcortical targets that in turn (1) project to centers that form the origin of peripheral nerves or (2) initiate a series of projections that feed back to the motor cortex through an organized thalamic relay. Therefore, indirect pathways involve a *series of intervening projections* that occur within the central nervous system between the projection arising from motor cortex and the origin of peripheral nerves.

DIRECT CORTICAL PATHWAYS. *Corticospinal projections* arise from a subpopulation of pyra- midal neurons in all the motor cortices, except from their face representations and from the FEF.[20,21,35] Ingrained in the classical literature was the belief that the only part of the *frontal lobe* giving rise to corticospinal axons was the primary motor cortex, or Brodmann's area 4. It is now clear that about half of the corticospinal contribution from the *frontal lobe* arises from the primary motor cortex and the remaining half from the premotor cortices (LPMC, supplementary motor cortex, and the cingulate motor cortex combined).[20] Accordingly, the direct and substantial contribution of the premotor cortices on spinal cord function must be taken into consideration. In addition, a large component of corticospinal projections also arises from several parts of the parietal lobe, such as the primary sensory cortex and superior parietal lobule.[35] They are thought to terminate dorsally in the spinal laminae and to be concerned with somatosensory regulation. The remainder of this discussion will focus on those projections involved in motor control.

Most corticospinal axons course through the internal capsule, cross the midline (or decussate) at the level of the lower medulla to form the lateral corticospinal tract, and then terminate in the gray matter of the spinal cord (Fig. 7–10; see Chapter 17). Some axons do not cross the midline at the level of the medulla, and these form the anterior corticospinal tract. A small percentage of anterior corticospinal tract fibers remains ipsilateral throughout their entire course, whereas a larger percentage eventually crosses the midline at or near spinal segmental levels that they innervate. The terminal distribution of the frontal lobe corticospinal projection involves the ventral and intermediate zones of the spinal gray

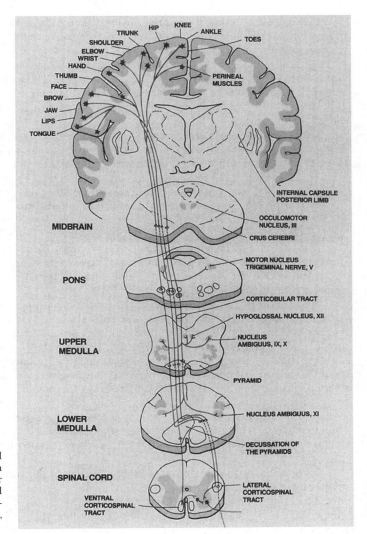

Figure 7-10. The corticospinal and corticobulbar pathways. (From Gilman, S and Newman SW: Manter and Gatz's Essentials of Clinical Neuroanatomy and Neurophysiology, ed 8. FA Davis, Philadelphia, 1992, p 77, with permission.)

matter. These projections terminate directly on motor neurons in the ventral horn of the spinal cord, forming a direct pathway that appears to originate primarily from the primary motor cortex. Although this motor tract innervates some motor neurons that innervate proximal muscles, most terminations of this tract are on motor neurons that control distal muscles. Corticospinal axons also terminate on interneurons in the intermediate zone and ventral horn, forming an indirect pathway that appears to arise from both the primary and premotor cortices.

These corticospinal projections from the frontal lobe are organized somatotopically.[20,21] For example, upper extremity representations in the cortex contain cell bodies that send their axons to the cervical enlargement of the spinal cord (which gives rise to the brachial plexus), whereas lower extremity representations project to the lumbosacral enlargement of the spinal cord (which gives rise to the lumbosacral plexus).

Because most corticospinal fibers cross in the medulla, a lesion in the primary motor cortex generally produces contralateral paresis that is more evident in the distal musculature. In addition, evidence suggests that ipsilateral signs and symptoms may be present due to the small portion of anterior corticospinal fibers that do not cross.[36]

Corticobulbar projections arise from the motor cortex and terminate directly in brainstem cranial nerve motor nuclei. It is surprising that the origin of cortical projections to brainstem motor nuclei has been poorly studied. The origins reported include projections to the facial nucleus of the cranial nerve VII, which innervates the muscles of facial expression; the hypoglossal nucleus of cranial nerve XII, which innervates tongue muscles; the nucleus ambiguus of cranial nerves IX and X, which innervates muscles in the pharynx and larynx; and the trigeminal motor nucleus of cranial nerve V, which innervates the muscles of mastication.

These nuclei generally receive a bilateral corticobulbar innervation. With bilateral innervation, a lesion above the nuclei in the corticospinal pathway or in the cortex of origin generally produces minimal or no clinical deficits. The major exception to this pattern of bilateral innervation is the facial motor nucleus located in the pons. Although the cortical projection to the part of the facial nucleus innervating the upper facial muscles is bilateral, the cortical projection to the part of the facial nucleus innervating the lower facial muscles is contralateral only. Therefore, a lesion in the primary motor cortex produces weakness in the muscles of facial expression in only the lower half of the face. In addition, even though the hypoglossal and trigeminal nuclei receive input from bilateral hemispheres, the input from the contralateral side predominates. Therefore, damage to the corticospinal pathways above the nuclei may produce slight and typically transient contralateral weakness in the muscles innervated by these nuclei.

INDIRECT CORTICAL PATHWAYS. *Corticoreticular projections* arise from all the motor cortices and terminate in the reticular formation of the midbrain and pons.[24,35,39] All motor cortices, except for the cingulate motor cortex and FEF, are known to project to the medullary and pontine reticular formation. In general, the corticoreticular projection from motor cortex is almost exclusively ipsilateral. The reticular formation of the pons and medulla in turn contain a subset of large neurons that project to the spinal cord via two reticulospinal tracts (see Fig. 6–6, and refer to Chapter 6). In the pons, the reticulospinal projection originates from the nucleus reticularis pontis oralis and caudalis and terminates ipsilaterally in the spinal cord. In the medulla, the reticulospinal tract arises from the nucleus reticularis gigantocellularis and projects bilaterally in the spinal cord. **The corticoreticular and subsequent reticulospinal pathways are involved primarily in the regulation of muscle tone.**

Corticopontine projections arise from all parts of the frontal lobe and terminate in the ipsilateral pontine nuclei.[10,37,38] Cells in the pontine nuclei in turn project to the contralateral cerebellum with their axons forming the middle cerebellar peduncle (see Chapter 8). This provides a critical pathway for the motor cortices to influence the cerebellum and its output. Cerebellar output is directed to several contralateral brainstem and thalamic nuclei. The red nucleus is one major brainstem target of cerebellar output. As discussed in the following text, the red nucleus projects to the contralateral spinal cord. Another major target of cerebellar output is the ventral lateral (VL) nucleus of the thalamus. Cerebellar projections to the thalamus constitute a critical link in a series of connections that converge eventually on the primary motor cortex.

Corticotectal projections arise from the FEF and prefrontal cortex and terminate in the ipsilateral superior colliculus of the midbrain.[10,39] Tectospinal fibers arise from cell bodies in the superior colliculus (see Chapter 6). The fibers cross the midline in the dorsal tegmental decussation and form the tectospinal pathway. This pathway is concerned with reflex neck and postural movements in response to visual and auditory-related stimuli.

Corticorubral projections arise from all the motor cortices and terminate in the ipsilateral red nucleus of the midbrain.[37,39,40] In turn, rubrospinal fibers arise from cell bodies in the magnocellular division of the red nucleus (see Chapter 6). They exit the nucleus and cross the midline in the ventral tegmental decussation to form the rubrospinal tract in the lateral funiculus (see Fig. 6–5). Rubrospinal fibers then terminate in all levels of the spinal cord.[41] Therefore, the overall effect of the corticorubrospinal system is contralateral, as is the effect of the more direct corticospinal system. The rubrospinal system is also organized somatotopically, so that projections from the upper extremity part of the red nucleus target the cervical enlargement and those from the lower extremity part target the lumbosacral enlargement.

Corticothalamic projections **arise from all parts of the frontal lobe and terminate in the ipsilateral thalamus.** [10,27,35,37,39] As a general rule, this connection is reciprocal. Although many thalamic nuclei are connected to the motor cortex, the major link is established with the ventral anterior (VA) and VL nuclei. The VA/VL complex has been termed the *motor thalamus.*[42] The prefrontal cortex is also connected preferentially with the adjacent medial dorsal thalamic nucleus.

Corticostriate projections **arise from all parts of the frontal lobe and terminate bilaterally in the caudate and putamen nuclei (striatum) of the basal ganglia.**[10,27,37,39] The projection from the motor cortices is primarily to the putamen, strongest ipsilaterally and somatotopically organized. Outflow from the basal ganglia is directed to topographic regions of the motor thalamus that involve primarily VA nuclei. Finally, projections from the motor thalamus are directed back to the motor cortex, in particular the premotor cortices, through topographically organized thalamocortical circuits. Recent information indicates that pathways arising from different parts of the motor cortex remain segregated as they course through the basal ganglia–thalamic loop (see Chapter 9).

Specific Connections and Functions of the Motor Cortices

Primary Motor Cortex

The primary motor cortex (M1) is located anterior to the central sulcus on both the lateral and medial surfaces of the hemisphere (see Fig. 7–4) and coincides with Brodmann's area 4. It projects subcortically to the basal ganglia, motor thalamus, red nucleus, reticular formation, pontine gray matter, and spinal cord (see Fig. 7–9). As previously mentioned, axons projecting from neurons in this motor area constitute a large portion of the corticospinal pathway.

The primary motor cortex is characterized by its restricted corticocortical connections, which involve a small set of relatively adjacent cortical areas. Generally, they include the premotor cortices, frontal operculum, primary (S1) and supplementary (S2) somatosensory cortices, and the anterior part of the parietal association cortex.[27] It has been shown that a subpopulation of small-sized pyramidal cells in the primary motor cortex is highly sensitive to somatosensory-related information.[18] The extensive anatomic affiliation between the primary motor cortex and the anterior parts of the parietal lobe may underlie this property.

Electrophysiologic stimulation experiments advance the proposal that the primary motor cortex plays an important role in the execution of contralateral movement occurring primarily around a single joint with emphasis on hand and finger movements.[7,8] This ability to isolate joint movement is referred to as **fractionated movement;** if it is confined to a single joint, it has been characterized as a **simple movement.**[8,43] *Contiguous movements,* referring to movements occurring about two adjacent joints,[8,43] and *complex movements,* referring to responses occurring at more than two joints,[8,43] rarely occur following stimulation of the primary motor cortex.[7,8] This evidence suggests that the predominant function of the primary motor cortex is to play a role in the execution of simple fractionated movements with emphasis on the distal musculature. Small hand and finger movements requiring finely graded responses appear to be directed from this area.[44] **In addition, single unit recording studies show that individual neurons in the primary motor cortex are concerned with parameters of movement such as force generation and modulation.**

As already discussed, stimulation experiments demonstrate that the primary motor cortex is organized somatotopically.[7,8,19,43] For example, the head representation is located ventrally on the lateral convexity of the hemisphere near the lateral fissure, and the upper extremity representation is immediately dorsal to the head representation (see Fig. 7–5). Both representations fall in the territory of the middle cerebral artery. The lower extremity representation is located on the dorsal convexity of the lateral hemisphere, extending onto the medial surface of the hemisphere. It falls primarily within the territory of the anterior cerebral artery. **Therefore, middle cerebral artery infarcts have a greater impact on head and upper extremity function, whereas anterior cerebral artery infarcts cause deficits that predominantly affect the lower extremity.**

Lateral Premotor Cortex

The LPMC is located rostral to the primary motor cortex and corresponds to Brodmann's area 6. Its anterior boundary is marked by the FEF (see Figs. 7–2 and 7–4). The LPMC is divided into dorsal and ventral components, and the main arterial supply to this area is the middle cerebral artery. The lateral premotor cortex projects subcortically to the same regions as does the primary motor cortex (see Fig. 7–9) and also contributes significantly to the corticospinal pathway.

The corticocortical connections of the lateral premotor cortex involve the primary and premotor cortices, the frontal operculum, the FEF, the supplementary somatosensory cortex (S2), and the anterior part of the parietal association cortex.[23,26,35] Also, the caudal part of the prefrontal cortex (multimodal association cortex) is linked to the very rostral parts of the LPMC.[23,26,31] The parts of the LPMC receiving prefrontal input do not appear to give rise to corticospinal output. Therefore, prefrontal influence on corticospinal neurons in the LPMC seems to be indirect.

The lateral premotor area appears to play a role in the planning and production of purposeful complex movements. Recordings of activity within the lateral premotor region indicate that a large number of neurons respond before and during the performance of complex movements[45] and that fewer neurons respond when executing simple movements. Physiologic evidence also indicates that activity in lateral area 6 is related to motor acts that are initiated by the presentation of sensory cues that include visual or somatosensory stimuli.[45,46] **This suggests that purposeful activities under the influence of sensory guidance are processed in this motor area.** In addition, neurons in the ventral part of lateral area 6 respond strongly during purposeful actions such as reaching, grasping, and bringing the hand toward the mouth.

There has been considerable debate regarding the influence of the LPMC on distal versus axial musculature. Face and upper extremity movements are heavily represented in the ventral part of the LPMC, and neurons in this area are active during reaching and grasping. It is interesting that **clinical evidence suggests that lateral area 6 lesions result in severe disturbance of postural support mechanisms, as well as in the inability to execute synergistically the proximal and distal muscle group.**[47] Recent intracortical stimulation experiments in monkeys indicate that the LPMC may influence proximal as well as distal movements.[48]

Supplementary Motor Cortex

The supplementary motor cortex (M2) is located on the medial wall of the cerebral hemisphere, along the superior frontal lobule and coincides with Brodmann's area 6m (see Fig. 7–4). The anterior cerebral artery supplies this cortical area, which projects to a number of important subcortical motor centers that include the basal ganglia, motor thalamus, red nucleus, reticular formation, pontine gray matter, and spinal cord (see Fig. 7–9).

The corticocortical connections of the supplementary motor cortex can be characterized as being moderately widespread, involving the primary and premotor cortices, FEF, primary (S1) and supplementary (S2) somatosensory cortices, parietal association cortex, medial parietal cortex, temporal association cortex of the superior temporal sulcus, cingulate gyrus, and lateral part of the orbitofrontal cortex.[24,34,35,49] Like the LPMC, area 6m is connected to the prefrontal cortex, and this connection involves primarily the rostral part of area 6m.[24,34] Since this part of the supplementary motor cortex coincides with the head representation and does not contain corticospinal neurons, prefrontal influence on corticospinal neurons in the supplementary motor cortex appears to be indirect.

The supplementary motor cortex participates in the planning, organization, and execution of complex movements with an emphasis on proximal and bilateral activities. In response to electrical stimulation, the supplementary motor cortex gives rise to simple, contiguous, and complex movements, with contiguous and complex movements predominating.[8,43] Contralateral as well as bilateral movements are expressed. The classical neurologic literature suggests a role in regulating whole-body movements.[50,51] Unit recording studies show that the supplementary motor cortex is active during stages that *precede* the onset of a learned motor task.[46] The supplementary motor cortex, therefore, **may play a role in the organizational or planning component of voluntary motor acts.** Behavioral studies suggest that the supplementary motor cortex may regulate the sequencing component of voluntary movements, as well as the bilateral execution of action.

Cingulate Motor Cortex

The cingulate motor cortex (M3) is located in the depths of the cingulate sulcus, along its lower bank and fundus on the medial surface of the hemispheres. Technically, it is in the limbic lobe, since it is located in the cingulate gyrus. However, it is somatotopically organized, and electrophysiologically excitable and projects to subcortical motor centers such as the spinal cord and red nucleus. A dual role is suggested at the interface between the emotional role of the limbic lobe and the motor-related activity of the frontal lobe. For purposes of this discussion, we will consider area 24c as the cingulate motor cortex, since the full extent of cortical territory occupied by the cingulate motor cortex has yet to be resolved. The cingulate motor cortex resides entirely within the territory of the anterior cerebral artery and its branches. Therefore, it is damaged with anterior cerebral artery infarcts.

The corticocortical connections of the cingulate motor cortex can be characterized as widespread, involving the primary and premotor cortices; FEF; supplementary somatosensory cortex; prefrontal, parietal, and temporal association cortices, several parts of the limbic lobe, and the orbitofrontal cortex[28,34,37,52] (Fig. 7–11). The widespread nature of these connections and the fact that strong links are formed with multimodal association cortex and limbic cortex distinguish the cingulate motor cortex from all other motor cortices.

A variety of key subcortical motor centers receive direct input from the cingulate motor cortex. These centers include the basal ganglia, motor thalamus, red nucleus, reticular formation, pontine gray matter, and spinal cord (see Fig. 7–11). The simple fact that the cingulate motor cortex receives powerful limbic and prefrontal input and gives rise to descending motor pathways establishes a unique relation between limbic and multimodal association cortices and subcortical motor targets such as the spinal cord.

With respect to function, events accompanying electrophysiologic stimulation of the anterior cingulate gyrus indicate that the cingulate motor cortex may mediate complex motor behaviors.[53–55] For example, **electrical stimulation of the anterior cingulate region elicits integrated combinations of movements that are adapted to environmental exploration. In the human, these movements involve primarily the face and upper extremity and are often goal-oriented.** Fluctuations in autonomic functions such as respiration, heart rate, and blood pressure also occur.

Unit recordings show that **neurons in the cingulate motor cortex are active *prior* to and during movement execution, and this activity is linked to a well-practiced motor response.**[56] Based on other studies, the change in neural activity appears to be expressed prior to substantial changes in unit activity occurring in the supplementary motor cortex. The exceedingly long lead time of activity detected in the cingulate motor region (greater

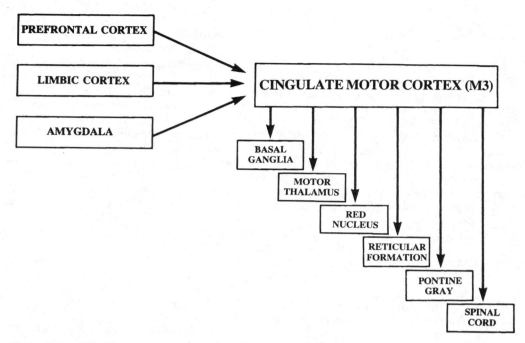

Figure 7–11. *Schematic Diagram Showing Prefrontal, Limbic, and Amygdalar Inputs to the Cingulate Motor Cortex.* This set of afferent projections *distinguishes* the cingulate motor cortex from all the other motor cortices. Also illustrated are basic subcortical outputs of the cingulate motor cortex. This set of efferent projections is *common* among the motor cortices in general.

than 2 seconds before movement onset) suggests that it may be involved in early organization of action and perhaps through its projections in "priming" other foci of the central motor apparatus for forthcoming motor commands. The widespread and powerful prefrontal and limbic projections that reach the cingulate motor cortex may represent a structural basis for the single unit observations.

Frontal Eye Field

The FEF is located on the lateral surface of the hemisphere between the prefrontal cortex rostrally and LPMC caudally (see Figs. 7–2 and 7–4). It is *not* classified as premotor cortex, because it has no direct connectional affiliation with the primary motor cortex. However, it plays an important role in visuomotor behavior and, by most contemporary standards, is classified as motor cortex. It coincides with Brodmann's area 8.

Corticocortical connections of the FEF involve several major regions of the cerebral cortex: the LPMC; supplementary and cingulate motor cortices; prefrontal cortex; parietal, temporal, and occipital multimodal association cortices; and the cingulate gyrus of the limbic lobe.[25,29,30] Studies have shown that nearly all these regions process distilled forms of visual stimuli.

Subcortically, the corticotectal projection from the FEF to the superior colliculus and pretectal nucleus may constitute an important pathway for regulating eye movement.[39] Fibers originating from the superior colliculus and pretectal nucleus project to neurons in the reticular formation, which in turn project to ocular motor centers throughout the brainstem. The FEF also projects directly to several subcortical motor centers, which include the basal ganglia, motor thalamus, red nucleus, reticular formation, and pontine gray matter.

Electrical stimulation of the frontal eye field produces saccadic eye movements that are directed contralateral to the stimulated hemisphere.[30] Saccadic eye movements are rapid and voluntary and are characterized by conjugate deviation of both eyes. Movements in the extremities are not evoked from this cortical field. Eye movements are paramount in directing attention to activity in the extrapersonal space and in tracking targets that are relevant to behavioral significance. A unilateral lesion affecting the FEF is accompanied by a useful clinical sign that can aid in diagnosing pathologic laterality. For example, **a manifestation of a unilateral FEF lesion is ocular deviation toward the side of the lesion.**

Prefrontal Influence on the Motor Cortices

The prefrontal cortex is situated in the rostral part of the frontal lobe, and its size is a landmark of primate evolution. Prefrontal function has long been associated with higher-order brain behaviors.[10,47,57–60] **Working memory, motor planning, decision making, problem solving, motivation, and attention all are functions mediated in part by the prefrontal cortex.** To appreciate the potential role of the prefrontal cortex in motor behavior, it is helpful to consider the basic cortical connections that may affect the activity of the prefrontal cortex.

The prefrontal cortex has widespread corticocortical connections that involve adjacent as well as distant parts of the cerebral cortex. Specifically, these connections involve isolated parts of the motor cortices, sensory association and multimodal association cortices of the parietal lobe, multimodal association cortex of the occipital and temporal lobes, and several parts of the limbic lobe.[10,31,33] For example, converging inputs from the posterior parietal, visual, and cingulate cortex project to the prefrontal cortex and provide it with information regarding spatial relation and body awareness in the environment.[61] Auditory input and information regarding form and object recognition are also directed to the prefrontal cortex from regions such as the lateral temporal cortex. These powerful inputs from the constellation of multimodal association cortices indicate that the prefrontal cortex can integrate information from different sensory modalities that has undergone a considerable amount of transformation. Limbic inputs may correlate with emotional and memory features that guide prefrontal function. Subsequently, **it appears that the prefrontal cortex engages in the complex distillation of this information that eventually influences the motor plan.**

Although neurons in the prefrontal area do not send projections into the corticospinal tract, they do project to other motor cortices that directly influence movements. The prefrontal cortex is linked directly to isolated parts of the motor cortices.[23,26,34,49] For example, the ventral part of the primary motor cortex, which corresponds to the head representation, the rostral lateral premotor cortex, and the supplementary cortex receive direct input from the prefrontal cortex. Of these prefrontal recipient areas, input appears not to directly involve corticospinal output zones. In contrast, the cingulate motor cortex receives strong prefrontal input which converges on parts of it, giving rise to the corticospinal pathway.

In summation, it appears as if the prefrontal area receives a wide variety of inputs that may influence motor planning and acts to synthesize this information and to project to other motor cortices to influence movement and motor control.

Limbic Influence on the Motor Cortices

It seems appropriate to consider in this chapter the effect of the limbic cortex on the motor cortex, since functions mediated by limbic structures bear heavily on all components of motor behavior from initiation to execution. **Motivation, emotion, olfaction, social** behavior, and memory all are functions linked to the limbic cortex. The limbic lobe forms a continuous ring of gray matter located on the medial edge of the cerebral hemisphere[62] (see Fig. 7–1). It consists of the cingulate gyrus dorsally, parahippocampal gyrus ventrally, posterior orbitofrontal cortex anteriorly, and retrosplenial cortex posteriorly. Generally, the limbic lobe is strongly interconnected with the multimodal association cortices, amygdala, and hypothalamus. It also projects to the basal ganglia (caudate and putamen nucleus) and pontine nuclei, therefore directly influencing major *subcortical* effector activities of the brain.

Except for the cingulate motor cortex, the motor cortices have a limited and primarily indirect connectional relation with the limbic lobe. For example, the primary motor cortex and LPMC are connected only with the dorsal part of the cingulate gyrus. Furthermore, it can be stated that nearly all parts of the limbic lobe are not directly connected to the primary, supplementary, and lateral premotor cortices and that what is established is limited to isolated parts of the anterior cingulate region. However, since widespread and powerful limbic lobe projections reach the anterior cingulate gyrus, this area may form an important relay station that advances limbic-related information to the motor cortices. In addition, portions of the anterior cingulate gyrus (area 24b) also send short but intense projections directly to the cingulate motor cortex. Presumably, this pathway represents the strongest link between the traditional limbic lobe and the corticospinal projection neurons.

Although the effects of limbic cortex on motor cortex are not well known, the recent finding of corticospinal axons arising from the dorsal part of the cingulate gyrus has reduced this gap and shed new light on potential cortical limbic-motor interactions. For example, the amygdala, an oval-shaped mass of gray matter in the temporal lobe, projects heavily to the more anterior parts of the cingulate motor cortex, a region that may correspond to the territory of the head representation. It is interesting that medial temporal lobe seizures in patients and experimental stimulation of the amygdala in humans and monkeys are often accompanied by pronounced facial movements related to different forms of facial expression. **The amygdala has been shown to be concerned with emotion and memory, and its projection to the cingulate motor cortex may lead to behavioral modification of planned motor acts. For example, voluntary movement may be influenced by a previous experience or event that is associated with fear, anger, happiness, sadness, embarrassment, or excitement.**

The FEF also receives some limbic lobe input.[29,30] Therefore, eye movements that involve a high level of motor integration may be influenced by a wide variety of emotional or motivational stimuli.

Language and the Frontal Lobe

Broca's area lies on the frontal operculum, rostral to the ventral part of the LPMC (Fig. 7–12). According to Brodmann's nomenclature, Broca's area is formed by areas 44 and 45. From a functional perspective, **Broca's area is involved with expressive language.** Electrical stimulation of the cerebral cortex in patients and nonhuman primates shows that other parts of the motor cortices, in addition to Broca's area, are involved in vocalization. These are the anterior part of the supplementary motor cortex and the anterior cingulate gyrus. Damage to Broca's area leads to a clinical condition known as **Broca's aphasia,** a language disorder characterized by a difficulty or inability to find words and express language in a smooth fashion with appropriate modifiers and connectors.

Synthesis

In the parietal, occipital, and temporal lobes of the cerebral cortex, basic sensory responses are received first at the level of the primary sensory area. This information is relayed to the primary association area and finally the multimodal association area. The

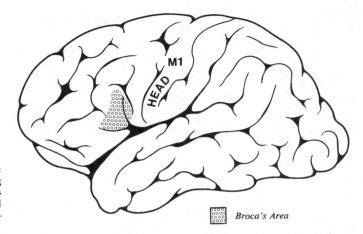

Figure 7–12. Lateral view of the human cerebral cortex illustrating the approximate location of Broca's area and its relation to the head representation of the primary motor cortex (M1).

Broca's Area

multiple elements that form a perception are thought to be recreated through a matrix of feedback and feedforward connections occurring across these areas. In this way, basic sensory stimuli are transformed and eventually have complex meaning related to present and past events. From the multimodal association region of the parietal, occipital, and temporal lobes, information is advanced to the prefrontal cortex for further analysis. Motor programming and complex regulation of the motor act are thought to take place in the province of the prefrontal cortex.

Subsectors located in the caudal half of the frontal lobe and lower bank of the cingulate sulcus form the motor cortices. These are the primary motor, lateral premotor, supplementary motor and cingulate motor cortices, and the FEF. The motor cortices share many fundamental features that support their common characterization. Generally, the motor cortex (1) is electrically excitable, (2) displays some form of somatotopic organization, and (3) projects to several key subcortical motor centers such as the spinal cord, reticular formation, pontine nuclei, red nucleus, motor thalamus (VA/VL complex), and basal ganglia. An exception is the FEF, because it sends no projection to the spinal cord.

The prefrontal cortex is reciprocally interconnected with the FEF, cingulate motor cortex, and isolated parts of the primary, supplementary, and lateral premotor cortices. These connections offer critical links through which prefrontal cortex can influence voluntary motor activity. The premotor cortices (lateral premotor, supplementary, and cingulate motor cortices) all are reciprocally interconnected with the primary motor cortex and therefore interact at the cortical level. Descending pathways emanating from the motor cortices to various subcortical, brainstem, and spinal cord targets provide a natural vehicle for the cerebral cortex to influence the peripheral motor apparatus.

Limbic influence on cortical motor control shapes the motivational status, emotional tone, and memory component of the motor response. Several important corticocortical pathways link the limbic and motor systems: (1) limbic lobe projections to the prefrontal cortex, (2) limbic lobe projections to the interhemispheric surface of the anterior cingulate gyrus, and (3) limbic lobe projections to the cingulate motor cortex, which constitutes a direct link between the limbic lobe and cortex giving rise to the descending motor pathways.

Since the motor cortices influence identical subcortical motor-related targets through their own set of descending projections, they can act in **parallel** and perhaps on a complementary basis. On the other hand, each motor cortex has its unique set of corticocortical connections. This distinguishing structural feature, combined with distinctive functional properties, suggests that the motor cortices can be organized on a **hierarchical** basis, with each motor cortex furnishing its unique influence on the motor act. Parallel and hierarchical components of the motor cortex are likely to collectively develop and produce elaborate and goal-oriented forms of voluntary movement.

RECOMMENDED READINGS

Brooks, VB: How Does the Limbic System Assist Motor Learning? A Limbic Comparator Hypothesis. Brain Behav Evol 29:29, 1986.

Damasio, AR: The Frontal Lobes. In Heilman, KM and Valenstein, ES (eds): Clinical Neuropsychology, ed 2. Oxford University Press, New York, 1985, p 339.

Freund, H-J: Abnormalities of Motor Behavior After Cortical Lesions in Humans. In Mountcastle, VB, Plum, F, and Geiger, SR (eds): Handbook of Physiology: The Nervous System, vol. V, Part 2. American Physiological Society, Bethesda, MD, 1987, p 763.

Fuster, JM: The Prefrontal Cortex; Anatomy, Physiology, and Neuropsychiatry of the Frontal Lobe, ed 2. Raven Press, New York, 1986.

Goldman-Rakic, PS: Circuitry of Prefrontal Cortex and Regulation of Behavior by Representational Memory. In Mountcastle, VB and Plum, F (eds): Handbook of Physiology: The Nervous System, vol. 5. American Physiological Society, Bethesda, MD, 1987, p 373.

Kalaska, JF and Crammond, CJ: Cerebral Cortical Mechanisms of Reaching Movements. Science, 255:1517, 1992.

Kuypers, HGJM: Anatomy of the Descending Pathways. In Mountcastle, VB, Brooks, VB, and Geiger, SR (eds): Handbook of Physiology: The Nervous System, vol II, Part 1. American Physiological Society, Bethesda, MD, 1981, p 597.

Van Hoesen, GW: The Modern Concept of Association Cortex. Curr Opin Neurobiol 3:150, 1993.

Weinberger, DR: A Connectionist Approach to the Prefrontal Cortex. J Neuropsychol 5:241, 1993.

Wiesendanger, M: Organization of Secondary Motor Areas of the Cerebral Cortex. In Mountcastle, VB, Brooks, VB, and Geiger, SR (eds): Handbook of Physiology: The Nervous System, vol II, Part 2. American Physiological Society, Bethesda, MD, 1981, p 1121.

Wiesendanger, M, and Wise, SP: Current Issues Concerning the Functional Organization of Motor Cortical Areas in Non-Human Primates. In Chauvel, P, et al (eds): Advances in Neurology, vol 57. Raven Press, New York, 1992, p 117.

Wise, WP and Evarts, EV: The Role of the Cerebral Cortex in Movement. In Evarts, EV, Wise, SP, and Bousfield, D (eds): The Motor System in Neurobiology. Elsevier Biomedical Press, Amsterdam, 1985, p 307.

Zilles, K: Cortex. In Paxinos, G (ed): The Human Nervous System. Academic Press, New York, 1990, p 802.

REFERENCES

1. Foerster, O: The Motor Cortex in Man in the Light of Hughlings Jackson's Doctrines. Brain 59:135, 1936.
2. Mills, CK: Cerebral Localisation in Its Practical Relations. Brain 12:358, 1889.
3. Jackson, JH: The Croonian Lectures on Evolution and Dissolution of the Nervous System. Lecture III. Br Med J 660, 1884.
4. Ferrier, D: Experimental Researches in Cerebral Physiology and Pathology. West Riding Lunatic Asylum Medical Reports 3:30, 1873.
5. Ferrier, D: Functions of the Brain. Smith Elder and Company, London, 1876.
6. Fritsch, G and Hitzig, E: Ueber die elektrische Erregbarkeit des Grosshirns. Arch Anat Physiol 37:300, 1870.
7. Huntley, GW and Jones, EG: Relationship of Intrinsic Connections to Forelimb Movement Representations in Monkey Motor Cortex: A Correlative Anatomic and Physiological Study. J Neurophysiol 66:390, 1991.
8. Luppino, G, et al: Multiple Representations of Body Movement in Mesial Area 6 and the Adjacent Cingulate Cortex: An Intracortical Microstimulation Study in the Macaque Monkey. J Comp Neurol 311:463, 1991.
9. Fuster, JM: Frontal Lobes. Curr Opin Neurobiol 3:160, 1993.
10. Goldman-Rakie, PS: Circuitry of Prefrontal Cortex and Regulation of Behavior by Representational Memory. In Mountcastle, VB and Plum, F (eds): Handbook of Physiology: The Nervous System, vol 5. American Physiological Society, Bethesda, MD, 1987, p 373.
11. Milner, B and Petrides, M: Behavioral Effects of Frontal Lobe Lesions in Man. Trends Neurosci 7:403, 1984.
12. Stamm, JS: The Monkey's Prefrontal Cortex Functions in Motor Programming. Acta Neurobiol Exp 39:683, 1979.
13. Van Hoesen, GW: The Modern Concept of Association Cortex. Curr Opin Neurobiol 3:150, 1993.
14. Weinberger, DR: A Connectionist Approach to the Prefrontal Cortex. J Neuropsychol 5:241, 1993.
15. Jones, EG and Powell, TPS: An Anatomical Study of Converging Sensory Pathways Within the Cerebral Cortex of the Monkey. Brain 93:793, 1970.
16. Pandya, DN and Kuypers, HGIM: Cortico-cortical Connections in the Rhesus Monkey. Brain Res 13:13, 1969.
17. Muakkassa, KF and Strick, PL: Frontal Lobe Inputs to Primate Motor Cortex: Evidence for Four Somatotopically Organized "Premotor" Areas. Brain Res 177:176, 1979.
18. Wise, SP and Evarts, EV: The Role of the Cerebral Cortex in Movement. In Evarts, EV, Wise, SP, Bousfield, D (eds): The Motor System in Neurobiology. Elsevier Biomedical Press, Amsterdam, 1985, p 307.
19. Woolsey, CN, et al: Patterns of Localization in Precentral and "Supplementary" Motor Areas and Their Relation to the Concept of a Premotor Area. Res Publ Assoc Res Nerv Ment Dis 30:238, 1952.
20. Dum, RP and Strick, PL: The Origin of Corticospinal Projections from the Premotor Areas in the Frontal Lobe. J Neurosci 11:667, 1991.
21. He, SQ, Dum, RP, and Strick, PL: Topographic Organization of Corticospinal Projections from the

Frontal Lobe: Motor Areas on the Lateral Surface of the Hemisphere. J Neurosci 13:952, 1993.

22. Brodmann, K: Beitrage zur histologischen Localisation der Grosshinrinde. III. Mitteilung: Die Rindenfelder der niederen. J Psychol Neurol 4:177, 1905.

23. Barbas, H and Pandya, DN: Architecture and Frontal Cortical Connections of the Premotor Cortex (area 6) in the Rhesus Monkey. J Comp Neurol 256:211, 1987.

24. Jürgens, U: The Efferent and Afferent Connections of the Supplementary Motor Area. Brain Res 300:63, 1984.

25. Künzle, H: An Autoradiographic Analysis of the Efferent Connections from Premotor and Adjacent Prefrontal Regions (Areas 6 and 9) in the Macaca Fascicularis. Brain Behav Evol 15:185, 1978.

26. Kurata, K: Corticocortical Inputs to the Dorsal and Ventral Aspects of the Premotor Cortex of Macaque Monkeys. Neurosci Res 12:263, 1991.

27. Leichnetz, GR: Afferent and Efferent Connections of the Dorsolateral Precentral Gyrus, (Area 4 Hand/Arm Region) in the Macaque Monkey, with Comparisons to Area 8. J Comp Neurol 254:460, 1986.

28. Morecraft, RJ and Van Hoesen, GW: Cingulate Input to the Primary and Supplementary Motor Cortices in the Rhesus Monkey: Evidence for Somatotopy in Areas 24c and 23c. J Comp Neurol 322:471, 1992.

29. Barbas, H and Mesulam, M-M: Organization of Afferent Input to Subdivisions of Area 8 in the Rhesus Monkey. J Comp Neurol 200:407, 1981.

30. Huerta, MF, Krubitzer, LA, and Kaas, LA: Frontal Eye Field as Defined by Intracortical Microstimulation in Squirrel Monkeys, Owl Monkeys and Macaque Monkeys: II. Cortical Connections. J Comp Neurol 265:332, 1987.

31. Barbas, H and Pandya, DN: Architecture and Intrinsic Connections of the Prefrontal Cortex in the Rhesus Monkey. J Comp Neurol 286:353, 1989.

32. Morecraft, RJ, Geula, C, and Mesulam, M-M: Cytoarchitecture and Neural Afferents or Orbitofrontal Cortex in the Brain of the Monkey. J Comp Neurol 323:341, 1992.

33. Morecraft, RJ, Geula, C, and Mesulam, M-M: Architecture of Connectivity Within a Cingulo-Fronto-Parietal Neurocognitive Network for Directed Attention. Arch Neurol 50:279, 1993.

34. Morecraft, RJ and Van Hoesen, GW: Frontal Granular Cortex Input to the Cingulate (M3) Supplementary (M2) and Primary (M1) Motor Cortices in the Rhesus Monkey. J Comp Neurol 337:669, 1993.

35. Kuypers, HGJM: Anatomy of the Descending Pathways. In Mountcastle, VB, Brooks, VB, and Geiger, SR (eds): Handbook of Physiology: The Nervous System, vol II, Part 1. American Physiological Society, Bethesda, MD, 1981, p 597.

36. Jones, RD, Donaldson, IM, and Parkin, PJ: Impairment and recovery of ipsilateral sensory-motor function following unilateral cerebral infarction. Brain 112:113, 1989.

37. Van Hoesen, GW, Morecraft, RJ, and Vogt, BA: Connections of the Monkey Cingulate Cortex. In Vogt, BA and Gabriel, M (eds): Neurobiology of the Cingulate Cortex and Limbic Thalamus: A Comprehensive Handbook. Birkhauser, Boston, 1993, p 249.

38. Brodal, P: Principles of Organization of the Monkey Corticopontine Projection. Brain Res 148:214, 1978.

39. Huerta, MF, Krubitzer, LA, and Kaas, JH: Frontal Eye Field as Defined by Intracortical Microstimulation in Squirrel Monkeys, Owl Monkeys, and Macaque Monkeys: I. Subcortical Connections. J Comp Neurol 253:415, 1986.

40. Humphrey, DR, Gold, R, and Reed, DJ: Sizes, Laminar and Topographic Origins of Cortical Projections to the Major Divisions of the Red Nucleus in the Monkey. J Comp Neurol 225:75, 1984.

41. Miller, RA and Strominger, NL: Efferent Connections of the Red Nucleus in the Brain Stem and Spinal Cord of the Rhesus Monkey. J Comp Neurol 152:327, 1973.

42. Ilinsky, IA and Kultas-Ilinsky, K: Sagittal Cytoarchitectonic Maps of the Macaca Mulatta Thalamus with a Revised Nomenclature of the Motor-Related Nuclei Validated by Observations on Their Connectivity. J Comp Neurol 262:331, 1987.

43. Mitz, AR and Wise, SP: The Somatotopic Organization of the Supplementary Motor Area: Intracortical Microstimulation Mapping. J Neurosci 7:1010, 1987.

44. Evarts, EV, et al: Motor Control of Finely Graded Responses. J Neurophysiol 49:1199, 1988.

45. Rizzolatti, G et al: Functional Organization of Inferior Area 6 in the Macaque Monkey II. Area F5 and the Control of Distal Movements. Exp Brain Res 71:491, 1988.

46. Okano, K and Tanji, J: Neuronal Activities in the Primate Motor Fields of the Agranular Frontal Cortex Preceding Visually Triggered and Self-paced Movement. Exp Brain Res 66:155, 1987.

47. Freund, H-J: Abnormalities of Motor Behavior After Cortical Lesions in Humans. In Mountcastle, VB, Plum, F, and Geiger, SR (eds): Handbook of Physiology: The Nervous System, vol V, Part 2. American Physiological Society, Bethesda, MD, 1987, p 763.

48. Gentilucci, M, et al: Functional Organization of Inferior Area 6 in the Macaque Monkey I. Somatotopy and the Control of Proximal Movements. Exp Brain Res 71:475, 1988.

49. McGuire, PK, Bates, JF, and Goldman-Rakic, PS: Interhemispheric Integration: I. Symmetry and Convergence of the Corticocortical Connections of the Left and Right Principal Sulcus (PS) and the Left and Right Supplementary Motor Area (SMA) in the Rhesus Monkey. Cerebral Cort 1:390, 1991.

50. Penfield, W and Welch, K: The Supplementary Motor Area of the Cerebral Cortex: A Clinical and Experimental Study. Arch Neurol Psychol 66:289, 1951.

51. Van Buren, JM and Fedio, P: Functional Representation on the Medial Aspect of the Frontal Lobes in Man. J Neurosurg 44:275, 1976.

52. Morecraft, RJ and Van Hoesen, GW: Convergence of Limbic Input to the Cingulate Motor Cortex in Rhesus Monkey. Soc Neurosci Abstr 18:324, 1992.

53. Kaada, BR, Pribaum, KH, and Epstein, JA: Respiratory and Vascular Responses in Monkeys from Temporal Pole, Insula, Orbital Surface and Cingulate Gyrus. J Neurophysiol 12:347, 1949.

54. Smith, WK: The Functional Significance of the Rostral Cingular Cortex as Revealed by Its Responses to Electrical Excitation. J Neurophysiol 8:241, 1945.

55. Talairach, J, et al: The Cingulate Gyrus and Human Behavior. Electroenceph Clin Neurophysiol 34:45, 1973.

56. Shima, K, et al: Two Movement-Related Foci in the Primate Cingulate Cortex Observed in Signal-Triggered and Self-Paced Forelimb Movements. J Neurophysiol 65:188, 1991.

57. Mesulam, M-M: Frontal Cortex and Behavior. Ann Neurol 19:320, 1986.

58. Mesulam, M-M: Large-Scale Neurocognitive Networks and Distributed Processing for Attention, Language, and Memory. Ann Neurol 28:597, 1990.

59. Roland, PE and Friberg, L: Localization of Cortical Areas Activated by Thinking. J Neurophysiol 53:1219, 1985.

60. Yajeya, J, Quintana, J, and Fuster, JM: Prefrontal Representation of Stimulus Attributes During Delay Tasks. II. The Role of Behavioral Significance. Brain Res 474:222, 1989.

61. Wilson, FAW, Scalaidhe, SPO, and Goldman-Rakic, PS: Dissociation of Object and Spatial Processing Domains in Primate Prefrontal Cortex. Science 260:1955, 1993.

62. Van Hoesen, GW: The Parahippocampal Gyrus: New Observations Regarding Its Cortical Connections in the Monkey. Trends Neurosci 5:345, 1982.

CHAPTER 8

■

Cerebellar Mechanisms

Christopher M. Fredericks, PhD

- ■ *Review of Superficial Anatomy*
- ■ *Internal Organization (Microscopic Anatomy)*
- ■ *Principal Connections with Extracerebellar Structures*
- ■ *Basic Cerebellar Circuitry*
- ■ *How the Basic Circuitry Works*
- ■ *Functional Systems*
- ■ *Role of the Cerebellum in Overall Motor Control*
- ■ *Motor Learning in the Cerebellum*
- ■ *Nonmotor Functions of the Cerebellum*

*T*he cerebellum is a small structure that lies on the dorsal side of the brainstem and comprises about 10% of the total mass of the brain. The cerebellum is a unique organ with many unusual properties. While it contains some of the most phylogenetically ancient motor control areas, it also contains some of the newest. Although the cerebellum is small and its circuitry is one of the simplest and most regimented of the brain, it contains approximately as many neurons as the rest of the brain put together and has a tremendous capacity for gathering and processing information. Despite its central and long-standing role in the control of movement, its destruction does not abolish movement and rarely causes muscle weakness. Instead, destruction of the cerebellum creates a certain incoordination or clumsiness of movement and sometimes abnormal muscle tone.

Despite the wealth of information that has accumulated regarding the anatomy and physiology of the cerebellum, there is little agreement on its precise role in the control of movement. We do know that the cerebellum has a huge afferent component, receiving inputs from proprioceptive and other somatic receptors in the periphery, from vestibular, visual, and auditory sense organs, and from motor and nonmotor areas of the cerebral cortex. In turn, the cerebellum has efferent projections to many areas of the brainstem, midbrain, and cerebral cortex.

Perhaps the simplest and most primitive function of the cerebellum is that mediated by brainstem connections involving regulation of vestibulo-ocular reflexes and other reflex components of equilibrium and balance. In addition, extensive connections with the sensorimotor cortex underly an important role for the cerebellum in the modulation of skilled voluntary movements involving the muscles of the distal extremities and of speech. Finally, its connections with prefrontal cortical areas may extend the functional domain of the cerebellum to the early stages of the planning and initiation of movement.

Apart from its role in somatic motor control, the cerebellum may also be involved in nonmotor activities, such as the regulation of certain vegetative functions and possibly in emotional and cognitive activities as well.

Review of Superficial Anatomy[1-4]

The cerebellum is the single largest structure in the posterior fossa of the skull. Although it is not part of the brainstem per se, it **lies just dorsal to the pons and medulla, forming the roof of the fourth ventricle** (Fig. 8–1). The surface of the cerebellum is extensively convoluted, with many transverse convolutions running from one side to the other. **Two deep transverse fissures** (the primary and posterolateral fissures) **divide the cerebellum into three major lobes** (Fig. 8–2). Moving from anterior to posterior, **these are the anterior, posterior, and flocculonodular lobes,** respectively. Shallower fissures subdivide each of these lobes into several lobules. **Viewed from side to side, the cerebellum is divided by two longitudinal grooves into medial (midline) and lateral regions.** The midline portion of the anterior and posterior lobes is called the *vermis,* whereas the lateral portions are the cerebellar hemispheres. Each hemisphere is composed of an intermediate (paravermal) and lateral zone, which, though not very distinct anatomically, are distinct in the afferent connections that they form and thus in their particular role in motor control.

The cerebellum is connected to the brainstem by three pairs of peduncles that contain all the afferent and efferent fibers transmitting information to and from this structure.

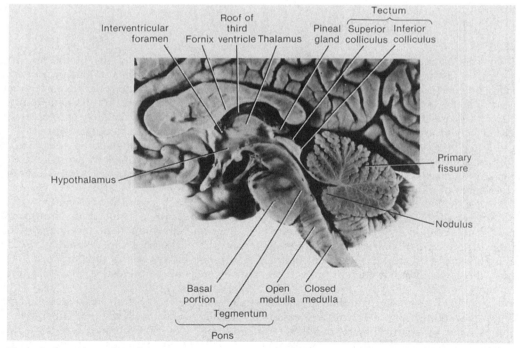

Figure 8–1. Relationship of the cerebellum to the major structures of the diencephalon and brainstem. (From Nolte, JA: The Human Brain: An Introduction to Its Functional Anatomy, ed 3. Mosby Year Book, St. Louis, 1993, p 23, with permission.)

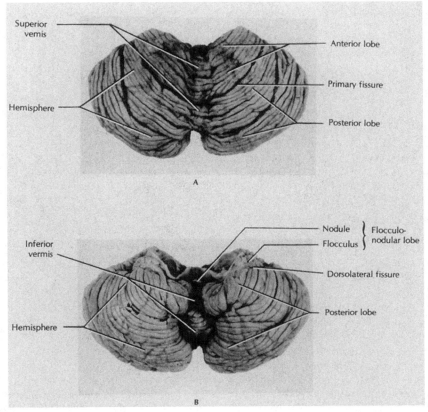

Figure 8-2. *Superficial Anatomy of the Cerebellum.* (A) Superior surface. (B) Inferior surface. The three major regions of the cerebellum (the flocculonodular, anterior, and posterior lobes) are clearly demarcated by the deep dorsolateral and primary fissures. (From Barr, ML, and Kiernan, JA: The Human Nervous System: ed 6. JB Lippincott, Philadelphia, 1993, p 161, with permission.)

Internal Organization (Microscopic Anatomy)[1-5]

The cerebellum is composed of an outer layer of gray matter (cerebellar cortex) containing neuronal cell bodies, **an internal core of white matter** containing primarily myelinated axons, **and three pairs of deep cerebellar nuclei** (fastigial, interposed, and dentate nuclei) (Fig. 8-3). **The cerebellar cortex is organized into three layers** (molecular, Purkinje cell, and granular cell layers) (Fig. 8-4) and is composed of five types of neurons (stellate, basket, Golgi, Purkinje, and granule cells) (Fig. 8-5). The outermost molecular layer consists primarily of granule cell axons and Purkinje and Golgi cell dendrites, along with a few scattered stellate and basket cells. The middle layer consists of a single row of the large ovoid cell bodies of Purkinje cells. These cells, which are the largest neurons in the brain, are the focal point of the cerebellar circuitry. Their dendrites project upward into the molecular layer, where they branch extensively. Their axons project downward through the third layer of the cortex to synapse on cells of the deep cerebellar nuclei and constitute the sole output of the cerebellar cortex. The innermost layer is composed primarily of densely packed small neurons called *granule cells* and a few larger Golgi cells. The granule cells send axons up to the molecular layer.

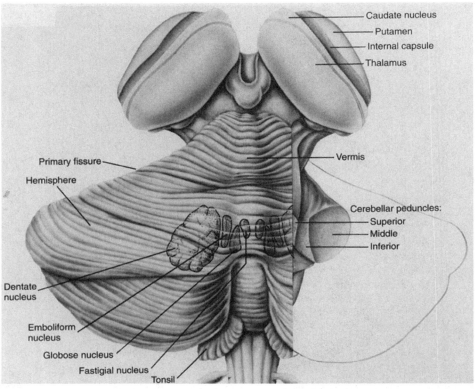

Caudate nucleus
Putamen
Internal capsule
Thalamus

Primary fissure
Hemisphere

Vermis

Cerebellar peduncles:
Superior
Middle
Inferior

Dentate nucleus

Emboliform nucleus

Globose nucleus

Fastigial nucleus

Tonsil

Figure 8–3. *Dorsal View of the Cerebellum.* In this drawing of the cerebellum, both superficial anatomy and deeper structures are represented. These include the globose nucleus, fastigial nucleus, and the dentate and emboliform nucleus which comprise the interposed nucleus. Part of the right hemisphere has been removed to reveal the underlying cerebellar peduncles. (From Kandel, ER, Schwartz, JH, and Jessell, TM (eds): Principles of Neuroscience, ed 3. Appleton & Lange, Norwalk, CT, 1991, p 628, with permission.)

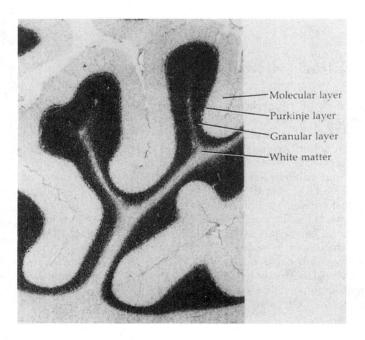

Molecular layer
Purkinje layer
Granular layer
White matter

Figure 8–4. *Cerebellar Cortex.* A low-power view of a section stained for myelin reveals the distinct layers of the cortex. (From Martin, JH: Neuroanatomy: Text and Atlas. Appleton & Lange, Norwalk, CT, 1993, p 252, with permission.)

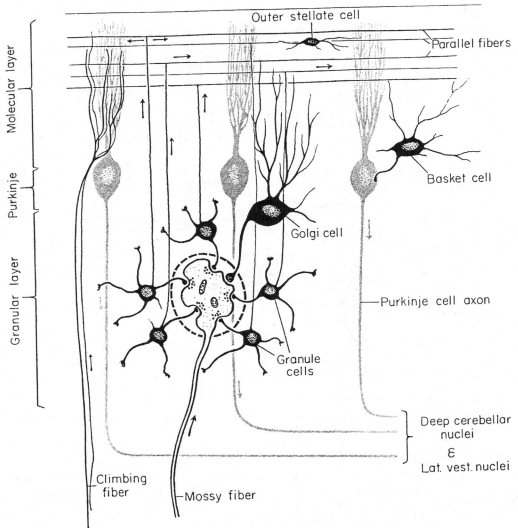

Figure 8–5. *Schematic Diagram of a Vertical Section of Cerebellar Cortex.* The cerebellar cortex is organized into three layers and contains five types of neurons. Excitatory inputs to the cortex are conveyed by climbing fibers and mossy fibers. The output is conveyed via the Purkinje fibers (Gray). Arrows indicate the direction of impulse conduction. (From Carpenter, MB: Core Text of Neuroanatomy, ed 4. Copyright © Williams & Wilkins, Baltimore, 1991, p 227, with permission.)

Principal Connections with Extracerebellar Structures[6-15]

One of the striking features of the cerebellum is the tremendous amount of afferent input reaching this organ. In fact, afferent fibers outnumber efferent by about 40 to 1 (Fig. 8–6). **Afferent inputs to the cerebellum originate in the spinal cord, as well as in many regions of both the cortical and subcortical brain.** The cerebellum receives both direct afferent inputs, as well as inputs that are relayed via various precerebellar nuclei in the brainstem. Afferents to the cerebellum terminate primarily within the cerebellar cortex. Within the cerebellar cortex, these fibers lose their myelin sheath and end either as mossy fibers or climbing fibers.

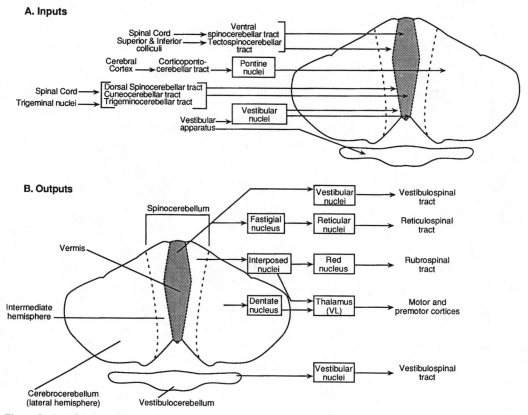

Figure 8–6. The three functional components of the cerebellum with their principle (*A*) inputs and (*B*) outputs.

The mossy fibers constitute the principal mode of termination of most cerebellar afferent systems. **Mossy fiber afferents originate in many regions outside the cerebellum, including the spinocerebellar tracts of the spinal cord, and the pontine, vestibular, and reticular nuclei of the brainstem** (Table 8–1).[8,11–13] Direct spinal afferents travel in the spinocerebellar and cuneocerebellar tracts, transmitting somatosensory input from proprioceptors and exteroceptors throughout the musculoskeletal and cutaneous systems. Vestibular apparatus afferents also project directly to the cerebellum via the mossy fiber system. These are accompanied by secondary projections from the vestibular nuclei. Many afferent inputs

Table 8–1. *Primary Mossy Fiber and Climbing Fiber Inputs*

Mossy Fibers

Spinocerebellar and cuneocerebellar tracts—Primary somesthetic afferents from periphery
Trigeminocerebellar tracts—Somesthetic afferents from face via trigeminal nuclei
Vestibulocerebellar tracts—Afferents from vestibular labyrinth and vestibular nuclei
Pontocerebellar tracts—Afferents from cerebral cortex via pontine nuclei
Reticulocerebellar tracts—Afferents from spinal cord as well as from cerebral cortex and other supraspinal
    structures via reticular nuclei

Climbing Fiber

Olivocerebellar tracts—Afferents from spinal cord as well as from cerebral cortex and other supraspinal
    structures via inferior olivary nuclei

are relayed to the mossy fiber system by precerebellar relay centers. Predominant among these are the pontine and reticular nuclei. The pontine nuclei form the main relay station for extensive inputs to the cerebellum that originate in the cerebral cortex, especially the frontal and parietal lobes.[8] The reticular nuclei receive and relay information converging from many sources, including the spinal cord, brainstem (e.g., vestibular and oculomotor nuclei), diencephalon (e.g., visual pathways and hypothalamus), cerebral cortex, and the cerebellar nuclei themselves. Information is not merely relayed by these nuclei, but considerable integration among the various input pathways occurs at these sites. It is interesting that the mossy fibers also provide a mechanism whereby the output of the cerebellar nuclei themselves can feed back to affect the activity of the neurons in the cerebellar cortex. These nucleocortical inputs terminate as mossy fibers in the granular layer of the cortex.

In marked contrast to the mossy fibers, **the climbing fibers mediate input from only one source, the inferior olivary nuclei of the medulla.**[8,14] These nuclei, in turn, receive a broad range of inputs from spinal, brainstem (e.g., trigeminal, vestibular, and reticular nuclei), diencephalon (e.g., visual pathways), and cortical areas. One of the most dense projections to the inferior olive is from the cerebellar nuclei themselves. Afferents to the olivary nuclei are precisely distributed within the nuclei, as are the olivary outputs very precisely distributed with the cerebellar cortex.

The only connections that exist between the cerebellum and extracerebellar structures are provided by the cerebellar peduncles (see Fig. 8–3). Cerebellar afferents arrive via all three peduncles, whereas efferent projections exit via only the inferior and superior peduncles. Most of the cerebellar input is channeled through the inferior cerebellar peduncle, except for the massive cortical input that is mediated by the middle cerebellar peduncle. Only a few fibers, including fibers from the ventral spinothalamic tracts, enter by way of the superior cerebellar peduncle. The primary efferent channel is the superior peduncle, although important vestibular and reticular projections course through the inferior peduncle.

Purkinje cell axons are the only output from the cerebellar cortex.[1–9,15] **Some of these axons,** arising in cells of the flocculonodular lobe and parts of the vermis, leave the cerebellum and **project directly to the vestibular nuclei.** This provides the only reasonably direct access the cerebellar cortex has to motor neurons of the spinal cord (i.e., via the vestibulospinal tracts). **All other Purkinje axons end in the deep cerebellar nuclei.** The various regions of the cerebellum project to specific cerebellar nuclei, with the most medial region (vermis) projecting to the most medial nucleus (the fastigial nucleus). The dentate and interposed nuclei constitute the source of most of the output. They send ascending fibers to innervate the red nucleus and other structures of the mesencephalon and thalamus, and they send descending fibers to reticular nuclei of the brainstem. Efferents of the dentate and interposed nuclei leave the cerebellum in the superior peduncle. Efferent connections of the fastigial nuclei constitute a much smaller proportion of the cerebellar output. These fibers exit by way of the inferior and superior peduncles, descending to terminate in vestibular and reticular formation nuclei of the brainstem or ascending to terminate in midbrain structures and the thalamus. **These efferent connections provide the cerebellum with access to reticulospinal, rubrospinal, vestibulospinal, and corticospinal tracts, as well as with the cerebral cortex via the thalamus.** In addition, there are projections from all three cerebellar nuclei back onto the cerebellar cortex itself.

Basic Cerebellar Circuitry[1,4,5,8,9,16–18]

The cerebellum is actually a relatively simple organ, composed of only a few different kinds of neurons. These neurons have very precise and complicated relationships with one another, forming a highly regimented neuronal circuitry (Fig. 8–7).

As we have seen, afferent fibers from numerous regions of the nervous system reach the cerebellar cortex through the underlying white matter, terminating as either mossy fibers or

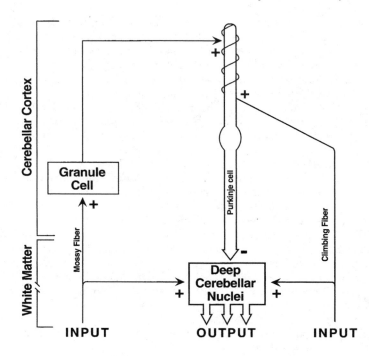

Figure 8–7. *Schematic Diagram of the Basic Input/Output Circuit of the Cerebellum.* Excitatory inputs arrive via the mossy fibers and climbing fibers. The only output cell of the cerebellar cortex is the Purkinje cell, which has strictly inhibitory connections with the deep cerebellar nuclei. The output of these nuclei is the net effect of these excitatory and inhibitory influences.

climbing fibers (see Fig. 8–5). Mossy fibers originate from a variety of structures in the central nervous system, whereas the climbing fibers arise from a single site in the medulla, the contralateral inferior olivary nucleus.

The **mossy fibers,** which constitute the majority (about two thirds) of the cerebellar afferents, **form excitatory synapses in the granular layer on the dendrites of granule cells** (see Fig. 8–5). **There is extensive convergence and divergence in this afferent system, such that each granule cell receives a large number of mossy fiber inputs and each mossy fiber synapses with a large number of granule cells.** The granule cells in turn send axons into the molecular layer, where they **form excitatory synapses on the dendrites of Purkinje cells** and several classes of interneurons. When the granule cell axons reach the molecular layer, they bifurcate as a T to run in opposite directions for several millimeters in longitudinal tracts of fibers, where they are termed *parallel fibers.*

Climbing fibers, on the other hand, show little divergence, synapsing on the cell body and dendritic tree of only a few (1 to 10) Purkinje cells. Moreover, each Purkinje cell receives input from only one climbing fiber. **Each climbing fiber,** however, **makes multiple synaptic contacts with their target Purkinje cell,** providing a powerful excitatory input. The climbing fibers get their name from the impression they give of climbing up the Purkinje dendritic tree.

In this way, the Purkinje cells receive direct input from both granule cells and climbing fibers, both of which are excitatory (see Fig. 8–7). Axons of the Purkinje cells then project to the deep cerebellar nuclei (primarily) or lateral vestibular nuclei. They also send collateral branches to other Purkinje cells and interneurons. **Although Purkinje cells are the sole output neurons of the cerebellar cortex, their synaptic actions are strictly inhibitory.** Both the mossy fibers and the climbing fibers also send collateral axonal branches to directly excite cells of the deep cerebellar nuclei.

In addition to the granule and Purkinje cells emphasized previously, three other types of neurons are present in the cerebellar cortex: the stellate, basket, and Golgi cells. Both stellate and basket cells are located in the molecular layer and cause inhibition of Purkinje cells. Golgi cells are located primarily within the granular layer (although their dendrites are within the molecular layer) and act to inhibit granule cells.

As complex as these cellular interconnections may appear at first glance, this physical arrangement creates a rather simple circuit for regulating the flow of information through the cerebellum (see Fig. 8–7). **The output from the cerebellum comes from the deep cerebellar nuclei.** The cells of these nuclei are tonically active but are continually affected by excitatory and inhibitory influences from the rest of the cerebellum. **Excitatory influences arise from direct connections with the mossy and climbing fibers,** which are bringing information to the cerebellum. **Inhibitory influences come from the Purkinje cells** of the cerebellar cortex. The level of output from the Purkinje cells is itself the net result of a variety of excitatory (i.e., from granule cells and climbing fibers) and inhibitory (i.e., from interneurons) influences. **The net output of the deep cerebellar nuclei, and hence the entire cerebellum, is thus determined by the balance among all of these opposing excitatory and inhibitory influences.**

Intermingled with this relatively simple, primary circuit are several types of inhibitory neurons affecting both granule and Purkinje cells. These interneurons are themselves stimulated by various factors, including both mossy and climbing fibers. Although this network of interneurons must serve to somehow modulate the activity of the cerebellar circuitry, the exact function of this interneuronal system is not known. Much like the lateral inhibition that is used in various sensory systems to heighten signal contrast, these interneurons may function to heighten the spatial and temporal definition of cerebellar information.[4,17]

The Monoaminergic System[8,9,14,19]

Although cerebellar afferent systems have been classically divided into mossy fibers and climbing fibers, **a third group of cerebellar afferent fibers has been identified, which cannot be strictly classified as either mossy or climbing. These are the (mono) aminergic afferent pathways.** These afferent fibers are characterized by fine axons that are distributed in both the molecular and granular layers of the cerebellar cortex. This afferent system contains well-developed noradrenergic and serotonergic fibers, as well as less well-defined dopaminergic fibers. These fibers originate primarily in certain brainstem nuclei (e.g., raphe nucleus and locus coeruleus), with a few arising in the hypothalamus. The physiologic actions of these afferents may be very different from those of the mossy or climbing fibers. One possibility is that they exert subtle effects on the excitability of cerebellar cortical neurons through the release of neurohumoral agents.

How the Basic Circuitry Works

The circuitry of the cerebellum may be the most uniform in the entire brain and the most phylogenetically persistent among vertebrates. The mossy fiber and climbing fiber systems are present in the cerebella of all species studied so far and in each case play an important role in the control of movement. Nonetheless, it is not at all clear how these two afferent systems contribute to overall motor control, or even how they interact to regulate the activity of the Purkinje cell on which they are focused.

What we do know is that the two systems are very different. In contrast to the simplicity that the climbing fiber system displays in its connectivity and distribution, the mossy fiber system is much more expansive and is among the most complex of the central nervous system. Whereas activation of a given set of climbing fibers creates an outcome in a few discrete cells, activation of a similar set of mossy fibers generates activity in a large group of Purkinje cells over wide areas of the entire cerebral cortex.

It has been suggested that the climbing fibers affect the ongoing processing of the cerebellar cortex, not so much by encoding detailed information about peripheral stimuli, but by modulating the responsiveness of the Purkinje cells to mossy fiber inputs. The mossy fiber system, on the other hand, provides a continuously upgraded description of both motor

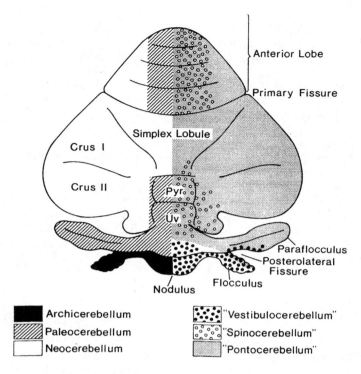

Figure 8–8. Diagram of the Cerebellum. Components of the cerebellum based on phylogenetic considerations (*Left*) and components of the cerebellum based on the sites of termination of major afferent systems (*Right*). (From Gilman,[10] p 38, with permission.)

command output and sensory input necessary for attuning premotor command signals to the existing functional context in which movement is occurring. Other theories ascribing different functions to these systems have also been proposed, each accompanied by its own supportive evidence. Others, for example, argue that the climbing fiber system is a true afferent system mediating a large variety of convergent inputs relayed by the olivary nuclei from the spinal cord, many regions of the brainstem, and from the motor cortex.

Functional Systems[2,4,5,7,9,10,20]

As vertebrate evolution occurred, the cerebellum evolved in structure and capacity,subserving increasingly diverse and complex motor activities. On phylogenetic grounds, the human cerebellum can be considered to be made up of three basic components: the archicerebellum, the paleocerebellum, and the neocerebellum, listed in order of their phylogenetic appearance[2,4,5,7,9,10,20] (Fig. 8–8). These three anatomic divisions correspond roughly to three *functional* regions of the cerebellum, each of which receives its main inputs from different sources and sends its primary outputs to different parts of the brain. These functional regions are the vestibulocerebellum, spinocerebellum, and cerebrocerebellum (pontocerebellum), respectively. These neuroanatomic and functional designations are often used synonymously, although they are not wholly congruent. A convenient way to discuss the function of the cerebellum, as well as the clinical aspects of its dysfunction (see Chapter 19), is in terms of the activities of each of these three functional systems (Table 8–2).

Archicerebellum (Vestibulocerebellum)

The **archicerebellum** is the earliest part of the cerebellum to evolve; it occupies the flocculonodular lobe. Because of its close ties to vestibular function, it is often referred to as

Table 8–2. *Principal Cerebellar Inputs and Outputs*

Functional Region	Anatomic Region	Origins of Principal Input	Deep Nucleus	Principal Descending Destination	Motor Function
Vestibulocerebellum	Flocculonodular lobe	Vestibular labyrinth and vestibular nuclei		Medial descending systems (vestibulospinal and corticospinal tracts)	Control of axial muscles in balance; coordination of head and eye movements
Spinocerebellum	Vermis	Spinal afferents (from proximal body); cranial nerve nuclei (from face); vestibular, auditory, and visual systems	Fastigial	Brainstem and cortical components of medial descending systems	Control of axial and girdle muscles
	Intermediate part of hemisphere	Spinal afferents (from limbs)	Interposed	Brainstem and cortical components of lateral descending systems	Control of distal limb muscles
Cerebrocerebellum	Lateral part of hemisphere	Wide areas of cerebral cortex, especially primary motor and somatosensory cortices; also premotor cortex	Dentate	Primary motor and premotor cortices to both lateral and medial descending systems; red nucleus	Programming and initiation of movement

Source: Modified from Ghez,[4] p 635, with permission.

the **vestibulocerebellum.** It receives its input exclusively from the vestibular system, receiving afferents from both the vestibular apparatus itself and the vestibular nuclei in the medulla. Its output is back to the vestibular nuclei. In humans, it retains its important relationships with the vestibular system and **functions in the coordination of head and eye movements and helps control equilibrium and balance through influences on axial muscles** mediated by medial and lateral vestibulospinal tracts. Its importance is seen in the maintenance of both normal stance and gait.

Paleocerebellum (Spinocerebellum)

The **paleocerebellum,** which was the next to develop in vertebrates, extends through the central portion of both the anterior and posterior lobes and longitudinally encompasses the vermis at the midline and the intermediate zone of the cerebellar hemispheres. Because of its association with spinal input, the paleocerebellum is also referred to as the **spinocerebellum.** The principal input to the spinocerebellum comes from spinocerebellar and cuneocerebellar tracts carrying somatosensory information from the body and limbs. This information is conveyed to specific parts of the cerebellum, which are somatotopically organized in much the same way that somatosensory information is represented in the sensory cortex[21] (Fig. 8–9). Sensory information also reaches the spinocerebellum from the head via cranial nerve nuclei mediating sensation in the face (i.e., trigeminocerebellar afferents) and from visual and auditory systems. The same somatotopic regions of the cerebellum can be activated by stimulating corresponding regions of the sensorimotor cortex.[3] This indicates that in addition to receiving sensory information directly from the periphery, the spinocerebellum receives information from the sensory and motor cortices themselves.

Although the arrangement of the somatosensory, visual, and auditory input to the cerebellar cortex has never actually been determined physiologically for the human brain, this is inferred from data derived from the study of monkeys and other animals. This mapping is not nearly as precise as in the sensory and motor areas of the cerebral cortex.[1] The spinocerebellum projects to regions of the deep cerebellar nuclei, which play a major role in controlling limb movements and muscle tone. These projections are somatotopically distributed within the nuclei.

Although included within the overall operation of the spinocerebellum, the vermis and intermediate hemispheres function very differently. Each receives different sensory inputs, while projecting to different deep nuclei and cortical regions, and thus controlling different descending motor systems. The *vermis* receives somatosensory input from the trunk

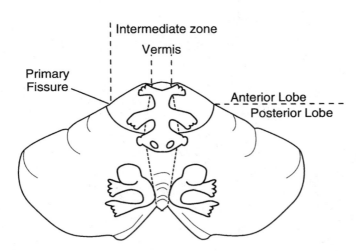

Figure 8–9. *Diagramatic Representation of the Topographic Organization of Inputs to the Spinocerebellum.* Somatic sensory projections are somatotopically organized. Representation is ipsilateral in anterior lobe and bilateral in paramedial lobules. Visual, auditory, and vestibular inputs project primarily to the "ear" and "eye" portions.

and the head. It also receives direct projections from the primary sensory neurons of the vestibular labyrinth, as well as visual and auditory input relayed by brainstem nuclei. The output of the vermis travels to the fastigial nucleus, which gives rise to many descending projections to the reticular formation and lateral vestibular nuclei of the brainstem, as well as a few ascending projections via the thalamus to the primary motor cortex. In this way, **the vermis controls** both the cortical (anterior corticospinal tracts) and brainstem (lateral and medial reticulospinal tracts and vestibulospinal tracts) **components of the ventromedial descending system and hence lower motor neurons to axial and girdle musculature.** The vermis is primarily involved in the regulation of posture and of stereotyped movements (e.g., rhythmic walking movements) that are largely programmed in the brainstem and spinal cord.

The *intermediate hemisphere* receives inputs from the extremities and projects to the interposed nuclei. From here, primary descending projections travel to the red nucleus, and ascending projections travel via the thalamus to the primary motor and supplemental motor cortex. In this way, **the intermediate zone controls** the cortical (lateral corticospinal tracts) and brainstem **components of the dorsolateral descending system (rubrospinal tracts) and hence lower motor neurons to the distal musculature of the extremities.**

Neocerebellum (Cerebrocerebellum)

The **neocerebellum** (the largest and newest component) occupies the lateral zone of the cerebellar hemispheres and receives extensive input from many areas of the cerebral cortex, especially the sensory, motor, and premotor cortices. These regions do not project directly to the neocerebellum but rather to the pontine nuclei that relay this information to the cerebellum. The bulk of the fibers arise in the ipsilateral frontal and parietal lobes. The pontocerebellar projection is massive and forms the bulk of the middle cerebellar peduncle. The neocerebellum is also called the **cerebrocerebellum,** or **pontecerebellum** reflecting its extensive interconnections with the cerebrum. The output of the neocerebellum is conveyed by the dentate nucleus to the thalamus and then to the primary motor and premotor cortices. These centers ultimately project descending efferent impulses through both the lateral and anterior (medial) corticospinal tracts, as well as reticulospinal tracts. Through its connections with the cortices, **the cerebrocerebellum is thought to contribute to the planning and timing of voluntary movements** (e.g., ipsilateral volitional limb movements), particularly learned, skillful movements that become more rapid, precise, and automatic with practice.[4,22-25]

The division of the cerebellum into these three functional units is somewhat misleading, since many interconnections exist among these units. All cerebellar zones receive direct or indirect input from both the spinal cord and cerebral cortex, and all project to some degree to both spinal cord and cortical structures.

Role of the Cerebellum in Overall Motor Control[4,5,10,26-29]

Despite extensive study of both the structure and function of the cerebellum, there is still no consensus regarding precisely how the cerebellar circuits contribute to motor control. We do know that the cerebellum receives a tremendous input from somesthetic, vestibular, visual, and auditory sensory systems defining the functional status of the body and the context in which movement is occurring. The cerebellum also receives information regarding motor commands being formulated and delivered by the motor system. This information is derived not only from the programming areas of the cerebral cortex but also from points along the chain of command nearer the final common pathway, such as collaterals from the corticospinal tracts and from spinal interneurons themselves. We also

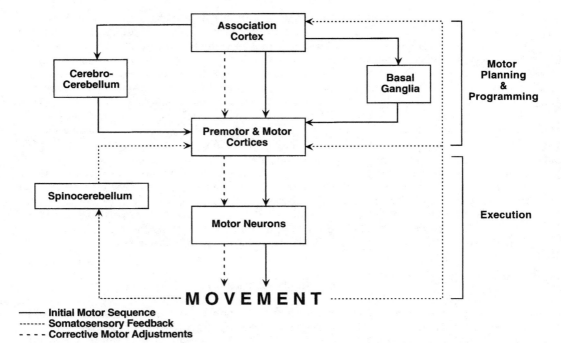

Figure 8–10. *Flow Diagram Representing the "Comparator" Role of the Cerebellum in the Planning and Execution of Voluntary Movement.* In coordinating rapid, phasic motor activity, the cerebellum (i.e., spinocerebellum) compares the movement plans formulated in the cerebral cortex and carried out through pyramidal and extrapyramidal pathways, with the actual evolution of movement. It then acts to correct any discrepancies (i.e., errors) between the intent and the actual movement as portrayed by unfolding somatosensory feedback. For simplicity, the thalamic relay of basal ganglia, cerebellar, and somatosensory input is omitted.

know that the cerebellum has extensive projections to brainstem motor nuclei (especially the red nucleus and reticular nuclei) and to the motor/premotor cortices, which provide access to the descending rubrospinal, reticulospinal, and corticospinal tracts. The cerebellar projections to the cerebral cortex are relayed in the thalamus, where additional connections are made with the basal ganglia and other structures involved in motor control.

The cerebellum has a tremendous capacity for processing information. **Using the feedback it receives from the sensory and motor systems, the cerebellum seems to be able to define the current status of the somatic systems, make predictions about how this will change in the context of ongoing motor activity, compare these outcomes with the intended outcomes of evolving motor activity, and issue its own directives to both descending and cortical elements of the motor system** (Fig. 8–10). The net result is greater synergy and accuracy in our movement. This role in the modulation and coordination of movement is important in the involuntary movements of posture and equilibrium, in simple rhythmic movement patterns such as walking, and in complex, skilled voluntary movements.

Posture and Equilibrium

Extensive interconnections exist between the human vestibulocerebellum and both the vestibular nuclei and the vestibular apparatus itself. These **vestibular interconnections mediate an important role for the cerebellum in coordination of head and eye movements, as well as in the maintenance of body equilibrium and posture.**[4,5,10,26-29] The cerebellum is particularly important in the maintenance of equilibrium during movement (e.g., locomotion). The cerebellum uses feedback from the vestibular system to determine changes occurring in the direction of motion and to institute—almost instantaneously—the corrections in postural motor signals necessary for maintaining equilibrium in the face of these changes in direction. Activity in the archicerebellum is assisted in this task by sensory feedback from the periphery received by the vermis.

Lesions in the flocculonodular lobes and portions of the vermis result in disturbances of equilibrium that are particularly evident during rapid changes in body position or in the direction of movement. Patients with such lesions may exhibit an unsteadiness of gait or an inability to stand or sit without swaying or falling. Note that destruction of the archicerebellum creates little change in muscle tone, and no tremor or dyssynergy is seen in the distal extremities.

The same portions of the cerebellum that are involved in the maintenance of equilibrium modulate the vestibular-ocular reflexes that coordinate head and eye movements. Damage to these areas results in abnormalities of eye movement such as nystagmus.

Skilled Voluntary Movement

The cerebellum plays important roles in the coordination and planning of skilled voluntary movements, most of which involve the musculature of the distal extremities.[4,5,10,26-29] These functions are highly dependent on the extensive interconnections that the cerebellum has with the cerebral cortex and have relatively little to do with the control of equilibrium and posture and the related axial and girdle muscles. As noted previously in this chapter, the intermediate zones of the cerebellar hemispheres receive considerable direct information from the premotor cortex regarding intended movements, as well as extensive feedback from the periphery regarding the actual movements being achieved (see Fig. 8–10). By comparing the intended with the actual motor activity, the cerebellum is able to detect discrepancies between the two and institute corrective measures to minimize these "errors." In this way, **the cerebellum promotes the kind of synchrony and accuracy of movements required for the performance of precise, purposeful movements.** The cerebellum in exerting its "corrective" influences on voluntary motor activity affects many aspects of movement, including rate, range, force, and direction. Distortion of each one of these parameters is evident among the characteristic clinical features of cerebellar dysfunction (see Chapter 19). If, for example, a limb is moving too fast (rate) and is destined to overshoot the intended target (range), the cerebellum will detect this and influence the appropriate agonists and antagonists to slow down the movement and prevent the overshoot. In cerebellar disease, the control of rate and range may be impaired, resulting in clinical presentations such as past-pointing and other forms of dysmetria.

In humans, the lateral zones of the cerebellar hemispheres are highly developed and have extensive interconnections with the cerebral cortex, most of which are with premotor and sensory portions of the cerebrum rather than with the primary motor cortex. Through these connections, the lateral portions of the cerebellar hemispheres may be involved in the planning and timing of sequential movements. The intent to perform a movement probably occurs in the motor association areas of the cerebral cortex, and evidence suggests that these areas act in concert with the lateral portions of the cerebellar hemispheres in the planning of movement. Consistent with this idea is the fact that most neurons in the dentate nucleus change their firing rates *before* voluntary movements occur, and many of them change firing rates even before activity in the motor cortex changes. Cooling or damaging the dentate nuclei may result in delays in the initiation of voluntary movement. One of the most important features of normal motor function is the ability to progress smoothly from one successive movement to the next. Moreover, the timing of each component movement in this progression must be appropriate; otherwise the entire orderly progression will be disrupted. Hore and Vilis[22] found that cooling the dentate nucleus in monkeys disrupted the precisely timed sequence of agonist and antagonist activity that occurs with normal rapid movements. The cerebellum seems to **play a central role in both the ordering and the proper timing of the initiation and termination of the many sequential motor steps**

required in most purposeful movements. Lesions of the cerebellum can result in an inability to progress in an orderly, timely fashion from one movement to the next, which becomes particularly evident in the disturbance of complex motor activities such as running, writing, or speaking. The lateral cerebellum may also perform a more general timing function that influences cognitive, as well as motor performance.[23-25] Not only do patients with lateral lesions show deficits in motor timing, but their ability to judge elapsed time in purely perceptual tasks may be severely impaired.[24]

Locomotion and Other Rhythmic Activities

In addition to the tonic motor adjustments associated with the maintenance of posture and the discrete phasic movement associated with volitional activity, **the cerebellum may play an important role in the control of certain primitive, rhythmic motor behaviors.**[30-32] Although rhythmic activities such as scratching, walking, and possibly writing are programmed as patterns in the spinal cord, they are strongly influenced by the cerebral cortex and the cerebellum.

In many animals, locomotion does not require the participation of the cerebral cortex. Dogs and cats whose spinal cord has been disconnected from the brain can emit patterns of gait as long as their weight is supported and the ground is moving under their feet.[31] Although a human with such a lesion would not demonstrate such motor behavior, it is notable that a stepping pattern can be elicited against a moving platform in normal human infants, well before they have learned to voluntarily ambulate (see Chapter 5). The cerebellum probably makes several different contributions to the control of locomotion, including adjustment of the timing of locomotive movements, modulation of interlimb coordination during locomotion, and coordination of various spinal reflexes with ongoing locomotor activity.[30] Medial (vermal) and intermediate regions of the cerebellum seem to be the most involved. The cerebellum provides important internal feedback to locomotor pattern generators in the spinal cord regarding the changing circumstances under which locomotion is taking place.

The involvement of the cerebellum in locomotion is attested to by walk-related rhythmic discharge in both cerebellar afferent and efferent connections. Rhythmic afferent activity is particularly evident in the mossy fiber input to the cerebellum (e.g., spinocerebellar and reticulocerebellar tracts).[32] The climbing fiber input from the olivary cells seems to be less involved and does not display any obvious fluctuations in activity related to the step cycle during locomotion. Walk-related output is evident in Purkinje cells, medial and intermediate outflow nuclei (i.e., fastigial and interposed nuclei), and vestibulospinal and reticulospinal tract neurons. Outflow in these tracts disappears when the limbs are forcibly stopped or the cerebellum is removed.[30] In addition, characteristic abnormalities in locomotion can be produced in experimental animals with cooling or ablation of specific regions of the cerebellum.[29] **Although the cerebellum influences locomotion, it is not essential for the generation of the basic movement patterns,** since locomotion (though clumsy) can still be carried out by a decerebellate animal, and stimulation of subthalamic or midbrain locomotor centers can still produce locomotion.[30,31]

Similar observations regarding cerebellar activity have been made in association with animal scratching behavior.[30] There is also a similarity between the pattern formed in walking and that in writing. Both are semiautomatic movements made at various cadences—one for legs and the other for the arm. It has been suggested that the central pattern generators and the cerebellum may be involved in writing as well.[31]

Muscle Tone[10,27-29,33,34]

Muscle tone is defined in terms of the ease with which a muscle may be passively stretched. Hypotonia specifically refers to a decrease in the resistance offered to passive stretch and is usually associated with a reduction in the amplitude of the deep tendon reflexes. When the entire cerebellum is removed from experimental animals, such as the monkey, hypotonia of limb muscles occurs.[27,29,34] **Hypotonia is also a common result of damage to the cerebellum or its projections in humans** (see Chapter 19). It is most evident shortly after acute cerebellar damage, but tends to resolve after several months. Hypotonia in man may lead to a number of distinct clinical signs (e.g., muscle flabbiness and pendular deep tendon reflexes) (see Chapter 12). Although it is not as conspicuous as the incoordination of movement associated with cerebellar dysfunction, hypotonia can exacerbate the symptoms of ataxia.

The response of skeletal muscle to passive stretch is mediated by muscle spindles in the context of the stretch reflexes[27,29,33,34] (see Chapter 5). Muscle tone is thus determined in part by the level of gamma (fusimotor) input to the muscle spindle. Increased gamma input increases the sensitivity of the spindle and thus the responsiveness of muscle to stretch (i.e., its tone). **Gamma efferent discharge is influenced by** various components of the central nervous system, one of which is **the cerebellum.** The cerebellum is thought to have a generally excitatory influence on the underlying gamma support of the stretch reflexes. **Cerebellar damage probably results in decreased excitation of gamma motor neurons, leading to reduced sensitivity of muscle spindles and hence decreased muscle tone.** In cats, for example, cerebellectomy significantly reduces muscle spindle sensitivity to stretch.[29,33] In addition, decreased muscle tone may reflect a loss of facilitation of the motor cortex and brainstem nuclei by tonic discharge of deep cerebellar nuclei.

Motor Learning in the Cerebellum[5,6,28,35–47]

One of the great challenges confronting neuroscientists has been to define the physical-anatomic correlates of learning—in other words, to discern the actual changes that occur in specific regions of the nervous system as learning progresses. The presumption is that the nervous system is to an extent "plastic" and that as reflexes, skills, or even memories of events and feelings are acquired, physical correlates of these acquisitions develop and persist. One type of learning that has been extensively studied is that involved in the acquisition or modification of motor behaviors. This is motor learning. A productive way to study motor learning has been to focus on a number of simple adaptive or conditioned motor responses and the role of specific nervous system regions in their learning or modification (adaptation). These techniques have been extensively applied to the cerebellum in the hope that this might prove to be a site at which irrefutable physical evidence of learning might be found.

Scientists have studied a wide variety of motor behaviors in an effort to define a role for the cerebellum in "learned" changes in these behaviors.[35–43] Perhaps the most widely studied models involve adaptive changes in the vestibulo-ocular reflex,[38] or conditioning of the eye blink response.[39–47] These studies have been carried out in both humans and various experimental animals, especially rabbits and monkeys. Lesion experiments have provided the strongest evidence that cerebellar circuits are important in motor learning. In this regard, the ablation of certain critical cerebellar regions often disrupts retention of a previously conditioned response in a trained subject, as well as prevents the adaptation or conditioning of a response in a naive subject. For example, adaptation of the vestibulo-ocular reflex is disturbed by removal of the flocculus or particular parts of the inferior olivary nucleus, whereas conditioning of the eye blink is disrupted by lesions to particular areas of the interposed nuclei or inferior olive. To proponents of cerebellar learning, **these kinds of findings support the notion that the cerebellum is the actual site of plastic changes associated with motor learning,** and various models of these changes have been proposed.

The debate regarding the role of the cerebellum in motor learning, however, is not settled.[44–47] Some investigators suggest that the cerebellum is not really the site of learning, but merely optimizes motor performance while learning takes place elsewhere. These opponents of cerebellar motor learning point to experiments in animals in which previously conditioned behaviors can still be executed after total removal of the cerebellum, or where naive animals can acquire a conditioned behavior following cerebellum removal or blockade with local anesthetic. These investigators suggest that the learning deficits caused by cerebellar lesions are more likely due to modifications in the performance of a reflex behavior than to the elimination of learning-related cerebellar mechanisms or critical storage sites for the underlying memory traces. Although cerebellar information processing may contribute to the time course and extent of learning, the most likely sites for the actual plastic changes are outside the cerebellum.

Motor learning is crucial to movement, because even the most routine motor behaviors require constant adaptation as circumstances change. While the role of the cerebellum in motor control is established, its role in motor learning remains to be determined.

Nonmotor Functions of the Cerebellum

Although the primary physiologic importance of the cerebellum resides in its involvement in somatic motor control and although the clinical sequelae of cerebellar dysfunction in humans are almost exclusively within the realm of disordered somatic activity, **considerable evidence suggests involvement of the cerebellum in a number of nonmotor aspects of human and animal function.**[6,35] These activities are nonmotor to the extent that they do not involve somatic systems directly and that they can be observed in the absence of somatic motor activity. The latter distinction is important, because it is well known that somatic activity itself can significantly affect nonmotor activity.

Visceral (Autonomic) Functions[6,35,48–51]

A growing body of evidence suggests that **the cerebellum may play an active role in the regulation of numerous visceral motor functions.** For example, the cerebellum has been shown to have anatomic connections with various visceral control centers in the brainstem, as well as reciprocal connections with the hypothalamus.[6,48–50] It was long thought that interaction between the cerebellum and the hypothalamus was mediated only by indirect multisynaptic pathways relayed through the reticular formation.[49,50] More recently, however, direct monosynaptic connections between the cerebellum and the hypothalamus have been identified. It is likely that cerebellar output directly to brainstem control centers, as well as cerebellar-hypothalamic pathways linked to descending hypothalamic projections to a variety of brainstem and spinal cord visceral centers, represent important circuits by which the cerebellum may directly influence or even regulate a wide variety of autonomic functions. It is also likely that the cerebellum receives afferent input directly from peripheral visceral structures, since electrical recordings in the cerebellum have demonstrated afferent connections to the cerebellum from at least the vagus and splanchnic nerves.[6,48]

Conclusions about the actual influence that the cerebellum may have on various visceral functions and, by implication, the role that it may play in their physiologic regulation have been largely drawn from experiments in which certain regions of the cerebellum have been either artificially stimulated (i.e., electrically or chemically) or destroyed (ablated).[6,48] Alterations in a wide range of autonomic responses and reflexes have been reported subsequent to experimental manipulation of cerebellar structures. Such responses include alterations in systemic blood pressure, heart rate, regional blood flow and the electrocardiogram; pupillary size (mydriasis and miosis) and reactivity to light; accommodation of the lens; respiratory rate and depth; urinary and gastrointestinal tract motility; and piloerection. The influence of the cerebellum on certain pupillary (e.g., the pupillary light reflex) and cardiovascular (the baroreceptor reflex) responses is perhaps the best established.[51]

Although cerebellar manipulation can produce significant and varied alterations in visceral function and although extensive anatomic connections exist by which visceral

regulatory areas might be influenced, the actual physiologic role of the cerebellum in the normal regulation of these systems in not known. Moreover, patients with cerebellar disease seldom show any clinical evidence of vegetative dysfunction directly attributable to the cerebellum.

Cognitive Functions[6,35,52–62]

As previously mentioned, it has been suspected for a long time that the cerebellum has a role in motor learning. Considerable evidence suggests that simple forms of associative learning, such as the conditioning of simple motor responses, are dependent on an intact cerebellum. **The question of whether the cerebellum has a role in more complex intellectual processes and cognition has more recently been raised.**[6,35,52,55]

Reciprocal anatomic connections do exist between the cerebellum and association areas and language areas of the frontal lobes of the human cerebral cortex.[6,53,54] Both mossy fibers and climbing fibers carry information to the cerebellum from association areas of the cortex, as well as from motor areas. Similarly, cerebellar projections travel to the frontal and parietal areas of the cortex.

It has been argued on phylogenetic grounds that the human cerebellum is prepared to undertake the information processing required for higher mental function.[53,54] With evolution, humans have developed a cerebellum that is larger than that of other animals, including other primates, thus providing the additional neuronal equipment necessary for more information processing. Also, the cerebellum has evolved extensive connections to the newest areas of the cerebral cortex. It is interesting that full growth of the cerebellum is not attained until a person reaches 15 to 20 years of age, which approximately parallels the maturation timetable for an individual's mental capabilities.

Perhaps the most revealing studies of cerebellar activity are those using the positron emission tomography (PET) scanner.[56–58] When normal subjects are asked to perform tasks that have no motor component, but that require significant mental processing such as thinking of words, silent speech, or doing mathematical calculations, PET scans show that during these activities metabolic or vascular changes occur in cerebellar areas that are highly developed in humans. The implication is that these areas are participating in the neuronal processes underlying these cognitive activities.

If these cognitive skills are being carried out by the cerebellum, one would expect them to be diminished as a result of disease or injury preventing interaction between the cerebellum and cortical association areas. Although some clinicians have noted an association between developmental disorders of the cerebellum and retarded intellectual development, cognitive abnormalities are usually not evident in patients with cerebellar disease or injury.[59] The conventional neurologic and neuropsychologic tests routinely used to assess these patients, however, provide only relatively gross measurement of these capabilities. Sophisticated neuropsychological tests have now shown subtle defects in verbal and nonverbal intelligence, in memory, and in "higher" functions in patients with cerebellar disease.[60–62] However, little evidence exists that the cerebellum is involved in conscious thought or sensation in man. Direct stimulation of the cerebellar cortex in alert man fails to arouse any conscious experience.

On balance, considerably more research remains to be done to conclusively determine whether the cerebellum has any role in higher mental processes.

Emotion[6,35,63–71]

Reciprocal anatomic connections have been shown between the cerebellum and the reticular formation, hypothalamus, and limbic system.[49,50] Although these are all areas involved in the perception of and reaction to emotion, **little is known of the role that the cerebellum may play in influencing the generation of emotions or in controlling emotional behaviors.** Both stimulation and ablation experiments in laboratory animals have resulted in alterations in various emotion-laden behaviors, such as rage, pleasure seeking, fear, and aggression.[6,35,63,64] Recently, certain structural abnormalities in the cerebella of patients with autism[65-67] and certain psychiatric disorders[68-70] (e.g., schizophrenia) have been revealed by computed tomography and magnetic resonance imaging scans, as well as by pathologic study. Also, cerebellar stimulation has been used with some limited success in the treatment of certain emotional disorders.[71]

RECOMMENDED READINGS

Barr, ML and Kiernen, JA: The Human Nervous System, ed 6. Chapter 10. Cerebellum. JB Lippincott, Philadelphia, 1993.

Bloedel, JR, Dichgans, J, and Precht, W (eds): Cerebellar Functions. Part 2, Cerebellum and Basal Ganglia. American Physiological Society, Bethesda, MD, 1981.

Brooks, VB: The Neural Basis of Motor Control. Chapter 13. The Cerebellum. Oxford University Press, New York, 1986.

Brooks, VB and Thach, WT: Cerebellar Control of Posture and Movement. Chapter 18. In Brookhart, JM and Mountcastle, VB (eds): Handbook of Physiology. Section 1. The Nervous System. American Physiological Society, Bethesda, MD, 1981.

Carpenter, MB: Neuroanatomy, ed 4. Chapter 8. The Cerebellum. Williams & Wilkins, Baltimore, 1991.

Dow, RS, Kramer, RE, and Robertson, LT: Disorders of the Cerebellum. Chapter 37. In Joynt, RJ (ed): Clinical Neurology, vol 3. JB Lippincott, Philadelphia, 1991.

Ghez, C: The Cerebellum. Chapter 41. In Kandel, ER, Schwartz, JH, and Jessell, TM (eds): Principles of Neural Science, ed 3. Appleton & Lange, Norwalk, CT, 1991.

Gilman, S: The Cerebellum: Its Role in Posture and Movement. In Swash, M and Kennard, C (eds): Scientific Basis of Clinical Neurology. Churchill Livingstone, New York, 1985.

Gilman, S: Cerebellum and Motor Dysfunction. Chapter 23. In Asbury, AK, McKhann, GM, and McDonald, WI (eds): Diseases of the Nervous System, ed 2. WB Saunders, Philadelphia, 1992.

Gilman, S, Bloedel, JR, and Lechtenberg, R: Disorders of the Cerebellum. FA Davis, Philadelphia, 1981.

Ito, M: The Cerebellum and Neural Control. Raven Press, New York, 1984.

King, JS (ed): New Concepts in Cerebellar Neurobiology. Alan R Liss, New York, 1988.

Martin, JH: Neuroanatomy: Text and Atlas. Chapter 10. The Cerebellum. Appleton & Lange, Norwalk, CT, 1989.

Noback, CR, Strombinger, NL, and Demarest, RJ: The Human Nervous System: Introduction and Review, ed 4. Chapter 18. Cerebellum. Lea & Febiger, Philadelphia, 1991.

Nolte, J: The Human Brain: An Introduction to Its Functional Anatomy, ed 2. Chapter 14. Cerebellum. CV Mosby, St. Louis, 1988.

Palay, S and Chan-Palay, V: Cerebellar Cortex Cytology and Organization. Springer-Verlag, Berlin, 1974.

Rothwell, JC: Control of Human Voluntary Movement. Chapter 9. The Cerebellum. Aspen Publishers, Rockville, MD, 1987.

Voogd, J, Feirabend, HKP, and Schoen, JHR: Cerebellum and Precerebellar Nuclei. Chapter 14. In Paxinos, G (ed): The Human Nervous System. Academic Press, San Diego, 1990.

REFERENCES

1. Nolte, J: The Human Brain: An Introduction to Its Functional Anatomy, ed 2. Chapter 14. Cerebellum. CV Mosby, St. Louis, 1988.

2. Martin, JH: Neuroanatomy: Text and Atlas. Appleton & Lange, Norwalk, CT, 1989.

3. Carpenter, MB: Neuroanatomy, ed 4. Chapter 8. The Cerebellum. Williams & Wilkins, Baltimore, 1991.

4. Ghez, C: The Cerebellum. Chapter 41. In Kandel, ER, Schwartz, JH, and Jessell, TM (eds): Principles of Neural Science, ed 3. Appleton & Lange, Norwalk, CT, 1991.

5. Gilman, S: Cerebellum and Motor Dysfunction. Chapter 23. In Asbury, AK, McKhann, GM, and McDonald, WI (eds): Diseases of the Nervous System: Clinical Neurobiology, ed 2. WB Saunders, Philadelphia, 1992.

6. Dow, RS, Kramer, RE, and Robertson, LT: Disorders of the Cerebellum. Chapter 37. In Joynt, RJ (ed): Clinical Neurology, vol 3. JB Lippincott, Philadelphia, 1991.

7. Noback, CR, Strominger, NL, and DeMarest, RJ: The Human Nervous System: Introduction and Review, ed 4. Chapter 18. Cerebellum. Lea & Febiger, Philadelphia, 1991.

8. Ito, M: The Cerebellum and Neural Control. Part III. The Cerebellar Control System. Raven Press, New York, 1984.

9. Brodal, A: Neurological Anatomy in Relation to Clinical Medicine, ed 3. Chapter 5. Cerebellum. Oxford University Press, New York, 1981.

10. Gilman, S: The Cerebellum: Its Role in Posture and Movement. Chapter 3. In Swash, M and Kennard, C (eds): Scientific Basis of Clinical Neurology. Churchill Livingstone, Edinburgh, 1985.

11. Gilman, S, Bloedel, J, and Lechtenberg, R: Disorders of the Cerebellum. Chapter 2. Inputs to the Cerebellum: Mossy Fiber Afferents. FA Davis, Philadelphia, 1981.

12. Dietrichs, E and Walberg, F: Cerebellar Nuclear Afferents: Where Do They Originate? Anat Embryol 177:165, 1987.

13. Bloedel, JR and Courville, J: Cerebellar Afferent Systems. In Brookhart, JM and Mountcastle, VB (eds): Handbook of Physiology: The Nervous System. Section 1. Vol II, Part 21. American Physiological Society, Bethesda, MD, 1981.

14. Gilman, S, Bloedel, J, and Lechtenberg, R: Disorders of the Cerebellum. Chapter 3. Inputs to the Cerebellum: Climbing Fiber and Aminergic Afferents. FA Davis, Philadelphia, 1981.

15. Gilman, S, Bloedel, J, and Lectenberg, R: Disorders of the Cerebellum. Chapter 6. Cerebellar Descending and Ascending Projections. FA Davis, Philadelphia, 1981.

16. Ito, M: The Cerebellum and Neural Control. Part I. Cerebellar Cortical Network. Raven Press, New York, 1984.

17. Eccles, JC, Ito, M, and Szentagothai, J: The Cerebellum as a Neuronal Machine. Springer-Verlag, New York, 1967.

18. Llinas, R: Functional Significance of the Basic Cerebellar Circuit in Motor Coordination. In Bloedel, JR, Dichgans, J, and Precht, W (eds): Cerebellar Functions. Springer-Verlag, Berlin, 1985.

19. Ito, M: The Cerebellum and Neural Control. Chapter 20. Monoaminergic System. Raven Press, New York, 1984.

20. Dichgans, J and Diener, HC: Clinical Evidence for Functional Compartmentalization of the Cerebellum. In Bloedel, JR, Dichgans, J, and Precht, W (eds): Cerebellar Functions. Springer-Verlag, Berlin, 1985.

21. Snider, RS and Stowell, A: Receiving Areas of the Tactile, Auditory, and Visual Systems in the Cerebellum. J Neurophysiol 7:331, 1994.

22. Hore, J and Vilis, T: Loss of Set in Muscle Responses to Limb Perturbations During Cerebellar Dysfunction. J Neurophysiol 51:1137, 1984.

23. Ivry, RB and Keele, SW: Timing Functions of the Cerebellum. J Cogn Neurosci 1:136, 1989.

24. Hallett, M and Massaquoi, SG: Physiologic Studies of Dysmetria in Patients with Cerebellar Deficits. Can J Neurol Sci 20(suppl 3): S83, 1993.

25. Roland, PE: Partition of the Human Cerebellum in Sensory-Motor Activities, Learning, and Cognition. Can J Neurol Sci 20(suppl 3): 575, 1993.

26. Ito, M: The Cerebellum and Neural Control. Part IV. Cerebellar Functions, Raven Press, New York, 1984.

27. Brooks, VB and Thach, WT: Cerebellar Control of Posture and Movement. In Brookhart, JM and Mountcastle, VB (eds): Handbook of Physiology: The Nervous System. Section 1, vol II, Part 2. American Physiological Society, Bethesda, MD, 1981.

28. Rothwell, JC: Control of Human Voluntary Movement. Chapter 9. The Cerebellum. Aspen Publishers, Rockville, MD, 1987.

29. Brooks, VB: The Neural Basis of Motor Control. Chapter 13. The Cerebellum. Oxford University Press, New York, 1986.

30. Ito, M: The Cerebellum and Neural Control. Chapter 29. Scratch and Locomotion. Raven Press, New York, 1984.

31. Brooks, VB: The Neural Basis of Motor Control. Chapter 10. Locomotion. Oxford University Press, New York, 1986.

32. Grillner, S: Control of Locomotion in Bipeds, Tetrapods and Fish. Chapter 26. In Brookhart, JM and Mountcastle, VB (eds): Handbook of Physiology. Section 1: The Nervous System, vol II, Motor Control. Part 2. American Physiological Society, Bethesda, MD, 1981.

33. Granit, R: Reconsidering the "Alpha-Gamma Switch" in Cerebellar Action. Chapter 12. In Rose, FR (ed): Physiological Aspects of Clinical Neurology. Blackwell Scientific Publications, Oxford, 1977.

34. Gilman, S, Bloedel, JR, and Lechtenberg, R: Disorders of the Cerebellum. Chapter 8. Cerebellar Hypotonia and Tremor. FA Davis, Philadelphia, 1981.

35. LaLonde, R and Botez, MI: The Cerebellum and Learning Processes in Animals. Brain Res Rev 15:325, 1990.

36. Thompson, RF: The Neural Basis of Basic Associative Learning of Discrete Behavioral Response. Trends Neurosci 11:152, 1988.

37. Glickstein, M and Yeo, C: The Cerebellum and Motor Learning. J Cogn Neurosci 2:69, 1990.

38. Nagao, S: Behavior of Floccular Purkinje Cells Correlated with Adaptation of Horizontal Optokinetic Eye Movement Response in Pigmented Rabbits. Exp Brain Res 73:489, 1988.

39. Knowlton, BJ and Thompson, RF: Conditioning Using a Cerebral Cortical Conditioned Stimulus Is Dependent on the Cerebellum and Brainstem Circuitry. Behav Neurosci 106:509, 1992.

40. McCormick, DA and Thompson, RF: Cerebellum: Essential Involvement in the Classically Conditioned Eyelid Response. Science 223:296, 1984.

41. Lincoln, JS, McCormick, DA, and Thompson, RF: Ipsilateral Cerebellar Lesions Prevent Learning of the Classically Conditioned Nictitating Membrane/Eyelid Response. Brain Res 242:190, 1982.

42. Yeo, CH, Hardiman, MJ, and Glickstein, M. Classical Conditioning of the Nictitating Membrane Response of the Rabbit. I. Lesions of the Cerebellar Nuclei. Exp Brain Res 60:87, 1985.

43. Lye, RH, et al: Effects of a Unilateral Cerebellar Lesion on the Acquisition of Eye-Blink Conditioning in Man. J Physiol (Lond) 403:58P, 1988.

44. Bloedel, JR, et al: Substrates for Motor Learning: Does the Cerebellum Do It All? Ann NY Acad Sci 627:305, 1991.

45. Yeo, CH: Cerebellum and Classical Conditioning of Motor Responses. Ann NY Acad Sci 627:292, 1991.

46. Thompson, RF: Neurobiology of Learning and Memory. Science 233:941, 1986.

47. Glickstein, M: The Cerebellum and Motor Learning. Curr Opin Neurobiol 2(6):802, 1992.

48. Ito, M: The Cerebellum and Neural Control. Chapter 31. Other Reflexes. Raven Press, New York, 1984.

49. Haines, DE, Deitrichs, E and Sowg, TE: Hypothalamo-Cerebellar and Cerebellar-Hypothalamic Pathways: A Review and Hypothesis Concerning Cerebellar Circuits Which May Influence Autonomic Centers and Affective Behavior. Brain Behav Evol 24:198, 1984.

50. Haines, DE and Dietreichs, E: On the Organization of Interconnections Between the Cerebellum and Hypothalamus. In King, JS (ed): New Concepts in Cerebellar Neurobiology. Alan R Liss, New York, 1987, pp 113–149.

51. Bradley, DJ, Ghelarducci, B, and Spyer, KM: The Role of the Posterior Cerebellar Vermis in Cardiovascular Control. Neurosci Res 12:45, 1991.

52. Schmahmann, JD: An Emerging Concept: The Cerebellar Contribution to Higher Function. Arch Neurol 48:1178, 1991.

53. Leiner, H, Leiner, A, and Dow R: Does This Cerebellum Contribute to Mental Skills? Behav Neurol 100:443, 1986.

54. Leiner, HC, Leiner, AL, and Dow RS: The Human Cerebro-Cerebellar System: Its Computing, Cognitive, and Language Skills. Behav Brain Res 44(2):113, 1991.

55. Irvy, RB, and Baldo, JV: Is the Cerebellum Involved in Learning and Cognition? Curr Opin Neurobiol 2:212, 1992.

56. Decety, J, et al: The Cerebellum Participates in Mental Activity: Tomographic Measurement of Regional Blood Flow. Brain Res 535(2):313, 1990.

57. Peterson, SE, et al: Position Emission Tomographic Studies of the Cortical Anatomy of Single-Word Processing. Nature 331:585, 1988.

58. Roland, PE, et al: Changes in Regional Cerebral Oxidative Metabolism Induced by Tactile Learning and Recognition in Man. Europ J Neurosci 1:3, 1989.

59. Sarnet, HB and Alcala, H: Human Cerebellar Hypoplasia. Arch Neurol 37:300, 1980.

60. Kish, SJ, et al: Cognitive Deficits in Olivopontocerebellar Atrophy: Implications for the Cholinergic Hypothesis of Alzheimer's Dementia. Ann Neurol 24:200, 1988.

61. Akshoomoff, NA, et al: Contribution of the Cerebellum to Neuropsychological Functioning: Evidence from a Case of Cerebellar Degenerative Disorder. Neuropsychologia 30(4):315, 1992.

62. Fiez, JA, et al: Impaired Non-Motor Learning and Error Detection Associated with Cerebellar Damage: A Single Case Study. Brain 115(pt 1):155, 1992.

63. Reis, DJ, Doba, N, and Nathan, MA: Predatory Attack, Grooming, and Consummatory Behaviors Evoked by Electrical Stimulation of Cat Cerebellar Nuclei. Science 182:845, 1973.

64. Supple, WF, Leaton, AN, and Fanselow, MS: Effects of Cerebellar Vermal Lesions on Species:-Specific Fear Responses, Neophobia, and Taste-Aversion Learning in Rats. Physiol Behav 39:579, 1987.

65. Murakami, JW et al: Reduced Cerebellar Hemisphere Size and Its Relationship to Vermal Hypoplasia in Autism. Arch Neurol 46:689, 1989.

66. Bauman, ML and Kemper, TL: Abnormal Cerebellar Circuitry in Autism. Neurology (suppl 3)39:141, 1989.

67. Holroyd, S, Reiss, AL, and Bryan, RN: Autistic Features in Jouberts Syndrome: A Genetic Disorder with Agenesis of the Cerebellar Vermis. Biol Psychiatry 29(3):287, 1992.

68. Snider, SR: Cerebellar Pathology in Schizophrenia: Cause or Consequence? Neurosci Biobehav Rev 6:47, 1982.

69. Volkow, ND, et al: Low Cerebellar Metabolism in Medicated Patients with Schizophrenia. Am J Psychiatry 149(5):686, 1992.

70. Sandyk, R, Kay, SR, and Merriam, AE: Atrophy of the Cerebellar Vermis: Relevance to the Symptoms of Schizophrenia. Int J Neurosci 57:205, 1981.

71. Heath, RG, Llewllyn, RC, and Roachell, AM: The Cerebellar Pacemaker for Intractable Behavioral Disorders and Epilepsy: Follow-Up Report. Biol Psychiatry 15:343, 1980.

CHAPTER 9

■

Basal Ganglia and Their Connections

George E. Stelmach, EdD
and
James G. Phillips, PhD

- ■ *Components of the Basal Ganglia*
- ■ *Connections of the Basal Ganglia*
- ■ *Topographic Organization of the Basal Ganglia*
- ■ *Parallel Circuits in the Basal Ganglia*
- ■ *Lesions of the Basal Ganglia*

*T*he basal ganglia are a group of nuclei located beneath the cerebral hemispheres (Fig. 9–1). Their relative inaccessibility has meant that much more is known about their structure and detailed neuroanatomy than about their function. This is offset by major therapeutic advances that have occurred as a result of a better understanding of the neuropharmacology of these structures. This chapter presents the structural anatomy of the basal ganglia with an overview of function; in Chapter 18, a more thorough discussion of basal ganglia function is presented.

Components of the Basal Ganglia

The term basal ganglia refers to a group of nuclei that develop from the telencephalon and diencephalon. Historically, the structures included in the basal ganglia have varied with our understanding of their connections and function.[1-3] **The five fundamental components of the basal ganglia are the caudate nucleus, putamen, globus pallidus, substantia nigra, and subthalamic nucleus** (Table 9–1). The globus pallidus may be further subdivided into an internal (globus pallidus internus [GPi]) and external (globus pallidus externus [GPe]) segment. The substantia nigra may be divided into anatomically and functionally discrete subdivisions, the substantia nigra reticulata (SNr) and the substantia nigra compacta (SNc). Some evidence suggests that **the nucleus accumbens and the ventral pallidum should also be classified among the basal ganglia.**

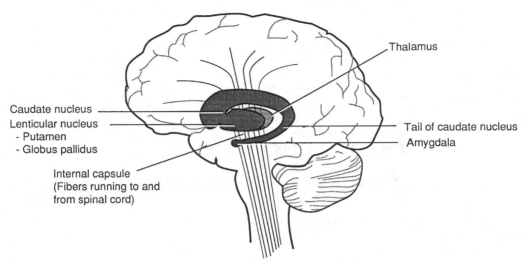

Figure 9–1. *Overall View of the Brain Showing the Relationships of the Basal Ganglia to Surrounding Structures.* The gray matter basal ganglia are located deep within the central white matter of the brain. Note that the many fibers of the internal capsule that course to and from the gray matter of the cerebral cortex pass between the putamen/globus pallidus and the thalamus.

The three largest nuclei of the basal ganglia are the caudate, the putamen, and the globus pallidus. These are often referred to as the *corpus striatum*. Phylogenetically, the caudate and putamen are more recent and are sometimes called the **neostriatum** (or simply the striatum). Myelinated fiber bundles crossing the internal capsule and connecting the caudate and putamen give these two nuclei their striated appearance. The phylogenetically older part of the corpus striatum is the globus pallidus, which is sometimes called the **paleostriatum.** The three nuclei of the corpus striatum are situated lateral to the thalamus and are separated from it by the internal capsule (Fig. 9–2). The caudate nucleus is shaped like a comma and follows the contours of the lateral ventricle. Its tail ends anteriorly in contiguity with the amygdala. The putamen and globus pallidus lie next to the caudate nucleus and thalamus under the insular cortex.

The functionally important basal ganglia nuclei which lie beneath the thalamus in the midbrain are the substantia nigra and the subthalamic nucleus.[1] The subthalamic nucleus (sometimes called the Luys' body) is situated ventral to the thalamus, whereas the substantia nigra is ventral and caudal to the subthalamic nucleus. Cells are more closely packed in the dorsal section of the substantia nigra, which is called the *pars compacta*. The ventral section is called the *pars reticulata*.

Table 9–1. *Terms Used to Refer to the Basal Ganglia*

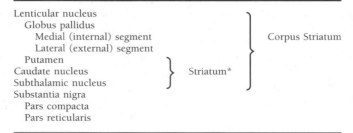

Lenticular nucleus
   Globus pallidus
      Medial (internal) segment
      Lateral (external) segment   Corpus Striatum
   Putamen
Caudate nucleus   } Striatum*
Subthalamic nucleus
Substantia nigra
   Pars compacta
   Pars reticularis

*The striatum is also referred to as the neostriatum.

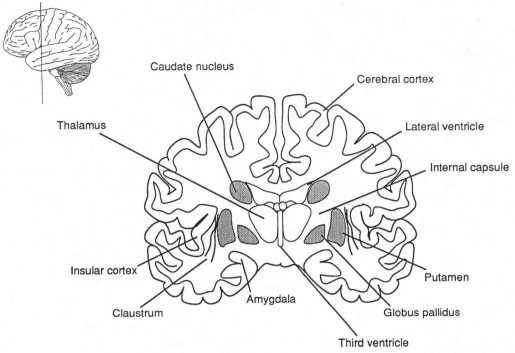

Figure 9-2. *Coronal Section of the Brain Through the Anterior Part of the Diencephalon.* This diagram shows the anatomic relationships between the basal ganglia and the cerebral cortex, internal capsule, thalamus, and other surrounding structures.

Connections of the Basal Ganglia

The components of the basal ganglia are often grouped according to their connections (Table 9-2). The **receptive components** receive afferent projections from central nervous system structures other than the basal ganglia. The **projection components** provide efferent connections to structures outside the basal ganglia, especially the thalamus. The **intrinsic components** receive input from and project to other basal ganglia. The main role of these intrinsic nuclei is to modulate the flow of information transmitted through the basal ganglia.

Table 9-2. *Components of the Basal Ganglia*

Receptive
  Caudate nucleus
  Putamen
  Nucleus accumbens
Projection
  Substantia nigra reticulata
  Globus pallidus internus
  Ventral pallidum
Intrinsic
  Globus pallidus externus
  Subthalamic nucleus
  Substantia nigra compacta

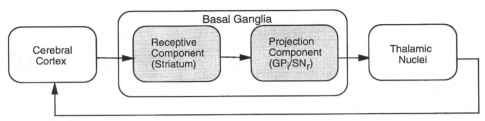

Figure 9–3. *Connections of the Basal Ganglia.* Schematic diagram representing the fundamental inputs and outputs of the basal ganglia.

The striatum is the major receptive component of the basal ganglia, receiving massive inputs from widespread regions of the cortex (Fig. 9–3). No part of the striatum is solely influenced by a single cortical area. The striatum in turn has projections to the GPi and the SNr. These two structures are the major projection components of the basal ganglia, projecting to the thalamus. The thalamus projects to more specific areas of the cerebral cortex. Although most of these connections are ipsilateral, there are bilateral contributions from the cortical projections to the motor components of the striatum.

Notably, there is a progressive reduction in the number of cells and afferent connections from cortex to striatum to GPi to thalamus. In other words, a tremendous amount of input convergence occurs from one component of this circuitry to the next. For example, there are about 50 million neurons in the human putamen. Approximately 50% of these are thought to project to output nuclei such as the GPi. Since the GPi has been estimated to have 0.15 million neurons and only two thirds appear to receive putaminal input, this means that there are about 200 putamen projections for every receiving neuron in the GPi.[4] These types of observations at one time led researchers to believe that the basal ganglia had an integrative or selective function.[5] The basal ganglia were thought to take diverse inputs from the cerebral cortex and to integrate and funnel these influences via the ventrolateral thalamus to the motor cortex. This viewpoint changed somewhat as reliable anatomic tracing techniques became available. **It became apparent that certain related cortical regions provided input to specific parts of the striatum and that such influences tended to remain segregated throughout the basal ganglia.** This contention is supported by the finding that **the striatum has a distinct topographic organization that tends to be maintained in other parts of the basal ganglia.**[6] This is to some extent confirmed both by observations of single cell activity and by the effects of lesions.[7,8] It is now thought that the basal ganglia consist of a number of relatively segregated parallel circuits that are topographically organized.[3,9]

Topographic Organization of the Basal Ganglia

The striatum receives massive inputs from all parts of the cerebral cortex, which appear to be excitatory in nature. Although this is a simplification (and there is some overlap), there is some initial segregation of the inputs into the striatum, with the sensorimotor cortex largely projecting to the putamen, association areas projecting predominantly to the caudate nucleus, and the limbic cortex mainly projecting to the nucleus accumbens.[6] Any of the overlap of projections has been thought to actually involve interdigitation rather than overlap.[10] Autoradiography indicates that the primary motor cortex projects *bilaterally* to the putamen, whereas premotor cortex projects ipsilaterally to caudate nucleus and putamen and prefrontal cortex projects ipsilaterally to the caudate nucleus.[11,12]

The afferents to the striatum have a topographic organization that tends to maintain the topology of the cerebral cortex. For example, the frontal lobe projects to the putamen and the anterior part of the head of the caudate nucleus; the visual cortex projects to the posterior part of the putamen and the posterior part (middle of the tail) of the caudate nucleus; and the temporal lobe projects to the ventral parts of the putamen and caudate

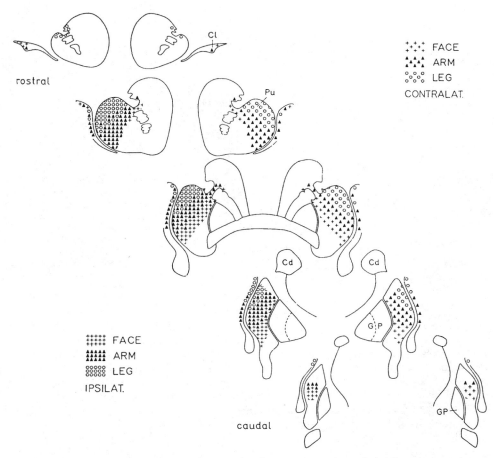

Figure 9–4. *Topographic Representation in the Putamen.* The motor cortex has orderly bilateral connections to the putamen. (From Kunzle,[11] p 205, with permission.)

nucleus.[13] More sensitive studies indicate that an even more discrete distribution of the cortical projections exists along the rostrocaudal axis of the striatum. The precentral cortex projects mostly to the putamen, where obliquely arranged strips maintain a somatotopic representation of face, arm, and leg,[11] with "leg-tail" motor cortex projecting bilaterally to dorsal and rostral parts of the putamen, and "face" areas projecting to ventral and caudal areas of the putamen (Fig. 9–4). Topographic organization is also maintained in the caudate nucleus. As in the putamen, the representations extend along the caudate nucleus's rostrocaudal axis. Contiguous longitudinal strips within the caudate nucleus, aligned along the mediolateral axis of the caudate, have been observed (Fig. 9–5).

This somatotopic organization may have significant clinical implications. **The specific disturbances seen in patients with focal dystonia or hemiparkinsonism in whom a specific limb is affected, for example, are potentially a product of this segregation of influences within the basal ganglia** (see Chapter 18). Moreover, the relative locations of areas within nuclei subserving specific functions can explain the spread of functional disturbance. Generalized dystonia tends to have a caudorostral progression, affecting the feet and working upward, whereas Tourette's syndrome tends to have a rostrocaudal progression, affecting face and then hands (see Fig. 9–4). **In addition, the relative contiguity of motor, sensory, and limbic territories can explain how a random lesion can have consequences not just for motor, but also for cognitive and emotional processes.**

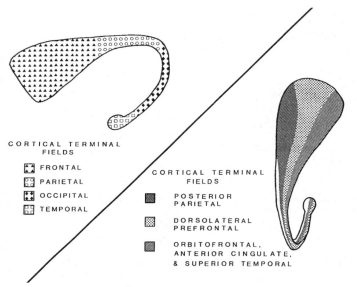

CORTICAL TERMINAL
FIELDS

▨ FRONTAL

▨ PARIETAL

▨ OCCIPITAL

▨ TEMPORAL

CORTICAL TERMINAL
FIELDS

▨ POSTERIOR
PARIETAL

▨ DORSOLATERAL
PREFRONTAL

▨ ORBITOFRONTAL,
ANTERIOR CINGULATE,
& SUPERIOR TEMPORAL

Figure 9–5. Topographic Representation in the Caudate Nucleus. Degeneration studies (*Upper Left*) suggested that the frontal lobes project to the head of the caudate nucleus. Autoradiography (*Lower Right*) reveals a finer grain longitudinal representation. (From Selemon and Goldman-Rakic,[10] p 791, with permission.)

In summation, the striatum is the receptive part of the basal ganglia, receiving excitatory inputs from the cortex, which are topographically organized. The striatum makes inhibitory projections to the globus pallidus and SNr. The striatum, subthalamic nucleus, globus pallidus, and substantia nigra are linked together in an orderly fashion along topographic lines. The basal ganglia makes its outputs from the GPi and SNr, which project to thalamic relay nuclei. These outputs are distinctive and do not appear to overlap in their effects on thalamic relay nuclei. The thalamic relay nuclei appear to project to premotor and supplementary motor areas rather than to primary motor cortex.[1]

Parallel Circuits in the Basal Ganglia

Studies of the effects of microstimulation and of single-cell activity have suggested that the *anatomic* somatotopy of the basal ganglia is maintained at a functional level. In this regard, microstimulation at specific depths of the primate putamen can elicit movement of different body segments (e.g., wrist, fingers, elbow, shoulder).[14,15] Functional somatotopy is also indicated by studies of single-cell activity. For example, neurons in the putamen, which receive inputs from sensorimotor cortex, respond to movement. This indicates that the putamen is part of a motor circuit.[7] On the other hand, neurons in the caudate nucleus, which receives inputs from the association cortex, respond to stimuli signaling the preparation or initiation of movement. This indicates a more cognitive circuit. Neurons in the ventral striatum, which receives inputs from limbic structures, respond to emotion-provoking or novel stimuli. This suggests the presence of a limbic circuit.[8] Neurons in the tail of the caudate nucleus, which receive inputs from the inferior temporal visual cortex, respond to changes in visual pattern.[7]

On the basis of the study of these connections, **Alexander and associates[9] have identified four parallel functional circuits within the basal ganglia. These are the motor, oculomotor, prefrontal and limbic circuits** (Fig. 9–6). Each circuit receives input from multiple functionally related cortical areas and appears in turn to modify the activity of a specific cortical area. The motor circuit is focused on precentral motor fields; the oculomotor circuit is focused on frontal eye fields; the prefrontal circuits are focused on the dorsolateral prefrontal and lateral orbitofrontal cortex; and the limbic circuit is focused on the anterior cingulate and medial orbitofrontal cortex (Figs. 9–6 and 9–7).[9]

Motor Circuit

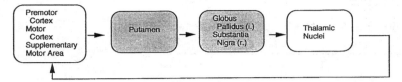

Oculomotor Circuit

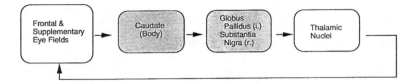

Prefrontal (Association) Circuits

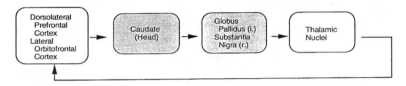

Anterior Cingulate (Limbic) Circuit

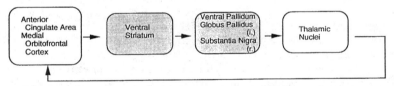

Figure 9–6. *Diagramatic Representation of Parallel Basal Ganglia–Thalamocortical Circuits.* Motor, oculomotor, prefrontal, and limbic circuits that are largely segregated from one another structurally and functionally appear to exist. i = internal segment, r = pars reticulata. (Adapted from Martin, JM: Neuroanatomy: Text and Atlas. Appleton & Lange, Norwalk, CT, 1989, p 272.)

Figure 9–7. *Frontal Lobe Targets of Basal Ganglia Output.* This figure illustrates schematically the cortical areas that receive the output of the separate basal ganglia–thalamocortical circuits. ACA = anterior cingulate gyrus; DLPC = dorsolateral prefrontal cortex; FEF = frontal eye fields; LOFC = lateral orbitofrontal cortex; MC = primary motor cortex; MOFC = medial orbitofrontal cortex; PMC = premotor cortex; SEF = supplementary eyefields; SMA = supplementary motor area. (From Alexander, Crutcher, and Delong,[9] p 120, with permission.)

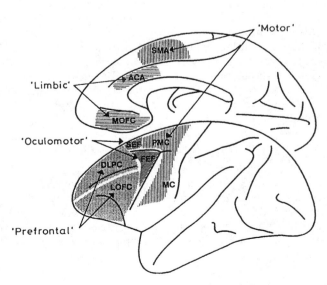

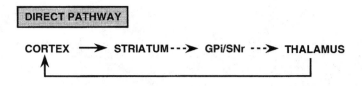

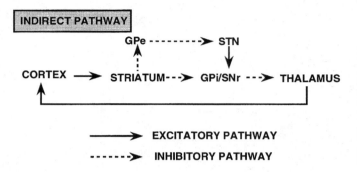

Figure 9–8. Direct and Indirect Pathways Through the Basal Ganglia. Diagram outlining direct and indirect pathways through the basal ganglia (with excitatory connections as *solid lines,* and inhibitory connections as *broken lines*). GPe = external globus pallidus; GPi = internal globus pallidus; SNr = substantia nigra pars reticulata; STN = subthalamic nucleus.

The Motor Circuit[9]

Organization

The primary components and connections of the motor circuit are illustrated in Figure 9–7. The motor cortex, primary motor cortex, arcuate motor area, and supplementary motor area provide excitatory glutamatergic inputs to the putamen. These projections are topographically organized, with the leg represented in the dorsolateral zone and the face represented in the ventromedial zone. There are two pathways by which the putamen eventually influences the thalamus and cortical areas (Fig. 9–8). In the simpler more *direct pathway,* the putamen exerts inhibitory influences (via γ-aminobutyric acid [GABA] and substance P), projecting topographically to the ventrolateral GPi and caudolateral SNr, which then influence the thalamus. In the *indirect pathway,* the putamen exerts inhibitory influences (via GABA and enkephalins), projecting topographically to the ventrolateral GPe. The GPe projects to the subthalamic nucleus, which then provides excitatory glutamatergic projections to the SNr, which then influences the thalamus.

In this way, the GPi and the SNr provide the outputs that influence the thalamus, although these outputs may be influenced by collateral and reciprocal projections with the pedunculopontine nucleus. This nucleus has been implicated in walking, and damage to these connections may be important in Parkinson's disease. The internal segment of the globus pallidus provides a tonic GABA-mediated inhibitory input to thalamic nuclei. The SNr also provides a tonic inhibitory GABA-mediated input to thalamic nuclei, which make excitatory projections (presumably glutamatergic) to the supplementary motor area, closing the motor circuit.

Functions

The motor circuit seems to provide positive feedback to specific areas of the motor cortex, reinforcing the activation of motor cortical areas. The *overall* function of the motor circuit involves the disinhibition of target nuclei in the thalamus, which activate specific cortical areas.[9] The GPi and the SNr provide a tonic inhibition of thalamic nuclei (see Fig. 9–8). This inhibitory effect is modulated by two pathways from the putamen to output nuclei in the GPi and SNr. In the simpler *direct* pathway through the basal ganglia, the cortex excites the putamen, which inhibits the output nuclei (GPi and SNr), which inhibit the thalamus, which in turn excites the supplementary motor area. This route, consisting of excitation-inhibition-inhibition-excitation and therefore containing a double inhibition, has an overall excitatory effect. In the more complex *indirect* route through the basal ganglia, the cortex excites the putamen, which inhibits the GPe, which inhibits the subthalamic nucleus, which excites the output nuclei (GPi/SNr), which inhibit thalamic nuclei, which in turn excite the supplementary motor area. This route, consisting of excitation-inhibition-inhibition-excitation-inhibition-excitation and therefore containing a triple inhibition appears to have an overall inhibitory effect. **It is thought that overall this motor circuit plays a part in motor control by disinhibiting the ventrolateral thalamus, which through its excitatory connections, facilitates cortically initiated movements.**[16]

As will be discussed further in Chapter 18, **dopamine appears to play a crucial role in basal ganglia motor function.** There are two classes of dopamine receptors (D_1, D_2). Dopamine tends to have an excitatory effect on the direct pathway from the striatum (via D_1 receptors) and an inhibitory effect on the indirect pathway (via D_2 receptors). Dopamine thus appears to have a net facilitory effect, both by activating the direct pathway (which has an excitatory effect overall) and by inhibiting the indirect pathway (which has an inhibitory effect overall).[16]

The motor circuit may play three general roles in the control of movement: (1) it may control slow changes in neural activity that is modulating the tonic amount of activity in a cortical area; (2) it may have a faster regulatory role in controlling the timing and sequencing of movement; (3) and since the extent to which parallel channels are maintained further along the motor circuit (e.g., in globus pallidus and substantia nigra) is not clear, there may be some regulation of the amounts of activity occurring simultaneously across motor subcircuits.

Studies of single-cell activity in the basal ganglia have found cells that respond to muscle activation and to direction of limb movement.[17] Movement-related neuronal activity occurs earlier in cortical than in subcortical areas of the motor circuit.[18] This indicates that cortical areas provide the input that activates the basal ganglia, which may in turn influence the supplementary motor area. However, the basal ganglia do not appear to have a simple integrative role. The somatotopic organization and indications of functional specificity have led Alexander and associates[4] to suggest that the motor circuit performs its task in parallel, not simply activating a specific muscle, but modulating activity over a massively parallel circuit. **Rather than activating one specific muscle at a time, the researchers suggest that the basal ganglia may activate many muscles at once.**

The role of the motor circuit can perhaps be understood by examining the behavior of its target structure, the supplementary motor area. Studies of the activity of single cells in the supplementary motor area suggest that it has a role in the preparation of movement. Alexander and Crutcher[18] found that more cells in the supplementary motor area (55%) were active *before* movement commencement than in the motor cortex (37%) or putamen (33%). **It has been suggested that the motor circuit of the basal ganglia provides a trigger for the outflow of the preparatory activity from the supplementary motor area.**[19,20] Studies of single cells in the globus pallidus (the output nuclei of the basal ganglia) indicate that neurons can discharge phasically to a movement. In monkeys trained to perform movement sequences, phasic discharges of globus pallidus neurons were related not so much to the beginning of a movement, but to the end of a component of a movement sequence. The definition and magnitude of the discharge depended on the predictability of the movement and were inversely related to its difficulty. **The basal ganglia may therefore provide the cue or trigger to enable the switching from one part of a behavioral sequence to the next in an automatic movement sequence.** These observations of single cells are confirmed by studies of cerebral blood flow.[21] During the initial phase of learning a manual skill, increases in cerebral blood flow have been observed in a number of areas (motor hand areas, premotor cortex, supplementary motor area, sensory hand area, supplementary sensory area, anterior lobe of the cerebellum). **However, while a subject is learning a new task, blood flow has** been found to rise significantly in the putamen and the globus pallidus, indicating that **the basal ganglia are involved in the automatization of movement.**[21]

The precise role that the basal ganglia play in the automatization of learned movements is still unclear. It may play a very specific role. For instance, the direct pathway from striatum to GPi/SNr may activate a motor pattern, and the indirect pathway (striatum to GPe to subthalamic nucleus to·GPi/SNr) may tune and smooth the motor pattern.[16] Alternatively, the direct pathway may activate a motor pattern, and the indirect pathway might inhibit conflicting motor patterns. Then again, the role of the basal ganglia may change. Although the basal ganglia may perform the same function (e.g., selection or activation) for each circuit, its eventual manifestation may depend on the precise function of the cortical areas it innervates.

It has been suggested that the motor circuit of the basal ganglia primarily terminates on, and is therefore associated with, the supplementary motor area rather than the primary motor cortex.[3] Although the primary motor cortex has specific direct control over movement, the supplementary motor area has less specific bilateral connections. **This implies that the basal ganglia have a more proximal/axial role in the coordination of movement.** As distinct from the distal manipulative role expected of motor cortex, the basal ganglia might be expected to have a more postural and supportive role.[22] Although the supplementary motor area does receive strong projections from the GPi via the thalamus,[23] there are suggestions that the basal ganglia may have wider efferent connections with cortical areas associated with movement. Using retrograde transneuronal transport of herpes simplex virus, Hoover and Strick[24] found that the dorsal GPi projects via thalamic nuclei to the supplementary motor area, whereas the ventral GPi projects via thalamic nuclei to the ventral premotor area, and other regions of the GPi project via the thalamic nuclei to the motor cortex. These multiple output channels of the basal ganglia imply that the basal ganglia may have a broader influence over the control of movement. Connections with the motor cortex may contribute to the control of specific movement parameters, whereas connections with premotor areas may be concerned with higher-order aspects of motor programming.[24]

The Oculomotor Circuit

Alexander and associates[9] also outline a basal ganglia circuit controlling eye movements (see Fig. 9–6). The posterior parietal cortex, dorsolateral prefrontal cortex, and frontal eye fields provide inputs to the body of the caudate nucleus. The caudate nucleus provides inputs to the GPi and SNr. These provide inputs to the thalamic nuclei, which project to the frontal eye fields in the cortex. The SNr also sends collateral projections to the superior colliculus. Since the portions of the oculomotor circuit are contiguous and parallel with those of the motor circuit and have similar neurotransmitters, it may perform a similar function to that performed by the motor circuit, but on a different set of cortical areas.

Both clinical and experimental evidence suggests that the oculomotor circuit has a role in the control of eye movement. Single cells in the frontal eye fields may discharge as a function of set (showing preparatory activity), visual fixation, or rapid (saccadic) eye movements. Similar observations have been made of single cells in the body of the caudate nucleus and ventrolateral SNr.[9] These observations of single cells are supported by studies of cerebral blood flow, which also indicated a role for the basal ganglia in the control of eye movement.[25] When humans engaged in voluntary, self-paced saccadic eye movements, there were changes in cerebral blood flow to specific regions of the cerebral cortex. Also occurring were increases in blood flow in traditional motor areas, such as the precentral gyrus, and areas corresponding to the supplementary motor area. More important, there were also the expected bilateral increases in cerebral blood flow in the putamen, globus pallidus, and thalamus. Patients with diseases affecting the basal ganglia such as Parkinson's disease and Huntington's disease exhibit characteristic oculomotor disorders that appear to be attributable to disruption of oculomotor pathways passing through the basal ganglia.[9]

Prefrontal Association Circuits

Two parallel circuits with primary connections between the frontal association areas and the caudate nucleus have also been identified, and evidence suggests that these circuits have a role in cognitive processing.[9] The first of these circuits is referred to as the *dorsolateral prefrontal circuit* and appears to play a role in spatial representation or attention (see Fig. 9–6). In this circuit, the arcuate premotor area, posterior parietal cortex, and dorsolateral prefrontal cortex all provide inputs to the caudate nucleus. The caudate nucleus provides inputs to the GPi and SNr. These provide inputs to the thalamic nuclei that project to the dorsolateral cortex. Lesions of the dorsolateral prefrontal cortex impair performance on spatial tasks, as do lesions of the dorsolateral caudate nucleus.[7] **This circuit may function to focus the attention in space on a signal by suppressing all other attention attracting events.**

The second prefrontal circuit is the lateral orbitofrontal circuit, which may play a role in attentional switching[9,26] (see Fig. 9–6). This loop begins with inputs from the lateral orbitofrontal cortex and projects through the caudate, GPi, and SNr and returns to the lateral orbitofrontal cortex to close the circuit. Lesions in the lateral orbitofrontal cortex or the projection zone within the caudate in monkeys result in perseveration or the inability to switch between behavioral sets.[9] Evidence suggests that these areas may be implicated in obsessive-compulsive disorders in which patients are unable to control ritualistic, repetitive behaviors.

The Limbic Circuit

The ventral striatum and ventral pallidum have been linked to limbic structures, so the basal ganglia may also have a limbic circuit (see Fig. 9–6). Although not as well differentiated as the other basal ganglia circuits, Alexander and associates[9] outline an anterior cingulate circuit involving limbic structures. Various limbic structures provide inputs to the ventral striatum. The ventral striatum provides inputs to the GPi, ventral pallidum, and SNr. These project to thalamic nuclei, which project to the anterior cingulate area. **Although the function of the limbic circuit remains uncertain, it appears as if these pathways play a role in emotional and motivational processes.** For example, neurons in the ventral striatum respond to novel visual stimuli, stimuli of emotional significance, and arousal.[7] These more cognitive circuits may function to focus attention and emotional participation on an event by suppressing all other attention-attracting events. There is also speculation that this limbic circuit may be involved in the behavioral manifestations associated with Tourette's syndrome (see Chapter 18).

Additional Connections and Circuits

The major putative basal ganglia circuits have been outlined. There are, however, some lesser nuclei that also have connections with the basal ganglia, creating circuits that may play a role in motor control or in the limbic functions of the basal ganglia. **Moreover, other parallel circuits have been proposed that are unrelated to these functions. For example, a unilateral language circuit which is based on the dominant basal ganglia, has been proposed by Crosson.**[27] This circuit involves the anterior and posterior language cortex, the caudate nucleus, globus pallidus, and ventral anterior thalamus. Evidence for a language circuit comes from lesion and electrical stimulation studies. For example, stimulation of the dominant ventral anterior thalamus can elicit language. Since the globus pallidus forms a part of an indirect inhibitory pathway, the effects of stimulation are somewhat different. Stimulation of the globus pallidus has been found to inhibit language. Nevertheless, although evidence for the existence of a language circuit remains tentative, it may be relevant in the context of disorders such as Tourette's syndrome in which disturbances of cerebral asymmetry have been observed (see Chapter 18).

Functionally Parallel Circuits

As previously outlined, **function appears to be segregated within the striatum.** As part of the motor circuit, for example, neurons in the putamen tend to respond to movement. Neurons in the caudate nucleus tend to be involved in more complex cognitive activity, responding to environmental stimuli signaling the preparation or initiation of responses. Neurons in the ventral striatum respond to novel visual stimuli or stimuli with emotional or motivational significance.[8] In this way, the activity of cells in each circuit appears to be primarily determined by activity in the specific cortical area innervating it. Most striatal cells do not show an unconditional response to stimulation or movement, implying that the striatum has a role-selecting, switching, or gating activity.

The apparent segregation of inputs and functions within the basal ganglia must be viewed with some caution. Most of our understanding of the connections of the basal ganglia and their parallel circuits has been based on the study of single cells. There are problems with such approaches, given the large numbers of neurons in the brain. A focus on cells that have simple identifiable functions in the context of a restricted number of specific tasks can present an overly selective and simplified picture of basal ganglia connections, activity, and function.[28] In addition, there has been an inherent difficulty dealing with between-cell connectivity when using single-cell techniques, which tends to emphasize or perhaps even exaggerate a sense of parallelism. To some extent, this is remedied by examining large samples of single cells. However, **the extent to which cells from parallel segregated circuits are linked by interneurons is still not clear.** For these kinds of reasons, we need to consider mechanisms of connectivity in more detail. In addition, studies dealing with larger masses of neural tissue are essential for an understanding of basal ganglia structure and function.

Lesions of the Basal Ganglia

Experimentally induced lesions in animals to some extent support the notion of parallel, segregated circuits. The basal ganglia are difficult to access, lying as they do beneath the cerebral hemispheres. This means that it is difficult to produce localized lesions without damaging nearby structures (such as the hypothalamus) or disturbing other pathways by damaging the internal capsule or surrounding white matter.[29] However, experimental damage to specific regions of the basal ganglia does produce consistent results. Damage to parts of the motor circuit can cause motor symptoms (although these effects are only clearly seen with bilateral lesions because some structures have bilateral connections). Lesions of the putamen or subthalamic nucleus produce an excess of spontaneous movement (hyperkinesia), whereas damage to substantia nigra or globus pallidus reduces the speed of voluntary movement (bradykinesia) and produces a lack of spontaneous movement (akinesia).[29] Damage to the circuits going through the caudate nucleus produces more complex cognitive changes, but even here the lesions confirm that there is functional specialization within the striatum. The effects of lesions within the caudate nucleus seem to reflect the particular function of the specific cortical area or limbic structures that project to that part of the striatum. For example, in the monkey, lesions of the anterodorsal part of the head of the caudate nucleus disrupt spatial alternation performance, as do lesions of the dorsolateral prefrontal cortex that projects to it.[7] On the other hand, lesions of the ventrolateral part of the head of the caudate nucleus produce impaired object reversal performance, as do lesions of the orbitofrontal cortex that projects to it. Lesions of other parts of the striatum or connecting cortical areas also show such parallel effects. Lesions of the tail of the caudate nucleus or the inferior temporal visual cortex that projects to it can produce a deficit of visual pattern discrimination. Damage to the ventral striatum or the ventral tegmental area that projects to it can impair motivational behaviors in the rat.[7]

Lesions in human beings produced by cerebrovascular accidents are much less precise than experimental lesions produced in animals, and they provide less concise information regarding the localization of function within the basal ganglia.[30–32] The warning signs preceding strokes in the internal capsule typically consist of motor, sensory, or sensorimotor symptoms affecting the face, arm, and leg simultaneously, with no cortical signs such as neglect, dyspraxia, or dysphasia.[30] However, in view of the parallel motor, cognitive, and limbic circuits within the basal ganglia, it is not surprising that strokes in this area can produce a variety of symptoms including cortical syndromes as diverse as spatial neglect, aphasia, agraphia, apraxia, and dementia.[31] It would be naive to locate all these disordered functions within the basal ganglia, since our understanding of the cognitive, motor, and limbic circuits indicates that the basal ganglia could play a part in *regulating* these cortical activities.[7] Since a study of lesions provides at best a very gross understanding of the connectivity and the functional importance of the basal ganglia, diseases of the basal ganglia continue to provide important converging information about the structure and function of the basal ganglia (see Chapter 18).

RECOMMENDED READINGS

Albin, RL, Young, AB, and Penny, JB: The Functional Anatomy of Basal Ganglia Disorders. Trends Neurosci 12:366, 1989.

Alexander, GE and Crutcher, MD: Functional Architecture of Basal Ganglia Circuits: Neural Substrates of Parallel Processing. Trends Neurosci 13:266, 1990.

Alexander, GE, Crutcher, MD, and DeLong, MR: Basal Ganglia-Thalamocortical Circuits: Parallel Substrates for Motor, Oculomotor, "Prefrontal," and "Limbic" Functions. Prog Brain Res 85:119, 1990.

Alexander, GE, DeLong, MR, and Strick, PL: Parallel Organization of Functionally Segregated Circuits Linking Basal Ganglia and Cortex. Ann Rev Neurosci 9:357, 1986.

Cote, L and Crutcher, MD: The Basal Ganglia. Chapter 42. In Kandel, ER, Schwartz, JH, and Jessell, TM (eds): Principles of Neural Science, ed 3. Elsevier, New York, 1991.

DeLong, MR and Georgopoulos, AP: Motor Functions of the Basal Ganglia. Chapter 21. In Brooks, VB (ed): Handbook of Physiology. Section 1. The Nervous System, Vol II. Motor Control, Part 2. American Physiological Society, Bethesda, MD, 1981.

Donnan, GA, et al: The Stroke Syndrome of Striatocapsular Infarction. Brain 114:51, 1991.

Graybiel, AM: Neurotransmitters and Neuromodulators in the Basal Ganglia. Trends Neurosci 13:244, 1990.

Parent, A: Extrinsic Connections of the Basal Ganglia. Trends Neurosci 13:254, 1990.

Rolls, ET: Experimental Psychology: Functions of Different Regions of the Basal Ganglia. In Stern, GM (ed): Parkinson's Disease. Chapman & Hall Medical, London, 1990, pp 151–184.

Rothwell, JC: Control of Human Voluntary Movement. Chapter 10. The Basal Ganglia. Aspen Publishers, Rockville, MD, 1987.

REFERENCES

1. Carpenter, MB: Interconnections Between the Corpus Striatum and Brain Stem Nuclei. In McKenzie, JS, Kemm, RE, and Wilcock, LN (eds): The Basal Ganglia: Structure and Function. Plenum Press, New York, 1984, pp 1–68.

2. Parent, A: Comparative Neurobiology of the Basal Ganglia. John Wiley & Sons, New York, 1986.

3. Alexander, GE, DeLong, MR, and Strick, PL: Parallel Organization of Functionally Segregated Circuits Linking Basal Ganglia and Cortex. Ann Rev Neurosci 9:357, 1986.

4. Alexander, GE, DeLong, MR, and Crutcher, MD: Do Cortical and Basal Ganglionic Motor Areas Use "Motor Programs" to Control Movement? Behav Brain Sci 15:656, 1992.

5. Kemp, JM and Powell, TPS: The Connections of the Striatum and Globus Pallidus: Synthesis and Speculation. Philos Trans R Soc Lond 262:441, 1971.

6. Parent, A: Extrinsic Connections of the Basal Ganglia. Trends Neurosci 13:254, 1990.

7. Rolls, ET: Experimental Psychology: Functions of Different Regions of the Basal Ganglia. In Stern, GM (ed): Parkinson's Disease. Chapman & Hall Medical, London, 1990, pp 151–184.

8. Rolls, ET and Johnstone, S: Neurophysiological Analysis of Striatal Function. In Vallar, G, Cappa, SF, and Wallesch C-W (eds): Neuropsychological Disorders Associated with Subcortical Lesions. Oxford University Press, Oxford, 1992, pp 60–97.

9. Alexander,GE, Crutcher, MD, and DeLong, MR: Basal Ganglia-Thalamocortical Circuits: Parallel Substrates for Motor, Oculomotor, "Prefrontal" and "Limbic" Functions. Prog Brain Res 85:119, 1990.

10. Selemon, LD and Goldman-Rakic, PS: Longitudinal Topography and Interdigitation of Cortico-Striatal Projections in the Rhesus Monkey. J Neurosci 5:776, 1985.

11. Kunzle, H: Bilateral Projections from Precentral Motor Cortex to the Putamen and Other Parts of the Basal Ganglia: An Autoradiographic Study in Macaca Fascicularis. Brain Res 88:195, 1975.

12. Kunzle, H: An Autoradiographic Analysis of the Efferent Connections from Premotor and Adjacent Prefrontal Regions (Areas 6 and 9) in Macaca Fascicularis. Brain Behav Evol 15:185, 1978.

13. Kemp, JM and Powell, TPS: The Corticostriate Projection in the Monkey. Brain 93:525, 1970.

14. Alexander, GE and DeLong, MR: Microstimulation of the Primate Neostriatum. I. Physiological Properties of Striatal Microexcitable Zones. J Neurophysiol 53:1401, 1985.

15. Crutcher, MD and DeLong, MR: Single Cell Studies of the Primate Putamen I. Functional Organization. Exp Brain Res 53:233, 1984.

16. Alexander, GE and Crutcher, MD: Functional Architecture of Basal Ganglia Circuits: Neural Substrates of Parallel Processing. Trends Neurosci 13:266, 1990.

17. Crutcher, MD, and Alexander, GE: Movement-Related Neuronal Activity Selectively Coding Either Direction or Muscle Pattern in Three Motor Areas of the Monkey. J Neurophysiol 64:151, 1990.

18. Alexander, GE and Crutcher, MD: Preparation for Movement: Neural Representations of Intended Direction in Three Motor Areas of the Monkey. J Neurophysiol 64:133, 1990.

19. Brotchie, P, Iansek, R, and Horne, MK: Motor Function of the Monkey Globus Pallidus: Neuronal Discharge and Parameters of Movement. Brain 114:1667, 1991.

20. Brotchie, P, Iansek, R, and Horne, MK: The Motor Function of the Monkey Globus Pallidus: Cognitive Aspects of Movement and Phasic Neuronal Activity. Brain 114:1685, 1991.

21. Seitz, RJ and Roland, PE: Learning of Sequential Finger Movements in Man: A Combined Kinematic and Positron Emission Tomography (PET) study. Eur J Neurosci 4:154, 1992.

22. Webster, KE: The Functional Anatomy of the Basal Ganglia. In Stern, GM (ed): Parkinson's Disease. Chapman & Hall Medical, London, 1990, pp 3–56.

23. Tokuno, H, Kimura, M, and Tanji, J: Pallidal Inputs to Thalamocortical Neurons Projecting to the Supplementary Motor Area: An Anterograde and Retrograde Double Labeling Study in the Macaque Monkey. Exp Brain Res 90:635, 1992.

24. Hoover, JE and Strick, PL: Multiple Output Channels in the Basal Ganglia. Science 259:819, 1993.

25. Petit, L, et al: PET Study of Voluntary Saccadic Eye Movements in Humans: Basal Ganglia-Thalamocortical System and Cingulate Cortex Involvement. J Neurophysiol 69:1009, 1993.

26. Thorpe, SJ, Rolls, ET, and Maddison, SP: Neuronal Responses in the Orbitofrontal Cortex of the Behaving Monkey. Exp Brain Res 49:93, 1983.

27. Crosson, B: Is the Striatum Involved in Language? In Vallar, G, Cappa, SH, Wallesch, C-W (eds): Neuropsychological Disorders Associated with Subcortical Lesions. Oxford University Press, Oxford, 1992, pp 268–293.

28. Fetz, EE: Are Movement Parameters Recognizably Coded in the Activity of Single Neurons? Behav Brain Sci 15:679, 1992.

29. Rothwell, JC: Control of Human Voluntary Movement. Croom Helm Limited, London, 1987.

30. Donnan, GA, et al, The Capsular Warning Syndrome: Pathogenesis and Clinical Features. Neurology 43:957, 1993.

31. Vallar, G, Cappa, SF, and Wallesch, C-W: Neuropsychological Disorders Associated with Subcortical Lesions. Oxford University Press, Oxford. 1992.

32. Donnan, GA, et al: The Stroke Syndrome of Striatocapsular Infarction. Brain 114:51, 1991.

CHAPTER 10

■

Theories of Motor Control

Patricia A. Burtner, PhD
and
Marjorie H. Woollacott, PhD

- *Reflex Hierarchical Theory of Motor Control*
- *Modular Theory of Motor Control*
- *Systems Theory of Motor Control*
- *Dynamical Systems Theory of Motor Control*

When rehabilitation services are requested for an individual with neurologic dysfunction, the therapist asks the question: How can I assist this person to gain greater control of body movements? The issue of disordered motor control is often central to the decrease in daily function the person exhibits. Traditionally, therapists have drawn information from basic science research to develop therapeutic models of treatment. The fields of anatomy, neuroanatomy, physiology, neurophysiology, neuropsychology, and, more recently, movement science (biomechanics, motor control, motor development, and motor learning) have been studied and applied to clinical practice to form the foundation of these models.

As new research in the basic sciences emerges, *therapeutic rehabilitation models change.*[1] The purpose of this chapter is to introduce the new reader in motor control theory to these changes. Previous chapters have focused on the central nervous system structures that assist in motor control functions. This chapter and the next chapter on motor learning form a bridge to the remaining text discussing pathology in motor control. To better understand the importance of motor control in therapy, a historic perspective on different theories is presented, with supporting studies that provide direction for theory formation. Within each theory, applied research for patient populations, adults and children with motor control deficits, is included. It is important to remember that our discussion is limited to only a portion of information available in motor control research.

For the purpose of this discussion, four specific theories are reviewed, representing established and emerging approaches to motor control. *Reflex hierarchical theory,* an established model in rehabilitation, is the first to be presented. This approach was based primarily on the contribution of central nervous system control to product-oriented motor output for specific movement patterns. The *modular theory* is also based on central nervous system function, but outlines a process-oriented organization with many motor functions sharing similar processes rather than a specific part of the brain controlling one movement process, a reflex hierarchical concept.

The major shift in thinking is represented in a more recent ecologic approach represented in *systems and dynamical systems* theories of motor control. Although these theories evolved from different disciplines—neurophysiology and physical science—they share a common origin and conceptual framework and therefore are often viewed as one theory. In this theoretical framework, no single system is considered to have priority in motor control; rather, the organization of many systems creates movement for successful task attainment. This concept is in direct contrast to the reflex hierarchical approach of higher to lower structural control.

Reflex Hierarchical Theory of Motor Control

In reflex hierarchical theory, motor control of an individual is considered to be the product of commands from the central nervous system to the periphery with modification by sensory inputs. Based on central nervous system organization as identified through animal and human pathology studies, the reflex hierarchical theory is conceptualized as a higher to lower center control of movement. The main concepts of the theory are that (1) sensory input is required for motor output, and (2) the central nervous system is organized hierarchically, with lower structures being controlled by higher cortical centers.

Motor Control Produced Through Reflex Chains

Research conducted by Sir Charles Sherrington[2] provides the basis of this motor control theory. In his scientific studies with cats, Sherrington removed brain structures above the midbrain and measured motor outputs following controlled sensory stimuli given to the remaining central nervous system structures. He demonstrated that stereotypical motor responses occurred following the sensory input, which he identified as "reflexes." A reflex was considered to be the basic unit of movement, with more complex movements assumed to be a chaining together of these reflexes (Fig. 10–1). Based on this concept of movement, therapists in clinics have provided sensory inputs to produce desired motor output using what could be called a "closed-loop" feedback system.

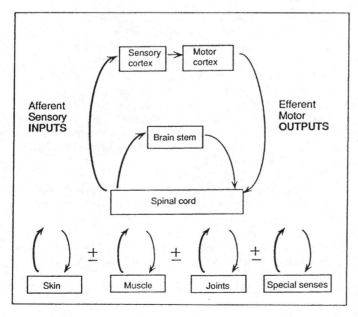

Figure 10–1. Chains of reflexes at spinal, brainstem, and cortical areas of the brain. (From Horak,[1] p 13. Reprinted with permission from the Foundation for Physical Therapy, Inc.)

Movement Without Reflex Chaining

Additional research has shown that closed-loop feedback systems are not required for movement. Polit and Bizzi[3] trained monkeys to reach for targets, with juice given as a reinforcer when they were accurate. Afferent roots to the spinal cord were cut to eliminate somatosensory stimuli to the motor units, and vision was occluded. In the absence of sensory input, the monkeys retained their accuracy in reaching the targets, even when the forearm position was moved prior to actual reaching tasks. The animals did not rely on closed-loop, sensory-based movement, but appeared to use the springlike properties of their muscles for successful aiming. However, when the shoulder area was moved, the monkey was unable to correct the perturbed arm movement if the displacement was made without sensory input. Why? Because this movement required that the monkey update the sensorimotor map of the body in space. The interaction of the biomechanical springlike properties of the arm with modulation of sensory input appears to be necessary to adjust to environmental conditions. Therefore, this evidence refutes the tenet of the reflex chaining model that sensory input is required for motor output.

Another major limitation of the closed-loop model is the significant time that is required for sensorimotor processing when movement relies on feedback signals alone. It has been shown that rapid and well-practiced movements, such as keyboarding, can be generated very quickly before feedback influence could occur.[4] **In more recent interactive movement models, the ideas of "open-loop" and "feedforward" control are incorporated.** Figure 10–2 outlines the schematic conceptualization of feedforward control, or control given without feedback signals available. In this model, the reference point or goal shown on the far left initiates the movement prior to sensory feedback. Feedforward signals are generated, which are based on previous experience or stored motor programs. This motor information of how the body previously moved in a similar situation is relayed to motor neurons to activate the appropriate movement, again without sensory feedback present. This motor output is corrected by external influence registered from the periphery (closed-loop feedback model) to produce the accurate force, position, and velocity needed for successful goal attainment. Internal feedback of this information (force, position, and velocity) is sent back to the comparator, which compares actual movement with the initial feedforward signal. When the two movement signals (feedforward versus actual) do not match, the difference or error is sent to the motor neurons to correct motor output for the next attempt.[1]

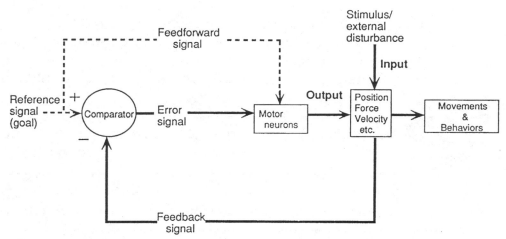

Figure 10–2. *The Closed Loop Feedback System* (Solid Arrows) *and Feedforward System* (Dashed Arrows) *for Motor Control.* Feedforward signals allow anticipatory movement prior to sensory feedback. (From Horak,[1] p 14. Reprinted with permission from the Foundation for Physical Therapy, Inc.)

This concept of feedforward control is important in therapy. Consider a patient who has recently suffered a stroke and has new paralysis of a limb (e.g., the arm). Previous movement information about the arm is available for use in feedforward control activities during retraining. It would therefore be important to have the patient use the affected arm as soon as possible in the rehabilitation program, using this feedforward control established by previous movement experience. If the patient is encouraged to use the nonparetic arm alone initially, new feedforward patterns are established that do not include the paretic arm. As a result, retraining of the affected limb after recovery may be more difficult.[5]

In pediatric therapy, accurate feedforward may not be initially available to the child with motor problems, since the actions required for the task have never been used or inaccurate patterns have been established. Refinement of motor patterns occurs with practiced interaction with the task itself, correction of error, and eventual establishment of accurate feedforward information. This approach reflects a systems approach to intervention for increasing an individual's motor control behaviors. In contrast, in the reflex chaining approach, sensory input is applied by the therapist to produce motor output for a specific movement, with little attention to the child's environment or the specific task context.

A Hierarchy Within the Central Nervous System

Associated with the concept of reflex chaining in movement has been the notion of a hierarchical organization within the central nervous system. This concept, first introduced by Sir Hughlings Jackson, outlines a lower to higher structural organization of movement.[6] **The spinal cord and brainstem are thought to be lower reflexive centers, which are controlled by higher centers in the subcortical and voluntary cortical areas of the brain** (Fig. 10–3). Central to this model is the hypothesis that there is a relationship between maturation in the developing brain and the emergence of behaviors seen during infant development. Through observations of infants in the early months of life, primitive reflex patterns were identified whose onsets were correlated with maturation of the spinal cord and brainstem pathways. After 4 to 5 months of age, righting and equilibrium reactions were present, whereas reflex behaviors were seen less often. These changes occurred as midbrain and cortical structures were maturing. The interpretation of this relationship between brain maturation and motor control changes has been that higher centers control the excitation and inhibition of lower central nervous system structures.[7]

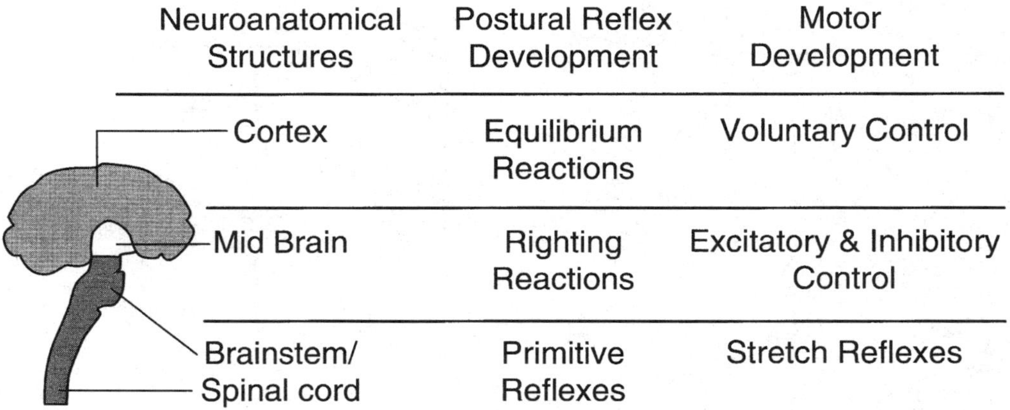

Neuroanatomical Structures	Postural Reflex Development	Motor Development
Cortex	Equilibrium Reactions	Voluntary Control
Mid Brain	Righting Reactions	Excitatory & Inhibitory Control
Brainstem/ Spinal cord	Primitive Reflexes	Stretch Reflexes

Figure 10–3. *Hierarchical Organization According to Neuroanatomical Structures.* Higher cortical centers are thought to control lower reflex centers. (Adapted from Shumway-Cook, A and Woollacott, MH: Theoretical issues in assessing postural control. In Wilhelm, I: Physical Therapy Assessment in Infancy. Churchill Livingstone, New York, 1993, p 163, with permission.)

When brain damage to higher centers occurs in adults and children, these individuals have a decrease or absence of voluntary control, whereas the presence of reflexive patterns coordinated at lower centers increases. The fact that such movement patterns occur with brain damage is well documented and still assists physicians in identifying where a lesion in the brain may be located and what prognosis the person may have for recovery. For example, the adult with unilateral cortical damage from a stroke exhibits less voluntary control in the limbs and trunk on the contralateral side of the body. Those individuals with spastic hemiplegia will have increased muscle tone and stiffness over time in the arm flexors and leg extensors. When head turning occurs in these patients, a tonic neck reflexlike response may be seen. Likewise, children with cerebral palsy often demonstrate tonic neck and primitive reflex patterns, such as the stepping reflex, beyond the time period that these reflex patterns can typically be elicited. Although observations of these patterns are helpful diagnostically, their usefulness in treatment is questionable. **Using a reflex hierarchical approach in therapy, the goal is to move the individual through patterns of reflex inhibition, while using facilitation techniques to establish righting and equilibrium reactions.** Traditional approaches by Bobath[8] and Brunnstrom[9] advocate forms of these reflex hierarchical concepts in rehabilitation.

Systems Control Replaces the Hierarchical Model

Recent studies in children and adults show that movement is a blending of reflexive and voluntary control, which is dependent on the demands of the environment or the task in which the individual is engaged. For example, very young infants demonstrate volitional movement control for prereaching as early as 4 to 5 days of age, when a brightly colored object is present; more random spontaneous movement patterns are noted when the object is absent.[10] This period of early development was previously thought to consist of only reflex movement patterns.

The idea that primitive reflexes disappear because of brain maturation has also been questioned. Infants who no longer demonstrated automatic stepping (i.e., the infant walking reflex) were studied by Thelen and colleagues.[11] It was noted that at the same time the stepping reflex disappears, infants have a significant increase in body weight. When investigators eliminated the effects of body mass by submerging the infants in water at chest height, automatic stepping movements increased. Thus, it appears to be the increase in body weight that affects the infant's ability to produce stepping movements in an upright position, rather than the increased maturation of higher brain structures and inhibition of lower reflex centers. The conclusion that Thelen and colleagues[11] reached was that reflexive behaviors are parts of nervous system pathways, which are refined for independent walking at 1 year of age. This concept suggests that rather than inhibit these reflex patterns, therapists may want to assist in their refinement.

Similarly, with adults who demonstrate increased muscle tone or spasticity in arm flexors and leg extensors, the focus of therapy has been inhibition of the reflexive behavior. Using electromyography (EMG), Sahrmann and Norton[12] recorded activity in the flexors (spastic) and primary mover extensor (agonist) muscles of the arm in patients with cerebral hemisphere lesions and multiple sclerosis. Results of this study identified the poor recruitment of the prime mover muscles, rather than spasticity in antagonist muscle as the cause of decreased motor control in the arm. Studies such as this suggest that the techniques based on reflex control theories may be ineffective.

Current therapeutic intervention focuses on active control of the weak primary mover muscle (arm extensors) by the patient rather than inhibition of the spastic muscle by the therapist. The goal of this intervention is to attain a balance between the agonist/antagonist muscles. Through initial isolated motor control activities using the prime mover, this muscle is strengthened. Then, repetitive functional reaching tasks, incorporating different distances, positions, and velocities are introduced to increase the timing between agonist and antagonist muscles. **This model of therapeutic intervention is task-oriented, in contrast to reflex inhibition/facilitation models.**[5] The hypothesized central nervous system organization for task-goal attainment within an environmental context is represented in Figure 10–4.

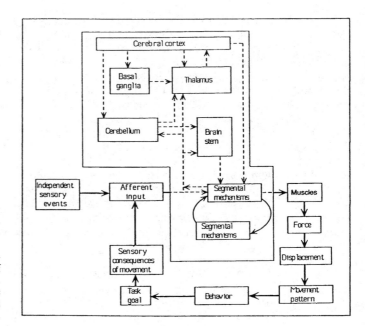

Figure 10–4. Anatomical connections considered to be the basis of motor control. (From Horak,[1] p 12. Reprinted with permission from the Foundation for Physical Therapy, Inc.)

Modular Theory of Motor Control

Another approach to motor control, the modular theory, addresses specific control processes such as motor timing or sequencing. Emerging from the area of neuropsychology, the modular theory incorporates cognitive components of movement with neurologic structures within the individual. **Although the modular theory is based on central nervous system structures, the *processes* of movement organization are considered rather than the production of individual movements. Specific processes of interest for the control of movement are timing, force regulation, and sequencing of motor tasks.**

Taking each computation separately, let us think of motor tasks in which one of these processes dominates. First, timing is seen in many effector muscle groups: in the legs for walking, skipping, or jumping; in the arms for bouncing balls and clapping; and in the mouth for drinking and tongue clicking. Likewise, force regulation is needed for kicking, pushing, and blowing. Motor sequencing is seen in hopscotch, writing, and speaking. Are there separate parts within the central nervous system for each of these body parts responsible for each of these motor skills? Proponents of the modular theory think these movement processes are organized in specific modules that are used in any motor or nonmotor task requiring the function.

The central nervous system, as conceptualized by Keele and colleagues,[13–15] is organized according to functions. Specifically, they hypothesize in their research that timing functions are particular to the cerebellum; force regulation is a function of the basal ganglia; and motor sequencing is supported in the supplementary motor cortex.

Timing Module

Many skills have an underlying rhythm to them. For example, the skills of typing, dancing, and speaking make use of very different muscle groups, but they share a common requirement—coordinated timing between muscles for successful movement production. In a series of studies by Keele and colleagues,[13–15] timing was investigated. First, subjects were asked to tap their fingers at a certain frequency using different body parts. Subjects who were better at tapping with their fingers were also found to be better with arm and foot tapping. Elite tappers, such as pianists, were found to be elite with all body parts, whereas children with motor dysfunction had difficulty with all tapping activities. The general mechanism for timing appears to have the same level of efficiency, despite the muscle groups used.

Subjects were then tested on general timing ability in a nonmotor task, auditory perception. For this test, two pairs of tones were presented and subjects were asked to identify which pair of tones had longer intervals between them. The subjects who had skill in tapping tasks were also more skilled in identifying the tone series with longer delays. These findings suggest that a timing function is shared in motor and perceptual nonmotor tasks.

Is this timing function located in a specific area of the brain? To identify which neural structure is responsible for timing abilities, these same tests were given to patients with cerebellar lesions, Parkinson's disease, and motor cortex lesions. These patients were compared with a control group of normal individuals. Patients with cerebellar lesions had the greatest deficit in motor and nonmotor timing tasks. This finding led to the theory that the cerebellum is related to timing functions.[13–15]

Force Module

Another key function in motor control is the ability to produce force accurately. Is this function specific to a different neural structure? To answer this question, the same groups of individuals with neurologic dysfunction were compared with a normal control group on measures of force production. Subjects were asked to isometrically generate forces on a force transducer, with the amount of force generated being compared with a target force displayed on a computer screen. When individuals had large variability in reaching the target, they were considered to have poor force regulation.[14]

Again, different effectors (fingers and arms) were used in the task. Those who accurately targeted force in fingers also did so with their arms. Patients with Parkinson's disease had the greatest difficulty with this task, and individuals with cerebellar and cortical dysfunction were more similar to normal subjects. These results suggested that a force regulation module exists and that the neural structure that supports this function is the basal ganglia.

Sequencing Module

If timing is a function of the cerebellum and force is particular to the basal ganglia, is motor sequencing a specific function of another brain component? On the basis of blood flow studies, Roland and colleagues[16] identified cortical activity in specific regions during different motor tasks. When subjects were asked to execute simple but rapid flexion/extension movements in the fingers, tasks that do not require sequencing, the contralateral primary sensory and motor hand areas of cortex had increased activity. A similar increase in blood flow was observed during execution of a sequence of ballistic movements. However, this time the supplementary motor cortex along with primary sensory and motor hand areas had increased activity[16] (Fig. 10–5A).

To further investigate sequencing in this area, Roland and associates[16] had the same group of subjects repeat the planning of the sequenced ballistic finger movements without actually moving the fingers (mental rehearsal). This time, increased cortical activity was seen only in the supplementary motor cortex (see Fig. 10–5B). These studies suggest that the supplementary motor area supports motor and nonmotor sequencing tasks.[16]

Clinical Application of the Modular Theory

To further test the hypothesis that motor processes are conducted by specific brain structures, children identified as clumsy were screened initially for neurologic signs of basal ganglia or cerebellar dysfunction and assigned to different groups.[17] Both groups were tested

Finger movement sequence
(performance)

Supplementary
motor area

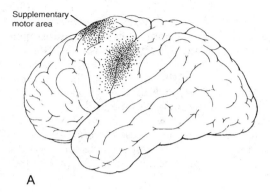

A

Finger movement sequence
(mental rehearsal)

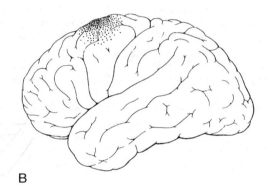

B

Figure 10–5. *Cerebral Flow Studies Conducted by Roland, et al.*[16] *(A) The subject performs a finger sequence with the activity in primary sensory and motor cortical areas as well as the supplementary motor cortex. (B) The same finger sequence is performed mentally (mental rehearsal); cortical activity is in the supplementary motor cortex only. (Adapted from Ghez, C: Voluntary movement. In Kandel, ER, Schwartz, JH, and Jessell, TM (eds): Principles of Neural Science, ed 3. Appleton & Lange, Norwalk, CT, 1991, p 621.)*

with tapping, time perception, and force regulation tasks. Performance on these experimental tasks were found to be specific to the subgroups of children. Children with cerebellar soft signs were found to be more variable in motor timing and time perception abilities, but force computation skills were intact. Force regulation difficulties were problematic in the group of clumsy children with basal ganglia soft signs.

Results of the series of studies presented suggest that therapeutic intervention may be most effective when context-related tasks are oriented to the neural mechanisms of dysfunction. Those individuals with cerebellar deficits may benefit from activities involving timing skill development, whereas patients with basal ganglia dysfunction may need specific force regulation training. This type of modular training is process-oriented in contrast to training each skill separately in a reflex hierarchical approach.

Systems Theory of Motor Control

While the modular theory demonstrates interactive processes within the central nervous system, do other body structures and the environment participate in movement outcome? This concept of increased ecologic involvement evolved with the systems theory.

Researchers conducting studies in Eastern Europe hypothesized that multiple subsystems contribute to successful motor control. Based on the research of Nicoli Bern-

stein,[18] **the systems theory of motor control has gained recognition.** Movement was considered by Bernstein to be organized by many elements or subsystems to solve problems or fulfill needs as an individual interacts in his or her environment. For example, an infant learning to walk requires experience and the maturation of both the nervous and musculoskeletal systems. Walking is considered to be a solution to the problem of the infant not being able to move freely to toys or people in the play area. This concept of problem solution is presented in contrast to the idea of the more simplistic perspective that, when the infant reaches a certain age, the cerebral cortex is mature enough to send out the specific command to walk.

To be successful in walking attempts, the child requires sufficient strength to move against gravity, good balance responses to maintain the upright posture, and enough coordination and force in the legs to propel the body weight forward. The goal of reaching a toy creates a meaningful context for all these elements to come together for movement. Coordinating the many elements or **degrees of freedom** (i.e., multiple muscle combinations; numerous planes of joint movement; available sensory information from visual, vestibular, and somatosensory systems; management of external forces in the environment) can be an overwhelming task for an adult, not to mention an infant. How does the body organize movement that will be successful to attain the goal?

These multiple elements or degrees of freedom, according to Bernstein,[18] **are constrained or reduced into single units of movement called** *synergies* **or** *coordinative structures.* Multiple systems act together for a common goal, in this case walking to a toy.

With the ideas of synergies in mind, the systems theorists, through postural studies, identified some units of movement.[19–21] They proposed that the individual subsystems interact and are constrained into functional units for postural stability, as depicted in Figure 10–6. In studies of balance, two processes are investigated: *motor coordination* (the combination of motor and musculoskeletal) and *sensory organization* (visual, somatosensory, vestibular systems) as they form units of postural control, also known as *synergies.* These synergies are used as needed in different environmental contexts. Sometimes "automatic postural responses" are needed, for example, when suddenly bumped while standing; at other times "anticipatory postural adjustments" are used, when reaching out while standing to answer the phone.

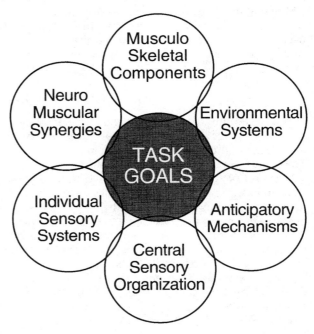

Figure 10–6. Systems theoretical components that interact for specific tasks and goals.

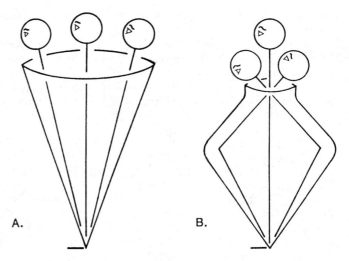

Figure 10–7. *Stability Cones.* Stability limits enclose areas of movement within which movement can occur without loss of balance. (*A*) Rotations about the ankles. (*B*) Movement around the hip joint in the hip strategy. (From Journal of Motor Behavior 21(3):225, 1989. Reprinted with permission of the Helen Dwight Reed Educational Foundation. Published by Heldref Publications, 1319 Eighteenth St, NW Washington, DC 20036-1082. Copyright © 1989.)

A.   B.

Systems Theory Applied to Postural Control

To identify the existence of system organization for automatic and anticipatory postural responses, Nashner and colleagues[19–21] developed research paradigms to test muscle response organization, sensory organization, and force regulation in balance. Postural control for balance was chosen as a behavior of interest, since developing and maintaining balance are critical for functioning in the environment.

Equilibrium is the control of the body's center of mass over its base of support. For example, in quiet stance, the base of support is the foot length of the person and stance width. We have small sway movements of the body as we maintain this position. Within this base of support, there is a *theoretical limit or cone of stability* within which we can move and still maintain our balance as shown in Figure 10–7.[22] When we move out of these limits of stability, a protective response occurs in the limb. In the case of standing, we step forward, backward, or to the side in a *stepping strategy* pattern. However, within the cone of stability, we use the *automatic* or *anticipatory postural adjustments,* depending on the context of our movement.[19,20]

Automatic Postural Responses

How do multiple systems organize their output into balance responses? By unexpectedly moving the base of support on which a person is standing and recording muscle responses to this perturbation, **automatic postural responses have been identified.**[19,21] **These muscle responses are predictable synergies, that is, multiple muscles constrained to act as a functional unit, with fixed timing and sequencing within the motor and subsequently the musculoskeletal system.** When a person experiences different balance demands according to changes in the base of support, different synergies are used. Automatic postural responses used are ankle and hip strategies of balance control. For example, when balance is disturbed while a person is standing on a normal base of support, with feet together, the ankle muscles are used in what has been termed an *ankle strategy* to maintain balance (Fig. 10–8A and B). When a person standing on a movable platform is suddenly displaced backward, the body sways forward. To compensate for this forward sway, the individual automatically uses the posterior muscles of the shank, upper leg, and trunk in a predictable distal-to-proximal sequence to regain the upright position. A similar ankle strategy is used when the platform is suddenly moved forward, producing backward sway of

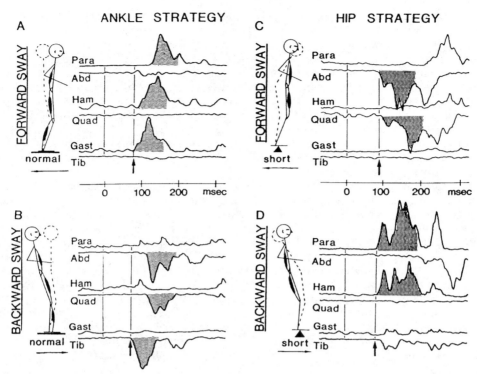

Figure 10–8.   *Ankle and Hip Synergies or Strategies in Response to Platform Perturbations.* Ankle synergy responses are distal to proximal in organization and directionally specific to the platform movement. Hip synergies involve upper leg and trunk muscles. (From Horak, FB and Nashner, LM: Central programming of postural movements: Adaptations to altered support surface configurations. JI Neurophysiol 55: 1369, 1986, with permission.)

the body. This time the anterior muscles are used to maintain standing. These ankle strategies are activated in a directionally specific manner according to forward and backward perturbation.[19–21,25]

When the base of support is reduced to standing on a narrow beam or when the base of support is moved quickly, a different strategy is used, with hip muscles providing the major control of postural stability.[19,20] During platform movements backward and forward, body sway again occurs, but this time sway is predominantly at the hips. The specific response is termed a *hip strategy* for balance control.[19,20] According to the researchers, in this strategy the proximal muscles (hip and trunk) on the opposite aspect of the body were used (see Fig. 10–8C and D).

Development of Automatic Postural Responses

The synergistic organization described for automatic postural responses is also seen in children. However, ongoing development occurs until 7 to 10 years of age, when adultlike responses are seen. In a series of studies by Woollacott, Shumway-Cook, and associates,[23–25] age-related changes in balance synergies have been documented.

Longitudinal studies of infants not yet walking (pulling to a standing position) were conducted, with muscle responses recorded monthly until they walked independently. Beginning organization of these postural synergies emerged in the ankle muscles during the pull-to-stand stage of development (7 to 9 months of age), whereas adultlike responses became organized at the time of independent walking. Although the adultlike responses of ankle to upper leg to trunk activation are present, timing of these muscles varies with slower recruitment of ankle muscles initially and longer duration of muscle responses.[24]

At 4 to 6 years of age, a child's muscle response characteristics regress, varying from trial to trial with initial muscle onsets being longer than in younger children and infants. This disorganization in 4- to 6-year-old children is followed by a reorganization in postural development with adultlike motor coordination responses established in 7- to 10-year-olds. Woollacott and colleagues[23] have hypothesized that 4- to 6-year-old children are going through transitional changes in postural stability, in which previous motor programs for controlling balance are no longer effective because of growth changes in height and weight. These changes in body morphology affect the center of mass over the base of support, which in turn affects equilibrium. During this transitional period, children learn to adapt sensory inputs to different contexts. By the end of this period, a restabilization of automatic postural responses occurs, resulting in the development of postural control strategies that they will continue to use through adulthood.

The automatic postural responses identified in adults and children support the concept of multiple degrees of freedom constrained into functional units or synergies. **Multiple subsystems (motor, sensory, and skeletal) contribute to balance control rather than the central nervous system solely controlling upright stance. Intervention for individuals with balance dyscontrol is therefore multisystem based rather than being specifically directed to central nervous system functions.**

The goal of therapy for persons with disordered motor control is to train them to use the right synergy response at the right time. Often these individuals move more slowly, are more unstable, and are more vulnerable to external balance threats (people and objects in the environment unexpectedly perturbing their base of support). In addition to training automatic postural responses, *anticipatory postural adjustments* are needed to create movement that is task- or goal-oriented. During these anticipatory postural adjustments, postural responses are combined with feedforward control for voluntary movement.

Anticipatory Postural Adjustments

Most movements in standing during routine daily activities include some type of voluntary movement. As we reach out overhead or pull a door closed, we adjust our body mass over our base of support or within our cone of stability to compensate for the arm movement we are initiating. Skilled movements such as these have both postural and voluntary components. The postural component provides the stabilizing support for the second component, the primary volitional or focal movement we need to accomplish a task.[25] This close relationship of postural and voluntary control has implications for patient populations we serve, since the lack of good postural stability decreases the number and the variety of movements these individuals perform.

Through research studies that focus on anticipatory postural adjustments, muscle activation patterns have been identified according to the movement context. Cordo and Nashner[27] recorded onsets of postural and arm muscles during arm flexion/extension tasks in which subjects pushed or pulled on a handle. When activation of the prime mover muscles (biceps) occurs in arm flexion (pulling) tasks, it is preceded by activation of the gastrocnemius, hamstrings, and trunk extensor muscles.[26,27] This sequence of postural muscle recruitment is the same organization used in automatic responses, with similar muscle onset recordings. Primary mover muscles—in this case arm biceps—follows the postural muscle activation.

Only with technologic advances such as EMG recordings have anticipatory postural adjustments been described. Because these responses occur quickly, the actual postural link to voluntary control is difficult to observe and identify. The implications of these findings to therapy are significant. In treatment, we now know that voluntary movement should not be trained separately from, but in conjunction with, the postural adjustment. **Developing treatment strategies that encourage postural adjustment prior to voluntary movement results in a more functional balance control for goal-directed tasks carried out during activities of daily living.**

Sensory Organization

Using a systems approach, the therapist evaluates both automatic and anticipatory postural adjustments. If both responses contributing to balance control appear to be intact for an individual, other systems are evaluated. **The second major component to consider in balance control is *sensory organization.***

Sensory information from visual, somatosensory, and vestibular systems form the basis of sensory organization needed for balance. Can a person compensate if one of these systems is not available (blindness) or if distorted sensory information is received? A research paradigm was established to test this question.[28-30] Using a platform for standing, six sensory conditions are presented systematically, as shown in Figure 10–9, to eliminate or distort the three postural senses.

Body sway, force changes through the feet, and actual loss of balance are measures of a subject's ability to resolve sensory conflict. Studies in normal adults have shown that increased sway occurs when vision and somatosensory information are not available.[28,29] However, these adults remained well within their limit of stability. Although children required up to three times longer than adults to demonstrate an adaptive attenuation of an inappropriate response, they were found to reweight sensory information within 15 trials.[23]

Throughout this overview of systems theory, postural studies in standing have been presented as a means of systematically reviewing this theoretical framework of multiple systems constrained into movement units or synergies. Additional studies, not reviewed in this chapter, have been conducted in sitting [31,33] and in gait,[34,35] which provide additional information for systems theory application in clinical practice.

Clinical Applications of Systems Theory

Using a systems approach, researchers have investigated individuals with a variety of neurologic conditions to determine whether motor coordination, sensory organization, or other processes are disturbed by damage to specific areas of the brain.[36-48]

The role of the basal ganglia was explored by Horak and colleagues.[36] Parkinsonian patients were compared with normal young and elderly adults to document automatic postural responses during platform perturbation tests previously described. Although ankle

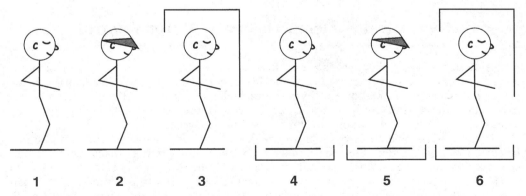

1   2   3   4   5   6

Figure 10–9. Six Sensory Conditions Used to Systematically Occlude or Alter Visual and Somatosensory Information. The six conditions are (*1*) normal standing, (*2*) standing with vision occluded, (*3*) standing with a visual surround that moves in direct proportion to the body, (*4*) sway servo standing that moves the supporting surface in direct proportion to body sway, (*5*) sway servo standing with vision occluded, and (*6*) sway servo standing with visual surround moving with the subject's body sway. In the last two conditions, the subject relies on vestibular information only. (Adapted from Peterka, RJ and Black, FO: Age-related changes in human posture control and sensory organization tests. Journal of Vestibular Research, 1:73, 1990.)

strategy recruitment in automatic postural responses was the same as in normal subjects, **nonmedicated parkinsonian patients used both hip and ankle strategies simultaneously.** In addition, excessive cocontraction of muscles (antagonistic muscle recruitment) was recorded (gastrocnemius contracted with tibialis anterior; hamstrings with quadriceps). These coactivation or cocontraction patterns increased stiffness around joints and may reflect the rigidity seen in these patients.

Sway measurements showed parkinsonian patients to be stiffer than the normal group, with a smaller sway area and slower adjustments to sway changes. Their actual limit of stability was smaller, because they stood rigidly in a small area. Although they were more stable, they lacked flexibility within their cone of stability. Once sway increased, the parkinsonian patients immediately lost their balance, giving an "all-or-nothing" approach to maintenance of the upright position. Such findings may explain the small steppage and shuffling gait patterns seen in patients with Parkinson's disease. **Anticipatory responses in parkinsonian patients are reported as absent or reduced**[40]; however, **their sensory organization is similar to normal subjects.**[35]

The focus in therapy for parkinsonian patients, based on the systems theory, would be to improve motor coordination parameters rather than sensory organization. Task-oriented intervention using both automatic and anticipatory postural adjustments would be included in the treatment protocol.

Other adult populations that have been studied using platform test conditions are patients with a history of cerebral vascular accident,[38,39] patients with traumatic brain injuries,[40] patients with cerebellar ataxia,[30,41,42] patients with vestibular dysfunction,[43] and elderly adults with a history of falling.[44] Motor control development has been studied in children with sensory and motor impairments as well, using the same platform conditions. To date, studies have included children with Down's syndrome,[45] children with different diagnoses of cerebral palsy, hearing-impaired children,[47] children with learning disabilities,[47] and children who are clumsy.[48]

When applying the systems theory to patient populations, therapists should be reminded of the ideas of Bernstein[18], who described movement as being carried out in an infinite number of ways, with an infinite number of combinations of muscle actions. In other words, in performing most skills there are an infinite number of solutions to a given problem, rather than a prescribed command from higher centers as outlined in the reflex hierarchical approach. The further evolution of this concept is demonstrated with the dynamical systems theory of motor control.

Dynamical Systems Theory of Motor Control

Although systems theorists interpret Bernstein's writings in terms of neural mechanisms, dynamical system theorists combine his concepts of human movement with the principles of pattern formation in physical and biologic systems. Although chaotic states have been observed in these natural systems, it has been proposed that specific patterns are formed through self-organization of elements within the system.[52]

Chaotic states actually have order, in which elements *organize and are constrained into functional units.* Consider cloud formations, a complex interaction of many elements into specific patterns. When ground moisture is warmed by the sun, air and heat elements form thermals, which rise because of instability in temperature. Stability is regained at the condensation level of the atmosphere. At this level, temperature and water vapor elements reach a critical level at which particles collide and are constrained into large droplets. The resulting pattern formation is a cumulus cloud, which is visible and functional. Depending on the characteristics of the system (density of the droplets, temperature, and wind patterns) the droplets become rain, snow, or hail.[49] This *self-organization* of elements provides multiple solutions leading to a common outcome, return of the water supply to the earth's surface. The process of pattern formation may be different (snow, rain, hail), but the end state is the same.

Likewise in movement, the goal may be walking, but different solutions to the problem of constraining multiple degrees of freedom for upright mobility may be exhibited. The organization of the multiple systems emerges as a variety of walking patterns by an individual, as well as between individuals. **Although it may be advantageous for the therapist to guide a patient in his or her movement patterns, the ultimate solution lies with self-organization of the degrees of freedom within the individual.**

Assumptions of the Dynamical Systems Theory

How does self-organization occur? To further understand the dynamical systems approach to motor control therapy, we will explore underlying assumptions of the theory as they relate to locomotion development. To explore these assumptions, a series of studies by Thelen and colleagues[50] and Heriza[51] will be presented. Although the elements of infant walking development are presented, an analysis of these elements and subsystems reveals that they are similar to those that therapists might consider during gait training in children and adults with movement disorders. Four major underlying assumptions are outlined as a conceptual framework for this theory.

Constraining Complexity into Simplicity

The *first* assumption of the dynamical systems model is that moving and developing organisms are complex, but cooperative systems. **The elements of movement (numerous muscle combinations, multiple planes of movement at joints, sensory information, inertial and external forces in the environment, and the individual's arousal level and motivation) are constrained through subsystem organization into a functional unit or** *coordinative structure* **to reach the goal** of independent walking. The concept of coordinative structure is similar to the synergy used in systems theory, with subsystems constrained into functional movement units.

Self-Organization Within Subsystems

The *second* **assumption of this approach is that behavior emerges from the self-organizing properties of many subsystems that are required for the function.** For example, Thelen and associates[50] and Heriza[51] identified eight subsystems that were considered to be involved in walking (Fig. 10–10). Taking each subsystem separately, these researchers hypothesized that if each subsystem was examined separately, it would be found that each developed at a different rate. They further hypothesized that as each subsystem matured, there was a critical time frame during which the skill level needed for walking emerged. However, until all eight subsystems acquired their individual critical level of skill, walking was not accomplished.

If you were asked to list the necessary components for walking, you may think of balance, reciprocal movement in the legs, and so on. These components are identical with some of the eight subsystems identified by Thelen and associates[50] and Heriza[51] (Table 10–1).

Nonlinear Development Within Subsystems

The *third* **assumption of the dynamical systems theory is that changes in the component or subsystem are asynchronous or nonlinear.** For example, some components develop early, such as pattern formation (alternating leg movements are seen at birth), whereas other components develop later (postural control in standing emerges at approximately 9 to 12 months). **These slower-developing components are considered to be** *rate-limiting* **factors.** In infant locomotion, Thelen and coworkers[50] hypothesized that specific elements—postural control, balance, and extensor strength—constrain the infant

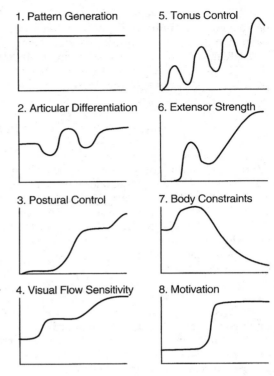

Figure 10–10. *Eight Hypothesized Components of Locomotor Development.* Each component is plotted over time, from birth to the onset of independent walking. (Adapted from Heriza.[51] Reprinted with permission from the Foundation for Physical Therapy, Inc.)

from independent walking. When maturation of these components occurs, the overall system, that is, the infant in the context of his or her environment, shifts into walking behavior. This abrupt shift or change from crawling in open space to independent ambulation reflects the nonlinear quality of the development of the behavior.[50]

Phase Shifts

Can we predict when these sudden shifts in behavior will occur? **The *fourth* assumption of the dynamical systems theory states that shifts from one qualitative behavior mode to another is discontinuous. Parameters that cause the shift from one mode to another, termed *control parameters*, disrupt the established preferred state and drive the system to seek a new attractor state.** Figure 10–11 presents a graphic representation of a *phase shift.*[50,51]

In the case of locomotion in open space, the infant may have established crawling as a preferred state of mobility. This state would be stable, much like the ball in the deep well in the left side of the figure. As more postural control for balance and extensor force are developed, crawling is disrupted. During this time period, the behavior may occur less often, may be more variable, or may be easily perturbed. Rather than always crawling, the infant may relax the timing of leg and arm alternating patterns and become less coordinated in actual reciprocal patterns. This period of instability of crawling is depicted as the shallow well in the diagram, a transiton period when the infant is attracted toward a new developmental stage. The actual phase shift is complete when a new stable attractor state is established, represented by the deep well in the right of Figure 10–11. The emergence of walking as a mode of locomotion becomes the preferred state, with crawling behaviors seen less and less frequently.

Table 10–1. *Subsystems Identified by Thelen*[50,51]

Subsystem	Contribution to Walking	Implications for Therapy
Pattern formation	Alternating pattern of the legs is required.	Alternating pattern may not be apparent due to poor postural control or increased stiffness in the legs.
Articulator differentiation	During walking, hip and ankle move separately from the knee.	Individuals with CNS impairment often display total flexion or extension of the limbs. Refinement of leg patterns may be a focus in therapy.
Postural control	To ambulate, the body must be held upright against gravity.	Poor postural control occurs in individuals with neurologic impairment.
Visual flow sensitivity	Individual must be able to differentiate his or her movement from environmental movement.	This component is particularly critical when power drive wheelchairs are prescribed.
Tonus control	Alternating timing of flexor and extensor muscle tone is needed in the legs before walking emerges.	Timing problems are characteristic of individuals with CNS impairment due to increased cocontraction/stiffness around the joints.
Extensor strength	To counteract the effects of gravity, extensor strength is required.	Decreased isolated strength of extensor muscle groups is often observed in those with CNS dysfunction.
Body morphology	At birth, the infant has a large head and proportionally small body. Increased weight gain occurs during the first year of life. These changes must be managed to produce upright postural control.	Sudden changes in height or weight may increase the energy requirement for walking.
Motivation	Interest in task goals often motivates the child to walk.	Lack of motivation by individuals.

The control parameter, shown as an arrow in Figure 10–11, is the component part that drives the infant to a new attractor state. No single subsystem has priority in being the driving force to shift the overall system into a new behavior mode. Thelen and coworkers[50] identified the *rate-limiting* components for walking to be postural control for balance and extensor strength; maturation of one or a combination of these may be the control parameter

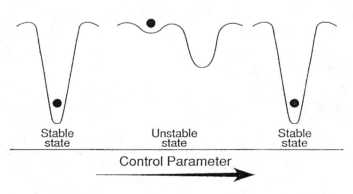

Stable state   Unstable state   Stable state

Control Parameter

Figure 10–11. *Phase Shifts in Dynamical Systems Theory.* Stable behaviors are like the ball in the deep well. As the system is disrupted by the control parameter, transition occurs shown as the shallow wells. During this time, the coordination pattern is unstable and easily perturbed. The phase shift is complete when a new stable attractor state is established, represented by the second deep well on the right. (From Heriza,[51] p 110. Reprinted with permission from the Foundation for Physical Therapy, Inc.)

for independent walking in an individual child. In children and adults with disordered motor control, only careful quantitative analyses over time can document the developmental changes in an individual to identify which subsystems may be considered to be control parameters.

Dynamical systems theory also applies to most movement patterns in adults. In the adult, the control parameter that causes a movement pattern to shift may be a velocity change within a rhythmic movement pattern rather than a developmental change. Let us consider a nondevelopmental example of dynamical patterning. In a classic study of movement, Haken and coworkers[52] asked subjects to move their index fingers rhythmically in an alternating *out-of-phase* pattern of flexion and extension. As one index finger flexed, the other extended. When the subjects were asked to move faster or increase the velocity of finger movements, there was a phase shift into a new preferred state.

In the new behavioral state, fingers flexed and extended together, an *in-phase* movement pattern. In this example, the control parameter to the change in behavior was increased velocity of finger movements. If the subjects were asked to begin the in-phase pattern slowly and increase speed, no phase shift was noted. The in-phase pattern was therefore the preferred state. At the time of transition from out-of-phase movement to in-phase movement, represented in the graph of finger cycles in Figure 10–11, there was a slowing of movement as reorganization occurred. Increased variability of actual control of finger flexion/extensor pattern was noted during this transition time. Haken and coworkers[52] suggested that these transition periods of high variability and instability are key to understanding complex behaviors.

Clinical Application of the Dynamical Systems Theory

The idea of phase shifts is important to therapists, who are always interested in making changes in movement conditions. **Since the period of instability during phase shifts is the time during which outside perturbations have the most impact, therapy may be more effective during transition periods.** By identifying control parameters that would cause phase shifts, the therapist would understand what component may be constraining a desired movement behavior from emerging. Increased focus on this particular subsystem may assist in the change to new pattern formations of movement.

Studies incorporating dynamical systems theoretical principles with atypical movement pattern formation are beginning to be conducted. The purpose of these studies is to identify control parameters that may be manipulated to assist in changing movement patterns. Preterm infant kicking patterns have been studied over time to determine when pattern formation of alternating leg movement is present and the characteristics of these patterns.[51] Leg pattern formation has also been documented in children with Down's syndrome.[53] Characteristics of reaching pattern formation are currently under investigation in normal infants, which will have implications for future studies using patient populations.[54] To determine the effects of increased stiffness on movement, the self-organization of crawling and gait patterns in children with cerebral palsy has been studied.[55,56] Perturbation conditions have been introduced to determine stability or instability within these patterns.[55]

Summary

Throughout this chapter, we have traced the evolution of motor control theories and their application to rehabilitation. This evolution is presented in Table 10–2. Research in movement science and other disciplines has demonstrated the importance of rehabilitation models based on systems theories. Although it was previously thought that the central nervous system hierarchical development and control dictated motor performance, new conceptual models suggest that many systems, including the motor, sensory, and musculoskeletal subsystems and the environmental context contribute to successful movement.

Table 10-2. *A Summary of Motor Control Theories*

Theory	Underlying Assumptions	Therapeutic Model	Strengths	Limitations
Reflex hierarchical	Sensory input is required for motor output. CNS is organized hierarchically with lower structures controlled by higher cortical structures.	To produce motor control, sensory stimulation is given. Therapist facilitates normal movement patterns to reduce spasticity, inhibit reflexes, and establish voluntary movement.	Therapist has control.	Patient is a passive recipient of movement. No evidence that reducing spasticity and reflex patterns increases voluntary movement patterns.
Modular	Motor control is not product-oriented, but process-oriented. CNS is organized according to specific functions (timing, force production, motor sequencing). Processes are used by many effector groups and in nonmotor tasks.	Intervention in motor control processes is emphasized rather than specific movement patterns. Intervention in these processes may affect a variety of motor and nonmotor tasks.	Intervention in specific processes may generalize to a variety of motor and nonmotor tasks.	Little evidence to date that carry over occurs to specific functional motor or nonmotor activities.
Systems	Movement is the organization and constraint of sensory, motor, musculoskeletal, and environmental systems into functional units. Movement is organized for successful task completion.	Emphasis is on practice of movement to achieve task goals. Motor problem solving is emphasized in different environmental contexts. Compensatory strategies are developed.	Patient has control of developing movement strategies through practice. Function is emphasized in the context of the environment. Other systems are considered (musculoskeletal) rather than a pure CNS focus.	Less control by therapist. Movement as cognitive-based approach is criticized as questionable when automatic reactions are required. Practice may be too time-consuming to be cost-effective. Quantitative studies needed.
Dynamical systems	Movement results from constraining complex cooperative subsystems into functional units of movement. Self-organization occurs within subsystems to meet the requirement of the task. Subsystems organize at different rates. The new movement will occur when all subsystems are mature or organized to meet the task requirement. Shifts into new behavior occur when the slowest rate-limiting subsystem is organized. This component acts as a "control parameter" to force a shift into a new movement pattern.	Emphasis on practice of movement to achieve task goals. Motor problem solving emphasized in different environmental contexts. During periods of instability, the movement pattern in state of reorganization, therapy may be more effective at this time. Control parameters identified to assist in the shift to new movement pattern formation.	Patient has control of developing movement strategies through practice. Function is emphasized in the context of the environment. Subsystems include not only sensory, motor, musculoskeletal systems, but also arousal, motivation, cognitive, and environmental systems. Identification of periods of instability, rate limiting factors, and control parameters provides a more specific focus in therapy.	More in-depth analyses of subsystem organization may be viewed as too time-consuming. Control parameters identified in the typical population may not be the same as those in atypical populations. Additional quantitative studies with patient populations are needed.

Within these systems, each component must be assessed separately to determine the specific subsystem to address in therapy. However, therapeutic intervention is based on the interaction of these components in a functional environmental context. The effectiveness of these theories in rehabilitation can be determined only with individual clients, using reliable, valid quantitative measures over time.

RECOMMENDED READINGS

Bernstein, N: Coordination and Regulation of Movement. Pergamon Press, New York, 1967.

Brunnstrom, S: Movement Therapy in Hemiplegia. Harper & Row, New York, 1970.

Carr, JH, Shepherd, RB, and Gordon, J (eds): Movement Science: Foundations for Physical Therapy in Rehabilitation. Aspen Publishers, Rockville, MD, 1987.

Diamond, A (ed): Developmental and Neural Basis of Higher Cognitive Function. New York Academy of Sciences, New York, 1990.

Horak, FB: Assumptions Underlying Motor Control for Neurologic Rehabilitation. In Foundation for Physical Therapy: Contemporary Management of Motor Control Problems: Proceedings of the II STEP Conference. Bookcrafters, Fredericksburg, VA, 1991.

Nashner, LM and McCollum, G: The Organization of Human Postural Movements: A Formal Basis and Experimental Synthesis. Behav Brain Sci 8:135, 1985.

Proceedings of the II STEP Conference. Bookcrafters, Fredericksburg, VA, 1991.

Talbot, RE and Humphrey, DR (eds): Posture and Movement. Raven Press, New York, 1979.

REFERENCES

1. Horak, FB: Assumptions Underlying Motor Control for Neurologic Rehabilitation. In Contemporary Management of Motor Control Problems: Proceedings of the II STEP Conference. Bookcrafters, Fredericksburg, VA, 1991.

2. Sherrington, CS: The Integrative Action of the Nervous System. Cambridge University Press, New York, 1947.

3. Polit, A and Bizzi, E: Characteristics of Motor Program Underlying Arm Movements in Monkeys. J Neurophysiol 42:183, 1979.

4. Lashley, KS: The Problem of Serial Order in Behavior. John Wiley & Sons, New York, 1951.

5. Gordon, J: Assumptions Underlying Physical Therapy Intervention: Theoretical and Historical Perspectives. In Carr, JH, Shepherd, RB, and Gordon, J (eds): Movement Science: Foundations for Physical Therapy in Rehabilitation. Aspen Publishers, Rockville, MD, 1987.

6. Walsche, FMP: Contribution of John Hughlings Jackson to Neurology. Arch Neurol 5:99, 1961.

7. Towen, B: Neurological Development in Infancy. Lavenham Press, Lavenham, England, 1976.

8. Bobath, K: The Motor Deficit in Patients with Cerebral Palsy. In Clinics in Developmental Medicine. No. 23. Lavenham Press, Lavenham, England, 1966.

9. Brunnstrom, S: Movement Therapy in Hemiplegia. Harper & Row, New York, 1970.

10. Hofsten, C von: Eye Hand Coordination in the Newborn. Dev Psychol 18:450, 1982.

11. Thelen, E, Fisher, DM, and Ridley-Johnson, R: The Relationship Between Physical Growth and a Newborn Reflex. Infant Behav Dev. 7:479, 1984.

12. Sahrmann, SA and Norton, BJ: The Relationship of Voluntary Movement to Spasticity in the Upper Motor Neuron Syndrome. Ann Neurol 2:460, 1977.

13. Keele, SW and Ivry, RI: Does the Cerebellum Provide a Common Computation for Diverse Tasks? A Timing Hypothesis. In Diamond, A (ed): Developmental and Neural Basis of Higher Cognitive Function. New York Academy of Sciences, New York, 1990.

14. Keele, SW, Ivry, RI, and Pokormy, RA: Force Control and Its Relationship to Timing. J Motor Behav 19:96, 1987.

15. Keele, SW, et al: Do Perception and Motor Production Share a Common Timing Mechanism? A Correlational Analysis. Acta Psychol 60:173, 1985.

16. Roland, PE, et al: Supplementary Motor Area and Other Cortical Areas in Organization of Voluntary Movements in Man. J Neurophysiol 43:118, 1980.

17. Lundy-Ekman, L, Ivry, RI, and Keele, SW: Timing and Force Control Deficits in Clumsy Children. Cogn Neurosci 3:367, 1991.

18. Bernstein, N: Coordination and Regulation of Movement. Pergamon Press, New York, 1967.

19. Nashner, LM and McCollum, G: The Organization of Human Postural Movements: A Formal Basis and Experimental Synthesis. Behav Brain Sci 8:135, 1985.

20. Horak, FB and Nashner, L: Central Programming of Postural Movements: Adaptations to Altered Support Surface Configurations. J Neurophysiol 55:1369, 1986.

21. Nashner, LM and Woollacott, MH: The Organization of Rapid Postural Adjustment of Standing Humans: An Experimental Conceptual Model. In Talbot, RE and Humphrey, DR (eds): Posture and Movement. Raven Press, New York, 1979.

22. McCollum, G and Leen, TK: From and Exploration of Mechanical Stability Limits in Erect Stance. J Motor Behav 21:225, 1985.

23. Woollacott, M, Shumway-Cook, A, and Williams, HG: The Development of Posture and Balance Control in Children. In Woollacott, M and Shumway-Cook, A (eds): Development of Posture and Gait Across a Lifespan. University of South Carolina Press, Columbia, SC, 1989.

24. Woollacott, MH and Sviestrup, H: Changes in the Sequencing and Timing of Muscle Response Coordination Associated with Developmental Transitions in Balance Abilities. Hum Mov Sci 11:23, 1992.

25. Woollacott, MH and Shumway-Cook, A: The Development of Motor Control. In Shumway-Cook, A and Woollacott, M (eds): Motor Control Theory and Practice Applications. Williams & Wilkins, Baltimore, 1995.

26. Inglin, B and Woollacott, MH: Age Related Changes in Anticipatory Postural Adjustments Associated with Arm Movements. J Gerontol 43:4, 105, 1988.

27. Cordo, PJ and Nashner, LM: Properties of Postural Adjustments Associated with Rapid Arm Movements. J Neurophysiol 47:287, 1982.

28. Peterka, RJ and Black, FO: Age Related Changes in Human Posture Control: Sensory Organization Test. Vestib Res 1:73, 1980.

29. Woollacott, MH, Shumway-Cook, A, and Nashner, LM: Postural Reflexes and Aging. In Mortimer, J (ed): The Aging Motor System. Praeger, New York, 1982.

30. Nashner, LM and Grimm, RJ: Analysis of Multiloop Dyscontrols in Standing Cerebellar Patients. In Desmedt, JE (ed): Progress in Clinical Neurophysiology, vol 4. Cerebral Motor Control in Man: Long Loop Mechanisms. Gasser & Cie AG, Basel, Switzerland. 1978.

31. Harbourne, RT, Guiliani, C, and MacNeila, J: A Kinematic and Electromyographic Analysis of the Development of Sitting Posture in Infants. Dev Psychobiol 26:51, 1993.

32. Moore, S, et al: Investigation of Evidence for Anticipatory Postural Adjustments in Seated Subjects Who Performed a Reaching Task. Phys Ther 72:335, 1992.

33. Forssberg, H and Hirschfeld, H: Postural Adjustments in Sitting Humans Following External Perturbations: Muscle Activity and Kinematics. Exp Brain 97:515, 1994 (submitted).

34. Hirschfeld, H and Forssberg, H: Phase Dependent Modulations of Anticipatory Postural Activity During Human Locomotion. J Neurophysiol 66:12, 1991.

35. Hirschfeld, H and Forssberg, H: Development of Anticipatory Postural Adjustments During Locomotion in Children. J Neurophysiol 68:542, 1992.

36. Horak, FB, Nashner, LM, and Nutt, JG: Postural Instability in Parkinson's Disease: Motor Coordination and Sensory Organization. Neurol Rep 12:54, 1988.

37. Forssberg, H, Johnels, B, and Steg, G: Is Parkinsonian Gait Caused by a Regression to an Immature Pattern? Adv Neurol 40:375, 1984.

38. Horak, FB, et al: The Effects of Movement, Velocity, Mass Displaced and Task Uncertainty in Associated Postural Adjustments Made by Normal and Hemiplegic Individuals. J Neurol Neurosurg Psychiatry 46:1020, 1984.

39. Pal'tsev, YI and El'ner, AM: Preparatory and Compensatory Period During Voluntary Movement in Patients with Involvement of the Brain in Different Locations. Biophysics 12:161, 1967.

40. Shumway-Cook, A and Olmscheid, R: A Systems Analysis of Postural Dyscontrol in Traumatically Brain-Injured Patients. J Head Trauma Rehabil 5:51, 1990.

41. Traub, MM, Rothwell, JC, and Marsden, CD: Anticipatory Postural Reflexes in Parkinson's Disease and Other Akinetic Rigid Syndromes and in Cerebellar Ataxia. Brain 103:869, 1980.

42. Horak, F: Comparison of Cerebellar and Vestibular Loss on Scaling of Postural Responses. In Brandt, T (ed): 10th International Symposium on Disorders of Posture and Gait. Thelme Press, Munich, Germany, 1990.

43. Nashner, L, Black, FO, and Wall, C: Adaptation to Altered Support and Visual Conditions During Stance: Patients with Vestibular Deficits. J Neurosci 2:536, 1982.

44. Woollacott, M: Aging, Posture Control, and Movement Preparation. In Woollacott, MH and Shumway-Cook, A (eds): Posture and Gait Across a Lifespan. University of South Carolina Press, Columbia, SC, 1989.

45. Shumway-Cook, A and Woollacott, MH: Dynamics of Postural Control in Down's Syndrome. Phys Ther 65:1315, 1985.

46. Nashner, LM, Shumway-Cook, A, and Marin, O: Stance Posture Control in Selected Groups of Children with Cerebral Palsy: Deficits in Sensory Organization and Muscular Coordination. Exp Brain Res 49:393, 1983.

47. Horak, F, et al: Vestibular Function and Motor Proficiency in Children with Hearing Impairment, or with Learning Disabilities and Motor Impairments. Develop Med Child Neurol 30:64, 1988.

48. Williams, HG and Woollacott, MH: Personal Communication.

49. Scorer, R and Verkirk A: Spacious Skies: The Ultimate Cloud Book. Resopal for David & Charles Publishers, Portugal, 1989.

50. Thelen, E, Ulrich, B, and Jensen, JL: The Developmental Origins of Locomotion. In Woollacott, MH and Shumway-Cook, A (eds): Posture and Gait Across a Lifespan. University of South Carolina Press, Columbia, SC, 1989.

51. Heriza, CB: Motor Development: Traditional and Contemporary Theories. In Contemporary Management of Motor Control Problems: Proceedings of the II STEP Conference. Bookcrafters, Fredericksburg, VA, 1991.

52. Haken, H, Kelso, JAS, and Bunz, HA: Theoretical Model of Phase Transitions in Human Hand Movements. Biol Cybern 51:347, 1985.

53. Ulrich, DA and Ulrich, BA: Spontaneous Leg Movements in Infants with Down's Syndrome: A Basis for Delayed Changes in Coordination and Control Child Dev (in press).

54. Thelen, E, et al: The Transition to Reaching: Mapping Intention and Intrinsic Dynamics. Child Dev 64:1058, 1993.

55. Sholz, JP: Dynamic Pattern Theory: Some Implications for Therapeutics. Phys Ther 70:827, 1990.

56. Holt, K and Jeng, SF: Advances in Biomechanical Analysis of the Physically Challenged Child: Cerebral Palsy. Pediatr Exer Sci 4:213, 1992.

CHAPTER 11

■

Motor Learning

Diane E. Nicholson, PT, NCS, PhD

- ■ *The Training-Learning Distinction*
- ■ *The Performance-Learning Distinction*
- ■ *Variables That Influence Motor Learning*
- ■ *Clinical Applications*

A primary goal of therapeutic intervention is to develop, or optimize, skilled movements. These movements consist of an enormous repertoire of coordinated, goal-directed actions in such varied situations as rolling over in bed to using a weakened upper limb to reach for a glass of water after a stroke. Therapy clients might be *learning* a skilled movement for the first time, or they might be *re-learning* an action, as is frequently the case in pediatric and adult populations, respectively. Re-learning occurs either by *recovery* (learning a strategy identical with that used prior to injury) or by *compensation* (learning a new strategy different from that used prior to injury).[1] However, regardless of whether a therapy goal is learning or re-learning, the focus is on optimizing physical function and skill.

The field of motor learning involves the investigation and discussion of the variables and principles that either enhance or inhibit a person's ability to learn a new skill. Although most of this text focuses on the anatomic and physiologic aspects of normal and abnormal motor control, it is equally important for anyone involved in the rehabilitation process to understand the principles that influence the acquisition or reacquisition of functional motor skills. The purpose of this chapter is to define some of the critical terms associated with motor learning, to describe the variables that influence a person's ability to learn a motor skill, and to discuss the application of motor learning principles in clinical situations.

The Training-Learning Distinction

It is important to differentiate between the process of learning a skill and the process of being trained in a skill.[2] *Training occurs when performers are provided with solutions to problems; for example, when a therapist encourages clients to memorize movement patterns by repetition. Learning occurs when performers are encouraged to develop their own solutions to problems.* Therapists, for example, may set up an environment in which clients need to propel a wheelchair on a level surface to reach a goal position. Therapists can demonstrate several patterns that the client is physically able to produce (two-arm drive, two-leg drive, or one-arm, one-leg drive), and the client is encouraged to select the appropriate strategy for a given situation. If goal success requires passing through a narrow doorway, a two-leg pattern may be optimal. If the environment consists of a wide hallway, a two-arm drive may be optimal. Note that, unlike training, learning encourages performers to select their own solutions to different environmental challenges. **Although cognitive impairments, as seen in clients with severe head injury, may mandate that therapeutic interventions focus on training, most therapeutic intervention in persons with neurologic impairment probably should focus on skill learning.**

The Performance-Learning Distinction

Performance or the ability to execute a task is influenced differentially by temporary and relatively permanent effects of several variables. For example, performance may improve transiently because of factors such as increased motivation. In contrast, sustained improvements in performance may be attributed to such factors as increased practice. *Motor learning* **refers to a process, due to practice or experience, which leads to a relatively** *permanent* **change in the capability to achieve a goal.**[3] The critical point with respect to motor learning is that the ability to perform the skill is retained over time. Because motor learning is a process, it cannot be measured directly, but must be inferred from observing relatively permanent changes in behavior or performance. **The distinction between temporary changes in performance and the relatively permanent changes in performance associated with learning is termed the** *performance-learning distinction.*

In studies of learning, groups of subjects practice under different experimental conditions, with a practice session termed *acquisition.* Practice conditions during acquisition have both temporary and relatively permanent influences on performance.[3-6] Temporary influences may include motivating or energizing effects of frequent feedback, or fatigue or boredom associated with long practice sessions. To measure the more permanent effects of variables, temporary influences must be allowed to dissipate, and re-emergence of differential temporary effects between groups must be minimized. A common experimental method for allowing temporary influences to dissipate is to provide a rest interval after acquisition, before measuring performance at a later session. **Testing after a prescribed rest interval allows one to examine the more permanent effects of the practice conditions or the amount of learning that has occurred.** Several studies have used a 5- to 10-minute rest interval, but because the duration of temporary effects is unknown, in more recent studies scientists have provided rest intervals spanning from 5 minutes to 4 months.[7]

To prevent the re-emergence of differential temporary effects between groups, after the rest interval all groups are usually evaluated under identical conditions in a retention or transfer session. In a retention session, performance is measured using the same task performed during the acquisition phase. **A retention session or test demonstrates the permanent or retained change in performance on a task practiced during acquisition.** However, in a transfer session, the task is different from that practiced by any group during acquisition. **The transfer tests demonstrate the amount of learning generalizability.**

In summation, practice during acquisition may produce both temporary and relatively permanent changes in performance. Retention or transfer sessions provide a measure of the more permanent effects of practice variables and represent the critical measures of motor learning. In addition, transfer sessions also provide a measure of the generalization of practice conditions to novel experiences.

Variables That Influence Motor Learning

A considerable research effort from various fields of study, including kinesiology, physiology, psychology, and engineering, has focused on understanding the variables and principles underlying skill learning. This section describes the potent variables that may be controlled by therapists (for a more comprehensive review, see Schmidt[3]) and will be followed by a discussion of the clinical applications.

Amount of Practice

The amount of practice and amount learned are often directly related. However, at least two variables interact with this relationship: feedback and intention to learn. For learning to occur, performers must receive information feedback about the relationship between their performances and the task goals, and they must be motivated or have an intention to learn.

Amount of practice has been studied most often with positioning tasks, in which blindfolded performers practice moving a handle along a linear slide to a predetermined goal position. Information about the goal position is often provided by having performers practice moving to a physical block that is placed at the goal. During presentation trials, performers are instructed to move to a physical block that is removed for the test trials.

Several studies have shown that performance on test trials is directly related to the number of preceding presentation trials, suggesting that repeatedly guiding performance to a goal position enhances learning.[8-10] However, the rest interval prior to the retention session (test trials) was less than 5 minutes' duration in each of these studies. Consequently, the temporary practice effects may not have dissipated, and it is difficult to accurately identify the more permanent change or amount learned. Although more research is necessary to confirm the relationship between amount of practice and learning, the literature supports the concept of a learning benefit directly related to amount of practice.

The continuation of practice after reaching a criterion level of performance is termed *overlearning* or *overpractice.* A question that has long been of interest to the army and is pertinent to therapists and companies that provide financial compensation for therapeutic intervention, is whether there are learning benefits when practice is continued *after* a task goal has been achieved. **Although it may be expensive to continue practice after reaching a criterion level of performance, evidence suggests that overpractice may help prevent forgetting and enhance the retention of skills.** This may prove to be especially valuable following a long delay without practice.

To study the benefits of overpractice, Melnick[11] instructed subjects to maintain their balance while standing in the center of an unstable platform surface that rotated freely in one plane (this platform is termed a *stabilometer,* which is similar to a shortened teeter-totter and is a commonly used apparatus in motor learning research). The goal criterion was to maintain standing balance for at least 28 seconds. There were four practice conditions: criterion (C), criterion plus 50% (C-50%), criterion plus 100% (C-100%), and criterion plus 200% (C-200%). During the acquisition phase, subjects in each condition practiced until they reached the criterion goal of 28 seconds. Subjects in the criterion condition received no further practice; subjects in the C-50%, C-100%, and C-200% conditions received 50%, 100%, and 200% additional trials of practice, respectively. Retention sessions were administered 1 week and 1 month after acquisition, when subjects practiced until the goal criterion was achieved. Average balance time on trial 1 and number of trials necessary to reach the criterion goal during the retention sessions were used as measures of amount learned.

The 1-week and 1-month retention sessions showed similar results. The mean balance time on trial 1 was reliably longer for the C-50%, C-100%, and C-200% groups than that for the criterion group. The average number of trials required to reach the criterion goal was reliably less for the C-200% group than for the criterion group. Although the C-50% and C-100% groups required fewer trials than the criterion group to reach the criterion goal on retention, these group differences were not significant. **These results suggest that compared to conditions in which performers practice only until they achieve a criterion goal, conditions that include overpractice enhance learning.** These beneficial learning effects seem to be especially potent when, after some time interval without practice, the first attempt at a response is critical. First responses seem especially important in avoiding falls or accidents. To balance the cost and benefits of overpractice, Magill [12] suggests that performers practice 100% beyond criterion.

The most common explanation for the positive effects of amount of practice on learning is that increased practice retards the forgetting of memory traces. Practice results not only in enhanced performance, but also in the formation of memory traces that are stored somewhere in the central nervous system. Although these memory traces have been given various names (e.g., motor program, schema, rule, coordinative structure, neural engram, and neural network), a common theme is that practice leads to the storage of some aspect of the action.

Trace decay **refers to a passive fading of a trace from memory; with little practice, or over time, the trace becomes weaker and weaker. Increasing the amount of practice results in a stronger trace, consequently the rate of decay or memory fade is retarded.** This results in the increased retention of learned motor skills. Unlike trace decay, interference is an active phenomenon in which other activities interfere with memory traces. There is little evidence that interference occurs in motor tasks, except when the controls of a task are reversed such that they produce an opposite action from that produced during original learning.

Information Feedback

Information feedback is often considered to be one of the most important variables influencing skill learning. In fact, amount of practice is the only variable considered to have a stronger effect on motor learning.[13-16] *Information feedback* **refers to information that is presented either before, during, or after an action, which informs performers about an action's correctness or effectiveness.** Information feedback is **intrinsic,** when it is produced by sensory feedback and is inherent in a task. An example of intrinsic feedback is the proprioceptive information received during ambulation on uneven surfaces. **Extrinsic feedback** is information provided by an external source and is not readily available in a task. An example of extrinsic feedback is information regarding task performance provided by a therapist.

Knowledge of results **(KR), a type of extrinsic information feedback that has been studied extensively, is defined as postaction information about the relation between an action and a predetermined environmental goal.** This extrinsic feedback may be provided in such forms as verbal information, graphic displays, and videotape replay and is frequently provided in clinical situations. For example, a client may be told that he or she is falling to the side when the goal is to stand unsupported. *Knowledge of performance* **(KP) is defined as extrinsic feedback providing information about the pattern of a movement that leads to a task goal.** An example of KP is when performers are told that they lack full knee extension in the terminal swing phase of gait.

Researchers have generally assumed that the various types of extrinsic feedback alter skill learning in a similar fashion. Therefore, although most feedback research has focused on KR, results are often generalized to situations in which other forms of extrinsic feedback are used.[3] In attempting to understand the principles of extrinsic feedback, investigators have altered numerous variables, including the scheduling, frequency, amount, temporal location, and the precision of KR.

Frequency of Feedback

In several experiments, the effects of frequency of KR have been studied.[17-22] Winstein and Schmidt[21] compared 100% and 50% practice conditions. In the 100% condition, KR was presented after each acquisition trial, whereas in the 50% condition, KR was withheld on half of the trials. Each group practiced a movement task for 2 days of acquisition, followed by no-KR retention sessions that were administered 10 minutes and 24 hours after the end of acquisition.

The task included both position and time accuracy demands. It consisted of moving a horizontal forearm lever through three reversals to produce a predetermined goal pattern that was displayed on a computer screen. The goal pattern was to extend the elbow to position 1, reverse directions and flex the elbow to position 2, make a second reversal and extend the elbow to position 3, then make a third reversal and return toward the start position. The movement was to be completed in 800 msec. A visual barrier was placed above the forearm lever, inhibiting subjects from viewing their movements. Prior to each action, the goal pattern was displayed on the computer screen. Feedback consisted of a graphic display of the performed pattern overlaid on the goal pattern, plus a numeric score of root–mean-squared error between the two patterns.

Figure 11–1 illustrates the mean root–mean-squared error for the 50% and 100% groups during acquisition and retention. Acquisition performance was similar for both groups. However, there were significant group differences during the retention phase. Errors in the 50% group were slightly smaller than that in the 100% group on the 10-minute retention session and significantly smaller on the 24-hour retention session. **These results suggest that when amount of practice is controlled relative to practice with KR on every trial, withholding extrinsic feedback (reducing feedback frequency) on some practice trials enhances learning.**

Scheduling of Feedback

Several schedules can be used to reduce the frequency of KR during acquisition. Winstein and Schmidt,[21] and Ho and Shea,[17] used a faded schedule of KR in their 50% conditions, in which feedback was presented frequently early in each acquisition session and less often as the acquisition session continued. Because both frequency and scheduling of KR were manipulated, these experimental designs confounded the effects of KR frequency and

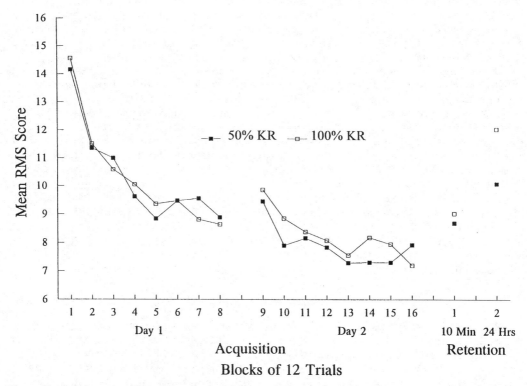

Figure 11–1. Mean root–mean-squared error for the 50% and 100% groups for two acquisition sessions and for the 10-minute and 24-hour no-KR retention sessions. (From Winstein, CJ and Schmidt, RA: Reduced frequency of knowledge of results enhances motor-skill learning. J Exp Psychol [Learn Mem Cogn] 16:677, 1990. Copyright © 1990 by the American Psychological Association. Adapted by permission.)

scheduling. To study the effects of KR scheduling, independent of KR frequency, Nicholson and Schmidt[19] contrasted three 50% practice conditions: constant, faded, and reverse- faded. The constant condition consisted of alternating feedback and no feedback on consecutive trials. In the faded condition, feedback was presented frequently early in acquisition and less often as acquisition continued. In the reverse-faded condition, feedback was presented seldom early in acquisition and frequently late in acquisition. Subjects participated in 2 days of acquisition followed by no-KR retention sessions, 10 minutes and 24 hours after the end of acquisition. The task was identical with that used by Winstein and Schmidt.[21]

Figure 11–2 illustrates the mean performance (mean root–mean-squared error) for the three groups during acquisition and retention. There were no reliable group differences during acquisition or during the 10-minute retention session. However, compared with practice with KR on every other trial, gradually increasing the frequency of KR across practice degraded performance during the 24-hour retention session and gradually decreasing the frequency of KR across practice enhanced it. **These findings suggest that gradually reducing the frequency of extrinsic feedback (faded schedule) across practice is more effective for skill learning than presenting feedback at a constant frequency throughout practice (constant schedule) or gradually increasing the frequency of KR across practice (reverse-faded schedule).**

Using other paradigms and tasks, several other scientists have demonstrated similar findings. For example, in *bandwidth-KR* conditions, quantitative feedback is withheld when errors are within a bandwidth of accuracy surrounding a target and presented when

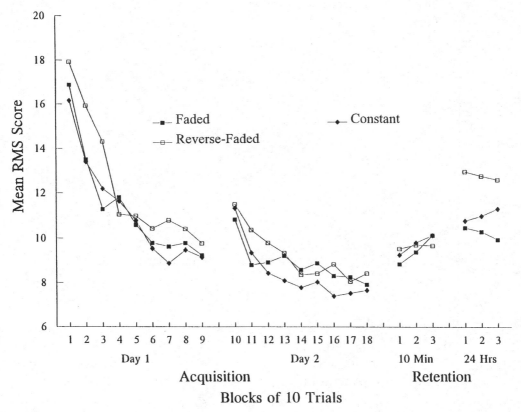

Figure 11–2. Mean root–mean-squared error for the constant, faded, and reverse-faded groups for two acquisition sessions and for the 10-minute and 24-hour no-KR retention sessions. (Adapted from Nicholson, DE and Schmidt, RA: Scheduling information feedback to enhance training effectiveness. Proceedings of the Human Factors Society 35th Annual Meeting 1991, p 1400.)

errors lie outside the bandwidth. Early in practice, because errors are usually large, performance is frequently outside the bandwidth, which results in frequent KR. Late in practice, because errors are relatively small, KR is often withheld. **Similar to practice with faded schedules of KR, practice with bandwidth KR is more effective for learning than practice with KR on every trial.**[23,24]

Timing of Feedback

When feedback is presented after an action, feedback can be presented instantaneously or delayed by some time interval. Swinnen and associates[7] examined the effects of feedback timing by having subjects practice a laboratory simulation of a *coincident-timing task* (similar to a back-handed tennis swing), in which a series of sequentially illuminated lights simulated a moving ball and a horizontal lever simulated a bat or racquet. After the first light in the sequence was illuminated, performers were to make a back swing past the light display and then reverse their movement such that the lever and light passed through a goal position simultaneously. Feedback, consisting of a numeric score directly related to the velocity and accuracy of a "hit" was presented on a computer screen after each practice trial.

Subjects practiced in either an instantaneous-KR or a delayed-KR condition. In the instantaneous-KR and delayed-KR conditions, feedback was presented 290 msec and 3.2 sec, respectively, after the lever passed through the goal position. Two days of acquisition were followed by no-KR retention sessions at 10 minutes, 24 hours, and 4 months after the end of acquisition. Average scores for the two groups during acquisition and retention are shown in Figure 11–3. Practice with KR withheld for as little as 3.2 sec after an action

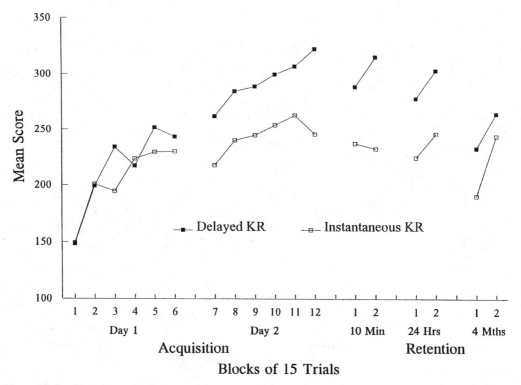

Figure 11–3. Mean scores for the instantaneous-KR and delayed-KR groups for two acquisition sessions and for the 10-minute, 24-hour, and 4-month no-KR retention sessions. (From Swinnen, S, et al: Information feedback for skill learning: Instantaneous knowledge of results degrades skill learning. J Exp Psychol [Learn Mem Cogn] 16:706, 1990. Copyright © 1990 by the American Psychological Association. Adapted by permission.)

was more effective for long-term retention than practice with KR presented instantaneously after an action. This result persisted even after 4 months without practice and suggests that delaying the presentation of feedback for a few seconds after practice action is more effective for learning than providing feedback immediately after each practice action.

The presentation of KR is also delayed in another KR manipulation termed *summary KR*. **In summary-KR conditions, KR is withheld until a predetermined set of trials are completed; then feedback about each trial in the set is presented simultaneously.** This manipulation results in practicing consecutive trials without an intervening KR presentation. **Similar to practice with KR delayed for a few seconds after completing an action, practice with summary KR is more effective in promoting learning than practice with feedback presented immediately after every action.**[25–28]

The Guidance Hypothesis

As illustrated in the preceding paragraphs, several lines of research suggest that practice with frequent, immediate, extrinsic feedback is less effective for learning than practice with feedback withheld or delayed on some trials, especially when feedback is withheld or delayed late in practice. **One hypothesis that provides a mechanism to account for these effects of KR frequency, scheduling, and timing is the guidance hypothesis.**[29] This hypothesis states that extrinsic feedback (KR) has both positive and negative effects on learning.

Positive effects of KR include (1) the provision of error information that "guides" performance toward the task goal, (2) the provision of motivating and energizing effects, and (3) the contribution of KR to the development of an association role in which performers learn a relationship between sensory feedback and movement outcomes.

Negative effects of KR are generally observed when KR is presented too frequently. These negative effects may be due to a "dependency" effect of KR, in which KR becomes a part of the "task," such that performers are unable to perform the task when the feedback conditions are changed or altered. Alternatively, frequent KR might interfere with processes that would normally occur when KR is withheld. For example, KR may discourage (or possibly prevent) performers from attending to intrinsic sensory feedback and developing a relationship between sensory feedback and movement outcomes. Consequently, when feedback is withheld on retention sessions, performers have a poor estimate of the relationship between sensory feedback and correct and incorrect actions. Essentially, they are unable to recognize their errors and performance is depressed.

Another possibility is that frequent feedback may discourage performers from practicing retrievals from long-term memory. Frequent feedback provides a solution for performing the next action; thus, performers do not need to plan their own solutions using experience or programs stored in long-term memory. Later when feedback is withheld, performers are required to generate their own solutions and because they have not practiced this process, performance is degraded.

Finally, frequent KR may encourage performers to alter their actions in response to even minimal errors, resulting in excessive performance variability.[30] In fact, recent findings suggest that KR forces performers to alter their actions, even when they are instructed to produce stable actions by repeating their previous action. One explanation for this phenomenon is that KR consists of at least two components: selection error (due to selection of an erroneous memory trace to produce a movement) and random variability or noise (due to unstable neuromuscular processes). The size of selection errors decreases across practice, but the size of neuromuscular variability remains roughly constant across thousands of practice trials. Consequently, frequent KR late in practice may encourage performers to alter their actions based primarily on neuromuscular noise, a process that is random and basically uncorrectable. These feedback-induced performance alterations, based on random processes, could account for the decreased effectiveness of frequent KR, especially when it occurs late in practice.

Guidance Versus Discovery Learning

Guidance refers to several methods of guiding performance toward a task goal, and the amount and type of guidance used during practice appear to influence the learning process. Guidance can consist of verbally or physically guiding performers to the goal, or it can consist of intermittent pushes or pulls to prevent errors. **Usually, guidance is considered to be the opposite of "discovery" learning, during which performers are given a problem and encouraged to discover their own solutions.**

In 1983, Hagman[31] examined the effects of guidance versus discovery learning. All subjects were instructed to move a lever to a goal position for each of 18 trials, which were either presentation or test trials. There were three practice conditions. A standard condition consisted of alternating presentation and test trials on consecutive trials, in which trial 1 was a presentation trial. A discovery condition consisted of one presentation trial followed by five test trials. The third condition was a guidance condition consisting of five presentation trials followed by one test trial. For the latter two conditions, the sequence was repeated three times. (Note that during acquisition the audience, standard, and discovery groups received 3, 9, and 15 test trials, respectively.) Three minutes and 24 hours after the end of acquisition, all subjects participated in retention sessions consisting of one test trial.

Figure 11–4 illustrates the mean absolute error on test trials for each group. During acquisition, the discovery group demonstrated reliably larger errors than either the standard or guidance groups. The discovery group also showed an increasing drift in performance away from the target as the number of consecutive test trials increased. However, note that a single presentation trial brought performance back toward the goal.

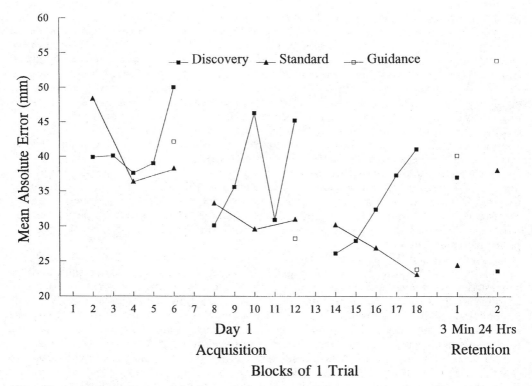

Figure 11–4. Mean absolute errors for the standard, guidance, and discovery groups for acquisition and for the 3-minute and 24-hour retention sessions. (From Hagman, JD: Presentation- and test-trial effects on acquisition and retention of distance and location. J Exp Psychol [Learn Mem Cogn] 9:334,1983. Copyright © 1983 by the American Psychological Association. Reprinted by permission.)

During the 3-minute retention session, the standard group demonstrated reliably smaller errors than the discovery or guidance groups, which performed equivalently. However, on the 24-hour retention session, compared with the standard group, the audience group demonstrated reliably large errors, and the discovery group demonstrated reliably small errors.

These results demonstrate several key principles concerning acquisition and retention during motor learning. First, the performance effects of variables can be remarkably different during acquisition and retention, probably because of the temporary and permanent effects of the practice conditions. Second, **practice conditions in which performers are allowed to make errors before being periodically guided back to the target are more effective for learning than conditions that prevent errors.** Third, **practice conditions that allow (or possibly force) performers to "discover" their own solutions to a problem are more effective for long-term retention than practice conditions in which performers are guided to a solution.**

Winstein and Pohl,[32] noting similarities between the effects of guidance and KR, argued that these variables influence underlying mechanisms and processes in a similar manner. To evaluate the relative effects of these variables, they designed an experiment that manipulated both the frequency of KR and guidance trials. Performers practiced a rapid arm movement to a goal position with high or moderate frequencies of guidance (presentation trials) or high or moderate frequencies of KR; then all performers participated in a delayed no-KR retention session consisting of test trials. The high-frequency guidance group demonstrated the smallest errors during acquisition, but larger errors than the other three groups during retention. **These data suggest that frequent on-target performance, achieved by physical guidance, is detrimental to learning.**

One explanation for the performance/learning effects of frequent guidance is that it acts like KR to the extent that it has both positive and negative effects on learning. Guidance is positive in that it is motivating and energizing, and it guides performance to the target. However, frequent guidance can act like a "crutch" whereby it interferes with processes that normally occur when guidance is withheld. Therefore, frequent guidance may discourage (or actually prevent) performers from engaging in the sensory encoding and retrieval processes that are necessary for learning. Based on this view, to optimize learning, frequent guidance during practice should be avoided.

Higgins[2] argued that guidance is closely associated with training, in which performers are given a solution. In contrast, skill learning focuses on the development of problem-solving capabilities. This interpretation suggests that to promote long-term retention, practice conditions should not involve frequent guidance and should promote situations in which performers are encouraged to process information and plan solutions. However, there are times when guidance may be appropriate. **Guidance may reduce fear and increase safety and is appropriate early in practice and periodically throughout practice to guide performance toward the goal.**

Part-Task and Whole-Task Practice

Nearly every therapist faces the decision of whether to teach a task in its entirety or to teach it by segments. **The issue of practicing an entire task as a "unit" or practicing components of a task separately, termed the *part-task versus whole-task dilemma*, has been the subject of several scientific studies.** One of the questions that arises when practicing partial tasks is whether the skill will be carried over when the whole task is attempted. For example, a common technique to encourage symmetry in weight-bearing during gait is to practice weight shift toward the weaker side in a stance posture. However, to determine whether this technique is effective, the relative amount of transfer or carryover from practicing stance weight shift and from practicing the "whole" task of gait should be compared. The most common conclusion is that beneficial transfer of part-task practice to the whole task is task-dependent.

Naylor and Briggs[33] suggested that amount of transfer depends on the coordination and information processing demands of a task. Coordination refers to the timing between each of the task's segments. **When segments of a task are linked to provide a coordinated continuous movement such as walking or swimming it is referred to as a *continuous task*. When practicing these continuous tasks in which the coordination, or "timing" that links segments is an integral part of the task to be learned, whole-task practice is more effective for learning than part-task practice.**

Serial tasks **often contain distinct information processing components that are not necessarily linked.** Serial tasks include mazes (such as the route from therapy to one's room), floor-to-stand transfers, and assembly line tasks. **These serial tasks benefit more from part-task than whole-task practice.** This is especially true when the whole task contains both difficult and relatively simple segments, which allow performers to concentrate on practicing the difficult segments without needing to repeat the relatively simple ones.

A prevalent "rule" for predicting the effects of part-task and whole-task practice is that movements governed by a single motor program should be practiced as a whole.[3] Continuous tasks, and short-duration (<200 msec) discrete tasks are often thought to be governed by a single motor program. In contrast, serial tasks, and longer-duration movements, are often governed by more than one motor program or by sensory feedback and may benefit from practice as discrete units.

When engaging in part-task practice the part must be an actual unit of the whole task. Several parts that appear to be units of a larger task may in fact not actually benefit learning of the larger task. At least one study demonstrated that practicing symmetric weight shift in stance did not influence gait characteristics.[34] One explanation for this finding is that symmetrical weight shift is not a unit part of gait.

Accuracy Versus Speed

A primary principle of motor control, termed the *speed-accuracy trade-off,* is that increasing the speed of an action will interfere with the spatial accuracy of the action. Because therapy clients often show deficits in both movement accuracy and speed, a therapist's task is to plan treatment programs that optimize both speed and spatial accuracy. At least one therapeutic approach suggests that accuracy should be acquired prior to attempts to increase speed.[41] However, **results from several lines of research suggest that if both speed and accuracy are important aspects of a task, both should be emphasized early in practice.**

Sage and Hornak[35] examined the learning effects of using one constant speed throughout practice versus gradually building up speed across practice. A group that practiced the criterion goal throughout practice demonstrated enhanced retention performance compared with a group in which the speed gradually increased across practice. These results suggest that gradually increasing speed across practice is less effective for learning than practicing the criterion speed throughout practice.

However, tasks practiced in therapy often have several—not one—criterion speed. For example, gait speed is different when crossing a crowded city street than when walking across a therapy gym. A pertinent question for therapists is what practice conditions optimize transfer to multiple criterion speeds.

This issue has been studied in what is termed the *variability-in-practice paradigm.* This paradigm usually consists of both constant and variable practice conditions, in which the number of practice trials is equated across groups. In *constant* conditions each subject practices only one speed, whereas in the *variable* condition each subject practices a task at several speeds. **Although constant and variable practice usually results in equivalent performance on retention sessions, variable practice usually results in more effective performance during transfer sessions when performers are practicing novel speeds.** These effects have been found in both laboratory and real-world tasks, including badminton and forearm tennis serves. Results from several studies, using different tasks and populations, suggest that compared with practicing a task at a single speed, practicing a task at several speeds enhances skill learning or the generalization of a task. (See Shapiro and Schmidt[36] for an excellent review of variability of practice.)

In summation, research findings suggest that the effects of emphasizing speed or accuracy early in practice are task-dependent. When speed and accuracy are both critical aspects of tasks, both speed and accuracy should be emphasized early in practice. When the task has solely one criterion speed, practice should focus on that goal speed, and when tasks have multiple criterion speeds, performers should practice numerous speeds in the same range as the criterion speeds.

Blocked Versus Random Practice Schedule

During a typical therapy session, several tasks are practiced. Often practice on one task is completed before beginning practice on a second task. An alternative way of scheduling the practice session is to intermingle the practice of various tasks, in which performers practice different tasks on consecutive trials. **Completing practice of one task before beginning practice on a second task is often termed** *blocked practice*, **whereas practicing a different task on consecutive trials is termed** *random practice*.

Random and blocked practice conditions have been studied in *contextual interference paradigms*. Usually, performers practice three tasks in either a random or blocked practice condition; then learning is measured by performance on either random or blocked no-KR retention sessions.

Figure 11–5 illustrates findings from a classic contextual interference experiment by Shea and Morgan.[37] The tasks in this experiment consisted of performing three movement

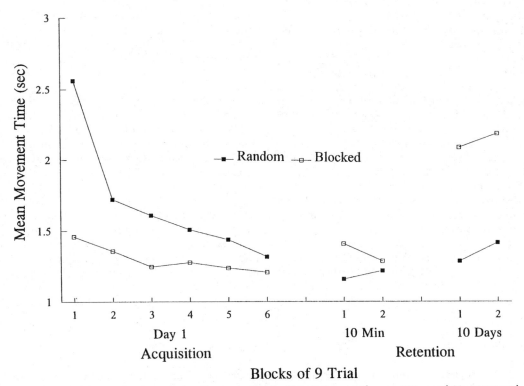

Figure 11–5. Mean total movement time for the random and blocked groups for acquisition and 10-minute and 10-day retention sessions. (From Shea, JB and Morgan, RL: Contextual interference effects on the acquisition, retention, and transfer of a motor skill. J Exp Psychol [Hum Learn] 5:179, 1979. Copyright © 1979 by the American Psychological Association. Reprinted by permission.)

sequences as rapidly as possible. During acquisition, the blocked group required less time to complete the tasks than the random group, suggesting that blocked practice enhances immediate performance. On the blocked retention sessions, there were no reliable group differences; however on the random retention session, the random practice group required less time to complete the tasks than the blocked group. **These results suggest that relative to practicing the same task over and over, intermingling different tasks throughout practice is beneficial for learning.**

Two explanations for contextual interference effects have been advocated. The first states that during random practice, performers forget the solution for the upcoming action and are thereby required to generate, or retrieve, a solution for each practice trial. These practiced retrievals are thought to be beneficial for learning.[38] The second explanation states that practicing different tasks on consecutive trials allows for more elaborate and distinctive encoding of tasks; consequently, the stored memory trace is stronger and clearer, and a strong memory trace is effective for learning.[37,39] (For an excellent review of contextual interference effects see Magill and Hall.[40])

Environmental Influences

Skill refers to the capability to consistently achieve a goal, in numerous environments, using multiple strategies, and with minimal energy expenditure. With the hypothesis that "normal" movement patterns are energy-efficient, therapy interventions (including the approaches of Bobath,[41] Johnstone,[42] and Voss and associates[43]) have focused on recovery of normal movement patterns for clients with neurologic impairment. These therapeutic approaches have largely neglected the influences of environment and multiple strategies on the consistency of achieving a goal. Consequently, although a client may demonstrate the ability to achieve a goal in a stereotypical fashion in a prescribed environment (e.g., the physical therapy department), often his or her ability to adapt to a new environment (e.g., their home) or situation is limited. If the goal of therapy is to achieve a level of skill in movement and function, therapists must consider the interactive effects of energy efficiency, multiple strategies, and multiple environments.

For example, people do not use one "ideal" energy-efficient gait pattern to ambulate. Visualize the environmental influences associated with walking on a slippery or icy surface. The knee is flexed in initial contact, enabling the entire foot to make contact with the ground, and step length and gait velocity decrease. These alterations probably result from a trade-off between energy efficiency and the likelihood of reaching the goal without falling. Now visualize the gait differences when walking on a country path where the scent of fresh fruit blossoms fill the air versus walking across an intersection in New York City at 5 P.M. on a Friday afternoon. These different environments require vastly different ambulation skills and movement strategies. **The capability of achieving a goal (ambulation) using multiple strategies (or multiple joints, limbs, or kinematic patterns) is termed** *motor equivalence.* To optimize physical function and skill, clients should be practicing motor equivalence to achieve goals in multiple environments. An excellent clinical example that illustrates this point is the customary restriction of ambulation training to hospital therapy departments or hallways. Many clients may require ambulation practice with exposure to uneven surfaces, curbs, traffic, carpets, and so on, to acquire the skills and strategies necessary to function in a realistic environment.

Prepractice Variables

The previous sections in this chapter have focused on potent motor learning variables that therapists can control *during* practice. However, several motor learning variables operate before practice, that is, before the practice session even begins. These prepractice variables include motivation, modeling or demonstrations, goal setting, audience effects, and educating performers to understand the goals of tasks. Extensive research has focused on the effects of these variables (for a review of the performance-learning effects of prepractice variables, see Schmidt[3] or Magill[12]).

Clinical Applications

Motor learning principles, and results from experiments of motor learning, provide a theoretical basis for therapeutic intervention. However, experiments on motor learning have almost always used persons without apparent dysfunction performing single-joint or single-limb movements. In contrast, therapeutic intervention focuses on persons with physical impairment, often performing multiple-joint or multiple-limb actions. Therefore, generalizing findings from these experiments to clinical situations must be approached with caution. Experiments focusing on multiple-joint and multiple-limb actions in persons with physical impairment are needed to confirm the effectiveness of these variables in therapeutic settings. With this limitation in mind, the subsequent sections will discuss clinical applications of the major principles of motor learning.

1. Temporary and permanent effects of practice variables can have remarkably different effects on performance. Therapists frequently document clients' performance during therapy, when both temporary and permanent effects of variables are confounded. To measure learning, performance should be evaluated after temporary effects have dissipated, possibly at the beginning of the subsequent therapy session. Learning can also be measured by evaluating the generalization of tasks. Examples include altering movement speed or excursion, or evaluating performance in alternative environments (such as in the client's home or community, on a crowded street or in a darkened room, or in the presence of the client's loved ones acting as an audience). In summation, therapists need to determine whether a client's performance primarily reflects the temporary or more permanent effects of therapeutic intervention.

2. Practice conditions that encourage (or possibly force) performers to process information, or, engage in sensory encoding and memory retrieval processes, are more effective for learning than practice conditions that frequently provide solutions. A therapist is likely to be more effective if he or she provides environments that encourage information processing. Information processing should be enhanced by providing occasional, not frequent, guidance or KR or by intermingling tasks throughout the therapy session rather than completing one task before beginning practice on a second task. Certainly drills, in which performers repeat the same movement over and over to memorize a "normal" movement pattern, should be avoided. Learning is process-specific; performers are more likely to learn the processes they practice than the movement patterns they practice.

3. The task-dependent effects of part-task practice also illustrate the benefit of practicing processes. Part-task practice is thought to be more effective than whole-task practice only when movements governed by a single motor program are practiced as one part or unit of the action. Practicing part of a task that is a segment of a single motor program has not been shown to be effective for learning, compared with practicing the whole task. For example, in sit-to-stand transfers, there is a break in the velocity profiles after a person scoots to the edge of a chair and before the anterior and vertical shift of the trunk, suggesting that these two parts of the task will benefit from part-task practice. However, there is no break in the velocity profile of the anterior and vertical shift of the trunk, suggesting that these parts of the task should be practiced as one unit of the task. Therapists should analyze each movement task to determine whether it is a continuous task, requiring whole-task practice, or a serial and segmented task, which may benefit from part-task practice.

4. The amount learned is usually directly related to amount of practice; therefore, clients should be encouraged to increase their practice time. This can be implemented by giving clients exercises to perform outside the therapy session or by using group sessions to practice skills. These extended practice sessions might be especially beneficial in promoting overpractice or the generalization of skills to new situations.

5. Videotape replay is an effective method of providing extrinsic feedback about movement trajectories to clients. Verbal cues identifying critical aspects of movements should probably be provided in conjunction with the videotape replay. Similar to KR, the provision of this form of KP should be provided frequently early in practice and less often as practice continues.

6. Many functional tasks practiced in therapeutic environments use multiple criterion speeds. During therapy, clients should practice these skills at multiple speeds. When accuracy and speed are both critical components of a task, both speed and accuracy should be emphasized early in practice. Documentation of a client's performance should include performance at multiple speeds with multiple strategies and should include multiple environments.

7. Several findings suggest that practice conditions with extrinsic feedback withheld on some trials, or delayed for only a few seconds after an action, are more effective for learning than practice conditions with frequent feedback or those with feedback presented instantaneously after an action. These findings have not been incorporated into the design of equipment that is often found in therapeutic settings. Manufacturers frequently market equipment as providing immediate and frequent feedback to performers. Therapists need to be wary that this frequent, immediate feedback may enhance performance during therapy but may be ineffective for long-term retention.

8. To develop true skill and acquire the ability to function in multiple environments and adapt to different conditions, a client must develop multiple movement strategies. This ability can be enhanced if the same skill is practiced under varying environmental or contextual conditions. For example, a client learning bed-to-chair transfers should practice transfers to various chair or bed heights from different directions and from chairs with and without arm rests and to both firm and soft surfaces. This will allow the client to develop multiple strategies and generalize or adapt this skill to perform in "real world" situations.

In conclusion, motor learning principles provide a theoretical basis for therapeutic intervention. Several motor learning variables are under the control of therapists and are easily incorporated into therapeutic settings. Based on studies using persons without apparent physical dysfunction, practice conditions that encourage information processing, multiple variations of a task, and multiple environments are more effective for skill learning than practice conditions that focus on repetition of a normal movement pattern. A present challenge for therapists is to test the generalization of motor learning principles to actions performed by persons with physical dysfunction.

RECOMMENDED READINGS

Gentile, AM: A Working Model of Skill Acquisition with Application to Teaching. Quest 17:3, 1972.

Lister, M, (ed): Contemporary Management of Motor Control Problems: Proceedings from the II Step Conference. Foundation for Physical Therapy, Alexandria VA, 1991.

Magill, RA: Motor Learning: Concepts and Applications, ed 3. Dubuque IA; WC Brown, 1989.

Montgomery, PC and Connolly, BH (eds): Motor Control and Physical Therapy; Theoretical Framework

and Practical Applications. Hixson, TN, Chattanooga Group, 1991.

Schmidt, RA: Motor Control and Motor Learning: A Behavioral Emphasis, ed 2. Champaign, IL, Human Kinetics, 1988.

Winstein, CJ and Knecht HG (eds): Movement Science Series, Part 1. Phys Ther 70:759, 1990.

Winstein, CJ and Knecht HG, (eds): Movement Science Series, Part 2. Phys Ther 71:25, 1991.

REFERENCES

1. LeVere, ND, Gray-Silva, S, and LeVere, TE: Infant Brain Injury: The Benefit of Relocation and the Cost of Crowding. In LeVere TE, Almli, RB, and Stein, DG (eds): Brain Injury and Recovery: Theoretical and Controversial Issues. New York, Plenum Press, 1988.

2. Higgins, S: Motor Skill Acquisition. Phys Ther 71:123, 1991.

3. Schmidt, RA: Motor Control and Learning: A Behavioral Emphasis, ed 2. Human Kinetics, Champaign, IL, 1988.

4. Guthrie, ER: The Psychology of Learning. Harper & Row, New York, 1952.

5. Hull, CL: Principles of Behavior. Appleton-Century-Crofts, New York, 1943.

6. Tolman, EC: Purposive Behavior of Animals and Men. Century, New York, 1932.

7. Swinnen, S, et al: Information Feedback for Skill Learning: Instantaneous Knowledge of Results Degrades Skill Learning. J Exp Psychol [Learn Mem Cogn] 16:706, 1990.

8. Adams, JA and Dijkstra, S: Short-Term Memory for Motorresponses. J Exp Psychol 71:314, 1966.

9. Gentile, AM and Nemetz, K: Repetition Effects: A Methodological Issue in Motor Short-Term Memory. Mot Behav 10:37, 1978.

10. Wrisberg, CA and Schmidt, RA: A Note on Motor Learning without Post-Response Knowledge of Results. Mot Behav 7:221, 1975.

11. Melnick, MJ: Effects of Overlearning on the Retention of a Gross Motor Skill. Res Q 42:60, 1971.

12. Magill, RA: Motor Learning: Concepts and Applications, ed 3. WC Brown, Dubuque, IA, 1989.

13. Bartlett, FC: The Measurement of Human Skill. Occup Psychol 22:83, 1948.

14. Bilodeau, IM: Information Feedback. In Bilodeau, EA (ed): Acquisition of Skill. Academic Press, New York, 1969.

15. Newell, KM: Knowledge of Results and Motor Learning. Exerc Sport Sci Rev 1976.

16. Salmoni, AW, Schmidt, RA, and Walter, CB: Knowledge of Results and Motor Learning: A Review and Critical Reappraisal. Psychol Bull 95:355, 1984.

17. Ho, L and Shea, JB: Effects of Relative Frequency of Knowledge of Results on Retention of a Motor Skill. Percept Mot Skills 46:859, 1978.

18. McGuigan, FJ: The Effect of Precision, Delay, and Schedule of Knowledge of Results on Performance. J Exp Psychol 58:79, 1959.

19. Nicholson, DE and Schmidt, RA: Scheduling Information Feedback to Enhance Training Effectiveness. Proceedings of the Human Factors Society 35th Annual Meeting, 1991, p 1400.

20. Suddon, FH and Lavery, JJ: The Effect of Amount of Training on Retention of a Simple Motor Skill with 0- and 5-Trial Delays of Knowledge of Results. Can J Psychol 16:312, 1962.

21. Winstein, CJ and Schmidt, RA: Reduced Frequency of Knowledge of Results Enhances Motor-Skill Learning. J Exp Psychol [Learn Mem Cogn] 16:677, 1990.

22. Wulf, G and Schmidt, RA: The Learning of Generalized Motor Programs: Reducing the Relative Frequency of Knowledge of Results Enhances Memory. J Exp Psychol [Learn Mem Cogn] 15:748, 1989.

23. Lee, TD, White, MA, and Carnahan, H: On the Role of Knowledge of Results in Motor Learning: Exploring the Guidance Hypothesis. J Mot Behav 22:191, 1990.

24. Sherwood, DE: Effect of Bandwidth Knowledge of Results on Movement Consistency. Percept Mot Skills 66:535, 1988.

25. Lavery, JJ: Retention of Simple Motor Skills as a Function of Type of Knowledge of Results. Can J Psychol 16:300, 1962.

26. Lavery, JJ and Suddon, FH: Retention of Simple Motor Skills as a Function of the Number of Trials by Which KR Is Delayed. Percept Mot Skills 15:231, 1962.

27. Schmidt, RA, Lange, CA, and Young, DE: Optimizing Summary Knowledge of Results for Skill Learning. Hum Move Sci 9:325, 1990.

28. Schmidt, RA, et al: Summary Knowledge of Results for Skill Acquisition: Support for the Guidance Hypothesis. J Exp Psychol [Learn Mem Cogn] 15:352, 1989.

29. Schmidt, RA: Frequent Augmented Feedback Can Degrade Learning: Evidence and Interpretations. In Stelmach, GE and Requin, J (eds): Tutorials in Motor Neuroscience. Klüwer Academic Publishers, Dordrecht, Germany, 1991.

30. Nicholson, DE: Information Feedback Disrupts Performance Stability. Unpublished Doctoral Dissertation. University of California, Los Angeles, 1992.

31. Hagman, JD: Presentation- and Test-Trial Effects on Acquisition and Retention of Distance and Location. J Exp Psychol [Learn Mem Cogn] 9:334, 1983.

32. Winstein, CJ and Pohl, PS: Frequent On-Target Experience during Practice Degrades the Learning of Target Location More Than Frequent Knowledge of Results (KR). Sport Exerc Psychol 15:S92, 1993.

33. Naylor, J and Briggs, G: Effects of Task Complexity and Task Organization on the Relative Efficiency of Part and Whole Training Methods. J Exp Psychol 65:217, 1963.

34. Winstein, CJ, et al: Standing Balance Training: Effect on Balance and Locomotion in Hemiparetic Adults. Arch Phys Med Rehabil 70:755, 1989.

35. Sage, GH and Hornak, JE: Progressive Speed Practice in Learning a Continuous Motor Skill. Research Q 49:190, 1978.

36. Shapiro, DC and Schmidt, RA: The Schema Theory: Recent Evidence and Developmental Implications. In Kelso, JAS and Clark, JE (eds): The Development of Movement Control and Coordination. John Wiley & Sons, New York, 1982.

37. Shea, JB and Morgan, RL: Contextual Interference Effects on the Acquisition, Retention, and Transfer of a Motor Skill. J Exp Psychol [Hum Learn] 5:179, 1979.

38. Lee, TD and Magill, RA: The Locus of Contextual Interference in Motor-Skill Acquisition. J Exp Psychol [Learn Mem Cogn] 9:730, 1983.

39. Shea, JB and Zimny, ST: Context Effects in Memory and Learning of Movement Information. In Magill, RA (ed): Memory and Control of Action. North-Holland, Amsterdam, 1983.

40. Magill, RA and Hall, KG: A Review of the Contextual Interference Effect in Motor Skill Acquisition. Hum Move Sci 9:241, 1990.

41. Bobath, B: Adult Hemiplegia: Evaluation and Treatment, ed 3. Heinemann Medical Books, Oxford, 1990.

42. Johnstone, M: Restoration of Motor Function in the Stroke Patient: A Physiotherapist's Approach, ed 3. Churchill Livingstone, New York, 1987.

43. Voss, DE, Ionta, MK, and Myers, BJ: Proprioceptive Neuromuscular Facilitation: Patterns and Techniques, ed 3. Harper & Row, Philadelphia, 1985.

SECTION

III

CLINICAL MANIFESTATIONS OF MOTOR DYSFUNCTION

Overview

Motor control requires the integrated activity of a vast assortment of both segmental and suprasegmental motor neurons. The latter include neurons in the cerebral cortices, the basal ganglia, the thalamic nuclei, the cerebellum, and various nuclei of the brainstem. In addition, many aspects of motor activity require continual sensory feedback to each level of the neural axis. With such a large portion of the nervous system involved in the control of movement, it is not surprising that motor symptoms may be caused by virtually any disorder that damages central or peripheral nervous tissue.

There are, however, a group of disorders that *primarily* affect the function of the motor system. In general, each one of these creates a characteristic constellation of signs and symptoms associated with disordered motor control. The purpose of this section is to introduce the student to the most prominent and important of these clinical presentations.

A familiarity with these clinical features is useful to the health care student for a variety of reasons. First, the clinical definition of the majority of these diseases, whether neurologic or myologic, is largely based on the pattern of these presentations. Their diagnosis rests heavily on patient history, patient complaints, and physical examination. Second, an understanding of these clinical features provides insight into the pathophysiology underlying the disorders. Finally, in considering these signs and symptoms, the student will be introduced to much of the clinical terminology associated with motor dysfunction.

More detailed discussion of the clinical manifestations associated with disordered motor control and their pathologic origins will be presented in the following chapters on the major disease entities. It will become apparent that although lesions in the various functional elements of the motor system frequently give rise to characteristic patterns of signs and symptoms, countless variations in presentation are possible and will inevitably appear in the clinic.

CHAPTER 12

■

Clinical Presentations in Disorders of Motor Function

Christopher M. Fredericks, PhD
and
Lisa K. Saladin, BMR (PT), MSc

- ■ Disorders of the Motor Unit (Neuromuscular Disease)
- ■ Disorders of Central Motor Control

*D*isturbances of motor function are among the most common symptoms causing people to seek medical help. Since such a large portion of the nervous system is involved in the control of movement, motor defects can be caused by virtually any disease that damages the central or peripheral nervous system. The focus of this chapter, however, is on those disorders that primarily affect motor function and the signs and symptoms that they create. Although the signs and symptoms described in this chapter are limited to those emanating primarily from disordered motor function, it should be remembered that in many motor disorders other organ systems are also involved, giving rise to entirely different findings (e.g., skin rash of dermatomyositis, cataracts and baldness of myotonic dystrophy, and visual disturbances of multiple sclerosis).

Although the terms "signs" and "symptoms" are often used synonymously to refer to any functional evidence of disease or of a patient's condition, they differ somewhat in their connotations. The term **sign** implies an objective finding as might be revealed to a clinician by physical examination. **Symptom**, on the other hand, suggests functional components of a disease that are perceived by the patient and are expressed in the patient history and complaint. In this regard, "presenting" symptoms are those symptoms of greatest concern to the patient and from which he or she specifically seeks relief. "Cardinal" signs or symptoms are the findings of greatest significance to the clinician in identifying an illness and in understanding a patient's reasons for seeking medical attention.

For purposes of discussion, motor disorders are divided into those that primarily involve the peripheral motor system (motor unit and associated sensory connections) and those that primarily affect central pathways and control mechanisms. Some overlap between these large categories is inevitable. For example, the anterior horn cell is clearly located within the central nervous system anatomically, but as part of the motor unit, it shall be considered with the peripheral disorders. By the same token, disease processes do not necessarily make a distinction between central and peripheral processes and may well

257

disturb both. The following discussion focuses on the clinical presentations of these disorders and their functional consequences.

Disorders of the Motor Unit
(Neuromuscular Diseases)

Disorders of the peripheral motor system, which are often termed *neuromuscular diseases,* are those that revolve around defects in the motor unit itself. The locus of impaired function may be the anterior horn cell (or analogous cranial nerve nucleus), spinal root, peripheral nerve, neuromuscular junction, or skeletal muscle itself. Although these disturbances are most often distributed among spinal motor units, they may afflict bulbar pathways as well. Even though neuromuscular disorders are numerous, the clinical signs and symptoms to which they give rise are relatively few, with muscle pain and weakness being the most common.[1-5] The clinical manifestations described in the following sections vary tremendously in the extent to which they are perceived as uncomfortable or disabling— hence in the extent to which they appear as presenting complaints. They all contribute to an assessment of the patient's condition.

Muscle Pain and Tenderness (Myalgia)

Skeletal muscle pain or tenderness often accompanies neuromuscular disease and is a common presenting symptom or chief complaint.[1-4,6-9] In assessing this symptom, it is useful to distinguish between tenderness of the muscle itself, either at rest or with moderate exertion, and painful muscle hyperactivity such as cramps or spasms. It is often difficult for the patient to make this distinction. Moreover, in many instances both conditions are present. Muscle pain at rest is usually a dull ache, which may be accompanied by more severe discomfort on palpation. This occurs notably in inflammatory myopathies, but may also occur in neurogenic disorders such as the Guillain-Barré syndrome. Muscle pain on moderate exertion occurs mainly in certain metabolic myopathies (e.g., McArdle's disease) and in hypothyroidism.[1-4] Muscle hyperactivity states such as cramps and spasms can be extremely painful, ranging from benign muscle cramps associated with overexertion to the disabling (even life-threatening) seizures of tetanus or strychnine poisoning.[6,8,9] Prolonged muscle tenderness may follow these episodes.

Myalgia does not always imply muscle or neuromuscular disease and in seeking the origins of discomfort, one must rule out pain of psychologic origin and referred pain. Referred pain is defined as pain subjectively described in a location distant from the site of actual pathology.[2] For example, pain localized in the muscles of the lower extremity may be generated by pathology in the joints of the lumbar spine. By the same token, diseases of overlying subcutaneous tissue or fascia or of tendons, bones, and joints may also refer to muscle. The convergence of multiple sensory afferents at the same spinal segment and their ascent to the brain in the same spinal cord pathways are responsible for this phenomenon. The muscle is often tender to palpation in cases of referred pain, a misleading sign, since the cause of the pain is entirely outside of the muscle.

Muscle pain is an important symptom of neuromuscular disease, but it is also an everyday occurrence and may reflect nothing more than the aftermath of unaccustomed or overly vigorous physical activity. The significance of muscle pain is determined by the presence of associated signs and symptoms.

Muscle Weakness (Paresis and Paralysis)[1-4,10-13]

Muscle weakness, which may be defined as an inability to generate normal levels of tension or force, is a common manifestation of neuromuscular disease. Weakness ranges

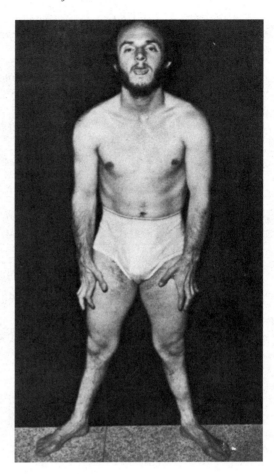

Figure 12–1. *Muscle Weakness and Atrophy.* Distal muscle wasting is apparent in all extremities in this case of inherited neuropathy. (From Vinken, PJ, and Bruyn, GW: Handbook of Clinical Neurology, vol 40. North-Holland Publishing Company, Amsterdam, 1979, p 320, with permission.)

from subtle deficiency, which can be revealed only by careful muscle testing, to a complete deficit. Although the terms **paralysis (plegia)** and **paresis** are often used interchangeably, they more accurately **distinguish between total or severe loss of voluntary contraction, and mild or partial loss, respectively.** Muscle weakness arising from peripheral neuromuscular dysfunction is most often accompanied by normal or diminished muscle tone, as distinct from the weakness of many central disorders, which is usually accompanied by spasticity or other forms of hypertonia.

It is important for diagnostic purposes and the identification of specific syndromes to carefully assess muscle weakness, not only in terms of some measure of its **severity,** but also its **onset, tempo,** and **distribution.** The onset of weakness can be defined by the age at which it occurs and whether its appearance is abrupt or slow and insidious. The tempo of a disease is the rate at which signs and symptoms progress with respect to time. In other words, does weakness progress rapidly or slowly? It is also important to note whether this progression is continual and relentless, or episodic with a course marked by periods of remission or exacerbation. The **distribution** of weakness also represents important diagnostic information. Muscle weakness may be defined as being proximal or distal, symmetric or asymmetric, and ascending or descending (Fig. 12–1). Many neuromuscular disorders present consistent and characteristic patterns of involvement, particularly in their early stages. Specific types of muscular dystrophy, for example, are largely defined by specific patterns of weakness. Common patterns of weakness are summarized in Table 12–1. Although these patterns are frequent, neuromuscular disease can affect almost any group of muscles, and a pattern of

Table 12–1. Patterns of Muscle Weakness

Type of Weakness	Definition	Common Cause
Hemiplegia (or paresis)	Paralysis (or weakness) of muscles of the arm, leg, and sometimes face on one side of the body	Internal capsule, cerebral hemisphere, spinal cord hemisection; rarely a high cervical spinal cord lesion
Monoplegia (or paresis)	Paralysis (or weakness) of all the muscles of one limb—arm or leg	Spinal cord lesion; lesion in a cerebral hemisphere; peripheral neuropathy
Paraplegia (or paresis)	Paralysis of muscles in both legs	Spinal cord lesion; peripheral neuropathy
Triplegia (or paresis)	Hemiplegia or paresis combined with paralysis (or weakness) of one limb on the opposite side of the body	High cervical spinal cord lesion or multiple lesions
Tetraplegia (or paresis), quadriplegia	Paralysis (or weakness) of all four extremities	Lesion in high cervical spinal cord, brainstem, or cerebral hemispheres; acute polyneuropathy or radioculopathy; myopathy

weakness that fits none of these descriptions may result. Although peripheral motor disease (e.g., a peripheral neuropathy) may produce weakness restricted to a single limb or even an isolated muscle group, other syndromes (e.g., familial periodic paralysis or adrenal insufficiency) are characterized by more generalized muscle weakness.

Although muscle weakness is a common symptom of neuromuscular disease, it is not as often a chief complaint. The significance of weakness to a patient and the extent of disability depend as much on the extent to which specific muscles are impaired as on the patient's particular lifestyle.[2] Patients can be entirely unaware of rather profound weakness if they do not ordinarily use the affected muscles to full capacity. Difficulty in walking, for example, is a common initial complaint, since few are able to avoid walking. On the other hand, subtle loss of function associated with facial weakness would go unnoticed by most, except perhaps by a trumpet player or glass blower. Patients with muscle weakness may not often use the word "weakness" to describe their symptoms, but rather characterize their motor problems in terms of the inability to carry out certain tasks or functional activities.

Accurate assessment of muscle strength may be made more difficult by concurrent musculoskeletal pain, which may prompt voluntary or involuntary curtailment of effort by the patient. In addition, nonorganic weakness of psychologic origins (e.g., caused by depression or hysteria), or resulting from purposeful malingering is a considerable problem, which is often revealed by inconsistent or incompatible findings. Total weakness, for example, would not appear genuine if unaccompanied by wasting, contractures, or changes in reflex activity.

Changes in Muscle Mass

Both decreases (atrophy) and increases (hypertrophy) in skeletal muscle mass are noted in association with various neuromuscular diseases.

Atrophy (Amyotrophy, Muscle Wasting)[1,2,4,14]

Although skeletal muscle **atrophy is a common manifestation of many neuromuscular disorders,** it is unusual for a patient to seek medical attention because of atrophy alone. When atrophy is accompanied by significant weakness or functional deficit, patients become concerned.

It is interesting that there is no invariable, proportionate correlation between atrophy of a muscle and weakness.[1] Severe atrophy, with relatively little weakness is a common feature of many systemic wasting diseases (such as cancer, tuberculosis, malnutrition) and aging. Old age may be accompanied by marked, generalized muscle atrophy, but surprisingly little decline in muscle strength. Conversely, profound weakness with relatively little atrophy is seen in several myopathies, such as polymyositis, myasthenia gravis, and periodic paralysis. Marked atrophy accompanied by proportionately severe weakness is characteristic of denervating conditions, such as the spinal muscle atrophies (e.g., polio, amyotrophic lateral sclerosis). This loss of muscle mass may reflect disruption of the trophic influences that are exerted by motor neurons on skeletal muscle and that are necessary for the maintenance of normal muscle mass. Severe atrophy may also be combined with severe weakness in the chronic muscular dystrophies.

Although muscle atrophy is generalized in the systemic wasting diseases, it can be focal in certain motor disorders, giving rise to characteristic appearances (e.g., wasted upper arm of fascioscapulohumeral dystrophy; gaunt face of myotonic dystrophy; storklike legs of peroneal muscle atrophy) (Fig. 12–1).

Hypertrophy[1,2,4]

Unaffected muscles adjacent to atrophied muscles often appear hypertrophied because of their normal muscle mass. These muscles must not be confused with those that are actually hypertrophied beyond their normal size. **True compensatory hypertrophy may occur in the synergists of weakened muscles as their workload increases.** These may be the muscles that normally act in synergy with the affected muscles or muscles on which new reliance has developed within the context of the existing disability. For example, in the early stages of Duchenne's muscular dystrophy, hypertrophy is often noted in the distal lower extremities (e.g., calves) in compensation for developing proximal weakness. These muscles are relatively strong and actually contain a high proportion of hypertrophied fibers. Later in the disease, replacement by fat and connective tissue may maintain the bulk in the face of the real loss of muscle fibers. This is the stage of **pseudohypertrophy.** Enlargement of muscles is also commonly seen in the limb girdle and Becker type of muscular dystrophy. Work-induced hypertrophy is observed in some myotonic disorders and may culminate in excessive generalized muscularity (Fig. 12–2). This may be a result of the excessive muscular activity accompanying these disorders.

Muscle Hyperactivity States

Skeletal muscle hyperactivity states are a common feature of many acute and chronic neuromuscular disorders.[2,4–6,8,9,15–17] These conditions all imply involuntary muscle activity, but vary tremendously in both form and intensity. Muscle hyperactivity may vary from the insensible twitching of fibrillation to the violent, excruciating spasms of tetanus. Although all these conditions may not constitute common presenting symptoms, they provide valuable diagnostic information. Involuntary muscular contraction in neuromuscular (peripheral) disease is distinct from the muscle spasticity and rigidity, as well as the involuntary movement disorders, associated with diseases of the central nervous system.

For discussion purposes, these muscle hyperactivity states may be divided by etiology into those arising primarily from disturbances of neuronal function (neurogenic), and those arising from primary disturbances of the muscle cell itself (myogenic) (Table 12–2). Patients may manifest signs and symptoms arising from both.

Neurogenic Origins

TWITCHINGS (FASCICULATIONS AND MYOKYMIA). Common among skeletal muscle hyperactivity states are various types of muscle twitchings, including fasciculations and myokymia. **Fasciculations are rapid, fine, painless contractions of groups of muscle fibers,** representing contraction of either part or all of a single motor unit.[2,4,15,16] Although

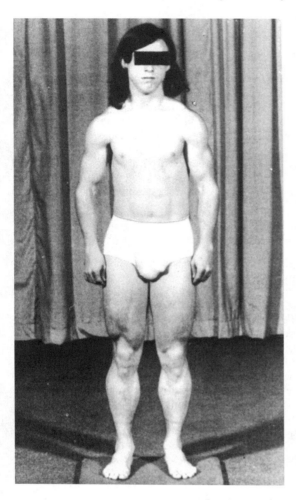

Figure 12-2. Muscle Hypertrophy. Generalized muscle hypertrophy has developed from excessive muscular activity in this case of myotonia congenita. (From Lovell, WW and Winter, RB (eds): Pediatric Orthopaedics, ed 3. JB Lippincott, Philadelphia, p 397.)

fasciculations vary in intensity, they are vigorous enough to be visible through the overlying skin and felt by the patient, but not strong enough to move the associated bones and joints. Fasciculations are most clearly viewed in superficial muscles, such as in the hands and tongue, and may often be precipitated by mechanical stimulation, such as percussion or pinching of the muscle. Fasciculations are thought to be due to the spontaneous activation of hyperirritable motor neurons and are most frequently seen in disorders of the anterior horn cells of the spinal cord (e.g., amyotrophic lateral sclerosis or progressive spinal muscular atrophy) and of the motor nuclei of the brainstem. Although spontaneous activity probably arises at irritable sites on the dying or degenerating nerve, the exact site is unknown. Fasciculations can be produced in healthy persons with the administration of anticholinesterases. Similarly, in patients with myasthenia gravis, frequent fasciculations can be an indication of overmedication with such agents. Most patients who present with fasciculations are healthy. These benign fasciculations are most often noticed in the calf, small hand muscles, and the eyelids in association with fatigue, cigarettes, and coffee.

Myokymia is a closely related form of spontaneous movement, which is somewhat slower, coarser, and more undulating than fasciculation.[2,4,15,16] Through the overlying skin, myokymia appears more like an undulating or rippling contraction of a small strip of muscle. Like fasciculations, myokymia is associated with motor neuron injury and may also occur in healthy persons after strenuous exercise or in association with fatigue. Myokymia is particularly common in facial muscles, especially the eyelid.

Table 12–2. *Muscle Hyperactivity States Associated with Peripheral Motor Disorders*

NEUROGENIC	
Fasciculation:	A brief muscle twitch, visible through the overlying skin, caused by the spontaneous activation of a group of muscle fibers innervated by the same motor neuron
Myokymia:	A coarse muscle twitch appearing as a wavelike or rippling contraction, visible through the overlying skin; slower and more persistent than fasciculation
Myoedema (mounding):	A localized contraction appearing as a rising lump or mound at the site of percussion of a muscle; usually seen in wasting, degenerating muscle
Spasm:	A sudden involuntary muscle contraction
Cramp:	A powerful spasmodic contraction of muscle, causing pain and muscle tautness, often persisting for minutes
Tetany:	A sustained spasmodic contraction of muscle associated with peripheral nerve hyperexcitability; most often occurring in distal extremities and facial and laryngeal muscles
MYOGENIC	
Fibrillation:	An extremely fine, rapid contraction of muscle resulting from the spontaneous activation of individual muscle fibers; not visible through the overlying skin
Myotonia:	A persistence of contraction after a voluntary activation of muscle, appearing as an involuntary delay of relaxation
Contracture:	An involuntary, often painful persistence of shortening, most often occurring after exertion in certain metabolic disturbances of muscle; muscle electrically silent on electromyography

POWERFUL MUSCLE CONTRACTIONS (CRAMPS AND TETANY). In contrast to the fine twitchings of muscle, such as fasciculations and myokymia, more powerful involuntary contractions of skeletal muscle may also occur in the context of neuromuscular disease. These contractions may actually be powerful enough to damage both muscle and the skeletal system. *Muscle spasm* **is a general term that denotes a forceful, involuntary contraction of a muscle or group of muscles** and implies interference with normal motor function and the production of involuntary movement. When such spasms are painful, they are often referred to as **cramps**; when they are violent and involve large groups of muscles, they are usually termed **convulsions**. Spasms can be clonic (alternating contraction and relaxation) or tonic (sustained contraction). The spasms associated with peripheral motor disorders are distinct in both form and pathogenesis from the muscle spasticity that often accompanies central nervous system dysfunction.

Cramps are powerful, involuntary contractions that are intense enough to be associated with pain, palpable tautness, and bulging of the affected muscle[3,6,8,9,15–17] (Fig. 12–3). Cramps often represent a level of contractile effort greater than even the most vigorous voluntary contraction. The muscle hardening of a cramp may wax and wane for several minutes or pass from one location to another within the same muscle. Although these contractions may occur spontaneously in a relaxed muscle, more often they are triggered by a brief voluntary contraction of the muscle involved. These powerful contractions are thought to be due to somatic neuron hyperirritability, probably originating in the distal portions of motor nerves, possibly the intramuscular (unmyelinated) portion of the nerve terminus.[8,9] Cramps are most effectively relieved by stretch, possibly reflecting the inhibitory effects of Golgi's tendon organ stimulation on the motor neuron. Pathologic cramps are most often associated with lower motor neuron disease, especially anterior horn cell disorders in which fasciculations are also common (e.g., amyotrophic lateral sclerosis). They also occur in spinal root disorders and peripheral neuropathies. Pathologic cramps are not typically associated with upper motor neuron lesions, extrapyramidal disorders, or

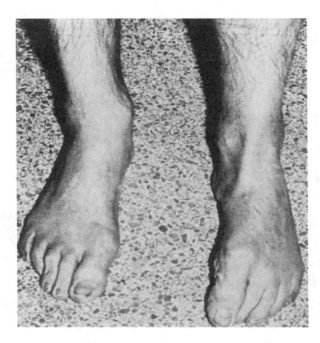

Figure 12–3. *Cramps.* This patient with an idiopathic cramp syndrome had sudden onset of a cramp in the left foot. Note the prominence of tendons over the dorsum of the ankle and plantar flexion of the big toe. (From Vinken, PJ and Bruyn, GW: Handbook of Clinical Neurology, vol 40. North-Holland Publishing Company, Amsterdam, 1979, p 327, with permission.)

myopathies. Benign cramps are also associated with a variety of nonprogressive disorders and conditions and are experienced by almost everyone at some point in their life. Ordinary cramps often occur at night (especially in the elderly), waking the person with painful contractions of the calf, causing plantar flexion of the ankles or toes.[2] A mild cramp subsides after a few seconds, but a severe cramp (charley horse) may last several minutes, leaving the muscle sore and tender for days. Benign skeletal muscle cramping is associated with such conditions as overexertion, sodium depletion (sweating), diuretics, water intoxication (miner's cramp), pregnancy, hemodialysis, psychogenic disorders, and numerous medications.

Tetany is a term used to specifically refer to the involuntary muscle spasms that frequently occur in a number of conditions characterized by hyperexcitability of peripheral nerve.[2,4,5,15–17] Tetany usually arises in the distal extremities (e.g., carpopedal spasm) and in the facial and laryngeal muscles. In severe cases, spasms may spread to more proximal muscles. In all forms of tetany, the peripheral nerves are abnormally excitable, as manifested by their sensitivity to percussion (Chvostek's sign) and ischemia (Trousseau's sign). Tetany most frequently develops with hypocalcemia, hypomagnesemia, and alkalosis (Fig. 12–4).

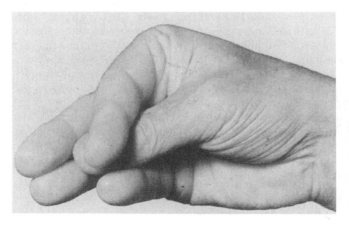

Figure 12–4. *Hypocalcemia Tetany.* Hypocalcemia may give rise to many signs and symptoms including carpopedal spasm, the Trousseau's sign. (From Colour Atlas of Endocrinology, ed 2, by R Hall and DC Evered, Mosby-Wolfe, an Imprint of Times Mirror International Publishers, Ltd, London, UK, 1990.

Myogenic Origins

FIBRILLATION.   **Fibrillations are small, asynchronous contractions occurring in single skeletal muscle fibers.** Although these contractions are too fine to be seen through the intact, overlying skin or to be felt by the patient, they can be revealed by recording their action potentials. This activity reflects involuntary activation of single or even parts of single muscle fibers in response to spontaneous action potentials arising from some hyperirritable segment of the sarcolemma itself—most likely in some area distinct from the motor end plate. Fibrillations are seen in increased numbers following denervation and in persons with certain myopathies.

MYOTONIA.   **Myotonia is a delayed capacity for relaxation in skeletal muscle.**[1,2,4,15] This is manifested as a persistence of shortening that lasts for a few seconds after voluntary contraction or after excitation by mechanical or electrical stimulation. This difficulty is probably due to some abnormality in the muscle membrane, which results in alterations in the membrane potential and heightened irritability. During the period of delayed relaxation, repetitive muscle action potentials can be recorded. Myotonic contractions are usually painless but may disable a patient by interfering with fine hand movements or by slowing ambulation. A patient with myotonia may find it difficult to release his or her grip after shaking hands or forcefully grasping an object. Myotonia is usually made worse with cold, so that the symptom in the hands can be precipitated by chilling the hands in cold water. Myotonia of the tongue can be elicited by percussing the edge of the tongue with an applicator stick. An indentation will remain after this stick is removed. Percussion of larger muscles, such as the deltoid, may cause contraction of a strip of muscle (Fig. 12–5). Eyelid myotonia can be demonstrated by having the patient rapidly look down. The eyelids will stay up exposing the sclera. Similarly, if the patient squeezes the eyelids tightly closed, he or she may need several seconds to open them. Myotonia of the hands and tongue is characteristic of myotonic dystrophy, whereas more diffuse myotonia can be demonstrated in myotonia congenita.

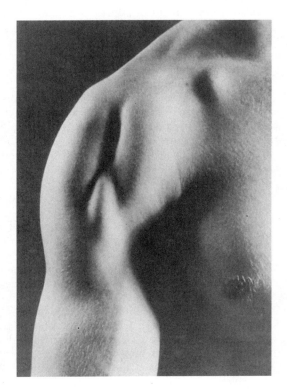

Figure 12–5. Percussion Myotonia. A persistent, involuntary contraction may often be elicited by percussion of myotonic muscle (in this case deltoid muscle). (From Engel, AG and Franzini-Armstrong, C: Myology. Basic and Clinical, ed 2. McGraw-Hill, New York, 1994, p 760, with permission.)

CONTRACTURE.[2,4,6,9,15] The term **contracture** is usually used to refer to a tightness or restricted range of motion across a joint. Contractures arise most frequently as a consequence of a lack of mobilization of a joint and may reflect deleterious changes in the joint itself, as well as in the associated muscles and adjacent soft tissues (see Chapter 23).

Contracture also **refers to a type of skeletal muscle hyperactivity characterized by involuntary, often painful shortenings of muscle, which occur in the absence of sarcolemma depolarization and excitation.**[2,4,6,9,15] In other words, they are observed in electrically quiet muscles. Contractures are not typically spontaneous, but are triggered by exercise, with their severity, and the resultant discomfort varying with the intensity of the exercise. Especially severe, long-lasting contractures can be provoked with ischemic exercise, such as that of the forearm muscles. Contractures occur most often in myopathies involving metabolic defects of glycogen or glucose metabolism, which limit the production of high-energy phosphates (i.e., glycogen storage diseases). When working muscle is depleted of adenosine triphosphate (ATP), actin and myosin remain bound together in "rigor" causing a persistence of contraction. In addition, low ATP may impair the ability of the sarcoplasmic reticulum to sequester Ca^{2+}, so that contractures may result from the increased concentrations of intracellular calcium activating further binding of actin and myosin. Physiologic contractures may occur in healthy persons following repetitive stimulation of muscle. This may likewise reflect an exhaustion of ATP and impaired muscle relaxation.

Muscle Fatigability (Myasthenia)[1,3,4,9]

Muscle fatigue **refers to the performance decline or decremental response that occurs with repetition of a muscular activity.**[1,3,4,9] Fatigability denotes the ease with which such a decline in performance develops. It can be distinguished from muscle weakness by the fact that the patient does not lack the ability to perform a task, but lacks the ability to perform it repetitively. Nonetheless, fatigability may be confused with muscle weakness or with voluntary curtailment of effort due to discomfort such as pain or stiffness. Climbing stairs, repeated extension or abduction of the arm against a resistance, repeated clenching of the fist, or the maintenance of a maximal upward gaze all are useful clinical maneuvers for evoking this sign. Abnormal fatigability occurs in many muscle-wasting conditions, both myopathic and neurogenic, possibly because weak or wasted muscles are compelled to work harder, nearer their metabolic limits, in performing normal motor activities. Excessive fatigability, however, is particularly evident in diseases of neuromuscular transmission and is a cardinal feature of myasthenia gravis. Patients with certain metabolic disorders of muscle also show an increased susceptibility to fatigue during ischemic exercise, but their daily activities are limited more by muscle pain and cramps than by fatigue. Myasthenia is also a major problem in many patients with serious renal, hepatic, cardiac, or pulmonary disease.

Abnormal Muscle Tone (Hypotonia)[2,4,18-20]

Normal muscle offers a certain amount of resistance to passive stretch; this is **muscle tone.** In disorders of both peripheral and central motor systems, abnormalities in this tone are common. Increased muscle tone or hypertonia is seldom a feature of peripheral disease. However, **a reduction in muscle tone (hypotonia)—with or without hyporeflexia—is frequently evident in patients presenting with weakness from neuromuscular disease.**[2,4,18-20] This is particularly true of those with lower motor neuron disorders and certain myopathies. Hypotonic muscles may feel soft and flabby and will produce less than normal resistance when passively stretched. The reduction in tone may be generalized or localized to specific muscles or limbs. Although changes in muscle tone can be detected by physical examination and contribute to functional difficulties, patients rarely complain specifically of decreased muscle tone. Mild degrees of hypotonia may be ignored by the

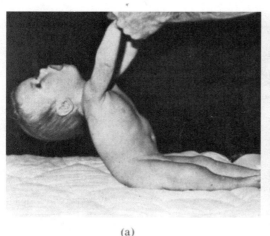
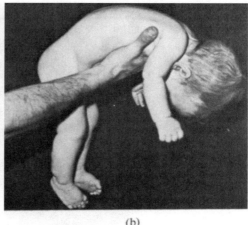

(a)   (b)

Figure 12–6. *Hypotonia.* In this infant with myotonic dystrophy, (*A*) the head lags with no attempt to flex the neck and (*B*) there is little attempt to straighten the back or flex the extremities. (From Vinken, PJ and Bruyn, GW: Handbook of Clinical Neurology, vol 40. North-Holland Publishing Company, Amsterdam, 1979, p 333, with permission.)

patient and have minimal functional consequences. Moderate-to-severe hypotonia manifests as an increased ease of passive movement, sometimes to the point of allowing excessive mobility at joints. Patients with severe hypotonia are at risk for developing joint subluxations, especially at the shoulder, and for developing postural deformities such as scoliosis because of the inability of the muscles to resist the effects of gravity.[2,18,20]

In infants and young children, hypotonia is one of the earliest and most important indications of neuromuscular disease. Hypotonia manifests in the newborn as limpness (floppy infant syndrome) (Fig. 12–6), or later as a delay in the development of postural control.[2,18] Early signs of hypotonia are poor head control and a lack of physiologic flexion at birth. This results in resting positions of extension, abduction, and external rotation, rather than the flexed, adducted, and internally rotated position seen in normal newborn infants. Later in childhood, the hypotonia may contribute to delays in the achievement of motor milestones, difficulty in controlling active movements, and abnormal resting postures. It is important to note that many central nervous system disorders also present with hypotonia, and a thorough evaluation is required to differentiate between these and neuromuscular disorders.

Abnormalities of Sensation[1,19,21–26]

Sensory abnormalities can occur with disease at any level of the nervous system, but **are a characteristic feature of peripheral neuropathy and are often an early presenting complaint** (Table 12–3).[1,19,21–24] In fact, in many neuropathies, motor symptoms are less evident than sensory symptoms, especially in the early stages of the disease. Sensory changes can be an important diagnostic tool in neuromuscular disease. If sensory abnormalities accompany paralysis, mixed motor and sensory nerves, or both, anterior and posterior roots are likely involved. If sensory changes are absent, the lesion must be situated in the gray matter of the spinal cord, in the anterior roots, in a purely motor branch of a peripheral nerve, or in motor axons alone.

In most neuropathies, there is a distal impairment of sensation, which is typically found in a "glove-and-stocking" distribution.[22–24] In some cases, paresthesias (e.g., tingling or "pins-and-needles" sensations) may be experienced. These sensations may become uncomfortable (dysesthesias), or even painful, especially when the feet or fingers make prolonged

Table 12–3. *Major Sensory Abnormalities*

Abnormality	Definition
Anesthesia	Loss of feeling or sensation, especially the loss of pain
Hypesthesia	Decreased sensitivity to sensory stimulation; also hypoesthesia
Paresthesia	Abnormal sensation such as burning, pricking, tickling, or tingling, especially occurring spontaneously
Dysesthesia	Unpleasant abnormal sensation produced by ordinary stimuli, including feelings such as itching, pins and needles, electric shock
Hyperesthesia	Exaggerated unpleasant sensitivity to touch or other non-noxious sensory stimuli
Hypalgia	Diminished sensitivity to painful stimuli; also hypoalgia
Hyperalgia	Excessive sensitivity to painful stimuli
Causalgia	Sensation of persistent, severe burning of the skin, often accompanied by hypersensitivity to touch and temperature and trophic skin changes
Hyperpathia	Exaggerated unpleasant response to painful stimuli, often persisting after removal of stimuli

contact with hard surfaces. Certain neuropathies present characteristic sensory abnormalities (e.g., the burning, painful feet associated with alcoholic neuropathy). The distribution of sensory disturbances corresponds to the distribution of the nerves affected. Sensory disturbances do not accompany disorders of the neuromuscular junction or muscle itself.

Peripheral sensory dysfunction may impair a patient's touch and position sense and may produce serious functional consequences. Although the effects of sensory disturbance on motor function are not entirely understood, impairments in coordination[25] and balance[26] frequently occur subsequent to pure sensory lesions. In certain peripheral neuropathies, in which only sensory fibers are affected, significant motor dysfunction may develop as a result of lost tactile and proprioceptive feedback. Gait and balance are particularly affected with disturbances in the feet and lower leg, whereas fine, manipulative tasks are markedly affected by impairment of sensory function in the hands. In addition, the inability to sense heat or other potentially damaging stimuli may make a patient vulnerable to injury.

Reduced or Absent Muscle Stretch Reflexes[19,23,27,28]

One of the most important elements of the neurologic examination is assessment of spinal cord and cranial nerve reflexes. Most of the clinically important reflexes involve skeletal muscle responses. These reflexes provide a convenient tool for assessing the functional integrity of both peripheral and central components of the somatic nervous system. Preeminent among these reflexes are the muscle stretch reflexes or so-called "tendon jerks."

A *tendon reflex* or *jerk* is a sharp muscular contraction evoked by sudden stretch of a muscle.[19,23,27,28] Tapping the tendon provides a convenient way of producing this stretch, but these reflexes may also be elicited by sudden displacement of the limb segment to which the muscle is attached. Although the reflex contraction is most evident in the specific muscle stretched, it is not necessarily confined to that particular muscle. Table 12–4 describes the principal tendon reflexes.

Each tendon reflex is dependent on the integrity of its neural arc (see Chapter 5). **Any lesion that interrupts this arc may diminish or abolish the reflex response.** Diminution of the response results when conduction is impeded through some component of the arc, whereas abolition of the response occurs when the arc is disrupted or conduction is otherwise totally blocked. Accordingly, neuromuscular disorders are typically associated with reduced or absent tendon reflexes. Muscular disease (myopathy), for example, may decrease or abolish a tendon reflex by rendering the muscle incapable of responding to the

Table 12–4. *Principle Muscle-Stretch (Tendon) Reflexes*

Reflex	Mode of Elicitation	Response	Nerve	Spinal Segment
Biceps reflex	Tapping the biceps tendon	Flexion of the elbow	Musculocutaneous	C-5–6
Brachioradialis reflex (radial periostial reflex; supinator jerk)	Tapping the brachioradialis tendon at the distal end of the radius	Flexion of the elbow	Radial	C-5–6
Triceps reflex	Tapping the triceps tendon	Extension of the elbow	Radial	C-6–8
Finger flexor reflex	Tapping the palmar surface of the semiflexed fingers	Flexion of the fingers and thumb	Median and ulnar	C-7–T-1
Quadriceps reflex (patellar reflex; knee jerk)	Tapping the quadriceps tendon	Extension of the knee	Femoral	L-2–4
Gastrocnemius-soleus reflex (Achilles reflex; ankle jerk)	Tapping the Achilles tendon	Plantar flexion of the ankle	Tibial	S-1–2

nerve impulse. The afferent component of the arc may be impaired by lesions of the sensory nerve or spinal root, whereas the efferent pathway may be similarly affected by lesions of the anterior horn cell or peripheral motor neuron. Both sensory and motor fibers may be impaired by peripheral neuropathy. Although reduced tendon reflexes are characteristic of neuromuscular disease, it should be remembered that disorders at higher levels of the nervous system, such as neural shock or deep coma, may also depress these reflexes.[27,28] Moreover, neurologic disorders with marked rigidity, spasticity, or muscle contracture, or joint disorders with ankylosis (stiffness) or contracture, may physically prevent these reflex movements from occurring.

Disorders of Central Motor Control

The characteristic presentations resulting from damage to the central nervous system are in many respects different from those of neuromuscular disease.[29–32] As previously discussed, the signs and symptoms of the peripheral disorders result from failure of some component of the motor unit; some kind of depression of motor activity (e.g., weakness, fatigability, hypotonia, or hyporeflexia) is common. In the case of the central disorders, the motor effector unit is usually intact, whereas control of this unit is impaired. As a result, the consequences of central lesions are often various forms of heightened (e.g., spasticity, rigidity, hyperreflexia) or disordered movement (e.g., unusual activation patterns, ataxia).

Abnormal Muscle Tone

Muscle tone refers to the resistance encountered when a muscle is passively lengthened or stretched. Both the intrinsic elastic properties of muscle and tendon and the active contraction of muscle (reflexive or voluntary) may contribute to this resistance. **The abnormal tone associated with central nervous system damage may occur in the form of hypertonia or hypotonia.**

Hypertonia

Central nervous system lesions frequently give rise to increased muscle tone.[19,33,34] These syndromes of muscle hyperactivity, which are manifested as spasticity, clonus, and rigidity, are distinct from the muscle hyperactivity states that accompany neuromuscular disease (e.g., cramps, myotonia, and contractures).

SPASTICITY. Disruption of upper motor neuron inhibitory pathways characteristically gives rise to spasticity. **Spasticity may be defined as a velocity dependent increase in muscle tone accompanied by hyperactive tendon reflexes.** Although spasticity takes a variety of clinical forms, it is typically manifested as increased resistance to passive movement.[35-37] When an involved muscle is stretched rapidly, the limb may move freely for a short distance followed by a rapid increase in muscle resistance opposing the movement. If the stretch is maintained, at some point the resistance may abruptly disappear (clasp-knife phenomenon). Spasticity may also have a tonic component. An increased resistance to passive movement throughout the range of movement has been documented in response to continuous slow elongation in patients presenting with spasticity. However, it is likely that this tonic resistance is due to compensatory changes in connective tissue rather than to neural hyperexcitability.

The form and intensity of spasticity may vary markedly, depending on the extent and site of the central nervous system damage. In general, the lower the level of the central nervous system injury, the more complete the lesion is apt to be and the more profound the spasticity. For example, stroke-induced spasticity is usually less severe than that caused by spinal cord injury. It is interesting that patients with incomplete spinal lesions may actually have greater spasticity than those with complete lesions, owing to the sparing of some descending facilitory fibers. Furthermore, the degree of hypertonia may temporarily fluctuate within each individual. **The degree of spasticity may, for example, transiently increase in response to changes in the position of the body,**[38] **psychologic excitation,**[39] **sensory stimulation, and voluntary effort involving the affected muscle groups.** This variability in the degree of spasticity impedes the reliable quantification of this clinical sign.[40]

In most neurologic patients, spasticity predominates in the antigravity muscles, particularly the flexors of the arms and the extensors of the legs (Table 12–5). Because of the resultant discrepancy in muscle tone in opposing muscle groups, the involved limbs tend to assume a typical resting posture and to retain this posture following passive displacement. An alternate pattern of spasticity that occurs occasionally in patients with multiple sclerosis, spinal cord injury, and traumatic brain injury consists of flexor spasticity of the lower extremities. This often results in a flexed resting posture and subsequent contractures. (Fig. 12–7).[41] The distribution may be either unilateral or bilateral, depending on the extent of neurologic injury.

The pathophysiology of spasticity is complex and is incompletely understood. It was once believed that spastic hypertonia was due primarily to hyperactivity of the gamma

Table 12–5. *Classic Distribution of Spasticity*

Upper Extremity	Lower Extremity
Shoulder	Hip
Adductors	Extensors
Internal rotators	Internal rotators
Elbow	Adductors
Flexors	Knee
Hand	Extensors
Wrist flexors and adductors	Ankle
Finger flexors	Plantarflexors
Forearm	Invertors
Pronators	

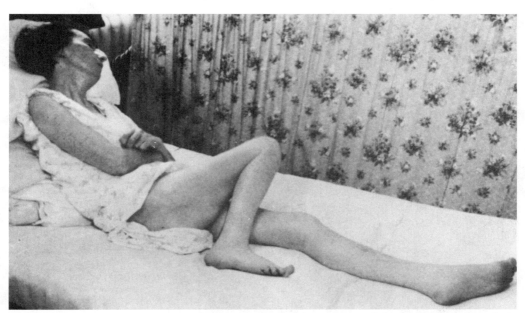

Figure 12–7.   Flexor Spasms. In this patient with multiple sclerosis, repeated flexor spasms of the right leg ultimately resulted in the limb remaining in the flexed position. (From Spillane, JD: An Atlas of Clinical Neurology. Oxford University Press, New York, 1968, p 346.)

efferent system (increased fusimotor activity), which caused an increased sensitivity of the muscle spindle to stretch. However, research has failed to support this hypothesis. Recent theoretical models of spasticity propose two possible underlying mechanisms[42]; the net result of either is increased motor neuron excitability. Hypertonia may be due to increased afferent input to the alpha motor neuron producing an enhanced stretch-evoked excitation, or there may be a lower threshold of excitability in the alpha motor neuron related to a loss of supraspinal and/or spinal interneuron inhibition. It is probable that multiple neural mechanisms interact to produce spasticity.

Many rehabilitation models for the patient with central nervous system dysfunction have been based on the assumption that loss of coordinated voluntary movement was primarily due to the presence of spasticity. It was postulated that spasticity induced antagonist restraint during voluntary activities. **However, the extent of the impact that spasticity has on volitional movement remains to be fully defined.** A correlation does exist between the presence of spasticity, as assessed by determining the passive resistance to stretch, and an impairment of voluntary motor control.[43] Furthermore, the presence of spasticity-induced antagonist restraint during voluntary activity has been observed in selected patients.[44–46] In these patients, it appears as if excessive co-contraction or the inability to inhibit the spastic antagonist may interfere with movement. However, the *absence* of spastic restraint during the execution of voluntary movements has also been documented in patients presenting with spasticity in both the lower[44,47] and the upper extremity.[48–50] In these patients, inadequate recruitment of the agonist, which resulted in the inability to generate adequate force, appeared to be responsible for the disordered voluntary motor control. In addition, **spastic hypertonia has not been shown to correlate significantly with impairment of specific functions such as gait**[51,52] **or upper extremity tasks.**[53,54] Recent models of neurologic rehabilitation propose that muscle weakness and abnormal patterns of muscle recruitment, rather than spasticity, may be the primary mechanisms responsible for the disordered voluntary motor control present in many central nervous system disorders.[55]

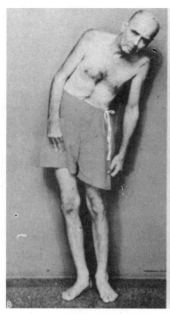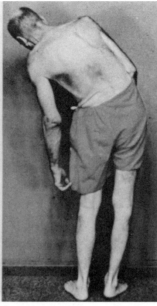

Figure 12–8. Muscle Rigidity. Rigidity in truncal muscles causes these postural flexion deformities characteristic of advanced parkinsonism. (From Cooper, IS: Involuntary Movement Disorders, Harper & Row, New York, 1969, p 4, with permission.)

RIGIDITY.   Pathologic conditions affecting the basal ganglia and other extrapyramidal systems typically cause a disturbance of muscle tone called muscle rigidity.[37,56,57] **Rigidity is a heightened resistance to passive movement of a limb that is independent of the velocity of stretch and relatively uniform throughout the range of motion of that limb.** This has been likened to the resistance noted in bending a lead pipe (hence the term, **lead pipe rigidity**). A special type of rigidity, which is common in parkinsonism, is called the **cogwheel phenomenon.** In this case, when the hypertonic muscle is stretched, a rhythmic, interrupted resistance is encountered. This might be manifested as a ratchetlike feeling when the wrist or arm is quickly flexed.

Although muscle rigidity superficially resembles spasticity to the extent that they both reflect increased muscle tone, they are different in form and pathophysiology. Rigidity tends to be most prominent in muscles that maintain a flexed posture (i.e., the flexor muscles of the trunk and limbs) (Fig. 12–8). However, it may be present in all muscle groups, including flexors and extensors. Spasticity usually involves the extensor muscles of the legs and the flexors of the arms. In contrast to spasticity, in muscle rigidity there is no initial period of low resistance to stretch nor sudden release of resistance later in the stretch, the tendon jerks are not hyperactive, and there is no clonus. When a rigid limb is released, it does not resume its original position as may happen in spasticity. In contrast to rigid states, spastic muscle at rest may be flaccid and electrically quiescent.

Rigidity typically affects muscles of the head and trunk as well as those in the extremities, manifesting as difficulty with speech, eating, and ambulation. Rigidity in the trunk musculature may result in numerous functional impairments, ranging from difficulty rolling over in bed to reduced pulmonary vital capacity. Similar to the complications experienced with spasticity, the continuous hyperactivity in rigid muscles and the associated reduction in mobility frequently produce adaptive muscle shortening with a subsequent loss of range of motion and function.

As with spasticity, the pathogenesis of rigidity is only superficially understood. Rigidity has less to do with hyperactivity of segmental reflexes. It is probably due primarily to the excessive supraspinal facilitation of alpha motor neurons themselves, resulting from disinhibition of cerebral structures that are normally inhibited by the basal ganglia.

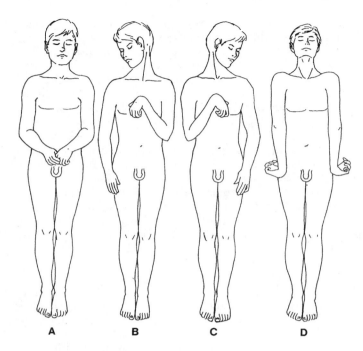

A   **B**   **C**   **D**

Figure 12–9. Decorticate (A to C) *and Decerebrate Rigidity* (D). (*A*) The decorticate patient is lying supine with the head unturned. (*B*) and (*C*) The tonic reflexes are elicited by turning the head to the right or left. (*D*) Decerebrate rigidity. (From Berne and Levy,[57] 1988, p 249, with permission.)

DECORTICATE AND DECEREBRATE RIGIDITY.[37,56,57] **Extensive midbrain or bilateral forebrain lesions commonly result in the onset of extreme forms of hypertonus referred to as** *decorticate* **and** *decerebrate rigidity,* **both characterized by marked hyperreflexia (Fig. 12–9).** Decorticate rigidity is a consequence of extensive damage to only cortical structures, and the rigidity that ensues is characterized by rigid extension of the lower extremities and flexion of the upper extremities. More caudal lesions that include either the diencephalon or midbrain may cause decerebrate rigidity, which manifests as extension of both the arms and legs with arching of the back and dorsiflexion of the head. Both decorticate and decerebrate rigidity are perhaps more akin to spasticity than to muscle rigidity because hyperreflexive deep tendon reflexes are present and because this form of hypertonus is not equally distributed between flexors and extensors. These syndromes are frequently observed immediately following traumatic brain injury and are indicative of extensive central nervous system damage. Evaluation reveals such a marked resistance to passive movement that only minimal passive movement may be possible.

In the patient with a central nervous system injury, either or both of these syndromes may occur spontaneously, or they may be evoked by various forms of stimulation. Posturing refers to strong involuntary movements that thrust the body into the decerebrate or decorticate positions in response to internal or external stimuli. **Stimuli such as changes in limb or body position, loud noises, and pain may induce posturing and increase the subsequent rigidity of the extremities.** One of the goals of management in the acute phase may be to reduce any stimulation that exacerbates the posturing or to use different positions to diminish this involuntary activity. For example, positioning the patient in a prone position may assist in reducing extensor hypertonus. An alternative approach would be to desensitize the patient to the stimuli through a process of accommodation.

Posturing and rigidity that persist are correlated with a poor prognosis for functional recovery. In patients whose neurologic recovery is evident, these manifestations gradually diminish over a period of days, weeks, or months. During this time, the rigidity may be replaced by spasticity.

FUNCTIONAL CONSEQUENCES OF HYPERTONIA.   **The most significant functional consequence of hypertonia is muscle contracture,** which in turn results in reduced joint range of
motion, altered biomechanics, musculoskeletal deformity, and functional disability (see
Chapter 23). Hypertonia is associated with a tonic state of muscle contraction and persistent
muscle shortening. Contractures develop as the muscles adapt to the shortened position and
modify joint alignment and muscle function. The most common site of contracture is at the
ankle plantar flexors in association with severe hypertonia in the gastrocnemius muscle. The
resultant reduction in passive ankle dorsiflexion influences standing alignment, balance
reactions, and ambulation. Other common sites of muscular contracture associated with
spasticity are the elbow flexors, shoulder internal rotators, and wrist and finger flexors.
Frequently, in the case of rigidity, the hypertonia is so severe that only minimal passive
movement is possible and functional activities such as sitting upright may be impossible.
The presence of contractures may seriously impede rehabilitation efforts and limit patient
self-sufficiency. Treatment is often focused on the prevention of secondary reductions in
joint range of motion associated with hypertonic muscle groups. Aggressive stretching,
casting, and mobility exercises are often required to minimize the potential for contracture
formation.

Hypotonia

Hypotonia **is a decrease in the normal resistance offered by muscle to passive
elongation and is usually associated with a reduction in the amplitude of deep tendon
reflexes (hyporeflexia).**[18-20] The affected extremity feels limp and heavy when moved
passively. Hypotonia and hyporeflexia typically occur immediately following disruption of
upper motor neuron pathways associated with cerebral shock. This period of hypotonia may
last from one day to several weeks, but is routinely followed by progressively increased
muscle tone or spasticity. **Persistent hypotonia is not particularly common in central motor
disorders** but may occur if the damage is limited to corticospinal pathways or if there is
damage to the cerebellum or its connections.

The presence of significant hypotonia is associated with joint instability, particularly
when dynamic muscle activity contributes to joint integrity. The glenohumeral joint is a
good example and is particularly susceptible to subluxation when severe hypotonia is
present. Normally, the upward orientation of the glenoid fossae is an important factor in
preventing downward dislocation of the humerus. Loss of tone in the scapular elevators
allows the glenoid fossae to slope downward, predisposing the humerus to subluxation. The
rotator cuff muscles, which play a pivotal role in maintaining the head of the humerus in the
fossae, become ineffectual when severe hypotonia is present and further contribute to
downward dislocation of the humerus. Consequently, management of a patient with
significant hypotonia should include protection of unstable joints to prevent further
musculoskeletal damage.

Hypotonia also appears to influence the control of voluntary movements. It is
associated with decreased postural control, difficulty initiating movements, weakness,
decreased endurance, and decreased coordination. **Movements of the extremities and trunk
that require sustained holding against gravity are most affected.** These deficits may
seriously impair a person's ability to ambulate independently.

Muscle Weakness[19,58-63]

In contrast to peripheral neuromuscular disorders in which weakness is due to
dysfunction of the motor unit, **weakness arising from central lesions reflects impaired
activation of the motor unit.** The selective postinjury loss of motor units and decreased
motor unit firing rates may also contribute to this type of weakness. Weakness emanating
from central nervous system dysfunction may be accompanied by the hypotonia typical of
lower motor neuron disorders or, as is more frequently the case, by heightened stretch

reflexes and spasticity. Significant atrophy is rare, since muscle innervation has been maintained. However, if the weakness persists, atrophy may occur because of disuse.

As observed in neuromuscular dysfunction, **weakness may range in severity from mild paresis to total paralysis, depending on the extent of the lesion** (see Table 12–1). Upper motor neuron lesions create characteristic patterns of weakness that are different from those often associated with peripheral motor deficits. Unilateral upper motor neuron lesions commonly produce hemiparesis with a predilection for upper extremity flexors and lower extremity extensors. This weakness is usually greater in the distal muscles because of the degree of bilateral cortical control over the proximal musculature. Lesions of the corticospinal pathways above the medulla typically result in contralateral weakness due to the decussation of the pathways at the junction of the medulla and the cervical cord. However, **some evidence exists that *ipsilateral* motor function may also be impaired following unilateral cerebral damage.** Jones and colleagues[63] investigated the performance of the ipsilateral limb on 12 computerized tests. Although no impairment was noted on clinical evaluation, **there were significant reductions in arm strength, reaction time, speed, steadiness, and tracking in the ipsilateral limb of stroke subjects compared with a group of controls.**

Quadriparesis often accompanies supraspinal bilateral lesions, whereas paraplegia or quadriplegia accompanies complete spinal lesions, according to the level of injury. Isolated weakness in one limb or in an individual muscle group, as might be observed in a peripheral neuropathy, or the selective patterns of weakness noted in the muscular dystrophies are rare.

Loss of Muscular Endurance

One element of motor function that is often associated with strength is muscle endurance or the ability to sustain a force over time. Sufficient endurance is particularly critical in the musculature involved in postural control or proximal stabilization. **Increased fatiguability has been observed in both hypertonic and hypotonic muscles following both traumatic brain injuries and strokes.** Low-intensity/high-repetition functional exercises should be incorporated into the overall treatment plan to improve muscular endurance.

Altered Muscle Activation Patterns

Most volitional movements require the coordinated activation and relaxation of many muscles and the proper control over multiple joints. Abnormalities in the coordination, timing, and sequencing of muscle contractions often result from central nervous system damage and produce a variety of abnormal muscle activation patterns. Some of these patterns may be discerned by clinical observation. Others are subtle and may be confirmed only by tests such as electromyography.

Loss of Fractionation[64,65]

Fractionation **is the ability to move a single joint without simultaneously producing unnecessary movements in other joints.** The ability to produce fractionated movements requires the precise coordination of muscles at many joints, even when actual movement may occur at only one joint. Flexing a finger, for example, requires the activation of wrist extensors to stabilize the wrist so that the finger flexor, which crosses the wrist joint, will not also flex the wrist. Therefore, fractionation requires the accurate selection of all the muscles necessary to produce an isolated movement and the modulation of the force within those muscles.

Loss of fractionation is a characteristic motor impairment associated with stroke and traumatic brain injury, as well as other neurologic disorders such as cerebral palsy. This is manifested as an inability to independently control joint movements in isolation. For

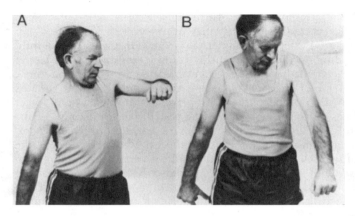

Figure 12–10. Loss of Fractionation. (*A*) A patient demonstrating active flexor synergy of the upper extremity. As he attempts shoulder flexion with an extended arm, his shoulder abducts (flexor component) and he is unable to extend his elbow. (*B*) A patient demonstrating active extensor synergy of the upper extremity. He is unable to extend his elbow without simultaneous shoulder internal rotation and forearm pronation. (From Davies,[64] p 26, with permission.)

example, a patient may not be able to isolate shoulder flexion without also producing elbow flexion, shoulder elevation and abduction, and wrist flexion. This inability to isolate individual joint movements contributes to the presence of the abnormal stereotypical movement synergies frequently observed.[64] **Dominant muscle synergies are those that emerge when voluntary activation of one joint movement is invariably accompanied by predictable movements at other joints forming a specific pattern or synergy** (Fig. 12–10). The typical dominant active movement synergies are described in Table 12–6.

The exact mechanisms accounting for the presence of these stereotypical abnormal motor patterns associated with brain lesions remain to be determined. However, one factor that may contribute to these patterns is a decreased short-term synchronization between

Table 12–6. *Dominant Active Synergies*

	Flexor Synergy	**Extensor Synergy**
Upper Extremity		
Scapular	Elevation	Protraction
	Retraction	
Shoulder	Abduction	Adduction
	External rotation	Internal rotation
Elbow	Flexion	Extension or flexion
Forearm	Supination	Pronation
Wrist	Flexion	Extension
Fingers	Flexion	Flexion
	Adduction	Adduction
Thumb	Flexion	Flexion
	Adduction	Adduction
Lower Extremity		
Pelvis	Elevation	Retraction
	Retraction	
Hip	Abduction	Adduction
	External rotation	Internal rotation
Knee	Flexion	Extension
Ankle	Dorsiflexion	Plantarflexion
	Supination	Inversion
Toes	Dorsiflexion	Plantarflexion
		Adduction

synergist motor neuron pools observed in stroke patients.[65] The reduced synchrony of firing between motor units in muscles that normally act as synergists may manifest as an inability to activate muscles in appropriate functional groups.

Movement Timing[66–75]

The **timing of a movement** has three basic components: the reaction time, the speed of the actual movement or movement time, and the time necessary to stop the movement. The reaction time is the time between the signal or command to move and the initiation of movement. **An increased reaction time has been documented in patients diagnosed with traumatic brain injury**[66,67] **and stroke,**[68–70] even on simple tasks that require minimal cognitive processing.[68] **This impairment has been demonstrated in the nonparetic ipsilateral limb, as well as in the paretic limb,**[68,71] **and appears to be more prevalent and severe in patients with right hemisphere lesions.**[69] This delay in reaction onset has significant clinical implications, especially for balance tasks in which fast reactions are required to prevent falls. However, it is one parameter of movement that is often not evaluated or treated during rehabilitation, even though data exist that support the effectiveness of training to reduce reaction times.[66,72]

Movement times or the time taken to complete a task after it has been initiated may also be increased in patients with central nervous system damage.[73,74] This may be reflected in the inability to achieve high velocities of movement or the sacrifice of accuracy to attain normal velocities.[75] Impaired movement velocity has the potential to interfere with coordination, balance, and the speed of functional movements. **To improve this motor impairment, treatment should incorporate fast-paced activities that demand variable movement times.**

Finally, **the time necessary to halt a movement in progress may be increased.** This contributes to difficulties in checking rapid movements and in performing rapidly alternating movements that require fast termination of agonist activity prior to activation of the antagonist.

Involuntary Movements[76–79]

Involuntary movements are a common and dramatic manifestation of central nervous system disease.[76–79] Although involuntary muscular activities also accompany peripheral motor disease arising from lesions in the motor neuron or the muscle itself, these are distinct from the conspicuous involuntary movements that often accompany central dysfunction. When supraspinal motor systems are damaged or their connections to the motor unit are disrupted, the control that they normally exert over motor activity is diminished. Without this direction and restraint, an assortment of involuntary motor behaviors may arise, disturbing both movement and posture. Some of the more distinct and consistent forms of involuntary activity are described in Table 12–7. These movements take many forms, and the distinctions made between them are often vague and somewhat arbitrary. With some notable exceptions, these movements are usually evident when the patient is at rest, are frequently increased by action, and often disappear during sleep. Such movements are distinguished mainly by visual inspection of the patient.

It is particularly common to observe involuntary movements in disorders associated with abnormalities of the basal ganglia, including tremors, choreas, athetosis, dystonia, and hemiballismus, all of which are termed *involuntary movement disorders* (Fig. 12–11). This group of disorders also encompasses myoclonus and tics, maladies that probably arise most often from sites outside the basal ganglia. Involuntary movements such as tremor and nystagmus often accompany lesions in the cerebellum. Subtle damage at the cortical levels of motor control may give rise to patterns of involuntary motor activity that are difficult to categorize, including complex tics and other stereotypical behaviors, restlessness, and hyperkinesia.

Table 12–7. Involuntary Movements

Movement	Description	Common Site of Pathology
Simple, Purposeless Movements		
Athetosis	Writhing, twisting movements occurring without fixed postures; seen most often in limbs, trunk, head, face, or tongue	Basal ganglia
Dystonia	Powerful, sustained contractions of groups of muscles that cause twisting or writhing of a limb or of the whole body; fast or slow, often painful; may result in gross deformity	Basal ganglia
Chorea	Sudden, brief, irregular movements most often seen in distal muscles; usually random in character; not repetitive or rhythmic	Basal ganglia
Dyskinesia	Certain choreic movements occurring repetitively at the same site, especially lingual-facial-buccal movements	Medication side effect
Hemiballismus	Large amplitude flinging or flailing limb movements, on one side of the body; ballismus if bilateral	Basal ganglia
Tremor	Rhythmic oscillating movement frequently seen in fingers or wrists; vary in form; occur at rest, while maintaining a posture of the hand or wrist, or during voluntary activity	Many; especially basal ganglia and cerebellum
Nystagmus	Recurring tendency of the eyes to slowly drift in one direction and then quickly correct back again	Many; especially cerebellum and peripheral labyrinth
Opsoclonus	Brief chaotic movements of eyes often seen in children	Brainstem, especially pons
Myoclonus	Repetitive, brief, shocklike contractions of a single muscle or group of muscle; may occur sporadically or regularly	Many; including cortex, brainstem, and spinal cord
Complex, Semipurposeful Movements		
Tics	Repetitive, stereotyped movements, commonly occurring in the face and proximal limbs; occasionally simple but usually complex	Higher centers; basal ganglia; largely unknown
Rhythmias	Repetitive compound movements; usually side-to-side and to-and-fro movement of trunk, head, or neck	Cerebral cortex
Akathisia	Movements of restlessness such as crossing and uncrossing legs, pacing, squirming in chair	Medication side effect
Hyperkinesia	Excessive motor activity; impulsive, impatient, and labile behavior, especially in children	Cerebral cortex

Associated Reactions[80]

An *associated reaction* is the unintentional movement of one limb that often occurs during the intentional movement of another limb (Fig. 12–12). Associated reactions are frequently observed in hemiplegic extremities, especially during activities that require significant force production. These reactions may also occur in the nonparetic extremities.[80] One explanation for this phenomenon is that there may be a natural coupling of certain movements, which is normally suppressed to allow independent movement. Damage to the supraspinal inhibitory mechanisms responsible for this suppression enhances these coupled movements, causing the associated reactions to occur.[80]

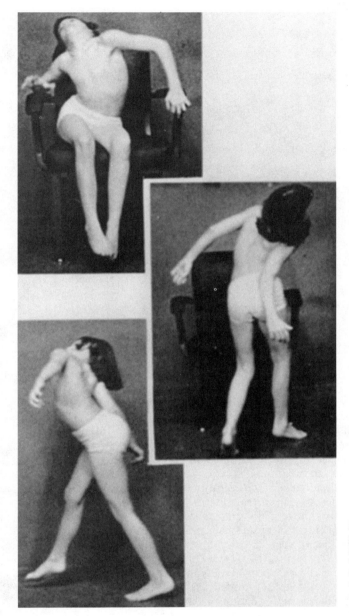

Figure 12–11. Advanced Dystonic Kyphoscoliosis in a Child. In this young girl, powerful, involuntary contractions of proximal muscle groups cause grossly distorted postures and disability. (From Cooper, IS: Involuntary Movement Disorders. Harper and Row, New York, 1969, p 148, with permission.)

Abnormalities of Coordination (Ataxia)[19,33,81,82]

The term *ataxia*, which is derived from the Greek word for "lack of order," **refers to an unsteadiness, incoordination, or clumsiness of movement** and is used most often in the context of intended or volitional movement. As a result of ataxia, motor acts requiring the smoothly coordinated activity of several muscles become halting, jerky, and imprecise. Patients with ataxia may have difficulties in regulating the force, range, direction, velocity, and rhythm of movements and in maintaining the synergy that normally exists among the various muscles contributing to a motor behavior. Ataxia is a general term and may be manifested in any number of specific clinical signs, depending on the site and extent of the nervous system involvement.

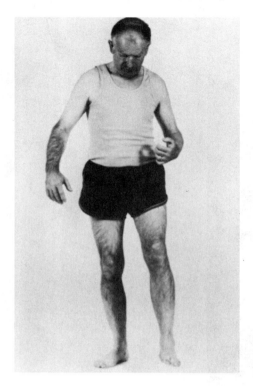

Figure 12–12. *Associated Reactions.* Associated reactions in the left upper extremity are evident as the patient actively attempts to dorsiflex the foot. (From Davies,[64] p 26, with permission.)

The movement disturbances related to the ataxic syndrome include dysmetria, **dyssynergia,** and **dysdiadochokinesia** (see Chapter 19). **Dysmetria** refers to errors in distance estimation that result in undershooting or overshooting a target. Intention tremor refers to the tendency for an extremity to oscillate as it approaches a target. This is thought to result from attempts to overcorrect dysmetria in alternating directions as the target is reached. **Dyssynergia** refers to errors in the timing or sequencing of muscle activation and is manifested as movements of individual limbs or of the entire trunk, which are jerky and lack fluidity. **Dysdiadochokinesia** manifests as abnormal rhythm and incoordination during an attempt to perform rapidly alternating movements such as fast alternation of pronation and supination of the hand. This poor control of onset/offset timing of muscle activations also often appears during functional activities such as running and jumping, which require fast agonist/antagonist reversals.

Ataxia may have more than one cause. **Motor ataxias** include conditions in which the sensory pathways are intact, but the integration and processing of motor commands are defective. Motor ataxia is usually due to malformation or damage to the cerebellum where much of this processing takes place, and it is often associated with hypotonia (see Chapters 8 and 19). This type of ataxia is often poorly compensated for by visual input. **Sensory ataxias** include conditions in which motor performance is faulty, not because motor control centers are dysfunctional, but because sensory pathways are disrupted resulting in inadequate transmittal of somatosensory and equilibratory sensory information to these centers. This type of ataxia can frequently be compensated for by using visual input to guide limb position. Thus sensory ataxia is often worse in the dark or when the eyes are closed. Patients with sensory ataxias generally have difficulties with vestibular function or with proprioception as a result of peripheral nerve or spinal cord disease. Coordination of movement may also be adversely affected by muscle weakness, pain, involuntary movements, and joint disorders.

Ataxia may be evident in the movement of individual limbs, but is usually most prominent as abnormal gait (Fig. 12–13). Ataxic patients are unsteady and stabilize

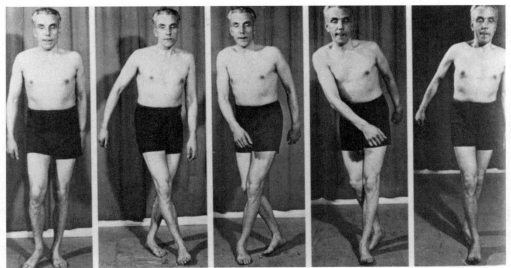

Figure 12–13. ***Ataxia of Gait.*** Incoordination in this multiple sclerosis patient is partly cerebellar and partly sensory. In the upper limbs, it was primarily cerebellar; in the lower limbs, there was marked proprioceptive sensory loss exacerbating any cerebellar ataxia. (From Spillane, JD: An Atlas of Clinical Neurology. Oxford University Press, New York, 1968, p 314, with permission.)

themselves with a broad-based gait. Their steps are uncertain and irregular, and they may stagger or veer from side to side. Over 90% of all patients with cerebellar disease have some form of gait ataxia. Abnormal gait may also result from disruption of the proprioceptive feedback from the feet and lower limbs as a result of peripheral neuropathy or spinal cord disease. Because gait disturbance is such a common and prominent manifestation of ataxia, the term "ataxia" is often erroneously used to designate just difficulty in walking. Truncal ataxia appears as swaying of the trunk and contributes to both a staggering gait and to difficulties in sitting unsupported. Bulbar muscles may also be involved, leading to slurred speech and oculomotor disturbances.

The functional consequences of ataxia are significant and may lead to severe disability. The ataxic abnormalities in movement regulation affect the range, direction, and magnitude of force, as well as the timing of activation. **As a result, movements such as balance reactions are often excessive or exaggerated because of difficulty in regulating small ranges of movement and in properly grading muscle contractions.** Many patients attempt to compensate for this by holding their trunk stiffly, avoiding movement, or by fixating with their upper extremities to gain stability in the trunk. Although sitting balance is often achieved, standing balance and gait are frequently severely limited or impossible if severe ataxia is present. Ataxia of the upper extremities frequently results in difficulty with activities such as eating and writing.

Apraxia[83–90]

Apraxia **is the inability to perform a goal-directed motor activity in the absence of paresis, ataxia, sensory loss, or disturbance of muscle tone.** The traditional definition suggests that apraxia is a disorder of "learned" movements in which patients have difficulty performing tasks with which they have already become familiar. However, recent evidence suggests that apraxic patients also demonstrate impairments when learning a new task.[87,88] The patient generally has intact comprehension and the physical ability to produce movement, but has difficulty conceptualizing and organizing the necessary movement patterns and translating them into purposeful actions. Apraxia is classified as a cognitive

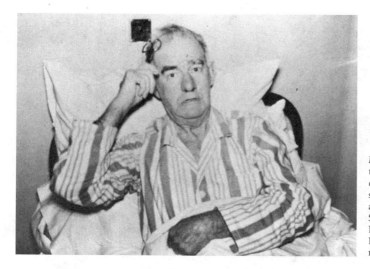

Figure 12–14. Apraxia. When this patient with a right parieto-occipital tumor was presented with scissors and asked to use them, he attempted to comb his hair. (From Spillane, JD: An Atlas of Clinical Neurology. Oxford University Press, New York, 1968, p 349, with permission.)

deficit that interferes with motor planning and is due to lesions in either the frontal or parietal lobes. **Most apraxic disorders result from lesions in the dominant hemisphere, which is usually the left in right-handed individuals.**[89,90] Apraxia may involve any of the motor activities, including speech and movement of the face, eyes, and limbs.

Although there are many different subtypes of apraxia, the two most common are ideational apraxia and ideomotor apraxia.[83–85] **Ideomotor apraxia** is associated with lesions in the premotor area of the frontal cortex. This is characterized by dyskinesia in which movements in response to commands are awkward and clumsy, and there is an inability to use sensory feedback to correct movement errors. Patients presenting with this form of apraxia understand the use of objects presented to them, but cannot sequence their movements to use them correctly. However, often the motor activities that cannot be elicited on command still occur automatically. For example, a patient may automatically reach for a tissue to blow his or her nose, but is unable to perform that same task when *asked* to do so. This deficit in motor planning is the most common form of apraxia. **Ideational apraxia** refers to a more severe disorder of motor planning typically associated with lesions of the frontal or parietal lobes. The most striking characteristic of this form of apraxia is the inability to recognize objects and their uses (Fig. 12–14). This is particularly evident when the patient is asked to use an object in an unaccustomed context. For example, when given a toothbrush and asked to use it, a patient will not understand the purpose of the toothbrush and may attempt to comb his or her hair with it. However, this patient could correctly brush his teeth when presented with the toothbrush in the bathroom.

The presence of apraxia may seriously interfere with self-care, mobility, and vocational activities. **Although automatic motor tasks that are performed habitually may remain intact, complicated or sequential tasks that require motor planning and an understanding of abstract concepts may be severely impaired.** In addition, the patients often have difficulty imitating movements and following commands, which may seriously interfere with rehabilitation efforts.

Hypokinesia (Akinesia and Bradykinesis)[33,34]

Hypokinesia **is a slowness or poverty of movement, which is independent of any disturbance of muscle power or coordination.** In contrast to paralysis, strength is not significantly diminished. Hypokinesia is also unlike apraxia, in which the patient has lost the memory of how to generate a pattern of movement. Akinesia and bradykinesia represent different degrees of the same pathologic phenomenon. **Akinesia** refers to extreme hypoactivity, whereas **bradykinesia** connotes a slowness rather than a lack of movement. A patient with hypokinesia is not only slow to initiate movement, but the velocity of the movement is slower than usual. Initial activation of the agonists involved in a motor activity is inadequate and gives rise to a low initial velocity. As a result, the patient typically moves to the point of aim slowly and usually undershoots (hypometria). The final position is often achieved by a repetitive series of small incremental steps. Particular difficulty is encountered in executing repetitive, concurrent, or sequential actions. The patient may find it especially difficult to execute two simultaneous motor acts or to switch from one motor act to another. He or she may actually "freeze" or reach a total standstill in the middle of a motor sequence. Skilled acts such as eating, dressing, washing, or walking may be delayed or interrupted, with the patient coming to a complete halt or being frozen in place. Poverty of movement may also be apparent in a variety of reflex motor activities that normally occur with little or no conscious awareness. Periodic blinking, facial movements, movement of arms while walking, and weight shifting during standing or sitting all may be impaired. Hypokinesia is manifested in voice disturbances, gait disorders (slow to start, shuffling), and difficulty in using the arms, especially in writing. It is interesting that akinesia may be episodic, raising questions about patient malingering or lack of motivation.

Akinesia and bradykinesia are characteristically found in association with certain disorders of the basal ganglia, especially Parkinson's disease. Although tremor and rigidity are the most dramatic aspects of this malady, the most disabling symptom is hypokinesia. The actual pathophysiology of this symptom is uncertain and probably involves defects in both the process of deciding how to act and in the accurate implementation of a complete plan of action. Complex actions requiring implementation of a number of sequential motor programs are most likely to break down. Most of what is known about hypokinesia has been derived from studies of patients with Parkinson's disease.

Abnormal Skeletal Muscle Reflexes[19,23,27]

The effects of central nervous system damage on the tendon reflexes are more varied than is the case in peripheral locomotor disturbances in which these reflexes are usually decreased or absent. **Certain central nervous system conditions are associated with hypoactive tendon reflexes, whereas others are associated with their exaggeration.** In conditions of generalized central nervous system depression (e.g., deep coma or spinal shock) as well as certain conditions causing hypotonia (e.g., cerebellar lesions), these reflexes are diminished. These reflexes become exaggerated with upper motor neuron lesions and are an important clinical sign of pyramidal tract damage. They may also be heightened by the loss of inhibitory influences from certain extrapyramidal (e.g., basal ganglia) and brainstem regions.[23,27] The hyperreflexia of the tendon reflexes may present in the form of **clonus,** a series of rapid involuntary muscle contractions occurring in response to abruptly applied stretch. Clonus is usually described in terms of the part of the limb that was stretched (e.g., ankle clonus). Innocuous stimuli such as the placement of the foot on a wheelchair foot plate or on the floor may elicit ankle clonus and interfere with functional abilities such as transferring from sitting to standing or ambulation.

Superficial or cutaneous reflexes are also important in the assessment of central nervous system function. These reflexes are responses of skeletal muscle elicited by stimulation of the skin or mucous membrane, rather than stretch. Many of these responses are altered by upper motor neuron dysfunction. **Perhaps the most important of the superficial reflexes** and possibly the most clinically important of all somatic reflexes **is the plantar reflex.** In this response in a normal individual, stimulation of the plantar surface of the foot is followed by plantar flexion of the toes, the small toes flexing more than the big toe. **In diseases of the pyramidal system, there is an inversion of the normal response,** consisting of dorsiflexion of the toes, especially of the big toe, together with a separation or fanning of the other toes (Fig. 12–15). **This response is termed** *Babinski's sign* **and is**

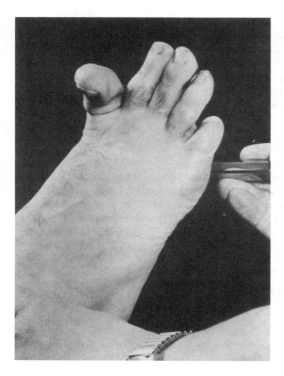

Figure 12–15. The Babinski's Sign. When the sole of the foot is stroked, the normal response is plantar flexion of the foot and toes. Babinski's sign is dorsiflexion of the big toe with fanning of the other toes. Babinski's sign is indicative of a pyramidal disorder. (From Spillane, JD: An Atlas of Clinical Neurology. Oxford University Press, New York, 1968, p 334, with permission.)

generally accepted clinically as strong evidence of damage to the pyramidal tracts. A bilateral extensor plantar response may also be observed during states of unconsciousness, such as deep sleep, coma, or anesthesia, and in the newborn in whom the corticospinal fibers are incompletely developed. This response persists in most children until 12 to 18 months of age.

Abnormal Balance[91–93]

Balance refers to the ability to maintain the body's center of gravity over the base of support. Human balance is a complex process that requires the integration of an ongoing flood of sensorimotor information within the central nervous system and the execution of an appropriate response mediated through the musculoskeletal system. Multiple factors may contribute to balance impairment. A central nervous system lesion that directly affects any component of the vestibular system may alter the integration of sensory input and motor commands necessary for balance and directly alter the balance response. Other direct effects of central nervous system lesions, such as weakness, sensory loss, or visual impairment, also may contribute to the impairment of the balance system. Furthermore, indirect effects of injury such as muscle contractures may place biomechanical constraints on the balance system and affect an individual's ability to execute an appropriate balance response.

Balance must be maintained during three primary conditions in order to prevent falls. First, one must be able to sit or stand statically without support. Second, one must be able to respond to displacement from an unexpected and external source. Finally, one must be able to accurately and safely adapt to self-imposed movements. Abnormal balance responses have been reported under all three conditions in patients with central nervous system injuries.[91–93] These abnormal responses may include delayed balance reactions, exaggerated or inappropriate balance reactions that overcompensate for the perturbation, and the absence of any observable balance response.

Significant balance impairment can be very disabling and in the extreme may prevent independent sitting or ambulation. One of the most serious consequence of balance impairment is the potential for falls and subsequent injury to the musculoskeletal system. Treatment of a balance dysfunction will vary according to which factors are contributing significantly to the disorder. Accurate identification of the underlying cause and effective treatment of balance dysfunction are critical in preventing the serious potential consequences of a fall.

Abnormalities of Senation[19,21,22,24]

The sensory deficits identified in Table 12–3 that may result from peripheral nervous system dysfunction may also occur as a consequence of lesions of the central nervous system. **Pain, temperature, touch, proprioception, and kinesthetic sense all may be impaired. The predominant feature that differentiates peripheral sensory deficits from deficits following central lesions is the distribution of impairment.** Sensory loss associated with disruption of the peripheral nervous system is often quite restricted, being localized to areas directly supplied by the nerve or nerves affected, and tends to occur in distinctive patterns (e.g., glove-and-stocking distribution). In contrast, sensory deficits secondary to central nervous system lesions are more diffuse. A lesion in the primary sensory area of the parietal cortex, for example, characteristically disrupts sensation in the face, trunk, upper extremity, and lower extremity on the contralateral side of the body.

Although controversy exists regarding the exact role that sensation plays in the control of voluntary motor activity, it is evident that sensory information is continually being received and used by motor systems. The preponderance of evidence suggests that although gross movements can occur in the absence of somatosensory feedback, fine motor control and the ability for movement error detection and compensation are impaired. Therefore, it is important to conduct a thorough evaluation of sensation in patients presenting with motor impairments.

RECOMMENDED READINGS

Adams, RD and Victor, M: Principles of Neurology, ed 5. Part II. Cardinal Manifestations of Neurologic Disease. McGraw-Hill, New York, 1993.

Bradley, WG, et al (eds): Neurology in Clinical Practice: Principles of Diagnosis and Management. Butterworth-Heinemann, Boston, 1991.

DeJong, RN and Haerer, AF: Case Taking and the Neurologic Exam. Chapter 1, In Joynt, RJ (ed): Clinical Neurology, vol 1, JB Lippincott, Philadelphia, 1991.

Gomez, MR: The Clinical Examination. Chapter 30. In Engel, AG and Franzini-Armstrong, C (eds): Myology: Basic and Clinical, ed 2. McGraw-Hill, New York, 1994.

Haerer, AF: DeJong's: The Neurologic Examination, ed 5. JB Lippincott, Philadelphia, 1992.

Haley, SM and Inacio, CA: Evaluation of Spasticity and Its Effect on Motor Function. In Glenn, MB and Whyte, J (eds): The Practical Management of Spasticity in Children and Adults. Lea & Febiger, Malvern, PA, 1990.

Lacote, M, et al: Clinical Evaluation of Muscle Function, ed 2. Churchill Livingstone, Edinburgh, 1987.

Layzer, RB: Neuromuscular Manifestations of Systemic Disease. Contemporary Neurology Series. FA Davis, Philadelphia, 1985.

Mayo Clinic, Department of Neurology: Clinical Examinations in Neurology, ed 6. Mosby-Year Book, St. Louis, 1990.

Pryse-Phillips, W and Murray, TJ: Essential Neurology, ed 4. Part 3. An Approach to Neurological Symptoms. Medical Examination Publishing Company, New York, 1992.

Ringel, SR: Clinical Presentations in Neuromuscular Disease. Chapter 8. In Vinken, PJ and Bruyn, GW (eds): Handbook of Clinical Neurology, vol 40. Diseases of Muscle. Part I. North-Holland Publishing Company, Amsterdam, 1979.

Rowland, LP (ed): Merritt's Textbook of Neurology, ed 8. Section 1. Symptoms of Neurologic Disorders. Lea & Febiger, Philadelphia, 1989.

Spillane, JD: An Atlas of Clinical Neurology. Oxford University Press, New York, 1968.

Swash, M and Schwartz, MS: Neuromuscular Diseases, ed 2. Chapter 1. Clinical Assessment. Springer-Verlag, London, 1988.

Walton, JN: Clinical Examination of the Neuromuscular System. Chapter 13. In Walton, JN (ed): Disorders of Voluntary Muscle, ed 4. Churchill Livingstone, Edinburgh, 1981.

REFERENCES

1. Swash, M and Schwartz, MS: Neuromuscular Diseases, ed. 2. Springer-Verlag, London, 1988.
2. Ringel, SP: Clinical Presentations in Neuromuscular Disease. Chapter 8. In Vinken, PJ and Bruyn, GW (eds): Handbook of Clinical Neurology, vol 40. North-Holland Publishing Company, Amsterdam, 1979.
3. Layzer, RB: Diagnosis of Neuromuscular Disorders. Chapter 1. In Layzer, RB: Neuromuscular Manifestations of Systemic Disease. FA Davis, Philadelphia, 1985.
4. Walton, JN: Clinical Examination of the Neuromuscular System. Chapter 13. In Walton, JN (ed): Disorders of Voluntary Muscle, ed 4. Churchill Livingstone, Edinburgh, 1981.
5. Gomez, MR: The Clinical Examination. Chapter 30. In Engel, AG and Franzini-Armstrong, C (eds): Myology: Basic and Clinical, ed 2. McGraw-Hill, New York, 1994.
6. Layzer, RB: Muscle Pains and Cramps. Chapter 31. In Bradley, WG, et al (eds): Neurology in Clinical Practice. Butterworth-Heinemann, Boston, 1990.
7. Roy, EP and Gutmann, L: Myalgia. Neurol Clin 6(3):621, 1988.
8. Pryse-Phillips, WEM and Murray, TJ: Muscle Cramps, Stiffness, and Pain. Chapter 27. In Pryse-Phillips, WEM and Murray, TJ: Essential Neurology, ed 4. Medical Examination Publishing Company, New York, 1992.
9. Layzer, RB: Muscle Pain, Cramps, and Fatigue. Chapter 66. In Engel, AG and Banker, BQ (eds): Myology: Basic and Clinical. McGraw-Hill, New York, 1986.
10. Brooke, MD: Motor Unit Weakness. Chapter 25. In Bradley, WG, et al (eds): Neurology in Clinical Practice. Butterworth-Heinemann, Boston, 1990.
11. Rowland, LP: Weakness: The Syndromes Caused by Weak Muscles. Chapter 10. In Rowland, LP (ed): Merritt's Textbook of Neurology, ed 8. Lea & Febiger, Philadelphia, 1989.
12. Pryse-Phillips, WEM and Murray, TJ: Weakness. Chapter 26. In Pryse-Phillips, WEM and Murray, TJ: Essential Neurology, ed 4. Medical Examination Publishing Company, New York, 1992.
13. Adams, RD and Victor, M: Motor Paralysis. Chapter 3. In Adams, RD and Victor, M (eds): Principles of Neurology, ed 5. McGraw-Hill, New York, 1993.
14. Bickerstaff, ER and Spillane, JA: Development and Wasting. Chapter 15. In Neurological Examination in Clinical Practice. Blackwell Scientific Publications, Oxford, 1989.
15. Layzer, RB: Motor Unit Hyperactivity States. Chapter 10. In Vinken, PJ and Bruyn, GW (eds): Handbook of Clinical Neurology, vol 4. North-Holland Publishing Company, Amsterdam, 1979.
16. Layzer, RB: Diagnostic Implications of Clinical Fasiculations and Cramps. In Rowland, LP (ed): Human Motor Neuron Diseases. Raven Press, New York, 1982.
17. Layzer, RB: Cramps and Stiffness. Chapter 133. In Rowland, LP (ed): Merritt's Textbook of Neurology, ed. 8. Lea & Febiger, Philadelphia, 1989.
18. Fenichel, GM: The Hypotonic Infant. Chapter 26. In Bradley, WG, et al (eds): Neurology in Clinical Practice. Butterworth-Heinemann, Boston, 1990.
19. Bannister, Sir R: Examination of the Limbs and Trunk. Chapter 3. In Bannister, Sir R: Brain and Bannister's Clinical Neurology, ed 7. Oxford University Press, Oxford, 1992.
20. Bickerstaff, ER and Spillane, JA: Muscle Tone. Chapter 16. In Bickerstaff, ER and Spillane, JA: Neurological Examination in Clinical Practice, ed 5. Blackwell Scientific Publications, Oxford, 1989.
21. Bickerstaff, ER and Spillane, JA: Common Patterns of Abnormal Sensation. Chapter 24. In Bickerstaff, ER and Spillane, JA: Neurological Examination in Clinical Practice, ed 5. Blackwell Scientific Publications, Oxford, 1989.
22. Pryse-Phillips, WEM and Murray, TJ: Patterns of Sensory Loss. Chapter 35. In Pryse-Phillips, WEM and Murray, TJ: In Essential Neurology, ed 4. Medical Examination Publishing Company, New York, 1992.
23. Dejong, RN and Haerer, AF: Case Taking and the Neurologic Examination. Chapter 1. In Joynt, RJ: Clinical Neurology, vol 1. JB Lippincott, Philadelphia, 1991.
24. Gordon, TR and Waxman, SG: Sensory Abnormalities of the Limbs and Trunk. Chapter 27. In Bradley, WG, et al (eds): Neurology in Clinical Practice. Butterworth-Heinemann, Boston, 1990.
25. Dobata, JL, Villanueva, JA, and Gimenez-Roldan, S: Sensory Ataxic Hemiparesis in Thalamic Stroke. Stroke 21:1749, 1990.
26. Nashner, LM: Sensory, Neuromuscular, and Biomechanical Contributions to Human Balance. In Duncan, P (ed): Balance: Proceedings of the APTA forum. American Physical Therapy Association, Alexandria, VA, 1989.
27. Bickerstaff, ER and Spillane, JA: The Reflexes. Chapter 25. In Bickerstaff, ER and Spillane, JA: Neurological Examination in Clinical Practice, ed 5. Blackwell Scientific Publications, Oxford, 1989.
28. Haerer, AF: DeJong's the Neurological Examination. Chapter 33. The Muscle Stretch Reflexes, ed 5. JB Lippincott, Philadelphia, 1992.
29. Bickerstaff, ER and Spillane, JA: Neurological Examination in Clinical Practice, ed 5. Blackwell-Scientific Publications, Oxford, 1989.
30. Bannister, Sir R: Brain and Bannister's Clinical Neurology, ed 7. Oxford University Press, Oxford, 1992.
31. Adams, RD and Victor, M: Principles of Neurology, ed 5. Part II. Cardinal Manifestations of Neurologic Disease. McGraw-Hill Information Services Company, New York, 1993.
32. Bradley, WG, et al (eds): Neurology in Clinical Practice: Principles of Diagnosis and Management. Butterworth-Heinemann, Boston, 1991.
33. Adams, RD and Victor, M: Abnormalities of Movement and Posture Due to Disease of the Extrapyramidal Motor Systems. Chapter 4. In Adams, RD and Victor, M: Principles of Neurology, ed 5. McGraw-Hill, New York, 1993.
34. Marsden, CD: Motor Dysfunction and Movement Disorders. Chapter 22. In Asbury, AK, McKhann, GM, and McDonald, WI: Diseases of the Nervous System: Clinical Neurobiology, vol II, ed 2. WB Saunders, Philadelphia, 1992.
35. Bodine-Fowler, SC and Botte, MJ: Muscle Spasticity. Chapter 26. In Nickel, VL and Botte, MJ: Ortho-

paedic Rehabilitation, ed 2. Churchill Livingstone, New York, 1992.

36. Burke, D and Lance JW: The Myotatic Unit and Its Disorders. Chapter 20. In Asbury, AK, McKhann, GM, and McDonald, WI: Diseases of the Nervous System: Clinical Neurobiology. WB Saunders, Philadelphia, 1992.

37. Little, JW and Massagli, TL: Spasticity and Associated Abnormalities of Muscle Tone. Chapter 32. In Delisa, JA (ed): Rehabilitation Medicine: Principles and Practice, ed 2. JB Lippincott, Philadelphia, 1993.

38. Hallenborg, SC: Positioning. Chapter 6. In Glenn, MB and Whyte, J (eds): The Practical Management of Spasticity in Children and Adults. Lea & Febiger, Philadelphia, 1990.

39. Burry, HC: Objective Measurement of Spasticity. Dev Med Child Neurol 14:508, 1972.

40. DeSouza, LH: The Measurement and Assessment of Spasticity. Clin Rehabil 1:89, 1987.

41. Johnstone, M: Restoration of Motor Function in the Stroke Patient. Churchill Livingstone, Edinburgh, 1983.

42. Katz, RT and Rymer, WZ: Spastic Hypertonia: Mechanisms and Measurement. Arch Phys Med Rehabil 70:144, 1989.

43. Sahrmann, SA: The Relationship of Voluntary Movement to Spasticity in the Upper Motor Neuron Syndrome. Ann Neurol 2:460, 1977.

44. Knutsson, E and Martensson, A: Dynamic Motor Capacity in Spastic Paresis and Its Relationship to Prime Mover Dysfunction, Spastic Reflexes and Antagonist Coactivation. Scand J Rehabil Med 12:93, 1980.

45. el-Abd, MA, Ibrahim, IK, and Dietz, V: Impaired Activation Pattern in Antagonistic Elbow Muscles of Patients with Spastic Hemiparesis: Contribution to Movement Disorder. Electromyogr Clin Neurophysiol 33:247, 1993.

46. Hammond, MC, et al: Co-Contraction in the Hemiparetic Forearm: Quantitative EMG Evaluation. Arch Phys Med Rehabil 69:348, 1988.

47. Rosenfalck, A and Martensson, C: Impaired Regulation of Force and Firing Pattern of Single Motor Units in Patients with Spasticity. J Neurol Neurosurg Psychiatry 43:907, 1980.

48. Colebatch, JG, Gandevia, SC, and Spira, PJ: Voluntary Muscle Strength in Hemiparesis: Distribution of Weakness at the Elbow. J Neurol Neurosurg Psychiatry 49:1019, 1986.

49. Fellows, SJ: Agonist and Antagonist EMG Activation During Isometric Torque Development at the Elbow in Spastic Hemiparesis. Electroencephalogr Clin Neurophysiol 93:106, 1994.

50. Gowland, C, et al: Agonist and Antagonist Activity During Voluntary Upper-Limb Movement in Patients with Stroke. Phys Ther 72:624, 1992.

51. Bohannon, RW: Gait Performance of Hemiparetic Stroke Patients: Selected Variables. Arch Phys Med Rehabil 68:777, 1987.

52. Norton, BJ, et al: Correlation Between Gait Speed and Spasticity at the Knee. Phys Ther 55:355, 1975.

53. Spaulding, SJ, et al: Wrist Muscle Tone and Self-care Skill in Persons with Hemiparesis. Am J Occup Ther 43:11, 1989.

54. Wilson, DJ, Baker, LL, and Craddock, JA: Functional Test for the Hemiparetic Upper Extremity. Am J Occup Ther 38:159, 1984.

55. Haley, SM and Inacio, CA: Evaluation of Spasticity and Its Effect on Motor Function. In Glenn, MB and Whyte, J (eds): The Practical Management of Spasticity in Children and Adults. Malvern, PA, Lea & Febiger, 1990.

56. Carey, JH, Crosby, EC, and Schintzlein, HN: Decorticate Versus Decerebrate Rigidity in Sub-Human Primates and Man. Neurology 21:738, 1971.

57. Berne, RM, and Levy, MN: Physiology, ed 2. CV Mosby, St. Louis, 1988.

58. Rowland, LP: Weakness: The Syndromes Caused by Weak Muscles. Chapter 10. In Rowland, LP (ed): Merritt's Textbook of Neurology, ed 8. Lea & Febiger, Philadelphia, 1989.

59. Adams, RD and Victor, M: Motor Paralysis. Chapter 3. In Adams, RD and Victor, M: Principles of Neurology, ed 5. McGraw-Hill, New York, 1993.

60. Goldblatt, D: Monoplegia. Chapter 22. In Bradley, WG, et al (eds): Neurology in Clinical Practice. Butterworth-Heinemann, Boston, 1990.

61. Monroe, C: Hemiplegic Syndromes. Chapter 23. In Bradley, WG, et al (eds): Neurology in Clinical Practice. Butterworth-Heinemann, Boston, 1990.

62. Thompson, PD: Paraplegia and Quadriplegia. Chapter 24. In Bradley, WG, et al (eds): Neurology in Clinical Practice. Butterworth-Heinemann, Boston, 1990.

63. Jones, RD, Donaldson, IM, and Parkin, PJ: Impairment and Recovery of Ipsilateral Sensory-Motor Function Following Unilateral Cerebral Infarction. Brain 112:113, 1989.

64. Davies, PM: Steps to Follow: A Guide to the Treatment of Adult Hemiplegia. Springer-Verlag, Berlin, 1985.

65. Powers, RK, Vanden Noven, S, and Rymer, WZ: Evidence of Shared, Direct Input to Motorneurons Supplying Synergist Muscles in Humans. Neurosci Lett 102:76, 1989.

66. Deacon, D and Campbell, KB: Effects of Performance on P300 and Reaction Time in Closed Head-Injured Patients. Electroencephalogr Clin Neurophysi 78:133, 1991.

67. Stuss, DT, et al: Reaction Time After Head Injury: Fatigue, Divided and Focused Attention, and Consistency of Performance. J Neurol Neurosurg Psychiatry 52(6):742, 1989.

68. Dickstein, R, et al: Reaction and Movement Times in Patients with Hemiparesis for Unilateral and Bilateral Elbow Flexion. Phys Ther 73:37, 1993.

69. Buonocore, M, Casale, R, and Arrigo, A: Psychomotor Skills in Hemiplegic Patients: Reaction Time Differences Related to Hemispheric Lesion Side. Neurophysiol Clin 20:203, 1990.

70. Harrington, DL and Haaland, KY: Hemispheric Specialization for Motor Sequencing: Abnormalities in Levels of Programming. Neuropsychologia 29:147, 1991.

71. Kaizer, F, et al: Response Time of Stroke Patients to a Visual Stimulus. Stroke 19:335, 1988.

72. Bitenski, NK, Mayo, NE, and Kaizer, F: Changes in Response Times of Stroke Patients and Controls During Rehabilitation. Am J Phys Med Rehabil 69:32, 1990.

73. Segal, RL and Youssef, EL: Wrist Movements in Able Bodied and Brain Injured Individuals. Arch Phys Med Rehabil 72:454, 1991.

74. Rosecrance, JC and Guiliani, CA: Kinematic Analysis of Lower-Limb Movement during Ergometer Pedaling in Hemiplegic and Non-Hemiplegic Subjects. Phys Ther 71:334, 1991.

75. Chaplin, D, Deitz, J, and Jaffe, KM: Motor Performance in Children After Traumatic Brain Injury. Arch Phys Med Rehabil 74(2): 161, 1993.

76. Adams, RD and Victor, M: Tremor, Myoclonus, Spasms, and Tics. Chapter 5. In Adams, RD and Victor, M: Principles of Neurology, ed 5. McGraw-Hill, New York, 1993.

77. Bickerstaff, ER, and Spillane, JA: Involuntary Movements. Chapter 19. In Bickerstaff, ER, and Spillane, JA: Neurological Examination in Clinical Practice, ed 5. Blackwell-Scientific Publications, Oxford, 1989.

78. Lang, AE: Movement Disorder Symptomatology. Chapter 28. In Bradley, WG, et al (eds): Neurology in Clinical Practice. Butterworth-Heinemann, Boston, 1990.

79. Jankovic, J (ed): Movement Disorders. Neurol Clin 2(3):415, 1984.

80. Lazarus, JC: Associated Movement in Hemiplegia: The Effects of Force Exerted, Limb Usage and Inhibitory Training. Arch Phys Med Rehabil 73:1044, 1992.

81. Harding, AE: Ataxic Disorders. Chapter 29. In Bradley, WG, et al (eds): Neurology in Clinical Practice. Butterworth-Heinemann, Boston, 1990.

82. Bickerstaff, ER and Spillane, JA: Co-ordination. Chapter 26. In Bickerstaff, ER and Spillane, JA: Neurological Examination in Clinical Practice, ed 5. Blackwell-Scientific Publications, Oxford, 1989.

83. Kirshner, HS: The Apraxias. In Bradley, WG, et al (eds): Neurology in Clinical Practice. Butterworth-Heinemann, Boston, 1990.

84. Geschwind, N: The Apraxias: Neural Mechanisms of Disorders of Learned Movement. Am Sci 63:188, 1975.

85. Freund, HJ: The Apraxias. Chapter 55. In Ashbury, AK, McKhann, GM, and McDonald, WI (eds): Diseases of the Nervous System: Clinical Neurobiology, ed 2. WB Saunders, Philadelphia, 1992.

86. Derenzi, E, Motti, F, and Nichelli, P: Imitating Gestures: A Quantitative Approach to Ideomotor Apraxia. Arch Neurol 37:6, 1980.

87. Motormura, N, et al: Motor Learning in Ideomotor Apraxia. Int J Neurosci 47:125, 1989.

88. Pistarini, C, et al: Multiple Learning Tasks in Patients with Ideomotor Apraxia. Riv Neurol 61:57, 1991.

89. Haaland, KY and Harrington, DL: Limb Sequencing Deficits After Left But Not Right Hemisphere Damage. Brain Cogn 24: 104, 1994.

90. Freund, HJ: Abnormalities of Motor Behavior after Cortical Lesions in Humans. Section 1. In Plum, F (ed): Handbook of Human Physiology. American Physiological Society, Bethesda, MD, 1987.

91. Lee, WA, Deming, L, and Sahgal, V: Quantitative and Clinical Measures of Static Standing Balance in Hemiparetic and Normal Subjects. Phys Ther 68:970, 1988.

92. Horak, FB, et al: The Effects of Movement Velocity, Mass Displaced, and Task Certainty on Associated Postural Adjustments Made by Normal and Hemiplegic Individuals. J Neurol Neurosurg Psychiatry 47:1020, 1984.

93. Newton, RA: Recovery of Balance Abilities in Individuals with Traumatic Brain Injuries. In Duncan, PW (ed): Balance. Proceedings of the APTA Forum. American Physical Therapy Association, Alexandria, Virginia, 1990.

SECTION

DISORDERS OF THE MOTOR UNIT

Neuromuscular Diseases

Overview

The purpose of this section is to describe the essential pathophysiologic and clinical features of the so-called **neuromuscular diseases**. This terminology is used to designate a large group of motor disorders, all of which arise from some pathologic disturbance of the motor unit or its associated sensory connections. In this regard, the site of dysfunction may be the anterior horn cell (or analogous cranial nerve nucleus), spinal root, peripheral nerve, neuromuscular junction, or skeletal muscle itself. Although these disorders most often involve spinal motor units, they may afflict bulbar motor systems as well.

Most of the neuromuscular diseases present a clinical picture dominated by the sequelae of diminished motor activity (Table IV–1). The most common features are muscle weakness, decreased muscle tone, and hypoactive stretch reflexes. In some instances, there is evidence of exaggerated or distorted motor activity (e.g., fasciculations, cramps, myotonia, or contractures). Sensory disturbances may accompany or in some instances occur in the absence of motor impairment. These range from mild paresthesias and disturbances of proprioception to complete anesthesia or severe pain. In addition, autonomic pathways may be involved in certain disorders, creating significant disturbances of autonomic function. Such disturbances range from relatively localized impairment of vascular control to gross disturbance of gastrointestinal, urogenital, or cardiovascular function.

The **myopathies** are disorders in which motor dysfunction arises from pathology in the muscle itself. The causes of myopathy are remarkably varied. Muscle function can be disturbed by exogenous influences impinging on muscle (e.g., physical trauma, toxic agents, infectious organisms, and systemic diseases), as well as by inherited defects in muscle structure or biochemistry (e.g., muscular dystrophies, congenital myopathies, and metabolic myopathies). Perhaps the most disheartening of the myopathies are the inherited muscular dystrophies. These incurable diseases are often relentlessly progressive, especially in children. The inherited metabolic myopathies, although rare, have been of particular interest to scientists studying muscle, because of what they have revealed about the relationship of muscle metabolism to contraction. The most widespread of the

Table IV–1. *Common Signs and Symptoms of Neuromuscular Disease*

Disease Location	Voluntary Strength	Atrophy	Stretch Reflexes	Muscle Tone	Involuntary Contractions
Muscle (myopathy)	Weak	Variable	Hypoactive	Diminished	Occasional myotonia, contractures
Neuromuscular junction	Weak	Slight	Hypoactive	Diminished	None
Lower motor neuron (peripheral neuropathy, radiculopathy)	Weak or paralyzed	Severe	Hypoactive or absent	Diminished (flaccid)	Occasional fasciculations, cramps
Lower motor neuron (anterior horn cell)	Weak or paralyzed	Severe	Hypoactive or absent (heightened with upper motor neuron involvement)	Diminished (increased with upper motor neuron involvement)	Fasciculations, cramps, spasticity, Babinski's response with upper motor neuron involvement

myopathies are those induced by infectious agents (e.g., the viral myositis of the flu) or by various drugs (e.g., intramuscular injection of antibiotics, vaccines, or analgesics).

Communication between the neural and muscular elements of the motor unit occurs at the **neuromuscular junction.** Disorders of this junction can significantly impair the transmission of excitation from the motor neuron to the muscle cell membrane, resulting in muscle dysfunction ranging from weakness and abnormal fatigability to complete flaccid paralysis. Relatively few disorders afflict the neuromuscular junction, but such disorders constitute some of the best understood of the neuromuscular diseases and have provided much insight into the function of the normal neuromuscular junction. These disorders are both acquired and inherited and reflect defects in both prejunctional and postjunctional processes. By far the most common are the acquired disorders. Notable among these are the autoimmune disease, myasthenia gravis, and conditions caused by the adverse effects of various toxic agents on the junction. The most severe of these is **botulism,** in which prejunctional motor nerve terminals are destroyed by a bacterial toxin, causing a flaccid (sometimes life-threatening) paralysis.

Normal motor activity depends on the functional integrity of both the lower motor neurons that activate skeletal muscle and the somatosensory fibers that provide proprioceptive feedback from the muscles and adjacent structures. Many disorders may impair the function of either or both of these neural systems. Unfortunately, the terminology used to classify these disorders is perhaps the most ambiguous of all the neuromuscular diseases. Classification problems begin with the fact that portions of each of these neurons reside within both the central and peripheral nervous systems. Not only does this have real functional implications, but it makes the distinction between central and peripheral disorders difficult and arbitrary. Although the motor neuron is a single cell, for example, a distinction is often made between central disorders of the anterior horn cell and peripheral disorders of the motor axon. Consider also that although pathology of the motor neuron cell body is within the central nervous system, that of the sensory or autonomic cell body is within the peripheral nervous system. Also, a distinction is often made between those disorders that affect primarily the motor neuron cell body (the neuronopathies) and those in which the cell processes are primarily involved (the peripheral neuropathies). This is, however, not always meaningful or even desirable. Both components of the neuron may be involved in the same disorder. Moreover, it is often impossible to differentiate between the primary sites of pathology and those that are secondary. To make matters worse, the term **motor neuron disease** is used by various authors to designate different things. "Motor neuron diseases" is often used to denote all disorders in which damage to the motor neuron cell body is the principal feature, whereas "motor neuron disease" often refers specifically to a group of idiopathic, adult-onset conditions typified by amyotrophic lateral sclerosis.

Many conditions adversely affect both the motor and sensory components of the **peripheral nervous system.** As diverse as the etiologies of these disorders are, the underlying pathologic reactions can be divided into those that primarily affect the axon (axonopathies) and those that primarily affect its myelin sheath (myelinopathies); the more common are the axonopathies. The peripheral neuropathies have many different causes, both acquired (e.g., trauma, infection, and inflammation) and inherited, and may be classified accordingly. Although emphasis is often placed on disorders of the peripheral spinal nerves, it should be remembered that the spinal roots (radiculopathies) and cranial nerves are susceptible to many of the same diseases. Their involvement is an important component of a number of peripheral neuropathies, and in some of these disorders may predominate.

There is also a group of disorders that primarily affect the **spinal or cranial motor neuron cell body,** causing degeneration and loss of the entire motor neuron. These cells may be adversely affected by a variety of infectious, metabolic, inflammatory, and toxic conditions. The archetype of motor neuron disease is amyotrophic lateral sclerosis, an idiopathic, adult-onset disorder characterized by progressive dysfunction of both lower and upper motor neurons. The spinal muscular atrophies are a group of inherited disorders, which constitute the most common disorder of the lower motor neuron in children. Despite its cloistered site within the central nervous system, the motor neuron cell body is also vulnerable to injury by a number of pathogens (e.g., the polio, herpes zoster, and rabies viruses) and toxins (e.g., tetanus). The clinical presentation of the neuronopathies reflects the loss of motor neurons and is usually one of skeletal muscle weakness and atrophy. However, in some of these disorders heightened or distorted contractile activity may be prominent.

CHAPTER 13

■

Disorders of Muscles: The Myopathies

Christopher M. Fredericks, PhD

- ■ *General Considerations*
- ■ *Muscular Dystrophies*
- ■ *Metabolic Myopathies*
- ■ *Specific Congenital Myopathies*
- ■ *Myotonias*
- ■ *Periodic Paralyses*
- ■ *Endocrine Myopathies*
- ■ *Toxic Myopathies*
- ■ *Inflammatory Myopathies*

Any disorder in which muscle dysfunction arises from some inherent defect in muscle itself or from damage directly to the muscle is termed a ***myopathy***.[1-9] Although disordered muscle function can also occur when the neural elements on which muscle is dependent are disturbed, it is those disturbances that directly afflict muscle that constitute the myopathies. Although the pathogenesis of most of the myopathies is not understood in any great detail, the primary muscle disorders can be classified according to general etiologic categories (Table 13–1).[1-9] It is apparent that muscle function can be disturbed by exogenous influences impinging on the muscle (e.g., physical trauma, toxic substances, infectious organisms, and endocrine and other systemic disorders), as well as by inherited defects in its structure and biochemistry (e.g., muscular dystrophies, congenital myopathies, and metabolic myopathies).

General Considerations

As diverse as the myopathies are, they are expressed clinically by relatively few signs and symptoms.[10-12] Myopathic disease is suggested by complaints of muscle weakness and fatigability, muscle pain, abnormal muscle tone, cramps, and discoloration of urine caused by the presence of myoglobin (myoglobinuria). Of these, the symptom of weakness is by far the most common. Patients usually describe weakness more in terms of its consequences on

Table 13-1. Classes of Human Myopathies

Disorders	Description
Muscular dystrophies	Inherited disorders of unknown etiology characterized by progressive muscular weakness and muscle fiber necrosis
Metabolic myopathies	Inherited disorders characterized by muscle weakness and exercise intolerance, each arising from a distinct enzymatic defect
Congenital myopathies	Inherited disorders presenting from birth with weakness and hypotonia, each defined by distinctive morphologic features
Myotonic myopathies	Inherited disorders characterized by difficulty in relaxing muscle; linked to abnormalities in sarcolemma ionic permeabilities
Periodic paralysis	Inherited and acquired disorders characterized by episodic weakness and flaccid paralysis; often associated with alterations of serum potassium; sarcolemma defects suspected
Endocrine myopathies	Most characterized by proximal muscle weakness and wasting; found in association with both excessive and deficient endocrine function
Toxic myopathies	Muscle weakness and other symptoms reflecting damage to muscle caused by drugs, pollutants, biologic agents, and other compounds; muscle fiber lysis and necrosis may lead to myoglobinuria
Inflammatory myopathies	Diverse group characterized by muscle weakness and evidence of an inflammatory reaction in muscle; precipitated by infectious agents and toxic compounds as well as unknown factors (idiopathic)

their daily activities than in terms of strength. Difficulty in performing common activities such as walking, running, climbing stairs; arising from sitting, kneeling, or reclining; placing objects above the head; and brushing the hair all provide evidence of muscle weakness. The relative scarcity of signs and symptoms in muscle disease makes diagnosis all the more dependent on other types of information, such as genetic history, laboratory findings, muscle biopsy, and electromyography.

The most direct information about whether a neuromuscular condition is primarily a myopathy and, if so, about what specific myopathy is involved, is provided by microscopic study of the structure of the affected muscles. Many basic pathologic reactions of muscle can be discerned by light microscopy, whereas ultrastructural alterations require examination with the electron microscope.[13-17] Compared with the range and diversity of muscle disorders, the specific pathologic changes that occur in the muscle fiber are relatively limited. **Alterations in muscle fiber structure may be grouped into three general categories.**[14,15] **Fiber necrosis** is probably the most common and is the complete destruction of muscle fibers, with intact supporting tissue (Fig. 13-1). As a result of this loss, a cumulative depletion of muscle occurs and less force can be generated when motor units are activated. **Fiber disfiguration** refers to conditions in which the muscle fibers are preserved, but undergo alterations in their morphology. These alterations include excessive numbers of vacuoles (vesicles), abnormal storage of materials such as glycogen or fat, and the deformation or hyperplasia of specific cellular organelles (mitochondria, nuclei, and myofilaments). In some cases, the specific structural abnormality gives the myopathy its name (e.g., glycogen storage disease or central core disease) (Fig. 13-2). Characteristic changes are also observed in **muscle fiber shape and size.**

Grosser abnormalities may also be discerned in the structure and composition of the whole muscle.[12-14] Common alterations are the loss of muscle fibers, changes in the proportion or distribution of specific fiber types (types I or II), an abnormal proliferation of connective tissue, the presence of inflammatory cells, and the deposition of abnormal materials.[13-17] As we shall see in the following discussion, each of these alterations may provide evidence of a specific disorder. Examples are fiber necrosis in the muscular dystrophies, abnormal cellular organelles in the congenital myopathies, accumulation of unused substrate material in the metabolic myopathies, and inflammatory cells in the inflammatory myopathies.

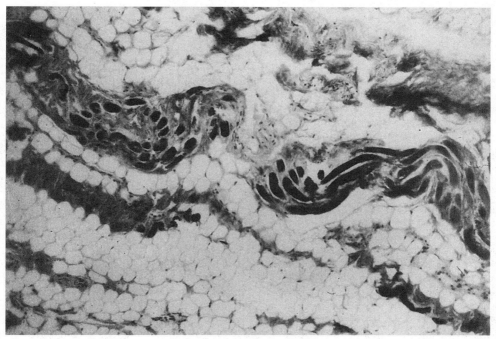

Figure 13–1. *Muscle Fiber Loss in Duchenne's Muscular Dystrophy.* In this longitudinal section of iliopsoas muscle acquired postmortem from a 17-year-old boy who suffered from Duchenne's muscular dystrophy, only a few muscle fibers (*diagonal band of dark cells*) remain in a muscle that has been almost completely replaced by fat (*many white cells*) (×100). Compare this with normal muscle in Figures 2–13 and 2–14. (From Adachi and Sher,[1] p 128, with permission.)

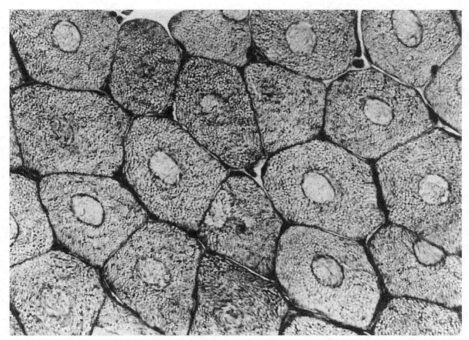

Figure 13–2. *Central Core Disease.* In this quadriceps biopsy specimen from an 11-year-old boy, almost all fibers contain a single central or peripheral "core" devoid of the normal fine sarcoplasmic network (×350). (From Adachi and Sher,[1] p 205, with permission.)

Although much is known about the characteristic pathologic changes that occur in muscle in association with various specific disorders, **relatively little is known of the actual link between these morphologic abnormalities and the physiologic abnormalities of muscle.** Although it is obvious, for example, that the necrosis and loss of muscle fibers that occur in the muscular dystrophies provide an explanation for the muscle weakness associated with these disorders, little is known of the functional significance of most of the morphologic abnormalities of the congenital myopathies. Although the destruction of muscle fibers is the most common process, other pathophysiologic alterations also occur in muscle.[17] For example, **abnormalities of the sarcolemma may prevent the generation of normal action potentials.** An inability to generate action potentials (as in periodic paralysis) may result in weakness, whereas excessive firing of action potentials (as in myotonia) may result in contractions that are excessive or prolonged. **The contractile process itself may be impaired,** in which case the muscle fiber may generate normal action potentials, but may be unable to produce normal contractions. In certain genetic disorders of muscle metabolism, muscle cells are unable to generate sufficient energy for contraction, leading to symptoms of exercise intolerance.

One of the interesting features of the myopathies is that despite the apparent similarity of their structure, **not all muscles are equally susceptible to disease.** In fact, practically no myopathy affects all muscles of the body, and each has as one of its features a selective distribution within the musculature. Even in the muscles involved, not all types of muscle fibers are affected to the same degree.[6,14–16,18] In a number of disorders, the atrophic process, for example, may predominate in either type I or type II muscle fibers.[6,14–16,19] Selective type I fiber atrophy is relatively uncommon, but is apparent in certain congenital myopathies and in myotonic dystrophy. Selective type II atrophy and loss is one of the most common findings in a variety of conditions including polymyositis, Duchenne's muscular dystrophy, various endocrine myopathies, and certain toxic myopathies.

The factors responsible for the selective vulnerability of certain muscles are not known. Often the largest, most proximal muscles are most affected. One might speculate that these muscles are more susceptible because they are used more often and are thus subject to greater metabolic demands. However, muscles innervated by cranial nerves are in constant use (e.g., ocular muscles), but are usually spared. Other possible factors influencing the susceptibility to disease are the size of motor units, metabolic differences (glycolytic versus oxidative), and differences in the pattern of vascular supply.[18]

Normal muscle possesses some capacity for regeneration; therefore, *acute* destructive processes of the muscle fiber (whether toxic, inflammatory, or metabolic) are usually followed by fairly complete regeneration of the muscle cells.[13–16] Unfortunately, many pathologic processes of muscle are *chronic* and progressive and end up destroying muscle fibers completely. Under these conditions, regenerative activity fails to keep pace with the disease, and the loss of muscle fibers is permanent and cumulative.

Muscular Dystrophies

The term **muscular dystrophy** refers to a heterogeneous group of disorders of unknown etiology, which have certain basic features in common.[4–8,20,21] **They are all genetic disorders characterized by simple, progressive weakness caused by degeneration and necrosis of skeletal muscle.** Typically, the muscle involvement is highly selective in the early stages, insidious in onset, and continuously progressive. These diseases are due to pathologic processes occurring almost exclusively in muscle tissue. They can be distinguished from other types of myopathies by the lack of associated conditions such as endocrine abnormality, inflammation, enzyme deficiency, or the specific morphologic changes found in the congenital myopathies.

The classification of the muscular dystrophies has historically been based on a mixture of clinical and genetic criteria (Table 13–2).[4–8,20,21] This method of classification

Table 13–2. *Features of the More Common Muscular Dystrophies*

Type	Features	Other Involvements
X-linked Recessive		
Duchenne's (30 per 100,000 male births)	Progressive weakness of girdle (especially pelvic) muscles apparent by age 4; enlargement of calves; inability to walk by age 11; kyphoscoliosis; respiratory failure in second to third decade	Cardiomyopathy, mental impairment
Becker's (3–6 per 100,000 male births)	Slowly progressive weakness of girdle muscles apparent in early to late childhood; marked enlargement of calves; mobility maintained into fourth decade; respiratory failure after fourth decade; resembles Duchenne's but more benign	Cardiomyopathy (occasional)
Autosomal Dominant		
Myotonic (>10 per 100,000)	Slowly progressive weakness of distal limb, eyelid, facial and neck muscles; onset any decade; myotonia.	Cardiac conduction defects, mental impairment, frontal baldness, cataracts, gonadal atrophy
Fascioscapulohumeral (0.5 per 100,000)	Progressive weakness of shoulder girdle and facial muscles apparent in second to fourth decade; highly variable rate of progression	
Oculopharyngeal (Uncommon)	Ptosis and dysphagia due to slowly progressive weakness of eyelid, extraocular, pharyngeal and tongue muscles apparent in fifth or sixth decade; death from starvation or aspiration pneumonia	
Autosomal Recessive		
Limb-girdle (Uncommon)	Slowly progressive weakness of shoulder and pelvic girdles apparent in early childhood to adult life; severe disability about 20 years after onset; probably encompasses several different recessively inherited disorders	Cardiomyopathy
Childhood (Uncommon)	Pelvic and pectoral girdle weakness similar to Duchenne's but milder and without muscle hypertrophy; apparent by age 5–10; inability to walk by end of second decade	
Congenital (Uncommon)	Present at birth with generalized hypotonic weakness and contractures; may be rapidly progressive (with early death), slowly progressive or stable	

is not entirely satisfactory because some cases do not fit into currently recognized groups and some dystrophies are heterogeneous by clinical, pathologic, and genetic criteria. Currently, increased emphasis is being placed on classification by purely genetic criteria, and as the specific genetic abnormalities underlying these disorders are defined in more detail, this type of classification is likely to predominate.[20] The most common dystrophies are Duchenne's, fascioscapulohumeral, and myotonic forms. The term "limb-girdle muscular dystrophy" is frequently used as a catch-all diagnosis encompassing a number of rather indistinct disorders.[7,20,21] Some syndromes that have been labeled limb-girdle muscular dystrophy have proved to be metabolic or inflammatory myopathies.

Because the inherited defects of dystrophic muscle have not been identified to any great extent, the pathogenesis of most of the muscular dystrophies is only superficially understood. **The decline in strength so characteristic of muscular dystrophies is due to a depletion of muscle fibers resulting from the cumulative necrosis of these cells.**[13–16,20,21] Despite a muscle's capacity for repair and regeneration, this necrotic process can eventually lead to the virtual disappearance of all muscle fibers and their replacement by fat cells and fibrous connective tissue (see Fig. 13–1). What actually causes muscle cell deterioration and death is not known.

Considerable insight into the pathogenesis of muscular dystrophy has been gained recently from extensive study of the closely related Duchenne's and Becker's muscular dystrophies.[4,14,20,22–27] It is now known that both of these forms of muscular dystrophy are caused by **genetic defects that lead to deficiency of a membrane protein called *dystrophin.*** Dystrophin is encoded by a large gene on the X chromosome. This protein is closely associated with the inner surface of the sarcolemma, particularly in the areas of the neuromuscular and musculotendinous junctions, and is necessary for sarcolemmal integrity. Immunocytochemical studies have shown that in almost all Duchenne's muscular dystrophy patients, dystrophin is markedly reduced or absent in nearly all muscle fibers. In patients with Becker's muscular dystrophy, dystrophin is present but is reduced or abnormal.[26] Electron microscopy reveals distinct lesions in the dystrophic sarcolemma, which ultimately lead to cellular necrosis. The exact link, however, between the dystrophin deficiency and the destruction of the muscle fiber is not known. Because dystrophin, together with other cytoskeleton proteins, provides mechanical support for the sarcolemma, a reduction in the amount of dystrophin or alterations in its properties may lead to structural weakness of the cell membrane and make the cell vulnerable to rupture under mechanical stress.[22,27] This relative fragility may explain the preferential involvement in these dystrophies of the muscles and muscle fiber types (i.e., fast-twitch) that are subject to the greatest mechanical stresses.

The basic clinical picture associated with all the muscular dystrophies is one of simple, progressive muscle weakness. The various specific forms of muscular dystrophy differ from one another largely in the distribution of this weakness, the age of onset rate of progression of the weakness, and the involvement of other organ systems. The predominant features of the most clearly defined syndromes are summarized in Table 13–2.[4–8,20,21] Among these, the most severe is Duchenne's muscular dystrophy, which is seen in very early childhood, is rapidly incapacitating, and is usually fatal by the late teens or early 20s (Fig. 13–3). Other dystrophies may be benign, with late onset, limited muscle involvement, and slow progression. These may result in little disability and not affect life span. In most of the dystrophies, the proximal muscles are the most noticeably involved, with sparing of distal and cranial nerve muscles. Myotonic dystrophy is a conspicuous exception, afflicting predominantly distal limb muscles, as well as eyelid, facial, and neck muscles. It is also notable in the extensive involvement of other systems.

Duchenne's Muscular Dystrophy

Duchenne's muscular dystrophy is by far the most severe of these dystrophic disorders. This disease presents early in childhood and is characterized by rapid, relentless progression to severe disability and early death.[4–8,21–24] After this disorder is clinically evident, patients require aggressive, lifelong treatment. Because Duchenne's muscular dystrophy requires so much rehabilitative effort and embodies so well the devastating functional consequences of progressive muscular weakness, it is useful to discuss it in some detail.

Although pathologic changes are evident within in utero and neonatal skeletal muscle, Duchenne's muscular dystrophy usually remains unnoticed until early childhood. Delayed motor development is common, and about 50% of affected patients are unable to walk at 18 months. Between 3 and 6 years of age, progressive muscle weakness becomes apparent in impaired motor activity; it may also be demonstrated by manual muscle testing. At this time, weakness is primarily proximal, with the muscles of the lower extremities and torso being more affected than those of the upper extremities. Early clinical features include difficulty with running, jumping, and climbing stairs, a lordotic waddling gait, toe walking, and a

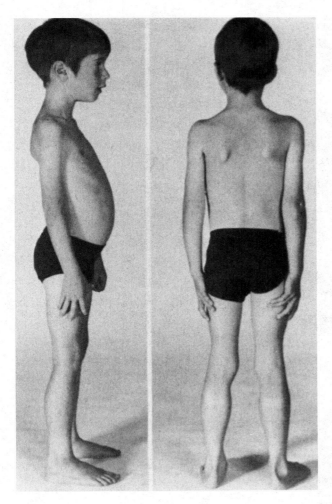

Figure 13–3. *Duchenne's Muscular Dystrophy in a 6-Year-Old Boy.* Note the typical lordotic posture, enlargement of the calves, and early winging of the scapulae. (From Asbury, AK, McKhann, GM, and McDonald, WI (eds): Diseases of the Nervous System. Clinical Neurobiology, vol 1, ed 2. WB Saunders, Philadelphia, 1992, p 167, with permission.)

tendency to fall. A valuable clinical sign is Gowers' maneuver (Fig. 13–4). In this maneuver, the child arising from a position on the floor turns into a prone position, assumes a quadriped stance, and gradually "walks" his or her hands up the legs to stabilize the quadriceps weakness before being able to extend the back. By the time the child is 5 or 6 years of age, calf hypertrophy is almost always present and other muscles such as gluteus, lateral vastus, and deltoids may also be enlarged. Later, calf enlargement is called **pseudohypertrophy**, since muscle is replaced by fat and connective tissue.

When the child is between 6 and 11 years of age, the strength of limb and torso muscles steadily decreases. Deterioration may be particularly rapid following immobilization in bed (even for short periods of time) because of respiratory infection, fracture, or orthopedic surgery. Walking usually requires the use of braces. With increasing but uneven weakness of agonists and antagonists, joint contractures develop, particularly in iliotibial bands, hip flexors, and heel cords. By age 12, most patients are dependent upon a wheelchair. During the second decade of life, and especially after ambulation is lost, all limb and torso muscles further deteriorate. Increasing weakness of the upper extremities also becomes apparent. This weakness may preclude crutch-assisted ambulation and eventually limits activities involving hand and forearm muscles. Paraspinal weakness produces progressive kyphoscoliosis (Fig. 13–5). The chest deformity associated with scoliosis further impairs

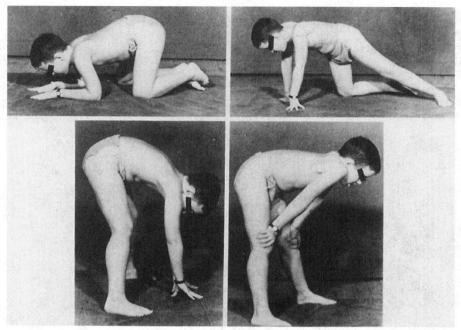

Figure 13–4.   *The Gowers' Maneuver.* The Gowers' maneuver is used to compensate for weakness in the pelvic girdle and is an important clinical sign in disorders creating proximal weakness. As the patient arises from the floor, he "walks" his hands up his legs thereby utilizing his upper body strength to stabilize his lower extremities. (From Lovell, WW and Winter, RB (eds): Pediatric Orthopaedics, ed 2. JB Lippincott, Philadelphia, 1986, p 265, with permission.)

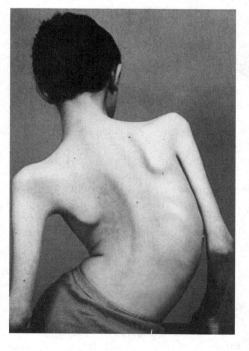
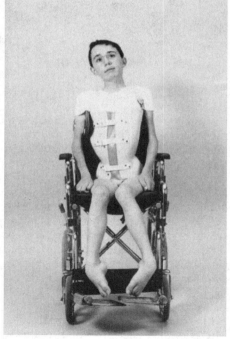

Figure 13-5.   *Advanced Duchenne's Muscular Dystrophy.* A 15-year-old boy with severe scoliosis and equinovarus deformity of the feet. Fair improvement in the scoliosis, which was still relatively mobile, was achieved with a well-fitting spinal brace. (From Dubowitz, V: Color Atlas of Muscle Disorders in Childhood. Year Book Medical Publishers, Inc., Chicago, 1989, p 23, with permission.)

pulmonary function, which is already diminished by weakness of the respiratory muscles. Death occurs in the late teens or early 20s. The most common cause of death is respiratory failure, although patients occasionally die from complications of cardiomyopathy.

The average IQ of patients with Duchenne's muscular dystrophy is 15 to 20 points lower than that of the normal population. Deficits are apparent in both verbal comprehension and expressive language.

Other Muscular Dystrophies

Other forms of muscular dystrophy also present with muscle weakness, but few are as severe or have as early an onset as Duchenne's muscular dystrophy. In **Becker's muscular dystrophy**, the genetics, clinical features, and management principles are basically the same as those for Duchenne's, except that the disease is milder and its progression is slower.[4-8,21-24,26] The incidence of Becker's is about 10% of that of Duchenne's. Most patients present between the ages of 5 to 25 years, with pelvic girdle weakness associated with a waddling gait and difficulty in running and climbing stairs. Significant contractures, scoliosis, and respiratory insufficiency are uncommon, and, except for those with fatal cardiomyopathy, the life span of a patient with Becker's muscular dystrophy is usually normal.

Fascioscapulohumeral muscular dystrophy, which is the most common of the dominantly inherited dystrophies, is a relatively slowly progressing disorder, which is extremely variable in its severity and age of onset.[4-8,21] Onset is commonly in the third or fourth decade. As the name implies, there is characteristic weakness of facial, shoulder girdle, and proximal arm muscles (Fig. 13–6). Muscle may be only mildly affected for many years. Scapular winging, sloping shoulders, and difficulty raising the arms over the head reflect weakness of serratus anterior, trapezius, rhomboid, and deltoid muscles. Facial weakness may be an early feature of the disease, causing an expressionless face and a sullen appearance. Except for early-onset cases, fascioscapulohumeral muscular dystrophy rarely leads to severe disability before the fourth or fifth decade and is associated with a relatively normal life span.

Myotonic muscular dystrophy, which is the most prevalent of the adult muscular dystrophies, is discussed later in this chapter in the section on myotonias.

Treatment of Muscular Dystrophies

There is no specific treatment for any of the muscular dystrophies. Therapy to prevent contractures and maintain ambulation, orthoses, and corrective orthopedic surgery can be used to maintain function and quality of life.[29-31] For management purposes, it may be useful to classify neuromuscular patients into three clinical stages, all of which are typically seen in Duchenne's muscular dystrophy (Table 13–3).[31] With proper treatment and support in each stage, these patients can remain active and have the most comfortable and productive life possible. The cardiac conduction defects in certain dystrophies may require medical treatment. The myotonia in myotonic dystrophy is rarely a clinical problem, but can be treated pharmacologically. Preventive treatment consists of prenatal diagnosis in families with known pedigrees, carrier detection, and genetic counseling. Discovery of the gene for the protein (dystrophin), which is lacking or abnormal in those with Duchenne's and Becker's muscular dystrophies, has raised the hope that **new therapeutic approaches may be developed which can restore the genetic capability of the dystrophic muscle cell.**[32-34]

There are two likely therapeutic approaches. The first involves the transfer of normal myogenic cells (myoblasts) into dystrophin-deficient muscle. The objective is to have the normal myoblasts fuse with the deficient muscle fibers. The dystrophin encoded by the

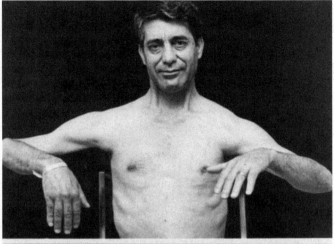
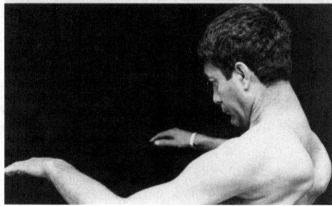

Figure 13–6. Fascioscapulo-humeral Muscular Dystrophy. This patient with fascioscapulohumeral muscular dystrophy has a typical shoulder girdle abnormality with elevation and winging of the scapulae on abduction of the arms, as well as facial weakness. (From Engel and Banker,[17] p 1254; with permission.)

Table 13–3. *Management Principles for Neuromuscular Disease*

Ambulatory Stage

Early establishment of the diagnosis and genetic counseling
Early and informed counseling and psychologic support to prevent counterproductive family psychodynamics, to encourage goal-oriented activities, and to prepare the patient and family for current and future therapeutic interventions (the advantages of early intervention during each stage should be stressed)
Early management of musculotendinous contractures and decreased pulmonary compliance
Appropriate use of supportive physical and occupational therapy and possibly splinting and therapeutic exercise
Prolongation of ambulation by the above plus possibly surgical musculotendinous releases and lower extremity bracing
Monitoring for and prevention of cardiac complications

Wheelchair-Dependent Stage

Facilitation of activities of daily living independence with assistive devices
Early prevention or correction of back deformity
Ongoing monitoring for and management of cardiac insufficiency
Maintenance of pulmonary compliance and alveolar ventilation

Stage of Prolonged Survival

Patient instruction and encouragement for taking responsibility for management decisions and directing his or her caregivers
Facilitation of activities of daily living independence with assistive devices
Early and appropriate introduction of noninvasive respiratory muscle aids to assist alveolar ventilation and clear airway secretions

From Bach and Lieberman,[31] p 1100, with permission.

normal nuclei might then rescue the dystrophic fibers. Although none of the patients treated to date with myoblast transplant therapy has suffered adverse reactions, the effectiveness of this treatment has been disappointing, as judged by muscle force generation or dystrophin content. Limitations are imposed on this form of therapy by immunologic and tissue barriers, the low fusion rate of implanted cells, and the inaccessibility of many muscles.[29–31] The second possibility is to bring about gene transfer through a viral vector. Retroviral or adenoviral vectors are current possibilities. The first experimental results in mice are encouraging, but the efficiency and safety of this technique will have to be carefully examined before human studies are attempted. As advances in our understanding of the genetic bases of these disorders are made, it is likely that effective genetic therapy will become available.

Metabolic Myopathies

The term *metabolic myopathy* **refers to a group of myopathies in which specific defects in muscle metabolism occur.**[4–8,35–42] **Typically, a single enzymatic defect is involved.** In most cases, **these are genetic disorders,** although the mode of genetic transmission and expression varies. While these are some of the rarest of all the disorders of muscle function, they are of great interest to muscle physiologists because of what they can reveal about the link between muscle metabolism and contraction.

Metabolic defects in skeletal muscle give rise to muscle weakness, as well as exercise-related symptoms.[35–42] Exercise-induced muscle pain, stiffness, contractures, and fatigue, which may be accompanied by myoglobinuria, are common features. The muscle weakness may resemble in its progression or distribution other neuromuscular disorders, such as muscular dystrophy, polymyositis, or neuropathy. The skeletal muscle signs and symptoms of these disorders manifest at varying ages. Symptoms vary markedly in their severity, with early onset often indicating the worst prognosis. In some infantile forms, metabolic defects are fatal. Death, as with other neuromuscular disorders, usually results from pneumonia and respiratory failure. Treatment of patients with metabolic myopathies revolves around offsetting the effects of muscle weakness and minimizing the debilitating effects of exercise. It is interesting that in some cases dietary supplementation with specific substrates seems to induce some clinical improvement. Although these metabolic defects are in some instances largely restricted to skeletal muscle, other organ systems are often affected. Cardiac, hepatic, and central nervous system pathologies are common, creating their own clinical problems.

The metabolic myopathies all are characterized by a deficiency of some critical enzyme of energy metabolism. Accordingly, the **histopathologic hallmark of these disorders is an abnormal accumulation within the cell of unmetabolized substrate, such as glycogen or lipid** (Fig. 13–7).[14–16] Although these substances often accumulate in abnormal cellular vacuoles, they may also accumulate in various cytoplasmic locations, such as between myofibrils or adjacent to the sarcolemma. Their accumulation may be great enough to compress and distort the myofibrils and other cellular structures. Specific enzyme deficiencies are revealed with special histochemical stains. Although ultrastructural (i.e., electron microscopic) studies are rarely needed for diagnosis, they are useful in revealing subtle abnormalities of cell morphology.

Diagnosis of the metabolic myopathies is made on the basis of clinical findings, enzyme assays, histologic findings, and special histochemical stains used to identify specific metabolites or the lack of particular enzymes. During the last decade, considerable progress has been made in defining the specific metabolic errors underlying these disorders. **With few exceptions, these involve key reactions in the pathways of muscle energy production.**[35–40] Defects have been revealed in the cytosolic and lysosomal enzyme systems, as well as within the metabolic processes of the mitochondria.

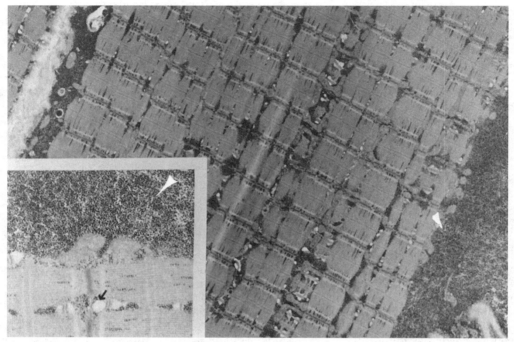

Figure 13–7. *Glycogen Storage Disease.* Electron micrograph of this phosphorylase-deficient muscle shows glycogen accumulation (*white arrow*) at the periphery of the muscle fiber (×600). Inset: sarcoplasmic reticulum (*black arrow*) is dilated in those fibrils next to a pool of glycogen (×20,000). (From Engel and Banker,[17] p 1591, with permission.)

Abnormalities of Glycogen Metabolism (Glycogenoses)

The metabolism of glycogen and glucose is a major source of energy for muscle contraction (see Chapter 2). Defects throughout this cascade of enzymes and substrates have been identified in a variety of tissues, including heart, liver, and muscle (Fig. 13–8). Skeletal muscle is affected to some extent in most of these disorders. In some of these, the enzymatic defect is found only in muscle (types V, VII, X, and XI).[35] In other disorders, the enzymatic defect is more generalized, and symptoms arising in other systems predominate, especially in the liver.

Specifically, **nine well-defined hereditary enzyme defects of glycogen metabolism or glycolysis are thought to affect muscle** (Table 13–4).[35,37,39,40] Of these, **six adversely affect glycogen breakdown or glycolysis.** Impaired energy production by carbohydrate metabolism is the usual consequence of these enzyme defects, and **the associated clinical picture is usually one of exercise intolerance with myalgia, cramps, and myoglobinuria.**

Abnormalities of Mitochondrial Metabolism

The oxidative metabolism of pyruvate, fatty acids, and amino acids that occurs in the mitochondria is an important source of energy in muscle. Mitochondria can quickly produce energy linked to adenosine triphosphate (ATP) from all the primary foodstuffs (carbohydrates, fats, and proteins) and can maintain the provision of this energy for long periods of time. The **mitochondrial myopathies are** a clinically and biochemically heterogeneous group of disorders **characterized by structurally or functionally abnormal mitochondria.**[5,6,35–41] The result is impaired mitochondrial energy production. Although such mitochondrial defects may be limited to a single tissue such as muscle, liver, or heart, multiple systems are often involved in creating diverse clinical findings. There is little consistent correlation

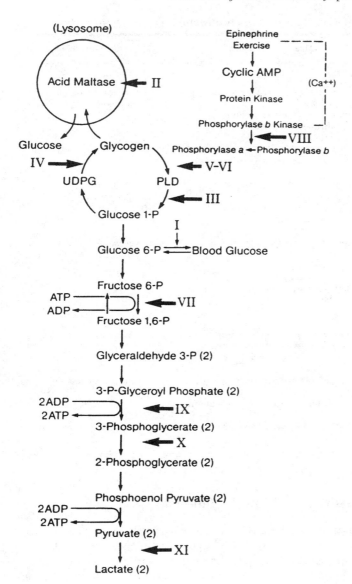

Figure 13–8. *Schematic Representation of Glycogen Metabolism and Glycolysis.* The arrows point to the sites of documented enzyme defects, and roman numerals refer to diseases. I: Glucose-6-phosphatase. II: Acid maltase. III: Debrancher. IV: Brancher. V: Muscle phosphorylase. VI: Liver phosphorylase. VII: Muscle phosphofructokinase. VIII: Liver and muscle phosphorylase kinase. IX: Phosphoglycerate kinase. X: Phosphoglycerate mutase. XI: Lactate dehydrogenase. (From Di-Mauro, S, et al: Metabolic myopathies. Am J Med Genet 25:635, 1986, with permission.)

between the clinical and biochemical features of the known mitochondrial disorders, so diagnosis rests strongly on morphologic evidence of abnormal mitochondria.[35] Increased size, excessive numbers, structural changes, and clumping of mitochondria all have been described.[5,6,13–16,35,36] Mitochondrial abnormalities have also been observed in an assortment of other muscular diseases, in which they may represent changes secondary to a primary pathology (e.g., muscular dystrophy, polymyositis, or other metabolic myopathies).

Although discussion of the details of mitochondrial oxidative metabolism is beyond the scope of this chapter, **the biochemical abnormalities of the mitochondrial myopathies can be divided into three broad categories.**[4,35,39–41] Defects in substrate utilization (e.g., lipid or pyruvate) predominantly affect the central nervous system, creating disturbances of motor control and seizures. The most severe deficits manifest in infancy as rapidly progressive and fatal encephalopathy. **Defects in the respiratory enzyme cascade** (respiratory chain) are probably the most common. Finally, a few cases have been described in which the primary **defect is in the phosphorylation system.**

Table 13–4. *Disorders of Glycogen and Glucose Metabolism Affecting Muscle*

Metabolic Defect	Muscle Involvement	Other Involvement
Acid maltase (type II)		
Infantile onset	Severe progressive weakness and hypotonia	Liver, heart; fatal due to cardiorespiratory failure
Childhood onset	Proximal weakness resembling Duchenne's muscular dystrophy; respiratory insufficiency	
Adult onset	Slowly progressive limb girdle (pelvic) weakness; respiratory insufficiency	
Debranching enzyme (type III)		
Infantile onset	Hypotonia and mild weakness	Liver; fasting hypoglycemia
Adult onset	Slowly progressive weakness of legs and hands; distal wasting	Heart
Branching enzyme (type IV)		
Infantile onset	Hypotonia, weakness, and muscle wasting	Liver pathology; may culminate in liver failure
Myophosphorylase (type V)		
Childhood onset	Exercise-induced cramps, myalgia, fatigue and myoglobinuria; mild weakness	
Phosphofructokinase (type VII)		
Childhood onset	Exercise-induced cramps, myalgia and fatigue; occasional myoglobinuria	Hemolysis
Phosphorylase kinase (type VIII)	Exercise intolerance and myoglobinuria	Liver
Phosphoglycerate kinase (type IX)	Exercise intolerance and myoglobinuria	Hemolytic anemia
Phosphoglycerate mutase (type X)	Exercise intolerance and myoglobinuria	
Lactate dehydrogenase (type XI)	Exercise intolerance and myoglobinuria	

Abnormalities of Lipid Metabolism

Fat is an important substrate for mitochondrial oxidative metabolism. In fact, at rest, fatty acid oxidation provides more than 50% of the energy needs of mammalian skeletal muscle. During fasting or prolonged exercise, fatty acid becomes even more indispensable. The transport of fatty acids into the mitochondria is dependent on their reaction with the substance carnitine—a reaction catalyzed by carnitine palmityl transferase. Carnitine is distributed in all tissues except the brain and is derived from both dietary sources and liver synthesis. **Several deficiencies in carnitine or carnitine palmityltransferase have been identified, which affect skeletal muscle.**[35–40] These myopathies are characterized morphologically by the accumulation of lipid droplets within the muscle fiber.[14–16,36] Lipid deposition may also occur in muscle fibers in a number of other neuromuscular disorders.

Carnitine deficiency occurs in both systemic and myopathic forms.[5,6,35,39,40] The myopathic forms usually present clinically in childhood and are characterized by slowly progressive muscle weakness, exertional myalgia, and episodic myoglobinuria. **Carnitine palmityltransferase** deficiency is associated with recurrent myalgia and myoglobinuria that may be precipitated by prolonged exercise (not necessarily of high intensity) or by fasting. Muscle weakness or fatigability is not a typical feature. This deficiency affects primarily type I fibers, whereas the pathology of the glycogenoses predominates among type II fibers. These carnitine defects might alternately be classified with the mitochondrial defects, since they disturb substrate (fatty acid) utilization by the mitochondria.

Abnormalities of Adenine Nucleotide Metabolism

Myoadenylate deaminase is a major enzyme of the purine nucleotide cycle and is important for muscle energy production. **Myoadenylate deaminase deficiency may be the most common of the known muscle enzyme deficiencies**, with an incidence in most studies of about 2%.[4,39,40,42] Most reported cases are first seen in childhood or early adulthood with exercise intolerance characterized by fatigability, cramps, or myalgia. Myoglobinuria is uncommon.

Myoadenylate deaminase deficiency has also been reported in association with an assortment of other neuromuscular disorders, including inflammatory myopathies, periodic paralysis, motor neuron disease, muscular dystrophies, other metabolic myopathies, certain congenital myopathies, and myasthenia gravis.[35,40] The association of this defect with such a diversity of clinical scenarios makes it somewhat difficult to determine its actual pathogenic significance.

Specific Congenital Myopathies

Strictly speaking, a congenital myopathy is any primary disease of muscle that is present from birth. Practically, however, the term *congenital myopathy* **refers to a group of rare disorders that present from birth with muscle weakness and hypotonia and may be defined by one or more distinctive morphologic features** (Table 13–5; see Fig. 13–2).[4–8,13–16,43–48] The congenital myopathy designation remains somewhat vague, and with the continued development of modern histochemical and electron microscopy techniques this group continues to expand. Although a number of these congenital myopathies have been repeatedly described and may now be considered firmly established clinical entities, others are based on a description of an individual patient or a few members of a single family and remain to be confirmed by additional observations.[44]

The congenital myopathies typically are seen in early childhood with muscle weakness and significant hypotonia.[43–46] This weakness is symmetric and affects predominantly the limb girdles and proximal limb muscles (Fig. 13–9), although in some infants, the weakness may be generalized. Weakness of the cranial nerve muscles is not a common feature, but there are instances in which these muscles are conspicuously affected. **Affected infants**

Table 13–5. *Principal Congenital Myopathies*

Myopathy	Characteristic Clinical Features	Muscle Biopsy Abnormalities
Central core disease	Dominant or sporadic trait; congenital dislocation of hip	Central area of fiber devoid of mitochondria; myofibril disruption variable
Multicore (minicore) disease	Nonprogressive proximal weakness; neck muscle weakness	Multiple small areas of severe filament disruption devoid of mitochondrial enzymes
Nemaline	Dominant or autosomal-recessive trait; skeletal dysmorphism; respiratory problems	Rodlike expansions of Z band
Myotubular (centronuclear)	Ptosis; weak external ocular muscles; usually dominant with variable penetrance	Most fibers with one or more central nuclei
Congenital fiber-type disproportion	Variable clinical features; muscle contractures; congenital dislocation of hips	Type I fibers smaller than type II; increased variability in fiber diameter

Adapted from Swash and Schwartz,[7] p 318, with permission.

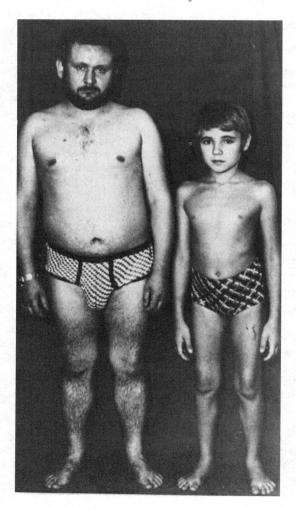

Figure 13–9. Central Core Disease. An 11-year-old boy and his 30-year-old father, both of whom are affected with central core disease. Each had proximal muscle weakness and biopsy specimens revealed multiple central cores (see Fig. 13–2). (From Adachi and Sher,[1] 1990, p 204, with permission.)

usually show reduced spontaneous movements (foreshadowed by reduced in utero activity), **and as these children mature their attainment of motor development milestones is often delayed.** Deep tendon reflexes are almost always decreased or absent. Muscle bulk is normal or somewhat diminished. In some cases, contractures may develop involving multiple joints. **The congenital myopathies are typified clinically by a nonprogressive or slowly progressive course,** with a generally benign prognosis. A few exceptions do exist in which the severity of muscle involvement is so great that patients succumb to respiratory failure. Often the congenital myopathies are accompanied by certain somatic features, such as ptosis, or skeletal deformities, such as kyphoscoliosis, pigeon chest, elongated facies, dislocated hips, and a high arched palate.[46–48]

Because the congenital myopathies have so many clinical features in common and share clinical features with other disorders, it is difficult to distinguish one from the other or from other motor disorders on clinical grounds alone.[45] The congenital myopathies may resemble, for example, an early-onset muscular dystrophy. Hypotonia and diminished spontaneous movements are also found in infants suffering from a number of nonneuromuscular problems, including asphyxia, systemic diseases, and developmental conditions of the central nervous system. The most accurate means of diagnosis of a congenital myopathy is is the study of muscle biopsy material with histochemical and electron microscopic techniques and the delineation of distinct morphologic abnormalities.[13–16,46–48] Even so, these morphologic features are not specific and may be evident in many diverse clinical conditions. Moreover, disease-related structural abnormalities may occur in one muscle of an affected patient, but not in others, or they may be encountered in one clinically affected patient, but not in another clinically affected member of the same patient's family. One of the conceptual problems with the congenital myopathies is that although many distinct morphologic features have been discerned, it is not yet possible to attribute any specific functional or pathogenic significance to these features. When the functional defects in these muscle fibers are better understood, a better scheme for their identification and classification will probably emerge.

Myotonias

Myotonia is defined as an involuntary, temporary stiffness of muscle, which may follow a voluntary contraction or contraction induced by electrical or mechanical stimulation.[4-8,49-55] Repeated use of a muscle ("warming up") generally leads to some relief of the stiffness, although after rest, the myotonia often returns. The severity of myotonia is heightened by cold and emotion, as well as by other factors, so the symptoms tend to vary considerably from day to day or even from hour to hour. Any muscle may be affected, including those of the trunk and face, and the degree of involvement can vary widely in different muscle groups. Patients with myotonia often show considerable muscle hypertrophy, possibly owing to excessive muscle use.

Clinically, myotonia is best demonstrated as a slowness in relaxation of the grip or by a persistent dimpling after percussion of a muscle belly. When an affected patient grasps an object, he or she has difficulty in letting go and the fingers uncurl slowly (Fig. 13–10). A brisk tap to muscle (e.g., to the thenar eminence or tongue) can evoke a persistent contraction or formation of a dimple, which slowly disappears (Fig. 13–11). Myotonia can be distinguished both clinically and electrophysiologically from such phenomena as tetany, the electrically silent contractures of McArdle's disease, or the prolongation of contraction in hypothyroidism. Considerable evidence suggests that the **myotonias are due to abnormalities in various ion channels and permeabilities in the muscle cell membrane, which result in the excessive firing of action potentials.**[50,52,55] In at least one distinct group of myotonias (e.g., recessive myotonia congenita), the fundamental electrophysiologic defect appears to be a reduction in membrane chloride conductance, which promotes T-tubular and sarcolemmal depolarization. In other disturbances, membrane hyperexcitability and repetitive action potentials probably arise from a number of abnormalities in sodium or potassium channels. Whatever the mechanism, myotonia is clearly caused by abnormality of muscle itself, since it persists after nerve or neuromuscular junction blockade.

Myotonia is a principal presentation in several disorders varying widely in their inheritance, pathology, and prognosis. These include myotonic dystrophy, myotonia congenita, and paramyotonia congenita. Myotonia, indistinguishable from that found in these disorders, also occurs as a reaction to several classes of drugs and other chemicals.

Myotonic Dystrophy

Myotonic dystrophy is the most common and most serious of the myotonic disorders. It is also the most prevalent of the adult muscular dystrophies, as well as one of the most common of all neuromuscular disorders. Its incidence is about 15 in 100,000 live births.[4-8,49,51,54,55] **Myotonic dystrophy is a multisystem disease affecting a variety of tissues in addition to skeletal muscle.** The disease is inherited in an autosomal-dominant pattern. Although the symptoms can become apparent in infancy, patients usually first present with myotonia and muscle weakness in early adult life. The **early involvement of cranial muscles and distal limb muscles** is very different from that observed in other

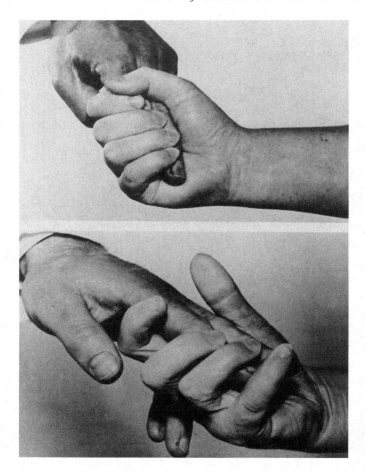

Figure 13–10. Grip Myotonia in Myotonic Dystrophy. A firm grip followed by an inability to let go rapidly will reveal active myotonia. (From Engel and Banker,[17] p 1270, with permission.)

muscular dystrophies. Weakness and atrophy of facial muscles, slurred speech, and ptosis may often be present for many years before diagnosis. Sternocleidomastoid weakness and wasting are prominent, especially in contrast to the well-preserved posterior neck muscles and shoulder girdle. Limb involvement in the early stages is usually slight and, in contrast to the other major muscular dystrophies, is most prominent distally.

The late occurrence of proximal limb weakness is a major factor enabling many patients with myotonic dystrophy to remain ambulatory throughout life. The myotonia accompanying the muscle weakness is perceived as stiffness but is seldom a source of patient complaint; it is most evident in the hands and the tongue. Generalized myotonia is unusual in myotonic dystrophy and is more common (and more severe) in myotonia congenita. Patients with myotonic dystrophy have a characteristic haggard appearance caused by frontal baldness, ptosis, sagging of the lower jaw, and marked atrophy of the temporal, masseter, and sternocleidomastoid muscles (Fig. 13–12). To one degree or another, this appearance may be shared by numerous family members (Fig. 13–13).

Few neuromuscular diseases involve such a variety of systems as does myotonic dystrophy. Associated abnormalities are cardiac conduction defects, respiratory insufficiency with esophageal and diaphragmatic involvement, dysfunction of smooth muscle throughout the gastrointestinal tract, testicular atrophy, cataracts, early frontal baldness, mental retardation, and personality abnormalities.[4–8,49,51–54]

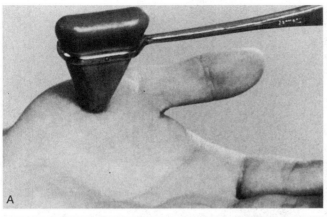

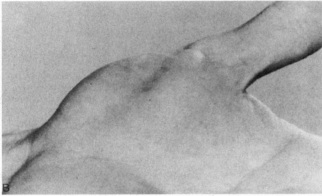

Figure 13–11. *Percussion Myotonia.* (A) When the thenar muscle group is percussed, (B) prolonged muscle contraction and delayed relaxation are evident. (From Riggs,[5] p 459, with permission.)

The disease is marked by slow, steady progression, with most patients becoming severely disabled and unable to walk by the fourth or fifth decade. Death usually occurs in the fifth or sixth decade due to cardiac failure, cardiac arrhythmias, or respiratory failure. Cardiac involvement as a frequent cause of death is not necessarily confined to patients with the most severe motor disability.

Myotonia Congenita

Myotonia congenita is an inherited disorder, which occurs in either an autosomal-dominant or recessive form.[4–8,49–53] In the **dominant form (*Thomsen's disease*),** the onset of myotonia is usually in infancy, but it may be delayed until late childhood. The myotonia is more widespread than in myotonic dystrophy and causes a generalized, painless stiffness accentuated by rest and cold and improved with use. Symptoms may be most prominent in the hands, legs, and eyelids. Diffuse muscle hypertrophy is common. Weakness is minimal. The myotonic symptoms do not progress and may improve as the subject ages. Life expectancy is normal, and no associated abnormalities are noted in other organ systems. In the **recessive form of myotonia congenita (*Becker's type*),** the myotonic symptoms are similar but somewhat later in onset (rarely before age 3 years), tend to be more severe, and are associated with mild muscle weakness and atrophy. Muscle hypertrophy may be striking (see Fig. 12–2) and is more marked than is seen in Thomsen's disease. In myotonia congenita, unlike in myotonic dystrophy, it is myotonia, not weakness, that can be disabling.

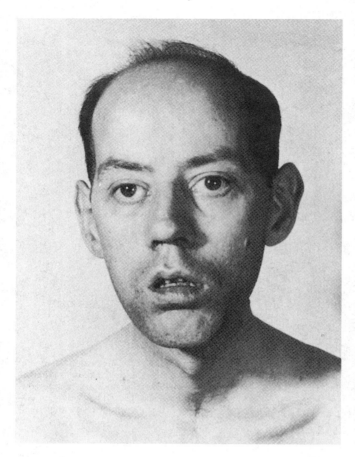

Figure 13–12. *Myotonic Muscular Dystrophy.* This 32-year-old patient demonstrates typical features of myotonic dystrophy, including frontal baldness; an elongated face; temporal, masseter, and sternocleidomastoid wasting; sagging of the jaw; and drooping of the lower lip. (From Asbury, AK, McKhann, GM, and McDonald, WI (eds): Diseases of the Nervous System. Clinical Neurobiology, vol 1, ed 2. WB Saunders, Philadelphia, 1992, p 172, with permission.)

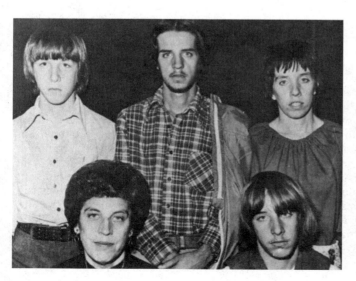

Figure 13–13. *Family with Myotonic Dystrophy.* This mother and her four children were all unaware that they had myotonic dystrophy until one of her sons (*Center*) sought medical attention for cramping of the hands. Typical features such as elongated face, temporal and masseter wasting, and a narrow neck are evident. (From Vinken, PJ and Bruyn, GW (eds): Handbook of Clinical Neurology, vol 40. Diseases of Muscle. Part I. North-Holland Publishing Company, Amsterdam, 1979, p 304, with permission.)

Paramyotonia Congenita

Paramyotonia congenita is an inherited (autosomal-dominant) condition that resembles myotonia congenita, but is unique in the extent to which the myotonia is induced or exaggerated by exposure to cold.[4-8,49-53,56] Paramyotonia is also aggravated rather than relieved by physical activity. Those affected also may suffer episodes of flaccid muscle weakness similar to the weakness seen in familial periodic paralysis. Generalized muscle hypertrophy and, in long-standing cases, permanent weakness may develop.

Periodic Paralyses

The periodic paralyses are a group of disorders characterized by recurrent episodes of weakness or flaccid paralysis often associated with alterations of serum potassium.[5,6,50,51,56-54] Although several different forms of this syndrome have been identified, they all have certain clinical features in common. Symptoms usually begin early in life, rarely after age 25; attacks typically follow rest or sleep and seldom occur in the midst of vigorous activity. Strength between episodes is usually normal or near normal, but after years of attacks a progressive weakness may develop. Although the various forms of periodic paralysis are similar, they differ somewhat in age of onset, the frequency and severity of attacks, and the factors precipitating their occurrence.

Although the pathophysiology of the periodic paralyses is not completely understood, it is evident that **the muscle cells are electrically inexcitable during an attack** and that the decrease in muscle strength is directly proportional to this loss of excitability.[50,56] **The immediate cause of this is a prolonged hypopolarization of the cell membrane,** which makes the cell unable to generate and propagate an action potential.[50,56-59] The exact physiologic events leading to this depolarization are not known and may vary among the different forms of this disease.

The periodic paralyses can be separated by etiology into *primary* **types that are genetic** (autosomal dominant), which are associated with shifts of potassium from one body compartment to another, **and** *secondary* **types, which are acquired** and which are associated with sporadic alterations of *total* body potassium.

Historically, **the primary (genetic) disorders have been divided into hypokalemic, hyperkalemic, and normokalemic forms,** depending on the changes in serum potassium that accompany the attacks.[5,6,8,56-59] In patients with **hypokalemic** periodic paralysis, the clearest link exists between muscle symptoms and alterations in serum potassium concentrations.[57] The drop in serum potassium accompanying the attacks primarily reflects a shift of potassium from the small extracellular pool into the cell. This may reduce serum potassium to as low as 1.5 mEq/L. Attacks may be initiated by factors that promote this shift, such as injection of insulin, epinephrine, glucocorticoids, or glucose, or they may follow ingestion of a meal high in carbohydrates. The attacks of periodic paralysis associated with **hyperkalemia** are briefer, milder, and less frequent than those associated with hypokalemia and are often accompanied by myotonia. The designation as hyperkalemic, however, is misleading, since patients' plasma values are often within normal limits or only slightly hyperkalemic during these attacks. Within this group, attacks may usually be provoked by potassium administration, so "potassium-sensitive" may better define these patients. Patients in the **normokalemic** group resemble the hyperkalemic group except that serum potassium is not increased even in the most severe attacks. Like the hyperkalemics, they are sensitive to potassium administration. The so-called hyperkalemic and normokalemic forms of this disorder may actually be the same disorder.[5,6,50,56]

Patients with **secondary acquired periodic paralysis** usually suffer from total body potassium depletion resulting from renal, endocrine, or gastrointestinal disease or induced by certain drugs (e.g., potassium-depleting diuretics). Hypokalemic patients usually have persistent weakness but occasionally experience periodic paralysis identical with the genetic forms and provoked by the same factors. In the secondary periodic paralyses, the serum potassium levels are always markedly abnormal when paralysis appears. In contrast, the paralytic episodes in the primary types can occur with relatively small changes in serum potassium levels.[8,56]

Attacks of periodic paralysis may also occur in paramyotonias provoked by exposure to cold or after exercise.

Endocrine Myopathies

Almost all classes of hormones affect the muscle cell to one extent or another. Hormones influence both cellular energetics and the synthesis of structural elements. **Myopathy is associated with a number of different endocrine disorders.** These are the endocrine myopathies (Table 13–6).[5,6,60–65] In addition to myopathies associated with endocrine disease, impaired muscle function may also occur when certain hormones are used therapeutically. In most instances, the muscle symptoms associated with an endocrine disorder constitute a minor part of the overall clinical picture, but sometimes, as in some patients with thyrotoxic (excessive thyroid hormone) myopathies, muscle symptoms may be a predominant feature of the disease. In general, **the endocrine myopathies are characterized by proximal weakness,** which is remedied by correcting the endocrine disorder. Pathologic changes are more evident in type II than in type I muscle fibers.[13–16,62]

Adrenal Dysfunction and Steroid Myopathy[60–65]

The **adrenal cortex produces three classes of hormones: sex steroid precursors, glucocorticoids, and mineralocorticoids.** Dysfunction of the gland can produce clinical signs related to abnormal activation of any or all of these hormones.

Table 13–6. *Endocrine Myopathies*

Primary Condition	Muscle Involvement
Adrenal dysfunction and steroid myopathy	
Glucocorticoid excess (e.g., Cushing's syndrome or excessive administration of glucocorticoid)	Proximal weakness and wasting—legs more than arms; myalgia common
Mineralocorticoid excess (e.g., primary hyperaldosteronism or Conn's syndrome)	Proximal weakness; tetany
Adrenal insufficiency (e.g., Addison's disease)	Generalized weakness and fatiguability; occasional cramps and contractions
Thyroid dysfunction	
Thyrotoxicosis (e.g., Graves' disease)	Weakness, especially of shoulder girdle and upper arms; atrophy
Hypothyroidism	Proximal weakness; muscle stiffness and pain; muscle cramping or myoedema; slowed muscle contraction and relaxation
Pituitary dysfunction	
Hyperpituitarism (e.g, acromegaly)	Mild proximal weakness and decreased exercise tolerance; muscle atrophy in advanced disease
Hypopituitarism (e.g., Simmonds' disease)	Marked weakness and fatigability with preservation of muscle mass
Parathyroid dysfunction and osteomalacia	
Hyperparathyroidism	Proximal weakness and atrophy; painful stiffness without myotonia
Hypoparathyroidism	Hypocalcemic tetany

The **adrenal sex steroids** exert their primary physiologic effects by being converted to active androgens or estrogens. Under normal circumstances, they contribute only a small percentage of the circulating sex hormones. This contribution can be markedly increased under pathologic conditions, contributing primarily to virilization of women. This may include increased muscle mass and strength. More common abnormalities of skeletal muscle, however, accompany abnormalities of glucocorticoid and mineralocorticoid secretion.

Glucocorticoid excess, whether due to excessive endogenous production by the adrenal gland (*Cushing's syndrome*) or to therapeutic administration (*iatrogenic steroid myopathy*) produces a characteristic syndrome of skeletal muscle weakness, which is one of the most common of the muscle disorders. Proximal muscle weakness and wasting are common in patients with Cushing's syndrome and to a lesser degree in patients treated with steroids for long periods of time.[64,65] Weakness is greatest in the hip and thigh muscles, and it may become difficult for patients to arise from a sitting, squatting, or kneeling position. In addition, walking may be impaired. The myopathy is usually gradual in onset, especially when associated with Cushing's syndrome. However, in some patients treated with steroids the muscle symptoms may develop rapidly, and wasting and muscle pain may be apparent in less than 1 month. Glucocorticoids have a catabolic effect on muscle, inhibiting the synthesis while enhancing the degradation of proteins; they also inhibit glycolytic metabolism, particularly in type II fibers. Microscopic examination of biopsy specimens usually reveals a more severe atrophy among type II fibers.[62] It is interesting that steroid myopathy is accelerated with inactivity and muscle disuse and may be partially prevented by exercise. Even passive range of motion may reduce steroid-induced atrophy. Therefore, physical therapy may be useful in preventing and treating muscle weakness and wasting in patients on long-term steroid therapy (as in treatment for asthma or rheumatoid disorders).

Excessive production of mineralocorticoid (as in primary hyperaldosteronism or Conn's syndrome) also has deleterious effects on skeletal muscle. In primary hyperaldosteronism, most patients **present with muscle weakness**, probably caused by chronic potassium depletion. Periodic attacks of marked weakness or paralysis lasting hours to weeks may be associated with periods of severe hypokalemia. Tetany may also be induced by the associated metabolic alkalosis.

Adrenal insufficiency due to destruction of the adrenal cortex is called **Addison's disease. Feelings of generalized weakness and easy fatigability are common complaints in hypoadrenal patients,** but are seldom accompanied by objective muscular weakness. Some patients may show wasting of proximal muscles. These symptoms probably reflect disturbances in plasma and muscle water content and electrolyte concentrations, since patients with Addison's disease are prone to hyponatremia, hypovolemia, and hyperkalemia.[60-65] The associated hypotension may also contribute. Adrenal insufficiency is frequently associated with anorexia and fasting hypoglycemia, as well as impaired muscle carbohydrate metabolism, all of which may further contribute to weakness and fatigue. In a few patients, severe, painful muscle cramps and rigidity may occur, involving mainly muscles of the lower trunk and thighs.

Thyroid Dysfunction[60-65]

Muscle is commonly affected in both hyperthyroidism and hypothyroidism. **In about 80% of untreated *hyperthyroid* (thyrotoxic) patients, a myopathy occurs in which mild or moderate muscle weakness and atrophy develop gradually,** predominantly in the shoulder girdle and upper arms.[64,65] In the lower extremities, proximal weakness may be restricted to the hip flexors. Atrophy of small periscapular and shoulder girdle muscles may be marked in some patients (Fig. 13–14). Thyrotoxic patients often have trouble climbing stairs, rising from a seated or lying position, and lifting their arms above their head. Although weakness can develop with relatively mild chronic thyroid excess, acute episodes are often accompanied by the most severe muscular symptoms, sometimes with striking involvement of bulbar

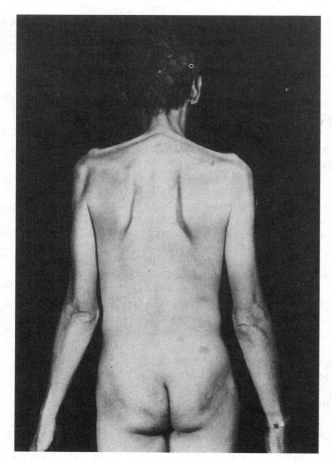

Figure 13–14. Thyrotoxic (Hyperthyroid) Myopathy. In this patient, there is severe wasting of the shoulder girdle muscles, which are preferentially affected in this condition. (From Becker, KL (ed): Principles and Practice of Endocrinology and Metabolism, ed 7. JB Lippincott, Philadelphia, 1990, p 1537, with permission.)

and external ocular muscles in addition to the more typical periscapular and upper limb weakness. The primary pathologic finding is nonselective muscle fiber atrophy.

Thyroid hormone stimulation of muscle metabolism and insulin resistance (impaired glucose uptake) may result in a depletion of muscle glycogen, ATP, creatine phosphate, and other energy stores and contribute to muscle weakness and atrophy. These direct effects on muscle energetics and contraction may be accompanied by impairment of neuromuscular junction transmission.[63–65] It may be significant that there is a greater incidence of thyroid disorders in patients with myasthenia gravis, and patients with myasthenia gravis have a relatively high prevalence of Graves' disease (hyperthyroidism).

Muscular symptoms are also common in *hypothyroidism* and revolve around a slowness of muscle contraction and relaxation, sometimes accompanied by mild proximal weakness. Muscle pain, stiffness, and cramps are common complaints. Gradual enlargement of muscle over months or years may be conspicuous in some hypothyroid children.[63–65] An interesting feature of hypothyroidism is myoedema, which is a localized electrically silent knot of contraction induced in a muscle by percussion. Myoedema is also seen in a variety of disorders associated with malnutrition and wasting (cachexia) and in aging.

The decreased velocity of shortening associated with thyroid hormone deficiency reflects a decreased rate of cross-bridge formation probably due to lower myosin ATPase activity and slower release and reuptake of calcium by the sarcoplasmic reticulum.[63–65] In addition, hypothyroidism leads to a reduction in the mitochondrial content of muscle and an impaired ability to oxidize carbohydrates and fats. This may limit the provision of energy for contraction and limit force generation similar to that seen in the glycogen storage diseases. Repair and replacement of myofibrillar protein may also be restricted, resulting in net protein catabolism. Biopsy specimens reveal type II fiber atrophy.[62]

Pituitary Dysfunction[60-65]

Excessive secretion of growth hormone by the pituitary gland causes the disease, *acromegaly,* which is characterized by enlargement of acral parts (ears, nose, jaw, hands, and feet), bony overgrowth, and multiple metabolic derangements. **Acromegaly in its earlier stages can give rise to muscular hypertrophy and increased strength,** especially if its onset precedes cessation of growth. **Later, many of the patients** with long-standing acromegaly will complain of decreased endurance and **present with an overt myopathy characterized by mild proximal weakness and muscle wasting.** Muscle atrophy is most evident in type II muscle fibers, whereas some hypertrophy may actually be evident among type I fibers.[62] A striking feature of acromegaly is that strength may be appreciably reduced despite normal or even increased muscle bulk.[63] This reduction in force-generating capacity may be due to decreased myofibrillar ATPase activity and reduced membrane excitability associated with prolonged growth hormone excess.

Pituitary failure (hypopituitarism) in adults causes severe weakness and fatigability without a loss of muscle mass.[63-65] This impairment of muscle function probably reflects primarily the loss of hormones from the thyroid gland and adrenal cortex. However, growth hormone synergizes with these hormones so that loss of growth hormone itself may also contribute to the weakness. Growth hormone plays a much greater role in muscle development than in maintaining muscle function. Hypopituitarism in children gives rise to dwarfism and poor muscular development.

Parathyroid Dysfunction and Metabolic Bone Disease (Osteomalacia)[60-65]

Hyperparathyroidism may result directly from the excessive production and secretion of parathyroid hormone by the parathyroid gland (primary hyperparathyroidism) or may develop as a consequence of some other condition such as renal failure or vitamin D deficiency (secondary hyperparathyroidism). **Patients with primary** *hyperparathyroidism* **often complain of proximal muscle weakness, fatigability, and stiffness,** although objective weakness may be difficult to demonstrate. Even with prominent weakness, only minimal muscle fiber atrophy is noted in biopsy specimens, although this is more marked in type II than in type I muscle fibers. Patients with chronic renal failure frequently develop a secondary hyperparathyroidism accompanied by a myopathy that closely resembles that seen in primary hyperparathyroidism.

Osteomalacia **is a disorder caused by vitamin D deficiency,** which is characterized by impaired bone mineralization and resulting softness, brittleness, and deformity of bones.[64,65] It is often grouped with these parathyroid disorders because of its clinical similarity. **About 50% of patients with osteomalacia develop proximal muscle weakness, wasting, and myalgia.** The muscle weakness is not readily explained by a loss of muscle bulk (which is minimal) but may reflect abnormalities in calcium transport within the muscle cell leading to abnormal excitation-contraction coupling.[64,65] The severity of the weakness is not directly correlated with serum concentrations of either calcium or phosphate. For example, plasma calcium may be elevated in primary hyperparathyroidism, decreased in secondary parathyroidism, and high or low in osteomalacia.

Hypoparathyroidism **leads to** hypocalcemia and frequently hypomagnesemia, which produce hyperexcitability of nerve fibers. **Sensory disturbances, such as numbness and paresthesias,** and **muscle tetany** result. Tetany of the facial muscles can be elicited by percussion of the facial nerve (**Chvostek's sign**) and carpopedal spasm (**Trousseau's sign**; see

Fig. 12–4) can be elicited by occluding venous return from an arm. Tetany is aggravated by systemic alkalosis (e.g., due to hyperventilation). In severe cases of tetany, laryngeal spasms can occur. The nerve hyperexcitability is caused by decreased serum calcium and magnesium concentrations.

Toxic Myopathies

A wide variety of chemical agents have been shown to have adverse effects on skeletal muscle, creating the so-called *toxic myopathies.*[15,66-71] This large group of compounds includes many commonly used drugs, environmental contaminants, and biologic agents. Perhaps the most widely studied and best defined are the drug-induced myopathies. Discussion of the injury produced by environmental pollutants and biologic agents, such as venoms, is beyond the scope of this chapter.

Drug-Induced Myopathies[66-72]

Many drugs may have deleterious effects on both the structure and function of muscle. These substances include agents in clinical use (prescription and nonprescription) and alcohol and other drugs of addiction.[72] Severe forms of drug-induced myopathy are uncommon, but when they do occur they may lead to severe disability and may even be fatal. The precise incidence of drug-induced muscle disorders is not known. With the exception of steroid myopathy, these disorders are usually considered rare. Given the widespread use of these agents, however, the incidence is almost certainly higher than is generally suspected, with many drug-induced reactions in muscle probably going unrecognized or being misdiagnosed.[67,68] One of the interesting facets of drug-induced myopathies is that most drugs that cause myopathy do so only in a very small proportion of the individuals who take the drugs. This suggests that there is some type of predisposition or heightened susceptibility in some people. Although all the factors that predispose a person to develop a drug-induced myopathy have yet to be defined, neural factors, impaired renal and hepatic function, nutritional abnormalities, and adverse drug interactions all have been implicated. As severe as they may be, most drug-induced myopathies are reversed by withdrawal of the offending agent. With extensive damage to muscle, recovery may be gradual and require extensive physical therapy and even surgery.

Drug-induced myopathy may result from a direct toxic effect of the drug on the muscle fibers themselves. This may be focal, when the drug is injected directly into or close to a muscle, or more diffuse, when the drug reaches the musculature as a result of systemic administration. In other instances, muscle damage is secondary to other disturbances caused by the drug. In addition, muscle effects may be accompanied (and exacerbated) by disturbances of peripheral nerve or neuromuscular junction function, since many of the drugs involved have adverse effects on both muscle and nerve. The specific cellular effects of most of these drugs on muscle are not well understood. The most common site of action is probably the cell membrane, at which drug effects may result in abnormal electrical properties and excitability or even disruption of basic membrane integrity.[67,69,70]

The deleterious effects of drugs on muscle are diverse and depend on the type of drug, the route of administration, the dose and duration of exposure, individual susceptibility, and a variety of aggravating conditions such as malnutrition or systemic disease. Drug-induced myopathies have been historically divided into a number of discrete categories, each with relatively distinct clinical features. However, these are somewhat arbitrary classifications, and a drug may not create all the features of a single syndrome or conversely may induce features of multiple syndromes simultaneously (e.g., chronic alcoholism). The most common form of drug-induced myopathy is a *subacute* or *chronic painless myopathy,* characterized by gradual development of proximal weakness and atrophy. This type of myopathy is created by steroid administration (see discussion of Endocrine Myopathies) and owes its high incidence to the frequent use of the glucocorticoid agents. Other drug-induced myopathies are described in the following sections.

Focal Myopathy

Localized areas of muscle damage, even muscle necrosis, can be produced by intramuscular injection of certain drugs. Almost any drug that is injected into muscle may occasionally produce such an effect, but certain drugs are particularly hazardous in this respect. Acute reactions include pain, swelling, hemorrhage, and sometimes abscess formation with repeated injections. More permanent changes in muscle may occur, including fibrosis, induration (hardening), and the development of contractures.[69] Contractures may be so severe that extensive physical therapy and even surgery may be required for their relief. Repeated injection of antibiotics, resulting in the involvement of the quadriceps or deltoid muscles in children, or the involvement of multiple limb muscles in adult addicts following repeated injection of narcotic drugs are common scenarios.[72] The chronic muscle damage in such cases is related to several factors, such as repeated needle trauma, recurrent infection (especially among drug addicts), hemorrhage, the extreme pH of injected material, and direct cytotoxic effects.

Necrotizing Myopathy and Rhabdomyolysis

Rhabdomyolysis is the term used to describe the breakdown of muscle cells that results in the release of myoglobin and its presence in plasma (myoglobinemia) and urine (myoglobinuria). **Muscle necrosis and rhabdomyolysis may occur after only a few days treatment with certain agents**, resulting in proximal or generalized muscle pain, tenderness, and weakness. In extreme cases with very rapid onset, the muscles may swell, flaccid paralysis may develop, and **myoglobinuria may be great enough to lead to acute renal failure**. Acute muscle necrosis has been reported, for example, after one heroin injection.[69,72] Muscle necrosis may also be delayed for weeks or months, in which case the symptoms are not usually as severe. Recovery occurs gradually, in weeks or months, depending on the severity of the injury. Treatment commences with withdrawal of the drug and may require extensive rehabilitation. Agents frequently associated with necrotizing myopathy are prescribed drugs, and abused substances such as alcohol, heroin, and phencyclidine.[67,70,72]

Hypokalemic Myopathy

Severe hypokalemia from any cause may adversely affect muscle. Drug-induced hypokalemic myopathy is due to potassium loss and occurs most often in patients taking purgatives (cathartics) or diuretics. Mineralocorticoids and excessive licorice ingestion may also promote potassium loss by disturbing renal potassium excretion. Most often hypokalemic myopathy is characterized by painless weakness of proximal muscles, but severe muscle necrosis and rhabdomyolysis with pain and myoglobinuria may occur. Potassium replacement and removal of the inciting agent result in complete recovery.

Inflammatory Myopathy

A number of drugs have occasionally been implicated in the development of an inflammatory myopathy.[66,69,70] The best known of these is D-penicillamine. Symptoms develop after weeks or even years of treatment with the drug. Although the symptoms are mild, recovery occurs slowly and may require steroid treatment in addition to drug withdrawal.

Table 13–7. *Inflammatory Myopathies*

Etiology	Comment
Infective	
Viral	Acute myositis following influenza most common
Bacterial	More common in tropical regions, but may accompany septicemia or localized contamination of muscle; none common
Fungal	May occur in immunodeficient person or by extension from local pleural or skin mycotic infection; uncommon
Parasitic	Linked to protozoa (toxoplasmosis), cestodes (cysticercosis), and nematodes (trichinosis); most common in less developed countries, arising from contaminated meat
Drug-induced (prescription or addiction/ abuse agents)	May produce focal or diffuse inflammation; penicillamine and alcohol are common examples
Idiopathic	Autoimmune origins suspected; often associated with connective tissue disorders or malignancy; polymyositis and dermatomyositis preeminent

Myasthenic Myopathy

A number of drugs, by adversely effecting acetylcholine release or motor end-plate receptors of the neuromuscular junction, may produce a "myasthenialike" syndrome.[67,69,70] These include certain antibiotics, cardiovascular agents, and psychotropic drugs. Patients with myasthenia gravis should use these agents with caution (see Chapter 14).

Malignant Hyperpyrexia or Hyperthermia

The term *malignant hyperthermia* **refers to a potentially lethal reaction characterized by muscle rigidity and myoglobinuria, hypermetabolism, and metabolic acidosis,** induced by exposure to certain anesthetic agents and muscle relaxants.[68,73] This reaction seems to be limited to certain susceptible persons, with predisposition usually running in families. Malignant hyperthermia may result from drug-induced release of excessive amounts of calcium ions into the muscle cells. This leads to sustained contraction, exhaustion of ATP, increased heat production, and deleterious effects on intracellular organelles and the cell membrane.

Inflammatory Myopathies[4–6,74–87]

Inflammatory myopathies constitute a diverse group of disorders characterized by muscle weakness and evidence of an inflammatory reaction in muscle (myositis) (Table 13–7).[74–77] Although not particularly common overall, the inflammatory myopathies are the most common of the *acquired* myopathies. **Some inflammatory myopathies are precipitated by known factors such as infectious agents (e.g., viruses, bacteria, or parasites) or toxic compounds (e.g., drugs or abused substances). In a larger group, no distinct cause can be identified (idiopathic),** but the inflammatory lesion is believed to be due, at least in part, to abnormal immune responses. The latter category is composed largely of the polymyositis-dermatomyositis complex, the most common of the inflammatory myopathies.

Skeletal muscle in all types of myositis appears relatively normal to the naked eye. At a microscopic level, **widespread degeneration and necrosis of muscle fibers are evident.**[74–77,79–81] Fibers may have disappeared altogether or may be present in varying stages of degeneration or regeneration. Inflammatory cell infiltrates are usually apparent, particularly around the vascular and connective tissue elements of the muscle (Fig. 13–15).

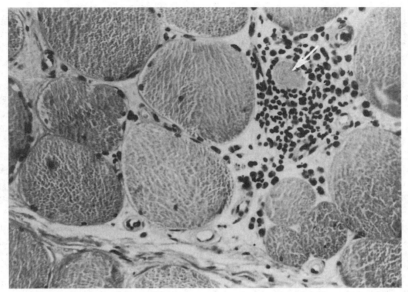

Figure 13–15. *Polymyositis.* This transverse section shows an infiltrate of inflammatory cells (*Small Dark Cells*) around an atrophic muscle fiber (*Arrow*). (From Kakulas and Adams,[15] p 494, with permission.)

In the later stages of disease, when all or nearly all of the muscle fibers have been lost and replaced by proliferating fibrous connective tissue, the muscle resembles that seen in the rapid forms of muscular dystrophy.[74–77]

The inflammatory myopathies are characterized by muscle weakness and sometimes pain. Muscle involvement is usually widespread, but may be focal. Acute, subacute, and chronic presentations may occur and the severity of symptoms may vary markedly even within a specific type of disorder, ranging from extremely mild to disabling or life-threatening. The most common cause of muscle inflammation is probably viral infection, particularly the influenza viruses. However, this inflammation is usually benign and short-lived and does not constitute a major clinical problem. On the other hand, the idiopathic inflammatory myopathies, polymyositis and dermatomyositis, are a relatively common complex of disorders, which may cause severe disability and even death. Fortunately, the inflammatory myopathies include some of the muscle disorders most successfully treated.

Infective Inflammatory Myopathies[67–81]

A number of viruses can cause an acute myopathy in human beings.[64–81] The resulting clinical syndromes vary from localized self-limiting forms of acute myositis (e.g., postinfluenza) to more severe forms with muscle necrosis. The inflammation of muscle that accompanies the flu is well known. In addition to the generalized myalgia that occurs during an attack of influenza, a postinfluenzal form of myositis may also occur. In a small proportion of children, the flu-like symptoms are followed within 1 week by myositis, presenting as muscle pain, tenderness, and sometimes swelling. The calf muscles are usually most severely affected, but the thigh muscles and other muscle groups may also be involved. Symptoms usually resolve spontaneously over a period of a week or so, with complete recovery. In adults, the syndrome is more variable and tends to be more severe. Occasionally severe damage to muscle may develop, with muscle cell lysis (rhabdomyolysis) and necrosis resulting in marked myoglobinuria.

Myopathies and other neuromuscular disorders develop in most patients with HIV infection. These conditions often occur concurrently with other AIDS-related medical illnesses and further increase the patient's disability. Myopathy and other neuromuscular conditions may also occur in isolation, providing the only indication of a chronic, silent HIV infection.[87]

HIV myopathy may manifest early in HIV infection, but is most often a complication of fully developed AIDS. This myopathy begins subacutely with proximal, often symmetric weakness and involves the arms and more often the legs.[87] Myalgia may be present. The myopathy is characterized histologically by inflammatory infiltrates in muscle and muscle fiber necrosis. It resembles clinically and histopathologically adult-onset polymyositis. Although the pathogenesis of HIV myopathy is poorly understood, it does not seem to be due to a direct viral infection of the muscle itself, since no electron microscopic evidence of viral particles in the muscle fibers or in the infiltrating lymphoid cells has been found.[87] More likely, it is caused by an autoimmune response against muscle antigens triggered by the virus's presence in cells other than muscle. This proposition is supported by the clinical, histologic, and immunopathological similarity between HIV myositis and polymyositis in HIV-negative patients. Other viral or infectious factors may also contribute to the myocytotoxicity observed in HIV myopathy. In addition, other factors contributing to the myopathy may include vitamin deficiencies due to long-standing infection and poor nutrition; disuse atrophy caused by prolonged immobilization; and the toxicity of various antimicrobial drugs.[87] It is also established that the drug zidovudine (AZT), which is used in the treatment of HIV, induces a unique myopathy that is caused by its mitochondrial toxicity.[87,88] The clinical features of the AZT myopathy include proximal muscle weakness, together with myalgia, predominantly in the thighs and calves. The symptoms are related to the dose of AZT and the duration of its use.

Muscle tissue does not provide a very favorable site for the growth of many bacteria, and consequently bacterial infections of muscle are uncommon. **Acute bacterial myositis may occur,** however, in the face of widespread systemic infection (such as septicemia) or by extension from locally infected arthritis, pleuritis, osteomyelitis, or skin decubiti.[74] It may also follow contamination of muscle by crushing or penetrating injury. For example, infection within muscles such as the deltoids or glutei may result from repeated intramuscular injections. The systemic symptoms of acute muscle infection are headache, fever, and malaise, followed by pain, tenderness, and edema of the affected muscle. Abscess formation may follow. Bacterial infections of muscle occur most frequently in tropical and subtropical regions.[83]

Fungal infections of muscle are uncommon.[79] Myositis may occur in patients with disseminated candidiasis who have impaired immune mechanisms (as in AIDS), and it may be associated with severe myalgia. Also, infection of muscle may occur by direct extension from a neighboring fungal infection, such as in pleura or skin.

Parasitic Inflammatory Myopathies

Muscle is susceptible to infection by relatively few parasites. The parasites invading muscle fall into three main groups: protozoa, cestodes (tapeworms), and nematodes (roundworms).[74,77,79,80,84] Muscle involvement may be focal, resulting in well-localized inflammation, or diffuse, resulting in polymyositis. Muscle symptoms are prominent only in cysticercosis (resulting from a cestode) and trichinosis (resulting from a nematode)—the latter being the most common parasitic infection of muscle. Although many of these parasites are distributed worldwide, parasitic infections are uncommon in developed countries. Most are transmitted by improperly prepared, contaminated meat and predominate in poorly developed countries with inadequate water and sewage management and primitive dietary customs. However, changing immigration patterns and an increased occurrence of immunodeficient states have contributed to an increased incidence of parasitic infections in Western society.

Drug-Induced Inflammatory Myopathies

Treatment with or abuse of certain drugs can result in varying degrees of muscle inflammation and the accompanying signs and symptoms.[69,70,77,79,80] Notable among these are D-penicillamine and alcohol. The drug-induced myopathies are discussed in this chapter under "Toxic Myopathies."

Idiopathic Inflammatory Myopathies

The idiopathic inflammatory myopathies are a diverse assortment of disorders grouped together because of the presence of inflammatory lesions in muscle and a lack of clear-cut etiology.[74-77,79-82,85,86] In Western society, where infective and parasitic forms of myosites are rare, most cases of myositis fall into this category. These disorders may occur in isolation or in association with other conditions, such as connective tissue disease or malignancy. Although disturbances of immune mechanisms have been implicated in the pathogenesis of most of these conditions, their diversity suggests that other factors (possibly genetic or environmental) may be involved as well. **Preeminent among the idiopathic inflammatory myopathies are polymyositis and dermatomyositis,** which occur in various forms. Polymyositis is characterized by a diffuse inflammation of muscle, frequently accompanied by degeneration and necrosis of muscle fibers. Dermatomyositis is a similar condition, involving the presence of inflammatory changes in the skin as well as in muscle.

Isolated Adult-Onset Polymyositis and Dermatomyositis

Adult-onset polymyositis and dermatomyositis in the absence of other major medical conditions constitute more than 50% of all myosites (inflammations of muscle). They occur most often in women and arise most often in the fifth and sixth decade.[74-77,79-82,85,86] In polymyositis, the onset of muscle weakness is usually insidious, gradually progressing over weeks to months (subacute form). Less often the muscle symptoms develop rapidly (acute form) or slowly over a period of years (chronic form). The proximal muscles, particularly of the pelvic and shoulder girdles, are most severely affected in a symmetric, nonselective fashion. Most patients have little or no involvement of distal muscles. Involvement of pharyngeal and upper esophageal muscles may lead to dysphagia. Respiratory involvement occurs in some patients and may contribute to respiratory insufficiency. In some instances, muscle fatigability is prominent. Muscle pain and tenderness may occur, particularly around the shoulder girdle and especially in the more rapidly progressing cases. Muscle atrophy is less than would be expected by the decline in strength, tends to develop later in the disease, and is never as pronounced as in muscular dystrophy or denervation. **Muscular weakness in dermatomyositis is indistinguishable from that of polymyositis, but is accompanied by characteristic inflammatory changes in the skin.** Typically, the patient has a dusky rash distributed in a butterfly pattern over the face, purplish discoloration over the eyelids, and edema around the eyes. Scaly patches may also be present over the knuckles, elbows, knees, and ankles. In more chronic forms and especially in the juvenile forms of dematomyositis, subcutaneous calcification may occur over heels, elbows, and knuckles, giving rise to subcutaneous nodules that may be disfiguring and cause pain, ulceration, or infection.

Cardiac involvement is present in most patients with polymyositis or dermatomyositis and presents as electrocardiogram changes, arrhythmias, and heart failure secondary to myocarditis.[77,79-82,85,86] Cardiac signs and symptoms are often evident prior to diagnosis of polymyositis or dermatomyositis. **Pulmonary complications** such as interstitial lung disease and fibrosis may occur, manifested by such symptoms as dyspnea and nonproductive cough. Respiratory insufficiency occurs in 5% to 10% of patients, and opportunistic respiratory infections may develop during immunosuppressive therapy. **Gastrointestinal**

tract complaints are also common. The most frequent problem is dysphagia due to pharnyngeal or upper esophageal weakness. Smooth muscle involvement has been shown throughout the tract.

Juvenile Polymyositis or Dermatomyositis

Dermatomyositis occurs more often than polymyositis in patients younger than 16 years old.[81] In the childhood or juvenile form, the typical rash is present much more often. As in adults, the muscle weakness is gradually progressive and is predominantly proximal. The Gowers' maneuver may be an important early feature (see Fig. 13–4). Cutaneous manifestations are similar, and cardiac, respiratory, and gastrointestinal tract complications may also occur. Vasculitis of the gastrointestinal tract is more common in children and may result in mucosal ulceration or perforation. In general, children with juvenile polymyositis respond well to therapy and have a good prognosis.

Polymyositis or Dermatomyositis Associated with Other Medical Conditions

About 20% of patients with polymyositis or dermatomyositis have an associated connective tissue disease.[77,79–82,85,86] The presumption is that most of these cases of myosites occur as a complication of these systemic disorders. Polymyositis or dermatomyositis may also be associated with other autoimmune disorders, such as myasthenia gravis and immune deficiency states such as AIDS. **An abnormally high incidence of malignancy is also associated with polymyositis or dermatomyositis.** The incidence of cancer is greatest in older, adult patients with dermatomyositis. The range of associated malignancies is extensive, but most common are carcinoma of the breast or ovary in women and of the lung or gastrointestinal tract in men. The association with malignancy is rare in cases of juvenile dermatomyositis or connective tissue disease.

Although the etiology of polymyositis and dermatomyositis remains uncertain, it is likely that abnormalities of both humoral and cell-mediated immune mechanisms are involved.[77,79–82,85,86] The factors that trigger these aberrant responses are not known. Although most patients experience no identifiable triggering factors, in some patients viral infection, vaccination, treatment with certain drugs, or the presence of malignancy may cause a temporary disturbance of immune mechanisms during which an autoimmune reaction directed against muscle is initiated. In the case of viruses, although a distinct link to the direct viral invasion of muscle has not been demonstrated, several mechanisms by which a virus might incite a self-perpetuating immune response against muscle are conceivable.[76,81] Antibodies to viral antigens might cross-react with muscle antigens, viral infection might alter the antigenicity of muscle, or viral infection may disturb broad immunoregulatory mechanisms. The diversity of the various inflammatory syndromes previously described may reflect differing underlying pathogenic mechanisms, as well as varying genetic and other predisposing factors.

Fortunately, **the polymyositis and dermatomyositis disorders are some of the few currently treatable diseases of muscle.**[79–82,85,86] Most forms of treatment are directed toward suppression of abnormal immune activity. Patients often respond favorably to corticosteroid (e.g., prednisone) therapy. Some patients who are unresponsive to steroids may improve on immunosuppressive drug treatment. Recent developments in the treatment of idiopathic inflammatory myopathy include the use of plasmapheresis and total body low-dose radiation in patients whose myopathy is resistant to corticosteroids and immunosuppressive agents or in those in whom side effects have curtailed treatment with these substances.[79–82,85,86,89] During very active disease when bed rest is required or in chronic polymyositis, rehabilitative therapy is useful in preventing contractures and other problems associated with immobilization.[75] During the active stage, passive exercise is recommended, but when the disease is in remission and inflammation has subsided more active strength-building exercises are encouraged.

RECOMMENDED READINGS

Adachi, M and Sher, JH: Neuromuscular Disease. Igaku-Shoin, New York 1990.

Adams, RD and Victor, M: Principles of Neurology, ed 4. Chapter 48. Principles of Clinical Myology: Diagnosis and Classification of Muscle Diseases. McGraw-Hill Information Services, New York, 1989.

Brooke, MH: Disorders of Skeletal Muscle. Chapter 83. In Bradley, WG, et al (eds): Neurology in Clinical Practice: The Neurological Disorders, vol II. Butterworth-Heinemann, Boston 1990.

Carpenter, S and Kapati, G: Pathology of Skeletal Muscle. Churchill Livingstone, New York, 1984.

Engel, AG and Franzini-Armstrong, C (eds): Myology: Basic and Clinical, ed 2. McGraw-Hill, New York, 1994.

Kakulas, BA and Adams, RD: Diseases of Muscle: Pathological Foundations of Clinical Myology, ed 4. Harper & Row, Philadelphia, 1985.

Mastaglia, FL and Detchant, Lord Walton (eds): Skeletal Muscle Pathology, ed 2. Churchill Livingstone, Edinburgh, 1992.

Morgan-Hughes, JA: Diseases of Striated Muscle. Chapter 14. In Asbury, AK McKhann, GM, and McDonald, WI (eds): Diseases of the Nervous System: Clinical Neurobiology, vol 1, ed 2. WB Saunders, Philadelphia, 1992.

Riggs, JE (ed): Muscle Disease. Neurol Clin 6(3):429, 1988.

Riggs, JE and Schocher, SS, Jr: Muscle Disease. Chapter 53. In Joynt, RJ (ed): Clinical Neurology, vol 4. JB Lippincott, Philadelphia, 1991.

Siegel, IM: Muscle and Its Diseases. Part III. Classification and Diagnosis of Neuromuscular Diseases. Year Book Medical Publishers, Chicago, 1986.

Squire, JM: Muscle: Design, Diversity, and Disease. Chapter 10. Muscle Diseases. The Benjamin/Cummings Publishing Company, Menlo Park, CA, 1986.

Swash, M and Schwartz, MS: Neuromuscular Diseases, ed 2. Section 5. Myopathies and Muscular Dystrophies. Springer-Verlag, London, 1988.

Vinken, PJ and Bruyn, GW (eds): Handbook of Clinical Neurology, vol 40. Diseases of Muscle. Part I. North-Holland Publishing Company, Amsterdam, 1979.

Vinken, PJ and Bruyn, GW (eds): Handbook of Clinical Neurology, vol 41. Diseases of Muscle. Part II. North-Holland Publishing Company, Amsterdam, 1979.

Walton, JN (ed): Disorders of Voluntary Muscle, ed 4. Churchill Livingstone, Edinburgh, 1981.

REFERENCES

1. Adachi, M and Sher, JH: Neuromuscular Disease. Igaku-Shoin, New York, 1990.

2. Engel, AG and Franzini-Armstrong, C (eds): Myology: Basic and Clinical, ed 2. McGraw-Hill, New York, 1994.

3. Mastaglia, FL and Detchant, Lord Walton (eds): Skeletal Muscle Pathology, ed 2. Churchill Livingstone, Edinburgh, 1992.

4. Morgan-Hughes, JA: Diseases of Striated Muscle. Chapter 14. In Asbury, AK, McKhann, GM, and McDonald, WI (eds): Diseases of the Nervous System: Clinical Neurobiology, vol 1, ed 2. WB Saunders, Philadelphia, 1993.

5. Riggs, JE (ed): Muscle Disease. Neurol Clin 6(3):429 1988.

6. Riggs, JE and Schocher, SS, Jr: Muscle Disease. Chapter 53. In Joynt, RJ (ed): Clinical Neurology, vol 4. JB Lippincott, Philadelphia, 1991.

7. Swash, M and Schwartz, MS: Neuromuscular Diseases. Section 5. Myopathies and Muscular Dystrophies, ed 2. Springer-Verlag, London, 1988.

8. Brooke, MH: Disorders of Skeletal Muscle. Chapter 83. In Bradley, WG, et al (eds): Neurology in Clinical Practice: The Neurological Disorders, vol II. Butterworth-Heinemann, Boston, 1990.

9. Munsat, TL: The Classification of Human Myopathies. Chapter 7. In Vinken, PJ and Bruyn, GW: Handbook of Clinical Neurology, vol 40. Diseases of Muscle. Part I. North-Holland Publishing Company, Amsterdam, 1979.

10. Vinken, PJ and Bruyn, GW (eds): Handbook of Clinical Neurology, vol 40. Diseases of Muscle. Part I. Chapter 8. Clinical Presentations in Neuromuscular Disease. North-Holland Publishing Company, Amsterdam, 1979.

11. Swash, M and Schwartz, MS: Neuromuscular Diseases, ed 2. Chapter 1. Clinical Assessment. Springer-Verlag, London, 1988.

12. Walton, JN: Disorders of Voluntary Muscle, ed 5. Chapter 13. Clinical Examination of the Neuromuscular System. Churchill Livingstone, Edinburgh, 1988.

13. Carpenter, S and Kapati, G: Pathology of Skeletal Muscle. Chapter 3. Major General Pathological Reactions and Their Consequences on Skeletal Muscle Cells. Churchill Livingstone, Edinburgh, 1984.

14. Cullen, MJ, Johnson, MA, and Mastaglia, FL: Pathological Reactions of Skeletal Muscle. Chapter 3. In Mastaglia, FL and Detchant, Lord Walton (eds): Skeletal Muscle Pathology, ed 2. Churchill Livingstone, Edinburgh, 1992.

15. Kakulas, BA and Adams, RD: Diseases of Muscle: Pathological Foundations of Clinical Myology, ed 4. Chapter 3. General Reactions of Human Muscle to Disease. Harper & Row, Philadelphia, 1985.

16. Banker, BQ and Engel, AG: Basic Reactions of Muscle. Chapter 35. In Engel, AG and Franzini-Armstrong, C (eds): Myology: Basic and Clinical, ed 2. McGraw-Hill, New York, 1994.

17. Engel, AG and Banker, BQ: Ultrastructural Changes in Disease Muscle. Chapter 36. In Engel, AG and Franzini-Armstrong, C (eds): Myology: Basic and Clinical, ed 2. McGraw-Hill, New York, 1986.

18. Dubowitz, V and Brooke, MH: Muscle Biopsy: A Modern Approach. Chapter 4. Definition of Pathological Changes Seen in Muscle Biopsies. WB Saunders, London, 1973.

19. Karpati, G and Carpenter, S: Small Caliber Skeletal Muscle Fibers Do Not Suffer Deleterious Conse-

quences of Dystrophic Gene Expression. Am J Med Genet 25:653, 1986.
20. Sher, JH: Muscular Dystrophy. Chapter 5. In Adachi, M and Sher, JH: Neuromuscular Disease. Igaku-Shoin, New York, 1990.
21. Engel, AG and Franzini-Armstrong, C (eds): Myology: Basic and Clinical, ed 2. Part 3. Diseases of Muscle. Section 1. Muscular Dystrophies. McGraw-Hill, New York, 1994.
22. Engel, AG, Yamamoto, M, and Fischbeck, KH: Dystrophinopathies. Chapter 41. In Engel, AG and Franzini-Armstrong, C (eds): Myology: Basic and Clinical, ed 2. McGraw-Hill, New York, 1994.
23. Love, DR, et al: Dystrophin and Dystrophin-Related Proteins: A Review of Protein and RNA Studies. Neuromusc Dis 3:5, 1993.
24. Specht, LA and Kunkel, LM: Duchenne and Becker Muscular Dystrophies. In Rosenberg, RN, et al (eds): The Molecular and Genetic Basis of Neurological Disease. Butterworth-Heinemann, Boston, 1993, pp 613–631.
25. Ohlendieck, K, et al: Duchenne Muscular Dystrophy: Deficiency of Dystrophin-Associated Proteins in the Sarcolemma. Neurology 43:795, 1993.
26. Bushby, KMD, et al: The Clinical, Genetic, and Dystrophin Characteristics of Becker Muscular Dystrophy. J Neurol 240:105, 1993.
27. Matsumura, K and Campbell, KP: Dystrophin-Glycoprotein Complex: Its Role in the Molecular Pathogenesis of Muscular Dystrophies. Muscle Nerve 17(1):2, 1994.
28. Scott, OM, et al: Prevention of Deformity in Duchenne Muscular Dystrophy. Physiotherapy 67:177, 1981.
29. Heckmatt, JZ, et al: Prolongation of Walking in Duchenne Muscular Dystrophy with Lightweight Orthoses: A Review of 57 Cases. Dev Med Child Neurol 27:149, 1985.
30. Rodillo, EB, et al: Prevention of Rapidly Progressive Scoliosis in Duchenne Muscular Dystrophy by Prolongation of Walking with Orthoses. J Child Neurol 3:269, 1988.
31. Bach, JR and Lieberman, JS: Rehabilitation of the Patient with Disease Affecting the Motor Unit. Chapter 52. In DeLisa, JA (ed): Rehabilitation Medicine: Principles and Practice, ed 2. JB Lippincott, Philadelphia, 1993.
32. Fardeau, M: Cellular Therapy and Gene Therapy: Perspectives in Neuromuscular Pathology. Pathol Biol 41(8):681, 1993.
33. Morgan, JE: Cell and Gene Therapy in Duchenne Muscular Dystrophy. Hum Gene Ther 5(2):165, 1994.
34. Law, RK, et al: Cell Transplantation as an Experimental Treatment for Duchenne Muscular Dystrophy. Cell Transplant 2(6):485, 1993.
35. DiMauro, S: Metabolic Myopathies. Chapter 10. In Adachi, M and Sher, JH(eds): Neuromuscular Disease. Igaku-Shoin, New York, 1990.
36. DiMauro, S, et al: Skeletal Muscle Storage Diseases: Myopathies Resulting from Errors in Carbohydrate and Fatty Acid Metabolism. Chapter 11. In Mastaglia, FL and Detchant, Lord Walton (eds): Skeletal Muscle Pathology, ed 2. Churchill Livingstone, Edinburgh, 1992.
37. Engel, AG and Franzini-Armstrong, C (eds): Myology: Basic and Clinical, ed 2. Part 3. Disease of Muscle. Section 5. Metabolic Disorders Affecting Muscle. McGraw-Hill, New York, 1994.
38. Cornelio, F and DiDonato, S: Myopathies Due to Enzyme Deficiencies. J Neurol 237:329, 1985.
39. Rowland, LP, Layzer, RB, and DiMauro, SD: Pathophysiology of Metabolic Myopathies. Chapter 12. In Asbury, AK, McKhann, GM, and McDonald, WI (eds): Diseases of the Nervous System: Clinical Neurobiology, vol 1, ed 2. WB Saunders, Philadelphia, 1992.
40. Swash, M and Schwartz, MS: Neuromuscular Diseases, ed 2. Chapter 17. Metabolic Myopathies. Springer-Verlag, London, 1988.
41. Morgan-Hughes, JA: Mitochondrial Diseases. Chapter 62. In Engel, AG and Franzini-Armstrong, C (eds): Myology: Basic and Clinical, ed 2. McGraw-Hill, New York, 1994.
42. Fishbein, WN: Myoadenylate Deaminase Deficiency. Chapter 60. In Engel, AG and Franzini-Armstrong, C (eds): Myology: Basic and Clinical. McGraw-Hill, New York, 1986.
43. Swash, M and Schwartz, MS: Neuromuscular Diseases, ed 2. Chapter 16. Benign Childhood Myopathies. Springer-Verlag, London, 1988.
44. Goebel, HH: Congenital Myopathies. Chapter 9. In Adachi, M and Sher, JH: Neuromuscular Disease. Igaku-Shoin, New York, 1990.
45. Bodensteiner, J: Congenital Myopathies. Neurol Clin 6(3):499, 1988.
46. Fardeau, M and Tome, FMS: Congenital Myopathies. Chapter 57. In Engel, AG and Franzini-Armstrong, C (eds): Myology: Basic and Clinical, ed 2. McGraw-Hill, New York, 1994.
47. Fardeau, M: Congenital Myopathies. Chapter 6. In Mastaglia, FL and Detchant, Lord Walton (eds): Skeletal Muscle Pathology, ed 2. Churchill Livingstone, Edinburgh 1992.
48. Kakulas, BA and Adams, RD: Diseases of Muscle: Pathological Foundations of Clinical Myology, ed 4. Chapter 5. Congenital Neuromuscular Defects and Intrauterine and Infantile Diseases. Harper & Row, Philadelphia, 1985.
49. Swash, M and Schwartz, MS: Neuromuscular Diseases, ed 2. Chapter 15. Myotonic Syndromes. Springer-Verlag, London, 1988.
50. Barchi, RL and Furman, RE: Pathophysiology of Myotonia and Periodic Paralysis. Chapter 13. In Asbury, AK, McKhann, GM, and McDonald, WI (eds): Diseases of the Nervous System: Clinical Neurobiology, vol 1, ed 2. WB Saunders, Philadelphia, 1992.
51. Nonaka, I and Satoyoshi, E: Myotonic Disorders. Chapter 8. In Mastaglia, FL and Detchant, Lord Walton (eds): Skeletal Muscle Pathology, ed 2. Churchill Livingstone, Edinburgh, 1992.
52. Barchi, RL: Myotonia. Neurol Clin 6(3):473, 1988.
53. Rudel, R, Lehmann-Horn, F, and Ricker, K: The Nondystrophic Myotonias. Chapter 49. In Engel, AG and Franzini-Armstrong, C (eds): Myology: Basic and Clinical, ed 2. McGraw-Hill, New York, 1994.
54. Harper, PS and Rudel, R: Myotonic Dystrophy. Chapter 43. In Engel, AG and Franzini-Armstrong, C (eds): Myology: Basic and Clinical, ed 2. McGraw-Hill, New York, 1994.
55. Harper, PS: Myotonic Dystrophy, ed 2. WB Saunders, London, 1989.

56. Lehmann-Horn, F, et al: Paralyses and Paramyotonia Congenita. Chapter 50. In Engel, AG and Franzini-Armstrong, C (eds): Myology: Basic and Clinical, ed 2. McGraw-Hill, New York, 1994.

57. Rudel, R., et al: Hypokalemic Periodic Paralysis: *In Vitro* Investigations of Muscle Fiber Parameters. Muscle Nerve 7:110, 1984.

58. Riggs, JE: The Periodic Paralysis. Neurol Clin 6(3):485, 1988.

59. Tome, FMS and Borg, K: Periodic Paralysis and Electrolyte Disorders. Chapter 9. In Mastaglia, FL and Detchant, Lord Walton (eds): Skeletal Muscle Pathology, ed 2. Churchill Livingstone, Edinburgh, 1992.

60. Ruff, RL and Weissman, J: Endocrine Myopathies. Neurol Clin 6(3):575, 1988.

61. Swash, M and Schwartz, MS: Neuromuscular Diseases, ed 2. Chapter 18. Endocrine Myopathies. Springer-Verlag, London, 1988.

62. Hudgson, P and Kendall-Taylor, P: Endocrine Myopathy. Chapter 1. In Mastaglia, FL and Detchant, Lord Walton (eds): Skeletal Muscle Pathology, ed 2. Churchill Livingstone, Edinburgh, 1992.

63. Kaminsky, HJ and Ruff, RL: Endocrine Myopathies (Hyper- and Hypofunction of Adrenal, Thyroid, Pituitary, and Parathyroid Glands and Iatrogenic Steroid Myopathy). Chapter 66. In Engel, AG and Franzini-Armstrong, C (eds): Myology: Basic and Clinical, ed 2. McGraw-Hill, New York, 1994.

64. Layzer, RB: Neuromuscular Manifestations of Endocrine Disease. Chapter 209. In Becker, KL (ed): Principles and Practice of Endocrinology and Metabolism, ed 7. JB Lippincott, Philadelphia, 1990.

65. Layzer, RB: Neuromuscular Manifestations of Systemic Disease. Chapter 3. Endocrine Disorders. FA Davis, Philadelphia, 1985.

66. Swash, M and Schwartz, MS: Neuromuscular Diseases, ed 2. Chapter 19. Drug-Induced and Toxic Myopathies. Springer-Verlag, London, 1988.

67. Mastaglia, FL: Adverse Effects of Drugs on Muscle. Drugs 24:304, 1982.

68. Kuncl, RW and Wiggins, WW: Toxic Myopathies. Neurol Clin 6(3):593, 1988.

69. Victor, M and Sieb, JP: Myopathies Due to Drugs, Toxins, and Nutritional Deficiency. Chapter 65. In Engel, AG and Franzini-Armstrong, C (eds): Myology: Basic and Clinical, ed 2. McGraw-Hill, New York, 1994.

70. Kakulas, BA and Mastaglia, FL: Drug-Induced, Toxic, and Nutritional Myopathies. Chapter 14. In Mastaglia, FL and Detchant, Lord Walton (eds): Skeletal Muscle Pathology, ed 2. Churchill Livingstone, Edinburgh, 1992.

71. Argov, Z and Mastaglia, FL: Drug-Induced Neuromuscular Disorders in Man. In Walton, JN (ed): Disorders of Voluntary Muscle, ed 5. Churchill Livingstone, Edinburgh, 1988.

72. DeGans, J, Stam, J, and Van Wijngarrden, GK: Rehabdomyolysis and Concomitant Neurological Lesions After Intravenous Heroin Abuse. J Neurol Neurourg Psychiatry 48:1057, 1985.

73. Gronert, GA: Malignant Hyperthermia. Chapter 63. In Engel, AG and Franzini-Armstrong, C (eds): Myology: Basic and Clinical, ed 2. McGraw-Hill, New York, 1994.

74. Kakulas, BA and Adams, RD: Diseases of Muscle: Pathological Foundations of Clinical Myology, ed 4. Chapter 7. Inflammatory Diseases (Myositis). Harper & Row, Philadelphia, 1985.

75. Swash, M and Schwartz, MS: Neuromuscular Diseases, ed 2. Chapter 13. Inflammatory Myopathies. Springer-Verlag, London, 1988.

76. Engel, AG and Franzini-Armstrong, C (eds): Myology: Basic and Clinical, ed 2. Part 3. Disease of Muscle. Section 3. Inflammatory Myopathies. McGraw-Hill, New York, 1994.

77. Mastaglia, FL and Walton, JN: Inflammatory Myopathies. Chapter 12. In Mastaglia, FL and Detchant, Lord Walton (eds): Skeletal Muscle Pathology, ed 2. Churchill Livingstone, Edinburgh, 1992.

78. Hays, AP and Gamboa, ET: Acute Viral Myositis. Chapter 53. In Engel, AG and Franzini-Armstrong, C (eds): Myology: Basic and Clinical, ed 2. McGraw-Hill, New York, 1994.

79. Mastaglia, FL and Ojeda, VJ: Inflammatory Myopathies. Part I. Ann Neurol 17(3):215, 1985.

80. Mastaglia, FL and Ojeda, VJ: Inflammatory Myopathies. Part II. Ann Neurol 17(4):317, 1985.

81. Kingston, WJ and Moxley, RT III: Inflammatory Myopathies. Neurol Clin 6(3):545, 1988.

82. Engel, AG, Hohlfeld, R, and Banker, BQ: The Polymyositis and Dermatomyositis Syndromes. Chapter 51. In Engel, AG and Franzini-Armstrong, C (eds): Myology: Basic and Clinical, ed 2. McGraw-Hill, New York, 1994.

83. Chiedozi, LC: Pyomyositis. Am J Surg 137:255, 1979.

84. Banker, BQ: Parasitic Myositis. Chapter 55. In Engel, AG and Franzini-Armstrong, C (eds): Myology: Basic and Clinical, ed 2. McGraw-Hill, New York, 1994.

85. Torii, J, Isonishi, K, and Adacui, M: Polymyositis and Dermatomyositis. Chapter 4. In Adachi, M and Sher, JH: Neuromuscular Disease. Igaku-Shoin, New York, 1990.

86. Plotz, PH, Moderator: Current Concepts in the Idiopathic Inflammatory Myopathies: Polymyositis, Dermatomyositis, and Related Disorders. Ann Intern Med 111:143, 1989.

87. Dalakas, MC: Retrovirus-Related Muscle Diseases. Chapter 54. In Engel, AG and Franzini-Armstrong, C (eds): Myology: Basic and Clinical, ed 2. McGraw-Hill, New York, 1994.

88. Pezeshkpour, GH, Illa, I, and Dalakas, MC: Ultrastructural Characteristics and DNA Immunocytochemistry in HIV and AZT-Associated Myopathies. Hum Pathol 22:1281, 1991.

89. Kelly, JJ, et al: Response to Total Body Irradiation in Dermatomyositis. Muscle Nerve 11:120, 1988.

CHAPTER 14

■

Myasthenia Gravis and Other Disorders of Neuromuscular Transmission

Christopher M. Fredericks, PhD

- ■ *Myasthenia Gravis*
- ■ *Transient Neonatal Myasthenia Gravis*
- ■ *Lambert-Eaton Myasthenic Syndrome*
- ■ *Congenital Myasthenic Syndromes*
- ■ *Botulism*
- ■ *Drug- and Chemical-Induced Myasthenic Syndromes*

*I*n a healthy individual, skeletal muscle is not spontaneously active, but is dependent on stimulation by the somatic nervous system. This stimulation is in the form of action potentials (impulses), which arise in cranial nerve nuclei of the brainstem or in anterior horn cells of the spinal cord and are then conducted to the muscle tissue in the periphery via cranial and spinal motor neurons, respectively (Fig. 14–1). These neurons do not terminate in actual contact with skeletal muscle, but are separated from it by a distinct synaptic gap. The specialized neuron terminus and the adjacent specialized portion of the muscle membrane, the motor end plate, constitute the neuromuscular junction.

Only by adequate neuromuscular junction transmission can skeletal muscle be activated by the somatic nervous system. As described in Chapter 3, transmission of excitation from motor neuron to muscle is mediated by neuronal release of the neurotransmitter, acetylcholine. The success of junctional transmission thus depends on both the adequacy of prejunctional release of acetylcholine and the postjunctional response to it.

In a normal neuromuscular junction, a single impulse reaching the motor neuron terminus provides more than enough stimulus for contraction. In fact, inherent in the response to a single impulse is a built-in "safety factor" reflecting excessive acetylcholine release and end-plate cholinergic receptor activity.[1] Although this safety factor protects skeletal muscle somewhat from deficiencies in junctional transmission, disorders of transmission can significantly impair motor neuron excitation of skeletal muscle.[1-11] Resultant muscle dysfunction may range from weakness and abnormal fatigability to complete flaccid paralysis. These disorders are both acquired and inherited and reflect defects in both prejunctional and postjunctional activity (Table 14–1).

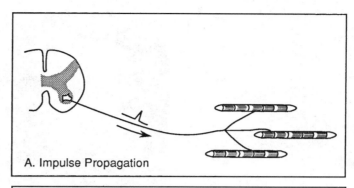

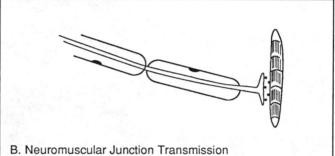

Figure 14–1. *Activation of Skeletal Muscle by the Somatic Nervous System.* The activation of skeletal muscle requires both (*A*) the propagation of impulses to the neuromuscular junction and (*B*) adequate neuromuscular junction transmission.

Table 14–1. *Disorders of Neuromuscular Transmission*

Defect	Disease	Etiology
Prejunctional		
ACh resynthesis or packaging	Familial infantile myasthenia	Inherited
	Congenital paucity of presynaptic vesicles and reduced quantal release	Inherited
	Black widow spider envenomation	Toxic
ACh release	Lambert-Eaton myasthenic syndrome	Autoimmune
	Botulism	Toxic
	Aminoglycoside antibiotics (Vibramycin)	Toxic
	Magnesium intoxication	Toxic
	Snake envenomation (β-bungarotoxin)	Toxic
Postjunctional		
AChR density	Myasthenia gravis	Autoimmune
	Congenital end-plate AChR deficiency	Inherited
AChR channel kinetics	Slow-channel syndrome	Inherited
	High-conductance, fast-channel syndrome	Inherited
Acetylcholinesterase	Congenital end-plate acetylcholinesterase deficiency	Inherited
	Organophosphate intoxication	Toxic
ACh:AChR binding	Congenital myasthenic syndrome with abnormal ACh-AChR interaction	Inherited
	Neuromuscular blocking agents (curare, succinylcholine, and others)	Toxic
	Snake envenomation (α-bungarotoxin)	Toxic

ACh = acetylcholine; AChR = acetylcholine receptors.
Modified from Gutmann,[3] p 2.

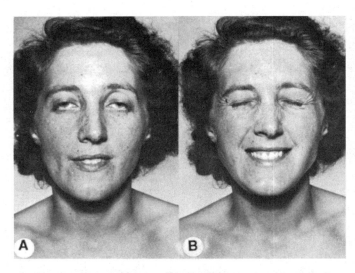

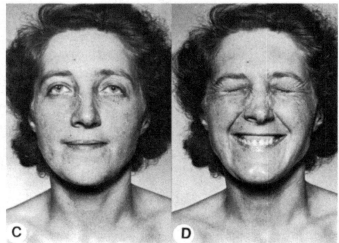

Figure 14–2. Bilateral Ptosis and Facial Weakness in Myasthenia Gravis. (A) and (B) are before injection of an anticholinesterase (neostigmine); (C) and (D) are 20 minutes after injection. In (A), note the ptosis and general lack of expression; in (B), note the failure to bury the eyelashes and the weak retraction of the corners of the mouth. These signs are all improved after inhibition of acetylcholine metabolism with an anticholinesterase (C and D). (From Spillane, JD: An Atlas of Clinical Neurology. Oxford University Press, New York, 1968, p 196, with permission.)

Myasthenia Gravis

Myasthenia gravis is an acquired autoimmune disorder characterized by fluctuating muscle weakness and fatigability, which is caused by deficient motor end-plate acetylcholine receptors.[3–16] It is the most common of all the human disorders of neuromuscular transmission. Myasthenia gravis is frequently not recognized, and its incidence is probably higher than that reported. Moreover, because patients are living longer with the disease, the prevalence of myasthenia gravis can be expected to increase.

The extraocular muscles are the first to be affected in about 50% of cases and are eventually affected in nearly all.[3–6,8–10,16] Ocular muscle involvement is usually bilateral, resulting in drooping eyelids (ptosis) and double vision (diplopia) (Fig. 14–2). Weakness of other muscles innervated by cranial nerves is also common and results in characteristic symptoms (Fig. 14–3). For example, facial weakness may result in loss of facial expression, everted lips, and a snarl-like smile. Oropharyngeal weakness may impair chewing, swallowing, and speaking. Eating may be progressively impaired by difficulty in biting, chewing, swallowing, and nasal regurgitation, and by choking on food and secretions. Together,

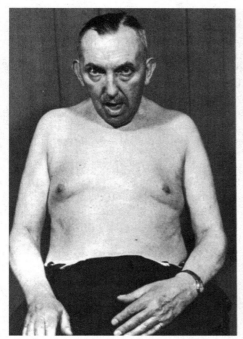 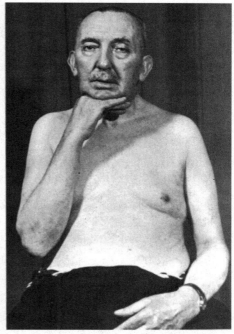

Figure 14–3. Muscle Weakness in Myasthenia Gravis. Weakness in this patient is evident in drooping of the eyelid, jaw, and head. (From Spillane, JD: An Atlas of Clinical Neurology. Oxford University Press, New York, 1968, p 199, with permission.)

oropharyngeal and ocular weakness occur in virtually all patients. Limb and neck weakness are also common, but usually in conjunction with cranial weakness; the limbs are seldom affected alone. When limbs are affected, proximal muscles are more affected than distal muscles. Weakness of respiratory muscles may result in shortness of breath, either at rest or on exertion. If myasthenia remains restricted to the ocular muscles beyond 2 to 3 years, generalized weakness is unlikely to develop. In 90% of the patients in whom the disease becomes generalized, this occurs within the first year. Myasthenia gravis does not involve cardiac or smooth muscle, nor are there alterations in coordination, sensation, or tendon reflexes.

Myasthenia gravis is unusual in the extent to which somatic signs and symptoms fluctuate.[3–6,8–10,16] Muscle weakness may vary over long periods of time, but may also vary from day to day or even hour to hour. Weakness is usually the least in the morning and worsens during the day, especially after prolonged exertion. Symptoms are provoked or exacerbated by many factors, including exertion, exposure to increased temperature, systemic illness (especially viral respiratory illness), menses, pregnancy, and emotional stress. Major prolonged variations are termed **remissions** or **exacerbations.** When an exacerbation involves oropharyngeal or respiratory muscles to the point of choking or inadequate ventilation, it is called a **crisis.** Such a crisis may be provoked by respiratory infection or surgical procedures, although it may occur with no apparent provocation. Prior to adequate respiratory care, myasthenic crisis was a life-threatening event. Now it is exceptional for patients to die of myasthenia gravis, except when cardiac, renal, or other disease complicates the picture. Spontaneous remissions lasting from weeks to years occur, although long-lasting remissions are not common.

The pathologic bases for the clinical findings in myasthenia gravis are perhaps the best defined of any neuromuscular disease. Considerable experimental and clinical evidence suggests that **myasthenia gravis is an autoimmune disorder in which circulating antibodies reduce the number of acetylcholine receptors (AChR) on the motor end plate,** thereby impairing neuromuscular junction transmission and the activation of skeletal muscle.[3–5,8,9,13,14] Evidence for this is drawn from the high titers of anti-AChR antibodies in myasthenic patients, and the clinical improvement associated with procedures such as thymectomy, immunosuppressive drug treatment, and plasmapheresis, which lower the levels of these antibodies. Circulating AChR antibodies are present in 85% to 95% of all patients, and immune complexes (immunoglobulin G and complement components) are deposited on the postjunctional membrane. Although a small percentage of these antibodies block the binding of acetylcholine to receptors, the major damage to the motor end plate results from an actual loss of functional receptors from the junctional folds. This probably results from both an acceleration of normal degradation of AChR, with inadequate replacement by new synthesis, and from complement-mediated lysis of the junctional membrane itself.[3–5,8,9,13,14]

Binding studies have shown that the number of AChR in the end-plate region of myasthenic muscle fibers may actually be reduced to 10% to 20% of normal. Immune-mediated alterations in the morphology of the junctions of myasthenic patients include a reduced postsynaptic region; sparse, flattened junctional folds; and shallow, sparse primary and secondary synaptic clefts (Fig. 14–4).[17] This reduction of AChR and these morphologic changes result in decreased effectiveness of neuromuscular junction transmission, with decreased amplitude of both miniature end-plate potentials and end-plate potentials. If transmission is decreased below threshold levels, it will fail to trigger muscle action

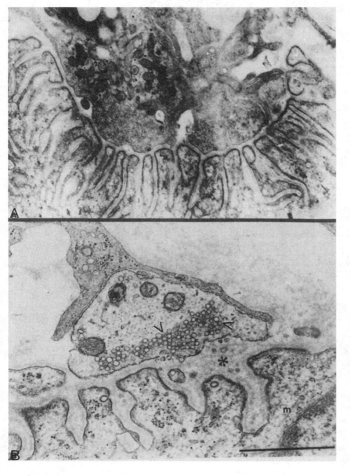

Figure 14–4. Ultrastructure of the Neuromuscular Junction. (A) In a normal specimen, the nerve terminal contains mitochondria and numerous presynaptic vesicles. The synaptic cleft is narrow and the postsynaptic clefts are deep with many secondary folds (EM ×28,000). *(B)* In a specimen from a patient with myasthenia gravis, presynaptic vesicles (v) are numerous, but the synaptic cleft (*) is widened and the postsynaptic folds are sparse with few secondary folds (EM ×39,600). The line is 1 μm long. (From Kakulas, BA and Adams, RD: Diseases of Muscle. Pathological Foundations of Clinical Myology, ed 4. Harper & Row, Philadelphia, 1985, p 677, with permission.)

potentials and muscle contractions. When transmission failure occurs at many junctions, the power of the whole muscle is decreased, which is manifested clinically as weakness.

What causes the appearance of the AChR antibodies is not known, but as in many other autoimmune diseases, a persistent viral infection has been suspected but not confirmed.[3–5,8,9,13,14,16] Considerable evidence suggests that the thymus plays an important role in the pathogenesis of myasthenia gravis in many patients. The thymus gland is almost always abnormal, with two thirds of patients with myasthenia gravis having thymic hyperplasia and 10% to 15% having a thymic tumor (thymoma). Thymectomy is beneficial in a high percentage of cases (Fig. 14–5). The thymus contains "myoid" or musclelike cells that have histologic characteristics of skeletal muscle and bear AChR.[3–5,8,9,13,14,16,18] It has been suggested that these cells act as antigenic sites that sensitize thymic lymphocytes to the AChR. In addition, it has been postulated that the thymus produces a hormone involved in initiating or perpetuating the immune response to AChR. Other autoimmune diseases have been noted in association with myasthenia gravis, including thyroid disease, ulcerative colitis, systemic lupus erythematosus, and rheumatoid arthritis. Whatever its origins, the heterogeneity of the disorder argues against any single etiologic factor.

The objectives of treatment are to relieve the symptoms by improving neuromuscular transmission and to prevent further immune-mediated destruction of AChR and other components of the neuromuscular junction.[3–5,8,9,15,19–21] **Anticholinesterase drugs** inhibit the enzymatic destruction of acetylcholine, allowing it to remain longer at the end plate. This increases the probability that enough receptors will be activated to generate a muscle action potential and hence contraction. These agents are effective in early symptomatic treatment in most patients (see Fig. 14–2). However, they do have some serious limitations. They produce only temporary improvement, are less effective over time, are prone to overdosage and underdosage, and produce frequent side effects even at therapeutic doses. Common side effects are gastrointestinal complaints (abdominal cramps, nausea, vomiting, and diarrhea) and increased oral or bronchial secretions.

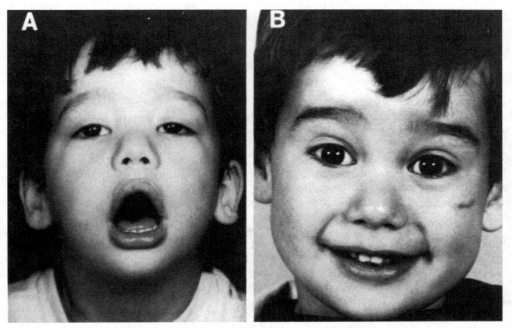

Figure 14–5. *A 2-Year-Old Boy with Severe Generalized Myasthenia Gravis.* (A) The patient shows bilateral ptosis and prominent facial and jaw weakness. (B) One year later after thymectomy, he has totally recovered without any medication. (From Gutmann,[3] p 5, with permission.)

Thymectomy is now recommended for almost all patients younger than 50 years of age, and almost all improve. The main disadvantages of thymectomy are operative complications and the long delay (often years) before improvement is complete. **Corticosteroid therapy** is the mainstay of therapy in older patients and in younger patients in whom anticholinesterase drugs and thymectomy have not been effective. The major disadvantages are corticosteroid side effects. Other **immunosuppressant drugs** are used in patients in whom corticosteroids are contraindicated or in patients who fail to respond to therapy with anticholinesterases, corticosteroids, or thymectomy. Virtually all patients improve at least temporarily following **plasmapheresis** (plasma exchange). This is used as adjunctive therapy in patients who have not responded to other forms of therapy to produce rapid improvement before thymectomy or other surgery, or it is used in myasthenic crisis. Although this procedure does result in a lowering of the AChR antibody titer and objective improvement within 48 hours in most patients, its effects are transient (lasting a few days to several months) and confer no greater long-term protection than immunosuppressant drugs alone.

Transient Neonatal Myasthenia Gravis

Transient neonatal myasthenia gravis develops in about 20% of infants born to myasthenic mothers.[3,9,22,23] The symptoms usually appear during the first few hours of life and may last for several weeks, after which the children are normal. Complete recovery is expected in less than 2 months in 90% of patients. The principal findings are generalized hypotonia, facial weakness, weak cry, poor sucking, and occasional respiratory difficulty. Neonates whose mothers have the highest levels of AChR antibodies are most likely to develop neonatal myasthenia gravis. Although the etiology of the disease is poorly understood, **it may be caused either by transfer of AChR antibodies across the placenta from the affected mother to the infant, or by independent antibody production by the infant.**[22,23] The latter may be caused by the transfer of immunocytes from the mother or by fetal AChR damaged by maternal antibodies, which trigger a transient immune response. These infants are very responsive to anticholinesterases.

Lambert-Eaton Myasthenic Syndrome

Lambert-Eaton Myasthenic Syndrome (LEMS) **is an acquired autoimmune disease associated with impaired nerve-evoked release of acetylcholine from the motor nerve terminal and a resultant syndrome of muscle weakness and fatigability.**[3,5–11,25–32] LEMS is most often diagnosed in patients older than 40 years, although much younger cases have been reported. In most cases (70% of men; 30% of women), the patient has had or will develop carcinoma, particularly small cell carcinoma of the lung. In about one third of cases, no carcinoma is evident. However, in many of these cases an autoimmune disorder such as thyroid disease, rheumatoid arthritis, or systemic lupus erythematosus or treatment with certain drugs such as the antibiotic, neomycin, has been noted.

LEMS is characterized by weakness and fatigability of proximal limb and torso muscles, with relative sparing of cranial nerve muscles. [3,5–11,24,25] The lower limbs are typically more involved than the upper limbs. Early symptoms may consist of aching of the proximal leg muscles and difficulty in walking or climbing stairs. In contrast to myasthenia gravis, the weakness in LEMS is present in rested muscle, but improves several seconds after the onset of maximal voluntary effort, before declining. This increase in strength probably results from facilitation of transmitter release at high rates of stimulation. The tendon reflexes are depressed or absent in most patients. **Notably, neuromuscular symptoms are often accompanied by autonomic manifestations,** such as dry mouth, sexual impotence, decreased sweating, orthostatic hypotension, and altered pupillary reflexes.

Most evidence suggests that LEMS, like myasthenia gravis, is an autoimmune disorder.[14,24–32] For example, patients with LEMS are responsive to immunosuppressant drugs and plasmapheresis, and nonneoplastic patients have other autoimmune diseases and organ-specific (thyroid and gastric) autoantibodies. Mice injected with immunoglobulin derived from patients with LEMS develop many of the morphologic and electrophysiologic features of the disease.[28,29,32] Unlike myasthenia gravis, **LEMS revolves around a *prejunctional* defect that results in a decrease in Ca^{2+}-dependent, nerve-evoked release of acetylcholine.**[24–32] Although acetylcholine synthesis and storage seem to be normal, actual release mechanisms are impaired. Electrophysiologic studies of LEMS skeletal muscle have shown that although the frequency and size of the miniature end-plate potentials are normal, the end-plate potentials themselves are small. This suggests that the spontaneous release of acetylcholine (which causes the miniature end-plate potentials) is normal, but the end-plate potential is diminished in amplitude because less total acetylcholine is released by each nerve impulse. **Clinical and experimental studies suggest that autoantibodies react with nerve terminal voltage–dependent Ca^{2+} channels,** thereby impeding the ingress of Ca^{2+}, which occurs when the terminal is depolarized by the nerve impulse.[24–32] This Ca^{2+} influx is required for transmitter-containing vesicle exocytosis and acetylcholine release. The antibodies eventually lead to the loss of the channels altogether. What triggers the development of such antibodies is not known. In carcinoma-related LEMS, it is possible that tumor Ca^{2+} channel antigens trigger the production of antibodies cross-reactive with antigen on the motor neuron terminus.[30]

Effective treatment of the associated carcinoma may induce remission.[26] Anticholinesterases are of benefit in some cases, but not to the same extent as in myasthenia gravis, probably because they do not improve acetylcholine release. Drugs that enhance the release of acetylcholine have been used with some success, but many produce serious side effects. Immunosuppression with corticosteroids and other drugs and plasmapheresis have been shown to be of value in both carcinoma-associated and noncarcinomatous LEMS.

Congenital Myasthenic Syndromes

Congenital myasthenia encompasses a diverse group of inherited disorders of neuromuscular transmission in which immunologic mechanisms are not implicated (Table 14–2).[1–3,5,9,33–44] AChR antibodies are not found in plasma nor have immune complexes been visualized in the neuromuscular junction. All these disorders are rare, and few cases have been discussed in the literature in any detail. This scarcity, however, may significantly underrepresent the true frequency of these disorders.[33] Congenital myasthenic syndromes are easily confused with myasthenia gravis, and extensive evaluation is required for their definitive diagnosis. Unfortunately, many of the sophisticated techniques used in evaluation of these disorders, such as muscle biopsy, electron microscopic analysis, and microelectrode studies, are available only in large medical centers.

In each of the congenital myasthenic syndromes, the safety factor built into neuromuscular transmission is compromised by one or more specific mechanisms, and this expresses itself clinically as muscle weakness and abnormal fatigability (Fig. 14–6 and 14–7).[1] In **each congenital myasthenic disorder, a primary, genetically determined abnormality either affects neuromuscular transmission directly or causes secondary derangements (e.g., junctional fold degeneration or loss of AChR), which eventually impairs transmission.**[33–44] These disorders (like the metabolic myopathies) are of particular interest to basic scientists for what they can reveal about normal junctional transmission. Detailed electrophysiologic studies reveal characteristic changes in miniature end-plate potentials, end-plate potentials, and muscle action potentials, alterations that are instrumental in both the diagnosis and understanding of the pathogenesis of congenital myasthenic syndromes. Light and electron microscopy reveal specific abnormalities in the morphology and ultrastructure of the neuromuscular junction—some reflective of the primary genetic defect, others more likely a

Table 14–2. Congenital Myasthenic Syndromes[1,2,36,37]

Syndrome	Inheritance	Clinical Features	Junctional Defects
Familial infantile myasthenia	Autosomal recessive	Intermittent ptosis, poor suck and cry, feeding difficulty, and secondary respiratory infections during infancy; periodic crises with markedly exacerbated weakness; symptoms tending to improve with age; responsive to anti-ChE	**Defect in acetylcholine resynthesis** or packaging into vesicles; vesicles smaller at rest
Congenital end-plate acetylcholinesterase deficiency	Autosomal recessive	Generalized weakness and abnormal fatiguability in multiple muscles from birth; particular involvement of axial muscles; unresponsive to anti-ChE	Total lack of acetylcholinesterase; smaller nerve terminals with **fewer releasable quanta and mild AChR deficiency** due to focal degeneration of junctional folds
Slow-channel syndrome	Autosomal dominant	Highly variable age of onset and pattern of progression; variable weakness in selected muscle groups; most severe in cervical, scapular, and finger extensor muscles; unresponsive to anti-ChE	Prolonged open time of AChR ion channels; resultant prolonged end-plate currents lead to calcium accumulation promoting **secondary degenerative changes in junctional folds, loss of AChR**, and myopathic changes
Congenital end-plate AChR deficiency	Autosomal recessive	Onset in infancy with signs and symptoms similar to autoimmune myasthenia gravis; responsive to anti-ChE	**Decreased AChR** on simplified junctional folds
Congenital paucity of synaptic vesicles and reduced quantal release	—	Fatigability and intermittent bulbar weakness since infancy; partially responsive to anti-ChE	Few synaptic vesicles in nerve terminal resulting in **fewer readily releasable quanta**
High-conductance, fast-channel syndrome	—	Mild, intermittent weakness of selected bulbar and limb muscles since infancy; unresponsive to anti-ChE	Functionally abnormal AChR ion channels; some **degenerative changes in junctional folds** and myopathic changes similar to slow-channel syndrome
Congenital myasthenic syndrome with abnormal ACh-AChR interaction	—	Severe generalized weakness and fatigability in multiple muscles since birth; unresponsive to anti-ChE	Possibly a **reduced affinity of AChR for ACh**; no morphologic or ultrastructural abnormalities apparent
Congenital AChR deficiency and short-channel open time	—	Hypotonia, bulbar weakness, and respiratory insufficiency since birth; with additional weakness and fatigability developing during first year; responsive to anti-ChE	Kinetic abnormalities in AChR ion channels and **decreased AChR**

Anti-ChE = anticholinesterase; ACh = acetylcholine; AChR = acetylcholine receptors.
Boldface type indicates most probable cause of reduced transmission safety factor.

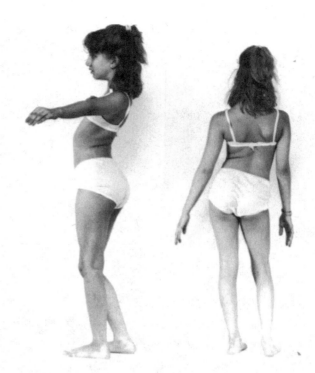

Figure 14–6. *Young Patient with Congenital Acetylcholinesterase Deficiency.* Lordosis and scoliosis due to axial muscle involvement worsened after a few seconds of standing. The lateral view shows maximal arm abduction after 15 seconds. Her younger sister had similar symptoms. In both, the symptoms were refractory to anticholinesterase drugs. (From Engel,[1] p 12. Reprinted with permission from Seminars in Neurology 10(1):12, 1990. Thieme Medical Publishers, Inc.)

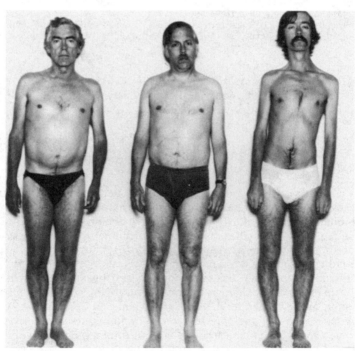

Figure 14–7. *Slow-Channel Syndrome in Two Generations.* From left to right. A 54-year-old patient with his 48-year-old brother and 29-year-old son. Note atrophy of shoulder and forearm muscles and mild asymmetric ptosis in the brothers. The son shows scoliosis, moderate to marked atrophy of cervical, shoulder, arm, and torso muscles, and pronounced ptosis. (From Engel, AG, et al: Recently Recognized Congenital Myasthenic Syndromes: [A] End-plate acetylcholine [ACh] esterase deficiency. [B] Putative abnormality of the ACh induced ion channel. [C] Putative defect of AChR synthesis or mobilization-clinical features, ultrastructure and cytochemistry. Ann NY Acad Sci 377:614, 1981, with permission.)

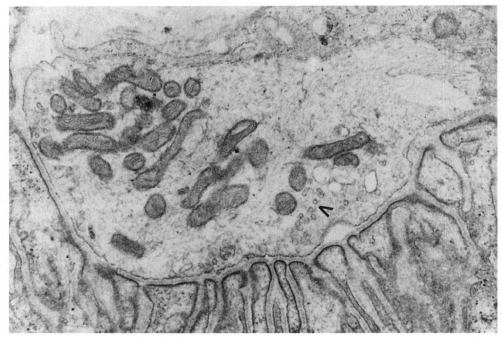

Figure 14–8. *Congenital Paucity of Synaptic Vesicles.* In this intercostal muscle specimen from a patient who had fatigability and weakness since infancy, the nerve terminal contains very few presynaptic vesicles (v) (compare with the many vesicles in Figure 14–4B). This was correlated with a reduction in the quantal content of the endplate potential. The junctional folds are normal (EM ×31,000). (From Engel,[36] p 125, with permission.)

complication of or a compensatory response to this defect (Fig. 14–8). Some of these myasthenic disorders are treatable, with varying responsiveness to anticholinesterases and other traditional forms of therapy for myasthenia.

Botulism

Botulism is a paralytic disease in which failure of neuromuscular junction transmission is caused by any one of several forms of a toxin produced by the bacterium, *Clostridium botulinum.*[3,5,9–11,45–48] Not all patients are equally affected; botulism may vary from mild illness requiring no medical assistance to fulminating disease resulting in death. Whether this variability is due to the specific form of toxin involved, the amount of toxin ingested, or individual susceptibility is not known.

The classic form of botulism occurs in adults after ingestion of toxin-contaminated food.[3,5,9–11,45] In this form of the disease, neuromuscular symptoms usually appear 12 to 36 hours after ingestion of the tainted food, although extremes of 3 hours to 14 days have been reported. In general, the earlier the appearance of symptoms, the more severe the disease. The first symptoms usually resemble those of food poisoning, including vomiting, diarrhea, abdominal pain, and dryness of the mouth, and may occur within a few hours of ingestion. However, the absence of these symptoms does not rule out botulism. Later, neuromuscular symptoms develop, with primarily bulbar findings such as diplopia, blurred vision, dysphonia, dysarthria, and dysphagia. Symmetric flaccid paralysis of the extremities may ensue, usually in a descending pattern of involvement. Weakness of respiratory muscles may necessitate assisted ventilation. Deep tendon reflexes are intact in milder cases, but if significant paralysis is present, these reflexes are reduced or absent. No pathologic reflexes or sensory disturbances are usually observed. Impairment of cholinergic transmission may also result in autonomic disturbances such as constipation, pupillary abnormalities, urinary retention, and reduced salivation and lacrimation. Once the symptoms appear, the disease may progress rapidly over several days. A period of stabilization is then followed by gradual recovery over weeks to months. Full recovery can usually be expected. Respiratory failure with septic complications still causes death in about 8% of patients.[45]

Although there were no reported **cases of infant botulism** prior to 1976, these **now constitute the majority of cases of botulism.**[46,47] It has been estimated that about 250 cases occur annually, but most probably go undiagnosed.[46] Infants with botulism are usually younger than 6 months of age, with an average age of onset of 6 to 12 weeks.[3,5,9–11,45–48] Symptoms almost always begin with constipation, followed by weakness. Constipation may actually precede weakness by up to 2 weeks. Once apparent, weakness typically progresses rapidly over a few days in a descending pattern to involve cranial nerve, trunk, and limb muscles. Affected infants end up with generalized weakness reflected in poor sucking, diminished gag, facial and ocular paralysis, ptosis, reduced spontaneous movements, lethargy, and respiratory difficulty.[45–48] The severity of involvement is highly variable, ranging from constipation, hypotonia, and poor feeding in mild cases, to cases of severe hypotonia and weakness requiring intubation, nasogastric feeding, and mechanical ventilation. Despite the severity of the motor deficit that may evolve, the prognosis in most cases is excellent with appropriate supportive care.[47,48] There is seldom any permanent neurologic deficit.

Wound botulism, although the rarest form of this disease, may result from toxin produced by *C botulinum* infecting a wound. Although wound botulism has historically been reported in patients with contaminated traumatic and surgical wounds, it has recently been reported in chronic drug users in whom minor wounds have been implicated. The clinical neurologic presentations of wound botulism closely resemble those of the more common form caused by contaminated food.

Botulism is caused by various analogs of a toxin that interferes with the release of acetylcholine from terminal axons of somatic motor neurons, as well as from autonomic cholinergic fibers.[3,5,9–11,45] This toxin irreversibly binds to presynaptic or prejunctional membranes, blocking the Ca^{2+}-dependent step of acetylcholine exocytosis. With decreased acetylcholine release, the end-plate potential in muscle that occurs in response to nerve stimulation diminishes in amplitude and finally disappears, at which point neuromuscular transmission ceases. Decreased spontaneous release of acetylcholine is reflected in decreased frequency and amplitude of miniature end-plate potentials. Parasympathetic transmission blockade explains anticholinergic signs such as dry mouth, constipation, urinary retention, and pupillary dilatation, which often accompany botulism. Central nervous system cholinergic pathways do not seem to be affected. Recovery occurs by sprouting of new terminal nerve filaments and the formation of new synapses.

***Clostridium botulinum* is an anaerobic, spore-forming bacterium, which is widely distributed in soil.** This bacterium produces an exotoxin (actually a group of immunologically distinct exotoxins) that constitutes one of the most potent poisons known. Adult humans are usually intoxicated by the ingestion of inadequately cooked food that has been contaminated by viable bacilli or spores, and hence by the toxin. The toxin is primarily absorbed in the stomach and upper part of the small intestine. Infantile botulism is somewhat different to the extent that the ingested or inhaled spores germinate, propagate, and produce the toxin within the gastrointestinal tract. Differences in the intestinal flora and a lack of *Clostridium*-inhibiting bile acids found in adults allow bacteria to multiply within the infant gastrointestinal tract.[46,47] The clinical manifestations of the infantile syndrome are relatively slow to develop, since the toxin is absorbed slowly as it is produced rather than all at once, as in the case of contaminated food. Honey has been the probable source of spores in a number of cases, and it is currently recommended that honey not be fed to children younger than 12 months old.[46,47] Honey has not been shown to contain toxin, so it is a safe food for older children or adults. There also seems to be a significant association between breast feeding and acquisition of this disease.[46,47] This may reflect differences in the intestinal environment of breast-fed and formula-fed infants. Why botulism occurs in some babies who ingest *Clostridium botulinum* spores and not in others is not known. These bacteria also thrive in dead or devitalized tissue, and toxin can be produced in even minor, anaerobic wounds.

Drug- and Chemical-Induced Myasthenic Syndromes

A wide variety of pharmacologic agents can directly interfere with neuromuscular junction transmission. These agents exert both prejunctional and postjunctional effects.[9,11,49-52] Prejunctional effects may prevent action potential propagation, impair the release of acetylcholine, or inhibit acetylcholine synthesis. Postjunctional actions may block acetylcholine from activating its motor end-plate receptors. Some agents, rather than exerting direct effects on the neuromuscular junction, seem to disturb immunologic mechanisms, resulting in antibody-mediated conditions similar to those found in myasthenia gravis. Although some of these agents are commonly used drugs, they seldom produce overt myasthenic symptoms in normal individuals unless their blood levels are excessively high because of overdose or impaired excretion by the kidney or liver.[49-52] **These agents may** create problems by potentiating the effects of neuromuscular blocking agents used during surgical procedures (see Chapter 3) or may **worsen or unmask preexisting disorders of the neuromuscular junction** (including myasthenia gravis and LEMS) in which transmission is already compromised (Table 14–3). Certain antibiotics and cardiovascular drugs account for most of these adverse reactions. The aminoglycoside antibiotics are well known for producing neuromuscular weakness. Specific drugs within this group act prejunctionally, postjunctionally, or both. Doxycycline (Vibramycin), for example, inhibits acetylcholine release, whereas neomycin blocks acetylcholine binding to its receptor. Among the cardiovascular drugs, certain antiarrhythmics and beta-blocking agents are capable of producing similar symptoms. The clinical manifestations of drug-induced disturbance of neuromuscular transmission resemble those of myasthenia gravis with varying degrees of ptosis and bulbar, respiratory, or generalized weakness. Because these agents may cause worsening of myasthenic weakness, they should be used with caution in myasthenic patients. **Therapists should be alert to any clinical worsening that occurs with the initiation of any new medication.**

Table 14–3. Drugs That May Worsen Myasthenic Weakness

D-Penicillamide

Aminoglycoside antibiotics, such as gentamicin, kanamycin, neomycin, and streptomycin

Cardiovascular drugs
  Antiarrhythmics, such as quinine, quinidine, and procainamide
  Beta-adrenergic blocking agents, such as oxprenolol, propranolol, practolol, and timolol
  Calcium channel blockers

Neuromuscular blocking agents, such as succinylcholine and D-tubocurarine

Ophthalmic drugs, such as beta-adrenergic blocking agents, timolol, and betaxolol

Local anesthetics (intravenous), such as lidocaine and procaine

Neuromuscular Blocking Agents

Note also that **there are a number of drugs called** *neuromuscular blocking agents,***which are used to intentionally block neuromuscular transmission** in order to produce muscle relaxation during anesthesia for surgery and certain other procedures (see Chapter 3).[49,52,53] Overdose, inadvertent administration, or poisoning with these agents may lead to junctional blockade and muscle paralysis. Moreover, these agents are more potent in patients with myasthenia gravis or LEMS and are potentiated by the concurrent administration of a number of different drugs including antibiotics, general anesthetics, local anesthetics, and antiarrhythmics.

D-Penicillamine

D-Penicillamine is used in the treatment of rheumatoid arthritis and certain other conditions.[9,17,49,50] A myasthenic state clinically and electrophysiologically indistinguishable from myasthenia gravis has been reported in a significant number of patients in long-term treatment with this agent. This disorder seems to occur only in susceptible individuals, however, who constitute a very small percentage ($<1\%$) of the patients treated with D-penicillamine. The myasthenic symptoms are usually mild and frequently restricted to ocular muscles. Rather than exerting some direct effect on the neuromuscular junction, D-penicillamine probably induces this condition by stimulating or enhancing an immune reaction against the neuromuscular junction.[9,49,50] In fact, increased titers of antibodies to AChR are found in many of these patients. The antibodies drop and the symptoms remit in most patients within 1 year of discontinuing the drug. Treatment with anticholinesterases is usually all that is necessary during this period.

Magnesium

Although rare, **marked elevations of plasma magnesium can cause neuromuscular junction blockade and a generalized flaccid paralysis.**[51,54,56] Because the physiologic mechanisms that regulate the plasma concentrations of magnesium are so effective, hypermagnesemia rarely reaches symptomatic levels without the intentional administration of magnesium-containing compounds.[54–56] Toxicity is usually associated with the use of magnesium-containing antacids or cathartics, in patients with chronic renal failure, excessive absorption of magnesium from retained enemas, or magnesium sulfate treatment for hypertensive crisis. Hypermagnesemia, for example, is intentionally produced during treatment of hypertension accompanying pregnancy and sometimes causes neuromuscular signs in pregnant women and newborns.

The signs of magnesium toxicity are correlated with the plasma levels.[54–56] The earliest effects consist of paralysis of smooth muscle and autonomic effects such as dry mouth, flushing, hypotension, pupillary dilatation, urinary retention, nausea, and vomiting. At higher concentrations, neuromuscular effects manifest as a flaccid paralysis with normal sensation and alertness. The neuromuscular manifestations of magnesium toxicity are very similar to those found in LEMS. In both conditions, there is relative sparing of the extraocular and other cranial muscles, early hyporeflexia, temporary relief of weakness with maximal voluntary effort, and evidence of abnormal autonomic activity. Magnesium can also potentiate the action of neuromuscular blocking agents and exacerbate preexisting disorders of the neuromuscular junction. Severe weakness after magnesium administration has been reported in both patients with myasthenia gravis and those with LEMS, despite normal or only mildly elevated plasma magnesium levels.[56]

Like calcium, magnesium acts at several different sites in the central and peripheral nervous system. The paralysis accompanying hypermagnesemia, however, is probably due entirely to neuromuscular junction blockade.[54–56] The junctional effects of magnesium have been extensively studied, and magnesium has proved to be a useful tool in the study of normal junctional activity. Junctional calcium is necessary for the evoked release of acetylcholine. Ca^{2+} is bound to specific binding sites on the outside of prejunctional calcium channels. With depolarization of the nerve terminal, these channels open and Ca^{2+} flows inward to activate acetylcholine release. The greater the influx of calcium, the more acetylcholine will be released by the nerve impulse, and hence the greater the amplitude of the end-plate potential. Magnesium and other metallic ions (such as strontium, manganese, cobalt, zinc, nickel, and cadmium) combine with the same membrane receptor as calcium and thus may competitively antagonize the entry of Ca^{2+} into the nerve terminal.[51,54,56] As the concentration of these metals increases in relation to that of calcium, transmitter release diminishes ultimately to the point of transmission failure. Hypermagnesemia does not impair the spontaneous release of acetylcholine, so that the amplitude and frequency of miniature end-plate potentials are not altered.

Magnesium blockade can be rapidly reversed by reducing the levels of magnesium and increasing the levels of calcium. Treatment includes discontinuation of magnesium, intravenous augmentation of calcium (e.g., calcium gluconate), and reduction of the magnesium overload by hemodialysis or peritoneal dialysis.

Biologic Toxins

Several biologic toxins, in addition to the botulinum toxin, can disrupt neuromuscular transmission.[51,52,57–63] For example, the venom of the black widow spider (α-latrotoxin) stimulates vesicle fusion and acetylcholine release while irreversibly inhibiting vesicle recycling in the nerve terminal.[59] This soon depletes nerve endings of releasable transmitter, so that transmission failure occurs and muscle paralysis develops. **The elapid snakes (e.g., cobras and kraits) produce toxins that have both prejunctional and postjunctional effects.**[51,52,57,58,60–63] The postsynaptic neurotoxins bind to the end-plate AChR, inhibiting their activation by acetylcholine. α-Bungarotoxin from the venom of certain kraits is the prototype of this class of neurotoxin and binds irreversibly to the AChR.[52,57,58,60] This characteristic has made this substance an invaluable tool in the study of the morphology, physiology, and pathophysiology of the neuromuscular junction. Presynaptic neurotoxins ultimately inhibit the release of acetylcholine, possibly through enzymatic effects on the nerve terminal membrane, resulting in irreversible changes in the release sites. The best-known toxin in this group is β-bungarotoxin.[51,57,58,60,62] Common clinical presentations resulting from poisoning with these neurotoxins revolve around paralysis of cranial nerve muscles (ptosis, ophthalmoplegia with blurred vision or diplopia, dysphagia, dysarthria, and facial weakness), neck flexors, and proximal limb muscles (Fig. 14–9). Respiratory paralysis and paralysis of all muscle groups may develop with a loss of tendon reflexes. Coma and convulsions may precede death. The prejunctional toxins tend to be associated with a more delayed onset, prolonged symptoms, poor response to antivenom, and they are more often lethal than the postsynaptically acting toxins. Although snake bites are relatively rare in the United States, snake envenomation is a major cause of death and disability in developing countries, particularly in India and southeast Asia.[61]

Organophosphates

The *organophosphates* are a class of compounds that irreversibly inhibit cholinesterases, including the acetylcholinesterase of the neuromuscular junction.[64–67] Organophosphates are most commonly used as insecticides, but they have also attracted some interest because of their potential for use in chemical warfare (i.e., nerve gases). These substances may be absorbed through the skin, mucous membranes, gastrointestinal tract, and lungs. Although organophosphate poisoning is relatively rare in the United States where these

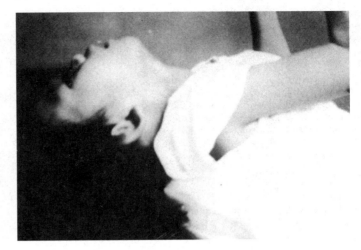

***Figure 14–9.** Snake Envenomation.* Muscular weakness with an inability to raise the head has been reported following bites by several species of snakes (e.g., cobras and kraits) with neurotoxic venoms. (From Minton,[60] p 58. Reprinted with permission from Seminars in Neurology 10(1):52, 1990. Thieme Medical Publishers, Inc.)

agents are not readily available, intoxication resulting from accidental (or even purposeful) ingestion is more common in other countries where their use as insecticides is widespread. The signs and symptoms of organophosphate poisoning may begin within a few hours of exposure, and death may follow within hours due to respiratory failure and cardiovascular collapse. **The clinical manifestations of intoxication reflect the ability of these agents to inhibit cholinesterase and cause the accumulation of acetylcholine within the neuromuscular junction, as well as within cholinergic synapses of the autonomic and central nervous system.**[64–67] This accumulation of transmitter causes a depolarizing blockade of junctional or synaptic transmission. At the neuromuscular junction, the organophosphates cause an initial stimulation of muscle followed by its paralysis. Involuntary twitches, fasciculations, and cramps are followed by muscle weakness or paralysis. Muscle weakness may be severe and life-threatening. Paralysis of respiratory muscles may lead to respiratory failure. Tongue and pharyngeal weakness may lead to airway obstruction and asphyxia. Autonomic effects may be numerous and include pupillary constriction, bronchoconstriction and increased bronchosecretion, sweating, diarrhea, and bradycardia. Central nervous system effects due to the accumulation of acetylcholine at central cholinergic synapses include anxiety, restlessness, tremor, confusion, ataxia, coma, and seizures. Treatment includes preventing additional exposure, respiratory support, and pharmacologic intervention directed at cholinergic blockade (e.g., atropine). In the absence of any significant complications, recovery usually occurs within 1 to 3 weeks. The return of cholinesterase activity depends on the synthesis of new enzymes.

RECOMMENDED READINGS

Bowman, WC: Pharmacology of Neuromuscular Function, ed 2. Wright, London, 1990.

Chou, SM: Pathology of the Neuromuscular Junction. Chapter 17. In Mastaglia, FL and Detchant, Lord Walton (eds): Skeletal Muscle Pathology, ed 2. Churchill Livingstone, Edinburgh, 1992.

Drachman, DB (ed): Myasthenia Gravis: Biology and Treatment. Ann NY Acad Sci 505:1, 1987.

Engel, AG: Acquired Autoimmune Myasthenia Gravis. Chapter 68. In Engel, AG and Franzini-Armstrong, C (eds): Myology: Basic and Clinical, ed 2. McGraw-Hill, New York, 1994.

Engel, AG: Myasthenic Syndromes. Chapter 69. In Engel, AG and Franzini-Armstrong, C (eds): Myology: Basic and Clinical, ed 2. McGraw-Hill, New York, 1994.

Engel, AG: Molecular Biology of End-Plate Diseases. Chapter 9. In Salpeter, MM (ed): The Vertebrate Neuromuscular Junction. Alan R Liss, New York, 1986.

Engel, AG, et al: Newly Recognized Congenital Myasthenic Syndromes. Chapter 14. In Aquilonius, SM and Gillberg, PG (eds): Progressive in Brain Research, vol 84. Elsevier, New York, 1990.

Graus, YMF and DeBaets, MC: Myasthenia Gravis: An Autoimmune Response Against the Acetylcholine Receptor. Immunol Res 12(1):78, 1993.

Gutmann, L: Disorders of Neuromuscular Transmission. Chapter 54. In Joynt, RJ (ed): Clinical Neurology, vol 4. JB Lippincott, Philadelphia, 1991.

Levin, KH and Richman, OP: Myasthenia Gravis. Chapter 11. In Adachi, M and Sher, JH: Neuromuscular Disease. Igaku-Shoin, New York. 1990.

Newson-Davis, J: Diseases of the Neuromuscular Junction. Chapter 15. In Asbury, AK, McKhann, GM and McDonald, WI (eds): Diseases of the Nervous System: Clinical Neurobiology, vol 1, ed 2. WB Saunders, Philadelphia, 1992.

Pascuzzi, RM (ed): Disorders of Neuromuscular Transmission. Semin Neurol 10(1): 1, 1990.

Penn, AJ, et al (eds): Myasthenia Gravis and Related Disorders. Ann NY Acad Sci 681:1, 1993.

Rowland, LP: Diseases of Chemical Transmission at the Nerve-Muscle Synapse. Myasthenia Gravis. Chapter 16. In Kandel, ER, Schwartz, JH, and Jessell, TM (eds): Principles of Neural Science, ed 3. Elsevier, New York, 1991.

Sanders, DB (ed): Myasthenia Gravis and Myasthenic Syndromes. Neurol Clin 12:231, 1994.

Sanders, DB and Howard, JF, Jr. Disorders of Neuromuscular Transmission. Chapter 82. In Bradley, WG, et al (eds): Neurology in Clinical Practice: The Neurological Disorders, vol II. Butterworth-Heinemann, Boston, 1990.

Swash, M and Schwartz, MS: Neuromuscular Diseases. Chapter 12. Myasthenia Gravis and Other Myasthenic Syndromes, ed 2. Springer-Verlag, London, 1988.

REFERENCES

1. Engel, AG: Congenital Disorders of Neuromuscular Transmission. Semin Neurol 10(1):12, 1990.
2. Engel, AG: Myasthenic Syndromes. Chapter 69. In Engel, AG and Franzini-Armstrong, C (eds): Myology: Basic and Clinical, ed 2. McGraw-Hill, New York, 1994.
3. Gutmann, L: Disorders of Neuromuscular Transmission. Chapter 54. In Joynt, RJ (ed): Clinical Neurology, vol 4. JB Lippincott, Philadelphia, 1991.
4. Levin, KH and Richman, OP: Myasthenia Gravis. Chapter 11. In Adachi, M and Sher, JH: Neuromuscular Disease. Igaku-Shoin, New York, 1990.
5. Newson-Davis, J: Diseases of the Neuromuscular Junction. Chapter 15. In Asbury, AK, McKhann, GM, and McDonald, WI (eds): Diseases of the Nervous System: Clinical Neurobiology, vol 1, ed 2. WB Saunders, Philadelphia, 1992.
6. Hopkins, LC: Clinical Features of Myasthenia Gravis. Neurol Clin 12:243, 1994.
7. Pascuzzi, RM (ed): Disorders of Neuromuscular Transmission. Semin Neurol 10(1):1, 1990.
8. Rowland, LP: Diseases of Chemical Transmission at the Nerve-Muscle Synapse: Myasthenia Gravis. Chapter 16. In Kandel, ER, Schwartz, JH, and Jessell, TM (eds): Principles of Neural Science, ed 3. Elsevier, New York, 1991.
9. Sanders, DB and Howard, JF, Jr: Disorders of Neuromuscular Transmission. Chapter 82. In Bradley, WG, et al (eds): Neurology in Clinical Practice: The Neurological Disorders, vol II. Butterworth-Heinemann, Boston, 1990.
10. Swash, M and Schwartz, MS: Neuromuscular Diseases. Chapter 12. Myasthenia Gravis and Other Myasthenic Syndromes, ed 2. Springer-Verlag, London, 1988.
11. Wyngaarden, JB, Smith, LH, Jr, and Bennett, JC (eds): Cecil Textbook of Medicine. Chapter 509. Disorders of Neuromuscular Transmission, ed 19. WB Saunders, Philadelphia, 1991.
12. Engel, AG: Autoimmune Myasthenia Gravis. Chapter 68. In Engel, AG and Franzini-Armstrong, C (eds): Myology: Basic and Clinical, ed 2. McGraw-Hill, New York, 1994.
13. Graus, YMF and DeBaets, MC: Myasthenia Gravis: An Autoimmune Response Against the Acetylcholine Receptor. Immunol Res 12(1):78, 1993.
14. Maselli, RA: Pathophysiology of Myasthenia Gravis and Lambert-Eaton Syndrome. Neurol Clin 12:285, 1994.
15. Grob, D, et al: The Course of Myasthenia Gravis and Therapies Affecting Outcome. Ann NY Acad Sci 505:472, 1987.
16. Oosterhuis, HJGH and Kuks, JBM: Myasthenia Gravis and Myasthenic Syndromes. Curr Opin Neurol Neurosurg 5:638, 1992.
17. Chou, SM: Pathology of the Neuromuscular Junction. Chapter 17. In Mastaglia, FL and Detchant, Lord Walton (eds): Skeletal Muscle Pathology, ed 2. Churchill Livingstone, Edinburgh, 1992.
18. Furuya, A, et al: Human Myasthenia Gravis Thymic Myoid Cells: De Novo Immunohistochemical and Intracellular Electrophysiological Studies. J Neurol Sci 101:208, 1991.
19. Verma, P and Oger, J: Treatment of Acquired Autoimmune Myasthenia Gravis: A Topic Review. Can J Neurol Sci 19(3):360, 1992.
20. Shah, A and Lisak, RP: Immunopharmacologic Therapy in Myasthenia Gravis. Clin Neuropharmacol 16(2):97, 1993.
21. Sanders, DB and Scoppetta, C: The Treatment of Patients with Myasthenia Gravis. Neurol Clin 12:343, 1994.
22. Eymard, B, et al: Anti-Acetylcholine Receptor Antibodies in Neonatal Myasthenia Gravis: Heterogeneity and Pathogenic Significance. J Autoimmunity 4:185, 1991.
23. Papazian, O: Transient Neonatal Myasthenia Gravis. J Child Neurol 7:135, 1991.
24. Pascuzzi, RM and Kim, YI: Lambert-Eaton Syndrome. Semin Neurol 10(1):35, 1990.
25. O'Neill, JH, Murray, NMF, and Newson-Davis, J: The Lambert-Eaton Myasthenic Syndrome. Brain 111:577, 1988.
26. McEvoy, KM: Diagnosis and Treatment of Lambert-Eaton Myasthenic Syndrome. Neurol Clin 12:387, 1994.

27. Nagel, A, et al: Lambert-Eaton Myasthenic Syndrome IgG Depletes Presynaptic Membrane Active Zone Particles by Antigenic Modulation. Ann Neurol 24:552, 1988.

28. Kim, YI: Lambert-Eaton Myasthenic Syndrome: Evidence for Calcium Channel Blockade. Ann NY Acad Sci 505:377, 1987.

29. Lambert, EH and Lennon, VA: Selected IgG Rapidly Induced Lambert-Eaton Myasthenic Syndrome in Mice: Complement Interdependence and EMG Abnormalities. Muscle Nerve 11:1133, 1988.

30. Leys, K, et al: Calcium Channel Autoantibodies in the Lambert-Eaton Myasthenic Syndrome. Ann Neurol 29:307, 1991.

31. Vincent, A, Lang, B, and Newson-Davis, J: Autoimmunity to the Voltage-Gated Calcium Channel Underlies the Lambert-Eaton Myasthenic Syndrome: A Paraneoplastic Disorder. Trends Neurosci 12:496, 1989.

32. Wray, DW, et al: Interference with Calcium Channels by Lambert-Eaton Myasthenic Syndrome Antibody. Ann NY Acad Sci 505:368, 1987.

33. Kaminski, HJ and Ruff, RL: Congenital Disorders of Neuromuscular Transmission. Hosp Pract 27(9):73, 1992.

34. Engel, AG and Lambert, EH: Congenital Myasthenic Syndromes. Electroencephalogr Clin Neurophysiol 39(Suppl):91, 1987.

35. Engel, AG: Congenital Myasthenic Syndromes. J Child Neurol 3:233, 1988.

36. Engel, AG, et al: Newly Recognized Congenital Myasthenic Syndromes. Prog Brain Res 84:125, 1990.

37. Engel, AG: Congenital Myasthenic Syndromes. Neurol Clin 12:401, 1994.

38. Mora, M, Lambert, EH and Engel, AG: Synaptic Vesicle Abnormality in Familial Infantile Myasthenia. Neurology 37:206, 1987.

39. Engel, AG, Lambert, EH, and Gomez, MR: A New Myasthenic Syndrome with End-Plate Acetylcholinesterase Deficiency, Small Nerve Terminals, and Reduced Acetylcholine Release. Ann Neurol 1:315, 1977.

40. Engel, AG, et al: A Newly Recognized Congenital Myasthenic Syndrome Attributed to a Prolonged Open Time of the Acetylcholine-Induced Ion Channels. Ann Neurol 11:553, 1982.

41. Oosterhuis, HJGH, et al: The Slow Channel Syndrome: Two New Cases. Brain 110:1061, 1987.

42. Vincent, A, et al: Congenital Myasthenia, Endplate Acetylcholine Receptors and Electrophysiology in Five Cases. Muscle Nerve 4:306, 1981.

43. Smit, LME, et al: A Myasthenic Syndrome with Congenital Paucity of Secondary Synaptic Clefts: CPSC Syndrome. Muscle Nerve 11:337, 1988.

44. Wokke, JHJ: Congenital Paucity of Secondary Synaptic Clefts (CPSC) Syndrome in 2 Adult Sibs. Neurology 39:648, 1989.

45. Cherington, M: Botulism. Semin Neurol 10(1):27, 1990.

46. Gay, CT: Infant Botulism. South Med J 81(4):457, 1988.

47. Schmidt, RD and Schmidt, TW: Infant Botulism: A Case Series and Review of the Literature. J Emerg Med 10:713, 1992.

48. Carriere, B and Broski, L: Infant Botulism: Diagnosis and Treatment. Clin Manage Phys Ther 9(1):20, 1989.

49. Kaeser, HE: Drug-Induced Myasthenic Syndromes. Acta Neurol Scand 70(suppl 100):39, 1989.

50. Howard, JF: Adverse Drug Effects on Neuromuscular Transmission. Semin Neurol 10(1):89, 1990.

51. Bowman, WC: Pharmacology of Neuromuscular Function, ed 2. Chapter 4. Pharmacological Manipulation of Prejunctional Events. Wright, London, 1990.

52. Bowman, WC: Pharmacology of Neuromuscular Function, ed 2. Chapter 6. Neuromuscular-Blocking Agents. Wright, London, 1990.

53. Taylor, P: Agents Acting at the Neuromuscular Junction and Autonomic Ganglia. Chapter 9. In Gilman, AG, et al (eds): Goodman and Gilman's: The Pharmacological Basis of Therapeutics, ed 8. McGraw-Hill, New York, 1993.

54. Krendel, DA: Hypermagnesemia and Neuromuscular Transmission. Semin Neurol 10(1):42, 1990.

55. Layzer, RB: Neuromuscular Manifestations of Systemic Disease. Chapter 2. Mineral and Electrolyte Disorders. FA Davis, Philadelphia, 1985.

56. Bashuk, RG and Krendel, DA: Myasthenia Gravis Presenting as Weakness After Magnesium Administration. Muscle Nerve 10:666, 1987.

57. Chang, CC: The Action of Snake Venoms on Nerve and Muscle. Chapter 10. In Lee, C-Y (ed): Snake Venoms: Handbook of Experimental Pharmacology, vol 52. Springer-Verlag, Berlin, 1979, p 309.

58. Senanayake, N and Roman, GC: Disorders of Neuromuscular Transmission Due to Natural Environmental Toxins. J Neurol Sci 107:1, 1992.

59. Meldolesi, J, et al: Mechanism of Action of α-Latrotoxin: The Presynaptic Stimulatory Toxin of the Black Widow Spider Venom. Trends Pharmacol Sci 7:151, 1986.

60. Minton, SA: Neurotoxic Snake Envenoming. Semin Neurol 10(1):52, 1990.

61. Nelson, BK: Snake Envenomation: Incidence, Clinical Presentation and Management. Med Toxicol 4:17, 1989.

62. Su, MJ and Chang, CC: Presynaptic Effects of Snake Venom Toxins Which Have A Phospholipase A_2 Activity (β-Bungarotoxin, Taipoxin, Crotoxin). Toxicon 22(4):631, 1984.

63. Warrell, WA, et al: Severe Neurotoxin Envenoming by the Malayan Krait *Bungarus Candidus* (*Linnaeus*): Response to Antivenom and Anticholinesterase. Br Med J 286:678, 1983.

64. Gutmann, L and Besser, R: Organophosphate Intoxication: Pharmacologic, Neurophysiologic, Clinical, and Therapeutic Considerations. Semin Neurol 10(1):46, 1990.

65. Besser, R, et al: End-Plate Dysfunction in Acute Organophosphate Intoxication. Neurology 39:561, 1989.

66. Senanayake, N and Karalliedde, L: Neurotoxic Effects of Organophosphorous Insecticides. N Engl J Med 316 (13):716, 1987.

67. Van den Neucker, K, et al: The Neurophysiological Examination in Organophosphate Ester Poisoning: Case Report and Review of the Literature. Electromyogr Clin Neurophysiol 31:507, 1991.

————■————

CHAPTER 15

Disorders of the Peripheral Nervous System: The Peripheral Neuropathies

Christopher M. Fredericks, PhD

- *Normal Peripheral Nervous System*
- *Pathophysiology of Peripheral Neuropathies*
- *Clinical Features of Peripheral Neuropathies*
- *Classification of Peripheral Neuropathies*
- *Disorders of Cranial Nerves*
- *Disorders of Spinal Roots (Radiculopathies)*

Motor function relies on an intact peripheral nervous system. Not only is the normal activation and coordination of skeletal muscle dependent on the integrity of the alpha motor neurons with which it is innervated, but it is also dependent on the afferent neurons transmitting sensory information from within the muscle and adjacent tissues to the central nervous system. All these fibers travel to and from muscle in what is termed the **peripheral nervous system.**

There are numerous pathologic conditions that adversely affect the peripheral nervous system, creating clinically significant deficits in sensory, motor, and autonomic function. In some cases, these deficits can be severe and even life-threatening. These are called the **peripheral neuropathies.**[1-6] Some affect the peripheral nervous system exclusively, whereas others affect the function of peripheral nerve fibers within the context of more widespread disease.

Without attempting to describe in any detail the dozens of specific syndromes that have been identified, **the purpose of the material presented in this chapter is to develop an understanding of the basic pathologic processes that may alter or disrupt peripheral nerve function and the characteristic clinical manifestations that result.**

Normal Peripheral Nervous System

The response of the peripheral nervous system to disease or injury reflects the complex morphology and physiology of this system. A brief review of the structure and function of peripheral nerves will make it easier to understand the response of this system to various pathogenic factors and the characteristic clinical features that arise from its dysfunction.

Organization of the Peripheral Nervous System

The *peripheral nervous system* is defined as those portions of the somatic and autonomic nervous systems that lie outside the pial membrane of the spinal cord and brainstem (Fig. 15–1).[3-10] As such, the peripheral nervous system includes the dorsal and ventral spinal roots, spinal and cranial nerves (except for the first and second), dorsal root and other sensory ganglia, sensory and motor terminals, and most of the autonomic nervous system. It is misleading, however, to consider this system anatomically distinct from the central nervous system, because the central processes of the dorsal root ganglion cells and the cell bodies and proximal axons of motor neurons and preganglionic autonomic neurons actually lie within the brain or spinal cord.

Spinal Nerves

The somatic component of the peripheral nervous system begins with the ventral and dorsal spinal nerve roots, which fuse in the intervertebral foramina to form the spinal nerves (Figs.15–1 and 15–2).[3-10] After leaving the foramina, the spinal nerves each divide into two main branches, the dorsal (posterior) and ventral (anterior) rami or divisions. In general, the dorsal rami pass posteriorly to innervate paraspinal muscles and the skin on the back of the neck, trunk, and buttocks. The larger ventral rami supply the ventral and lateral parts of these structures, as well as the upper and lower extremities and their girdles. In the cervical and lumbosacral regions, the ventral rami intermingle and form plexuses from which the major peripheral nerves emerge. Within each spinal nerve are both somatic sensory and motor fibers. The cell bodies of the motor fibers lie within the anterior horn of the spinal cord, whereas the cell bodies of the sensory neurons reside in the dorsal root ganglia.

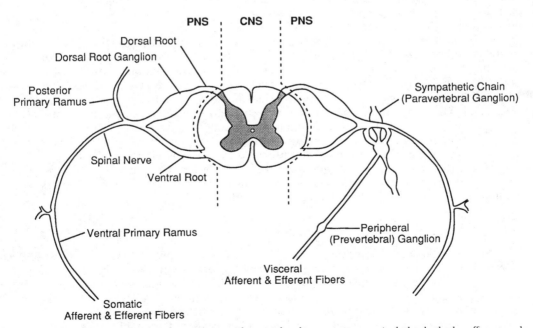

Figure 15–1. *The Peripheral Nervous System.* The peripheral nervous system includes both the efferent and afferent portions of the somatic and autonomic nervous systems that lie outside the pial membrane of the spinal cord and brainstem.

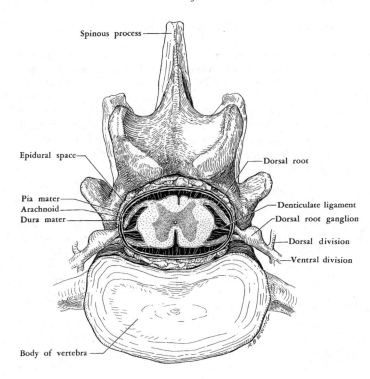

Spinous process

Epidural space

Dorsal root

Pia mater
Arachnoid
Dura mater

Denticulate ligament
Dorsal root ganglion
Dorsal division
Ventral division

Body of vertebra

Figure 15–2. Transverse Section of a Vertebra and Spinal Cord. The spinal root filaments pass through the thin pia mater of the cord, exiting and entering the vertebra via the intervertebral foramina as dorsal and ventral roots. The meninges of the cord fuse with the connective tissue sheaths of the peripheral nerve. (From Jenkins, TW: Functional Mammalian Neuroanatomy, ed 2. Copyright © Lea & Febiger, Philadelphia, 1978, p 99, with permission.)

Fibers of the autonomic nervous system accompany the somatic fibers to and from the periphery. Each autonomic fiber as it travels to its effector tissue in the periphery is interrupted by a single synapse. In the case of the **sympathetic** nervous system, which is distributed through spinal nerves of the thoracic and lumbar spinal cord, this synapse is usually located near the spinal cord. Specifically, sympathetic preganglionic fibers from the spinal cord usually synapse with postganglionic cells in paravertebral ganglia. Many of these postganglionic fibers then rejoin the ventral rami to travel to the periphery in individual peripheral nerves. Other postganglionic fibers reach their destination in the periphery by traveling along arteries. Sympathetic fibers innervate sweat glands and blood vessels in areas of the skin that correspond to the distribution of the sensory fibers with which they are associated. The sympathetic fibers in the ulnar nerve, for example, control sweating in the same part of the hand that derives its cutaneous somatic innervation from that nerve. Some sympathetic preganglionic fibers, such as those innervating intra-abdominal organs, pass through the paravertebral chain to synapse in remote prevertebral ganglia closer to the organs of destination. The **parasympathetic** nervous system is distributed through spinal nerves of the cervical and sacral spinal cord. Parasympathetic preganglionic fibers synapse with postganglionic cells in ganglia close to or within their effector targets.

Cranial Nerves

In many respects, the cranial nerves are similar to the spinal nerves.[11,12] Most of the cranial nerves leave the ventrolateral surface of the brainstem as cranial roots and pass through narrow bony foramina to extensively ramify in the periphery. As in the spinal cord, the cell bodies of motor and sensory neurons are found in different locations. The cell bodies of motor neurons are located in motor nuclei within the brainstem, and are analogous to anterior horn cells of the spinal cord. The cell bodies of afferent fibers lie outside the brainstem, either in ganglia analogous to the dorsal root ganglia or in specialized end-organs such as the eye. The peripheral cranial nerves are composed of an assortment of motor,

Table 15-1. *Classes of Motor and Sensory Neurons*

Neurons	Feature
Spinal Cord	
Somatic motor	Innervate skeletal muscle of the trunk and limbs
Visceral (autonomic) motor	Innervate autonomic ganglion cells regulating blood vessels, glands, and body cavity viscera
Somatic sensory	Innervate the skin, muscles, and joints of the trunk and limbs
Visceral (autonomic) sensory	Innervate the body cavity viscera
Brainstem	
Somatic motor	Innervate the extraocular and tongue muscles
Special visceral (branchial) motor	Innervate muscles of facial expression, jaw, and neck; larynx and pharynx; trapezius and sternomastoid; ear drum and middle ear
General visceral motor	Innervate parasympathetic ganglion cells regulating tear and sweat glands; blood vessels; smooth muscle of pupil and body cavity viscera
General somatic sensory	Innervate skin and skeletal muscles of head and neck; mucous membranes of mouth and sinuses; meninges; teeth
Special visceral sensory	Innervate the taste buds and olfactory epithelium
General visceral sensory	Innervate pharynx, larynx, and body cavity viscera
Special somatic sensory	Innervate cochlea and vestibular apparatus; retina

sensory, and autonomic fibers and are structurally similar to the peripheral nerves originating in the spinal cord.

The cranial nerves differ in several respects from the spinal nerves. They are attached to the brain at irregular rather than regular intervals, and they are not formed of dorsal and ventral roots. Because of the proximity of cranial structures, most of the cranial nerves are shorter than spinal peripheral nerves. Some have more than one ganglion, whereas others have none. Because of the presence of special sense organs and the mixed embryologic origins of the muscles of the head, the cranial nerves contain several more classes of motor and sensory neurons than do the spinal nerves (Table 15-1). Moreover, some cranial nerves are predominantly motor, sensory, or visceral, whereas spinal nerves are usually extensively mixed.

Structure and Composition of a Peripheral Nerve

Each peripheral nerve, regardless of whether it has spinal or cranial origins, is composed of nerve fibers, layers of connective tissue, and blood vessels (Figs. 15-3 and 15-4).[9,10,13-17] The nerve fibers include somatic motor neurons (alpha and gamma); somatic afferent fibers from muscle, skin, and joints; and afferent and efferent autonomic fibers. Each peripheral nerve thus contains both myelinated and unmyelinated neurons. The axons of myelinated fibers are covered with a sheath of myelin formed by many compacted layers of Schwann cell plasma membranes, interrupted only at the nodes of Ranvier (see Chapter 1). Each internodal segment of myelin is formed from an individual Schwann cell. The normal function of these nerve fibers depends on the integrity of the myelin sheath, which insulates and protects the neuron and increases the speed of impulse conduction. Proprioceptive and somatic motor fibers are the largest myelinated fibers, whereas sensory fibers that mediate diffuse, aching pain are the smallest.

Unmyelinated fibers are enveloped by whole Schwann cells, not myelin. These small fibers include autonomic fibers and sensory fibers mediating sharp, pricking pain and temperature. Unmyelinated fibers are dispersed among the myelinated fibers rather than being segregated within special compartments. The proportion of unmyelinated to myelinated fibers in a peripheral nerve trunk varies with the function of the nerve, but in most

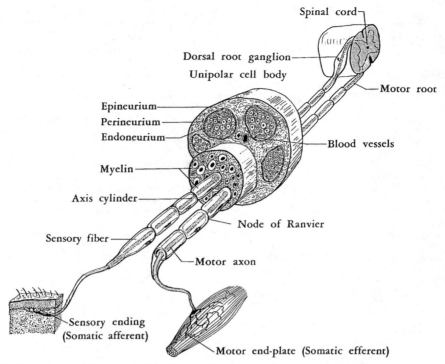

Figure 15–3. *Schematic Diagram of a Spinal Nerve.* This diagram illustrates the relationships between the neural, vascular, and connective tissue elements of a typical peripheral nerve. (From Jenkins, TW: Functional Mammalian Neuroanatomy, ed 2. Copyright © Lea & Febiger, Philadelphia, 1978, p 103, with permission.)

nerves about 75% of the fibers are unmyelinated.[10] Each peripheral nerve is thus composed of thousands of nerve fibers of many different types, each with its own particular morphologic and functional characteristics. In turn, the diseases and injuries that affect peripheral nerves may affect their constituent fibers differently, each causing its own distinct functional deficits.

   The nerve fibers that make up each peripheral nerve are surrounded by successive layers of connective tissue, which serve to protect and sustain them (Fig. 15–4).[16] Individual fibers are surrounded by the *endoneurium,* which provides support for the fibers and is important for the guidance of axons during regeneration. **Groups of fibers are closely packed in bundles called** *fasicles,* **each of which is surrounded by a strong connective tissue sheath, the** *perineurium.* This sheath provides great mechanical strength, in addition to serving as a perifascicular diffusion barrier.[9] The perineurium chemically isolates the nerve fibers from their surroundings, preserving a distinct fluid environment in the interior of the fascicles (i.e., the endoneurial fluid), much like the blood-brain barrier protects the environment of the central nervous system. The perineurium, by acting as a barrier to macromolecules, may protect nerve fibers from various disease-promoting substances such as certain toxins, antigens, and viruses. **Bundles of fascicles are in turn surrounded by an outermost layer of connective tissue, the** *epineurium.* This rather loose connective tissue layer serves as a cushion during movements of the nerve, protecting the fascicles from external trauma and maintaining the oxygen supply via the epineurial blood vessels. The tensile strength and elasticity of peripheral nerves reside predominantly in the epineurial connective tissues. The amount of epineurium varies among the nerves and at different sites along the same nerve. For example, where the nerve lies close to bone or joint, the epineurium is often more abundant, reflecting a greater need for protection at these locations. The spinal nerve roots have thinner, less well-defined connective tissue sheaths, and the nerve fibers in the nerve root may consequently be more susceptible to trauma.[18,19]

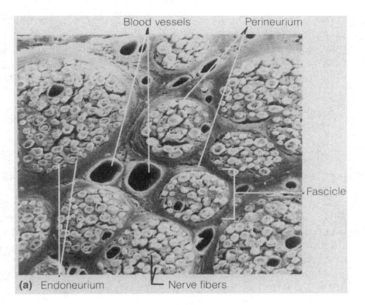

Figure 15–4. *Transverse Section of a Peripheral Nerve.* In this scanning electron micrograph of a transverse section of a peripheral nerve, the fasicles (fiber bundles), connective tissue layers, and blood vessels are clearly visible. The nerve fibers within each fasicle are both myelinated and unmyelinated (×400). (From Kessel, RG and Kardon, RH: Tissues and Organs: A Text-Atlas of Scanning Electron Microscopy. WH Freeman & Co., New York, 1979, p. 79, with permission.)

Nerve fibers are living cells and as such require a blood supply to meet their metabolic requirements and to remove metabolic waste products. **Peripheral nerves are well vascularized**, receiving their blood supply from numerous small arteries that enter at intervals along their length and form highly anastomosed networks of arterioles and venules within the connective tissue framework of the nerve.[17] The extensive interconnections within this network make nerves relatively resistant to vascular disease.

The internal environment of the nerve fasicles is thus determined jointly by the vascular endothelium and the perineurium.[9] Damage to these structures by trauma, toxins, ischemia, or metabolic disturbances may cause disturbance of this environment and interference with nerve function.

Axonal Transport[7,13,14,20,21]

Nerve fibers are unique in that the neuronal cell body must maintain a cellular projection, the axon, of enormous relative length and volume. The axon contains hundreds of times more cytoplasm than the cell body and its length may be thousands of times that of the cell body diameter. **Because the axon and nerve terminal lack the cellular apparatus (i.e., ribosomes) necessary for the synthesis of proteins and other essential cellular constituents, these materials must be produced in the cell body and supplied to axonal sites of utilization.** To this end, structural components, organelles, nutrients, and neurosecretory molecules all are transported along the axon from the cell body toward the nerve terminal in what is called **antegrade axonal transport.** Transport also occurs in a retrograde direction from the periphery toward the cell body. Spent neurotransmitter vesicles, for example, are returned to the cell body by **retrograde axonal transport** for recycling of their components. By the same token, a number of exogenous substances in the environment of the nerve terminal may be taken up and transported toward the cell body.[20] Natural substances such as nerve growth factor (necessary for neuronal growth and development) and foreign substances such as toxic and biologic agents (i.e., virus) can in this way gain access to the cell body and influence its function.

Defects in the transport of materials along the axon can significantly disturb neuronal function. Disruption of these transport processes probably underlies the disturbance of nerve function caused by many disorders of the peripheral nervous system. This is particularly evident in the rapid degeneration of the axon that occurs distal to the site of acute axonal injury. Although injury to the distal portion of the axon does not usually result in permanent damage to the nerve cell body, blockade of retrograde transport providing materials such as trophic factors to the cell body may also have deleterious effects on neuronal activity. Axonal transport may also contribute to neuronal dysfunction by dispersing the defective products of abnormal cell body synthesis to the axon.

Pathophysiology of Peripheral Neuropathies

Disease and injury can disturb peripheral nerve function in a number of ways, and the particular signs and symptoms that characterize a specific disorder will reflect the nature of these underlying disturbances, as well as the particular fibers disrupted. Despite the wide variety of factors that can cause peripheral neuropathy, the **pathologic processes afflicting peripheral nerve are few and can be divided into those that primarily affect the axon and those that primarily affect its ensheathments, the surrounding myelin or Schwann cells.** It should be remembered that although this categorization is useful for the purposes of discussion and provides insight into the conditions observed clinically, many neuropathies show major changes in both axons and their coverings. This makes sense, since the activities of the axon and its sheaths are intimately interrelated.

Axonopathies

The most common disorders of peripheral nerve are those that affect primarily the axon itself. These are the **axonopathies.** In this regard, the axon may be subject to either acute injury or chronic derangement of function.

Wallerian Degeneration

In acute traumatic lesions in which the axon is abruptly interrupted, a form of axonal disintegration occurs called *wallerian degeneration.*[14,15,21-28] Acute disruption of the axon may result from complete transection of the nerve (such as by laceration) or from severe local crushing, traction, or ischemia. In laceration, the connective tissue membranes of the nerve are destroyed; in the other lesions, they may remain more or less intact. In all these lesions, the functional continuity of the axon is disrupted. **Deprived of the irreplaceable materials that are synthesized in the cell body and transported along the axon, the nerve fiber distal to the site of injury rapidly deteriorates** (Fig. 15–5). Degenerative changes begin to occur in the nerve terminal within a matter of hours and synaptic transmission fails soon after injury, even before the first morphologic signs of degeneration are evident.[23] After about 2 weeks, the synapses formed by this distal segment have degenerated completely. Within a week or so after the initial injury, wallerian degeneration of the entire distal axon begins. The axon swells and ultimately breaks apart. In addition to disintegration of the axon, major changes occur in its coverings. In myelinated fibers, the myelin sheath fragments and is phagocytosed. In unmyelinated fibers, there is less proliferation of Schwann cells. Changes may also occur in the neuron proximal to the site of injury. If axonal disruption is close enough to the cell body, neuronal cell death may occur. Otherwise, **axonal degeneration may spread for a short distance proximally from the injury, while characteristic changes occur in the morphology of the cell body.**[14,15,21-26] Notably, the rough endoplasmic reticulum breaks apart and is repositioned in the periphery of the swollen cell body (chromatolysis). The rough endoplasmic reticulum is the site of protein synthesis, and its reorganization may occur in preparation for the massive synthesis of proteins necessary for regeneration of the axon. If regeneration is successful and proper synaptic connections are restored, chromatolysis ceases and the cell body usually regains its normal appearance in a few months. In human pathology, chromatolysis is most evident in large motor cells such as anterior horn cells and the motor nuclei of cranial nerves.

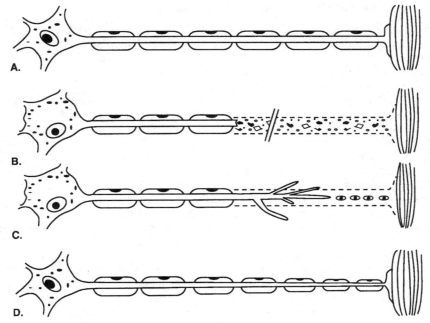

Figure 15–5.   *Wallerian Degeneration.* (A) Normal myelinated nerve fiber. (B) Focal injury has disrupted the continuity of the axon. Proximal to the injury, the axon and cell body respond with somal swelling, chromatolysis, and nuclear enlargement and migration. Distal to the injury, the axon and its myelin sheath undergo wallerian degeneration. The muscle fiber rapidly atrophies. (C) The proximal axon has begun to sprout new axonal branches. With successful connection of one sprout, the others will degenerate. (D) Regeneration is completed, usually with a thinner axon and myelin and shorter internodal segments.

Wallerian degeneration proceeds more rapidly in peripheral nerves, where degenerative changes are complete in a few weeks, than in the central nervous system, where degeneration proceeds over several months. More importantly, in the peripheral nervous system, regeneration of the nerve is possible if the parent cell body survives; this regeneration does not occur in the central nervous system.[23] Neurons with processes confined to the central nervous system cannot restore their proper synaptic connections and either degenerate entirely or remain in a state of severe atrophy.

After acute axonal disruption, recovery may occur through the growth of new axons, and under ideal circumstances function may be completely restored.[14,21–28] The rate and extent of this regeneration depend, however, on the nature and severity of the injury. **Regeneration is initiated by the growth of new branches or sprouts from the proximal segment of the interrupted axon** (see Fig. 15–5). After nerve transection, as many as 25 sprouts may arise from a single axon. One or more of these may succeed in growing along the original pathway to reinnervate the original destination. The regenerating nerve fiber seems to be guided to the proper destination by residual connective tissue elements and Schwann cells. Regeneration is quicker and more complete in crushing injury than with transection, since more of these nerve fiber components remain intact.[21–24,27] When a nerve is completely transected, reinnervation is poor because the axonal sprouts have no distinct pathway to follow to their original target. Many sprouts will follow aberrant routes to inappropriate destinations. For example, motor fibers may innervate muscle fibers other than those they originally supplied, resulting in movement of muscles other than those intended. Similar faulty regrowth also affects sensory nerve fibers, resulting in poorly or incorrectly localized sensation. Axonal sprouts that fail to form appropriate peripheral connections ultimately disappear. In most lesions other than laceration, not all axons are destroyed and some function remains. Smaller fibers are more resistant to such injuries and are more likely to be spared.

Axonal Degeneration (Distal Axonopathy)[4,14,15,21-28]

Axonal disintegration may also develop slowly in association with chronic disease or long-term insult to the nervous system. This is termed *axonal degeneration* or *distal axonopathy*.[4,14,15,21-28] Slowly progressive degeneration of the distal axon is probably the most common of the pathologic reactions of the peripheral nerve. This occurs most often in association with toxins and metabolic disorders and may also underlie certain hereditary neuropathies. Although the precise morphologic reactions of the nerve fibers vary with the nature and severity of the condition, **the degeneration typically starts in the most distal part of the axon and progresses toward the cell body** (Fig. 15–6). **This is termed** *dying back.* While the axon sheaths may be initially spared, dying back may ultimately be accompanied by deterioration of the myelin or Schwann cell coverings (secondary demyelination). Although the pathology of chronic axonal degeneration is not well understood, it is likely that abnormal cellular metabolism results in synthetic failure in the cell body or alterations in axonal transport, which deprive the distal axon of materials necessary for its survival. **The most distal regions of the longest, largest-diameter axons are the most vulnerable,** explaining the early clinical involvement of the most distal lower extremities in many of these disorders.

If the neuronal insult is temporary, the dying back of the distal axon will cease and can be followed by axonal regeneration and varying degrees of structural and functional recovery. On the other hand, if the neuronal derangement is prolonged or severe, the degeneration may extend to the nerve cell body and result in cell death. When regeneration and recovery occur, it takes months or years. As occurs with acute injury, muscle atrophy is evident.

Chronic axonal degeneration may also occur in the central nervous system, particularly at the distal ends of long, large fibers (e.g., corticospinal). Regeneration, however, is less effective and recovery of function less likely.

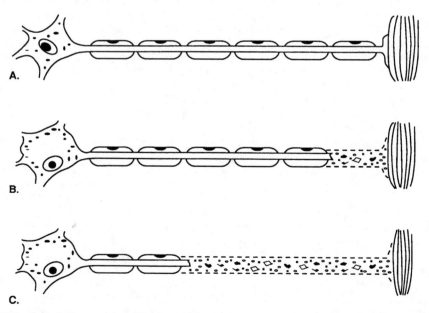

Figure 15–6. *Axonal Degeneration ("Dying Back").* (*A*) Normal myelinated nerve fiber. (*B* and *C*) Axonal degeneration progressing proximally from the most distal portion of the axon. This degeneration may extend to the nerve cell body producing cell death.

Effects of Axonopathy on Skeletal Muscle

Predictable changes occur in skeletal muscle when it is denervated, regardless of whether this is due to degeneration of the axon (i.e., an axonopathy) or malfunction of the cell body itself (i.e., a neuronopathy; see Chapter 16).[29] Denervation is followed by many changes in muscular physiology and biochemistry, the most conspicuous of which is gross muscle atrophy. **This atrophy characteristically develops rapidly during the first few weeks after injury,** then progresses more slowly to some maximal level. The permanent loss of muscle fibers in denervated human muscle begins after 6 to 9 months, with few fibers remaining after 3 years.[30] **As the muscle fibers decrease in size, they also tend to change shape,** becoming more angulated or elongated in cross section. In most neurogenic disorders, type II fibers tend to atrophy earlier and more rapidly than type I fibers.

In partially denervated muscle, the performance of a normal motor task imposes an exaggerated workload on the remaining functional fibers, causing their compensatory hypertrophy. Denervated muscle therefore becomes a mixture of atrophied and hypertrophied muscle fibers.

Muscle atrophy is accompanied by a decrease in the number of capillaries per muscle fiber and by proliferation of the connective tissue surrounding the muscle fibers.[31]

In many of the peripheral neuropathies, a significant amount of reinnervation may occur through the collateral sprouting of nearby intact motor axons. This results in transformation of muscle fibers and a characteristic reorganization of the overall pattern of fiber types. In normal, innervated skeletal muscle, the individual muscle fibers of separate motor units are extensively intermingled, creating a randomly distributed mosaic of fiber types (Fig. 15–7). With reinnervation, however, **greatly enlarged motor units may be created,** containing up to seven times as many muscle fibers. These giant motor units are

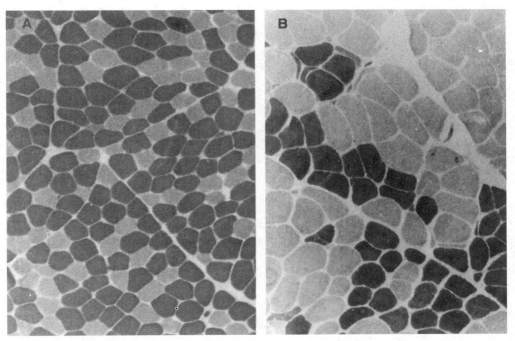

Figure 15–7. *Changes in Muscle Histology Associated with Denervation.* (A) In gastrocnemius muscle from a normal adult, the two types of muscle fibers are roughly equal in number and evenly distributed. (B) In gastrocnemius from a patient with a chronic sensorimotor polyneuropathy, the muscle fibers are grouped together in large motor units by fiber type as a result of denervation and reinnervation. (From Kandel, ER, Schwartz, JH, and Jessell, TM: Principles of Neural Science, ed 3. Appleton & Lange, Norwalk, CT, 1991, p 248, with permission.)

necessarily of one histochemical type of fiber. **This increases the likelihood that large groupings of closely packed fibers of the same type will be evident in muscle cross section,** rather than the usual "checker-board" pattern (see Fig. 15–7). This type of reorganization becomes more evident the longer the cycle of denervation and reinnervation continues, and it provides a built-in microscopic record of the period of denervation. Some evidence suggests that these giant motor units may impose undue stress on their motor innervation, ultimately resulting in its failure. This may underly the postpoliomyelitis syndrome of muscle weakness that is appearing with increasing frequency among long-term polio survivors (see Chapter 16).

Myelinopathies[14,15,25,26,29]

A variety of genetic, immunologic, and toxic disorders may adversely affect peripheral nerve, not by directly affecting the axon, but by primary destruction of the myelin sheath or the myelin-producing Schwann cells. The axon itself may be relatively intact. **These are the *myelinopathies*. In these disorders entire internodal segments of myelin are usually lost, a phenomenon called *segmental demyelination*** (Fig. 15–8). Although primary demyelination probably reflects direct injury to the myelin-producing Schwann cells, secondary demyelination may also occur as a result of axonal deterioration (e.g., in axonopathies).[21,22] In practice, primary demyelination occurs most often in acquired immune-mediated inflammatory conditions (e.g., diphtheritic neuropathy or Guillain-Barré syndrome) and occasionally in inherited disorders. In general, **the loss of myelin results in slowed impulse conduction and, when great enough, may lead to complete conduction block.** Even in fibers in which considerable impulse conduction (albeit slowed) continues to occur, prolonged stimulation may result in intermittent conduction block, which impairs the ability to transmit long trains of impulses.[32,33] In addition to alterations in conduction, demyelinated fibers may demonstrate abnormal spontaneous discharge, as well as abnormal interactions with other nerve fibers.[32,33]

In this regard, it is important to remember that each motor function is subserved by many more nerve fibers than the minimum necessary for performing that function. The impact of demyelination on that function depends on the proportion of fibers in which

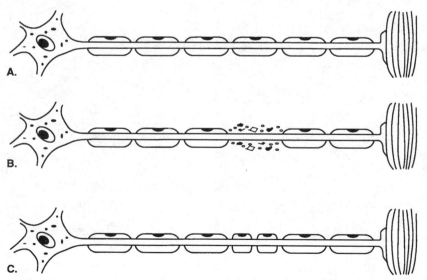

Figure 15–8. ***Segmental Demyelination.*** (A) Normal myelinated nerve fiber. (B) Loss of an internodal segment of myelin produced by one Schwann cell. (C) Remyelination with shorter, thinner internodal segments.

conduction is abnormal. For example, complete conduction block in large numbers of nerve fibers is a major factor in the production of severe paralysis or sensory loss seen in the acute stages of demyelinating neuropathy. Less severe deficits probably arise from conduction block in a smaller proportion of fibers. Mere slowing of conduction does not necessarily produce overt symptoms. [32,33] However, when the axons of a nerve begin to conduct action potentials at slightly different velocities because of varying degrees of demyelination among these axons, the normal synchrony among the impulses is loss. This slowing and temporal dispersion of action potentials may account for some of the early clinical signs of neuropathy. Two of the most frequently abnormal signs in peripheral neuropathy—depression of deep tendon jerks and impairment of vibratory sense—probably belong in this category. [32,33]

In each of the demyelinating disorders, the extent of damage done is highly variable, and different fiber types are selectively involved. In localized lesions, there is loss of function in the limited area supplied by the nerve. In more generalized disease, numerous sites are involved. **The areas most likely to lose function are the most distal regions supplied by the largest nerves.** For example, the myelinated axons of the sciatic nerve are the longest, the most heavily myelinated, and statistically the most likely to be involved in a random demyelinating process. The resultant distal clinical deficits are reminiscent of those accompanying axonal disorders.

Schwann cells survive in most of these conditions, and remyelination of demyelinated segments usually follows both primary and secondary demyelination. Following segmental demyelination, the internodal segments that were originally ensheathed by one Schwann cell are usually re-ensheathed by several cells, resulting in multiple, short internodes (see Fig. 15–8). The regenerated myelin sheath is also usually thinner than the original. In contrast to the slow recovery following axonopathies, the **recovery of function following segmental demyelination may be rapid** because the intact but denuded axon needs only to become remyelinated.

Since much of the trophic action of the demyelinated motor axon is maintained, skeletal muscle does not usually undergo the rapid changes associated with denervation. However, it may undergo disuse atrophy if paralysis is prolonged. Axonal loss may occur in primary demyelinating disease, in which case muscle atrophy is severe.

In contrast to the axonopathies, there is little central nervous system involvement in the myelinopathies. Most toxic and inflammatory peripheral myelinopathies spare the central nervous system. Many myelinotoxic agents are unable to cross the blood-brain barrier; also the immune-mediated response of the inflammatory neuropathies is directed specifically at substances present in peripheral myelin. Some hereditary metabolic diseases of myelin do, however, have extensive central nervous system involvement (see Chapter 22).

Neuronopathies[4,25]

A third group of conditions exists in which the primary morphologic or biochemical changes occur in the nerve cell body (see Chapter 16). **These are termed** *neuronopathies* **or perikaryal disorders.** These are a heterogeneous group of disorders, which may involve either motor neurons or primary sensory neurons. Primary cell body degeneration and loss is a finding in a variety of disorders, including conditions associated with infectious, hereditary, and toxic factors. One of the features of these disorders is the highly selective involvement of specific neuronal populations (e.g., affinity of the poliovirus for the anterior horn cell), although the mechanism of this selective vulnerability is not known. **The clinical expression of these disorders resembles that of the disorders that primarily affect the axon of the cell.**

In the case of sensory fibers and autonomic fibers, these disorders conform to our definition of the peripheral nervous system, since the primary site of involvement, the cell body, lies outside of the central nervous system. On the other hand, disorders of the somatic motor neuron cell body arise within the anterior horn of the spinal cord or in the brainstem and might be considered disorders of the central nervous system. Although a rigid distinction between anterior horn cell disease and peripheral neuropathy is not entirely defensible, for the sake of convenience diseases of the anterior horn cells will be considered in detail in Chapter 16.

Although the three pathologic processes discussed above are described as separate entities, they are not disease-specific and may be present in varying combinations in any given patient. Moreover, they may be directed at varying groups of nerve fibers and at varying sites along their individual courses.

Clinical Features of Peripheral Neuropathies

For purposes of discussion, **the neuropathies may be divided into several broad clinical categories depending on the pattern of nerve involvement.**[4,5,25,34-37] At one extreme, there are disorders emanating from focal involvement of a single nerve trunk. These are termed **mononeuropathies.** In other cases, a number of individual nerve trunks may be affected (simultaneously or sequentially) by multiple, focal lesions. These are termed **multiple mononeuropathies** or **mononeuropathies multiplex.** In either case, the lesions that underly the mononeuropathic disorders result from processes that produce localized damage. Nerve entrapment, compression, and direct trauma (e.g., crushing, traction, and laceration) are the most common causes; vascular lesions and granulomatous, neoplastic, or other infiltrations follow. These neuropathies may exist in isolation or may be associated with other pathologic conditions. Individual nerves already abnormal by virtue of a preexisting generalized condition (e.g., diabetes mellitus) may be particularly susceptible to damage. **In the mononeuropathies and multiple mononeuropathies, the motor and sensory manifestations are limited to the distribution of the nerve or nerves affected.** Tendon reflexes are usually preserved unless the reflex in question is dependent on the specific muscles supplied by the damaged nerve.

In **polyneuropathies,** damage to the peripheral nervous system is more diffuse, with equal involvement of many peripheral nerves and widespread clinical features. Although many patterns of involvement are possible, **the clinical manifestations of polyneuropathy are most often bilateral and symmetric, and usually start distally in the largest nerve fibers** (Fig. 15-9). The specific constellation of clinical features observed in polyneuropathy is determined by the location and severity of neural involvement, as well as by the nature of the underlying pathology. Patients with disorders in which the underlying pathology is predominantly demyelination present differently from those with pathology involving primarily axonal degeneration (Table 15-2). There are many neuropathies in which deleterious changes occur in both axons and their myelin coverings. **Although some of the polyneuropathies are purely motor, sensory, or autonomic, in most a combination of abnormalities occurs.** Polyneuropathies tend to be associated with conditions that act diffusely on the peripheral nervous system, such as toxic substances, deficiency states, systemic metabolic disorders, and certain immune reactions.[34] Some of these disturbances may be complicated by superimposed focal nerve damage. As the multiple mononeuropathies worsen, there is a tendency for the neurologic deficit to become more widespread, confluent, and symmetric, thereby resembling a polyneuropathy.[35]

Signs and Symptoms

A number of motor, sensory, reflexive, and autonomic manifestations are typical of peripheral nerve and spinal root disorders.[3-5,22,34-38] These signs and symptoms vary markedly, reflecting not only the basic type of disease process, but factors such as the types and location of the nerve fibers affected, the severity of their involvement, the involvement of other tissues, and the presence of other medical conditions. Nonetheless, certain clinical manifestations do consistently occur in the neuropathies and provide criteria for their diagnosis.

Loss of Motor and Sensory Function
(Negative Signs and Symptoms)

Persistent weakness is the most common motor symptom of peripheral neuropathy. In this regard, muscle weakness may be localized, as in focal involvement of a peripheral nerve in mononeuropathy, or more widespread, as in polyneuropathy or multiple mononeuropathy. **In most polyneuropathies, weakness begins symmetrically and distally, with muscles of the feet and legs affected first** and most severely, followed later by involvement of the hands and forearms ("glove-and-stocking" distribution) (see Fig. 15–9). In milder forms of polyneuropathy, only the lower extremities may be involved. Most of the nutritional, metabolic, and toxic neuropathies assume this pattern. In severe cases, the patient may become quadriplegic and respirator-dependent (e.g., Guillain-Barré syndrome). In the final analysis, muscle paralysis is due to an inability to conduct motor nerve impulses from the central nervous system to the periphery. **The degree of weakness is proportionate to the number of motor neurons affected,** although the motor deficit may be exacerbated by concurrent loss of sensory (proprioceptive) input.

Although all sensory modalities are often diminished by polyneuropathy, in some disorders certain modalities may be preferentially impaired.[34] Positional and vibratory sense may be affected in some, whereas pain and temperature perception may be diminished

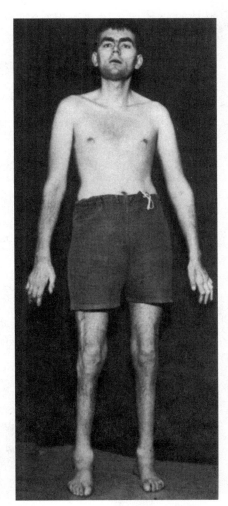

Figure 15–9. *Chronic, Progressive Idiopathic Polyneuropathy.* In this 35-year-old patient with a progressive polyneuropathy since aged 15, there was complete glove-and-stocking anesthesia and wasting of the distal musculature. Note the clawing of the fingers and toes. (From Spillane, JD: An Atlas of Clinical Neurology. Oxford University Press, London, 1968, p 107, with permission.)

Table 15–2. *Basic Clinical Findings in Polyneuropathies*

Findings	Axonopathy	Myelinopathy
Onset	Rapid following trauma, otherwise gradual and insidious; signs and symptoms preceded by prolonged subclinical disease	Often develops quickly, over hours to weeks; may be gradual
Initial clinical manifestations	Symmetric clinical involvement of distal arms and legs (glove-and-stocking) Earliest usually sensory Abnormalities and loss of ankle jerks; proximal tendon reflexes preserved	Symmetric, diffuse weakness and mild sensory loss in lower extremities and occasionally bulbar muscles; sensory loss may be limited to distal extremities; general impairment of tendon reflexes
Motor nerve conduction velocity	Normal or slight slowing	Marked slowing or complete conduction block
Recovery	Slow, reflecting slowness of axonal regeneration; months or years; residual disability common	Rapid, reflecting speed of segmental remyelination and restoration of impulse conduction; residual disability slight
Skeletal muscle	Denervation atrophy	Disuse atrophy if paralysis is prolonged; denervation atrophy if demyelination is accompanied by axonal loss
Central nervous system	Some involvement	Seldom involved
Common causes	Exogenous toxins; also metabolic and hereditary factors	Immune-mediated inflammation most common; rarely toxic, infectious, or hereditary factors

in others. Vibratory sense is often affected more than positional sense. These senses are mediated by different types of sensory fibers (see Chapter 4), and their selective loss is attributed to the selective involvement in various neuropathies of "large" and "small" classes of sensory fibers, respectively. **Sensory loss, even more than motor dysfunction, begins in the feet, gradually spreads upward to the knees, and then involves the fingers and hands.** As a polyneuropathy worsens, there may be a spread of sensory loss to more proximal parts of the limbs and sometimes to the abdomen and head.

Distorted or Exaggerated Motor and Sensory Activity (Positive Signs and Symptoms)

In addition to the diminished motor and sensory activity caused by degeneration or conduction block, **the signs and symptoms of neuropathy may include evidence of distorted or exaggerated activity, resulting from the abnormal generation of action potentials in motor or sensory neurons.** These "positive signs" may coexist with or succeed negative signs. **Involuntary activation of muscle may accompany muscle weakness.** Fasciculations and cramps of skeletal muscle are sometimes observed in peripheral neuropathies. Both, however, are more common and problematic in certain anterior horn cell disorders (see Chapter 16). **Asynchronous, repetitive activation of multiple motor units may also occur** (referred to as **neuromyotonia, myokymia,** or **continuous motor unit activity syndrome**) and may manifest as generalized muscle stiffness. This type of activity has been described in widely differing forms of neuropathy, including both demyelinating and axonal types, and is thought to result from abnormal impulses arising in the damaged regions of peripheral nerves. The origin of these impulses in the peripheral nervous system are attested to by the persistence of this activity during sleep and spinal anesthesia and its decrease with distal nerve blockade or blockade of the neuromuscular junction with curare.[22]

Abnormal sensations (paresthesias, or dyesthesias, if unpleasant) frequently accompany sensory or mixed sensory/motor neuropathies.[34] These sensations are usually described as numbness, tingling, prickling, or "pins-and-needles" sensations and tend to be most evident in the hands and feet. Although the mechanism producing these sensations is not well understood, they may arise from spontaneous ectopic impulses, distorted impulse conduction, or abnormal communication between nerve fibers.[32,33] **Pain may also constitute an unpleasant feature of a variety of focal and generalized neuropathies.**[22,34] This pain may be spontaneous or elicited by stimulation of the skin (e.g., hyperesthesia or hyperpathia). A particularly severe and persistent type of burning pain, termed **causalgia,** may result from acute injury to a nerve trunk and radiate beyond the territory of the injured nerve. As with the paresthesias, the precise mechanisms underlying these painful conditions are not known. Mechanisms that may contribute to the creation of pain are ectopic discharge in primary sensory fibers, abnormal interactions between sensory and autonomic fibers, and secondary changes in the central nervous system, which may by themselves cause pain.[22,34,35]

Tendon Hyporeflexia and Areflexia

Diminution or loss of tendon reflexes is common in peripheral nerve disease, although it may not develop until late in those disorders that initially affect primarily small nerve fibers. Early hyporeflexia or areflexia probably reflects an early loss of muscle spindle afferent fibers (axon degeneration) or a dispersion of afferent input to the spinal cord resulting from impaired conduction (demyelination).[22,32-34]

Ataxia and Tremor

In neuropathies with a predominant sensory component, muscle movements may be strong but distorted. **Loss of proprioceptive input with retention of a reasonable degree of motor function may result in sensory ataxia of gait and limb movements.** Sensory ataxia is particularly evident in cases with selective loss of the large fibers transmitting proprioceptive input. A tremor present during movement may also appear during certain phases of a polyneuropathy, likewise reflecting inadequate or distorted proprioceptive feedback.

Autonomic Dysfunction

Impaired sweat production (anhidrosis), disturbance of genitourinary function, and orthostatic hypotension are the most common manifestations of autonomic dysfunction and may be major features of certain polyneuropathies. These and other autonomic disturbances may occur without other evidence of neuropathy but are usually accompanied by somatic motor or sensory disturbances. In general, **sympathetic nervous system dysfunction is more common than parasympathetic.** Alterations in autonomic function are most evident in polyneuropathies in which small diameter nerve fibers are extensively affected. Autonomic disturbances are most frequently seen in diabetic polyneuropathy, although they may also occur in amyloid and certain hereditary neuropathies.

Deformity and Trophic Changes

Long-standing polyneuropathies frequently give rise to foot, hand, and spinal deformities, especially when the disease begins during childhood (Figs. 15-9 and 15-10). Cavus deformity of the feet with clawing of the toes is the most common abnormality. Kyphoscoliosis of the spine and clawing of the hands may also develop. Although the mechanism of these deformities is not entirely understood, muscle imbalance is surely a major contributor.

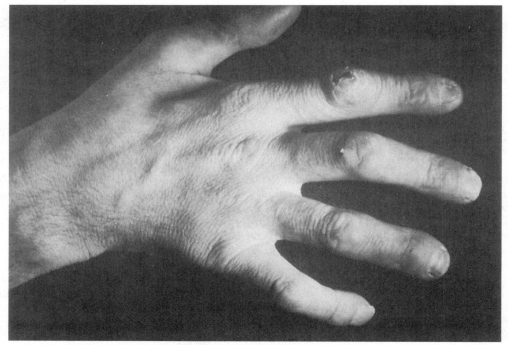

Figure 15–10. *Hand Deformity in Polyneuropathy.* Deformity (clawing) and scarring of the fingers is due to longstanding weakness and wasting of small hand muscles and distal anesthesia in the polyneuropathic patient in Figure 15–9. (From Spillane, JD. An Atlas of Clinical Neurology. Oxford University Press, London, 1968, p 107, with permission.)

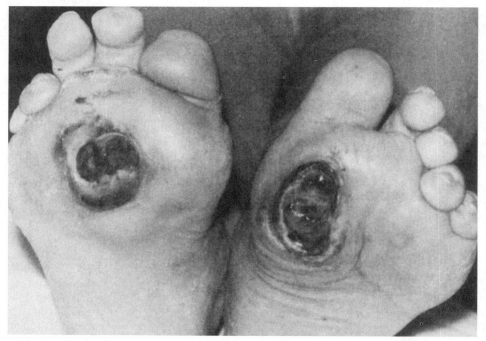

Figure 15–11. *Ulcerated Feet in Sensory Neuropathy.* In this patient with a sensory neuropathy, distal sensory impairment led to the development of painless perforating ulcers on the soles of both feet. (From Chadwick, Cartlidge, and Bates,[5] p 235, with permission.)

Trophic changes in a variety of tissues also frequently accompany neuropathy. These are most prominent when denervation occurs. Muscle atrophy can develop rapidly with denervation and is proportional to the loss of nerve fibers. In demyelinating diseases, muscle atrophy may develop from protracted disuse. Accompanying denervation are trophic changes in the nails, skin, and subcutaneous tissues, as well as deleterious changes in bone and joints. In an anesthetic and immobile limb, the skin becomes tight and shiny, the nails become curved and rigid, and subcutaneous tissues thicken.[3] Chronically traumatized joints may collapse and disintegrate. Repeated injuries and chronic subcutaneous and osteomyelitic infections may result in a painless loss of digits and plantar ulcer formation (Fig. 15–11). Although pathogenesis of these trophic changes is not fully understood, disuse, alterations in blood supply, and sensory loss all probably contribute. A critical factor is impaired neural regulation of the distal vasculature, which interferes with normal tissue responses to trauma and infection.[3] In diabetic neuropathy in which sores are common, distal anesthesia is compounded by ischemia and hypersusceptibility to infection.[34,35]

Classification of Peripheral Neuropathies

Because of the diversity and vagaries surrounding the pathogenesis of the peripheral neuropathies, it has been difficult to define a single practical classification scheme for these disorders. In some schemes, emphasis has been placed on the nature of the underlying pathology, focusing either on the anatomic or morphologic site of the pathology, or on the etiologic factors provoking it (see Table 15–3). In syndromic schemes, emphasis is placed on the nature and evolution of the clinical manifestations of these disorders.

Whatever criteria are used to categorize the peripheral neuropathies, it is beyond the scope of this discussion to describe the dozens of specific disturbances that are recognized clinically. The following descriptions are designed to provide the student with a practical overview of the etiologies and primary clinical features of the basic types of peripheral neuropathies.

Table 15–3. *Approaches to Classifying Peripheral Neuropathies*

Pathologic classification
    Axonal dysfunction
        Wallerian degeneration (secondary to acute disruption)
        Distal axonopathy
    Myelinopathy

Etiologic classification
    Acquired forms
        Mononeuropathy
            Entrapment or compression
            Traumatic
            Infectious/inflammatory
            Neoplastic
        Multiple mononeuropathy
            Vascular/ischemic
            Entrapment or compression
            Metabolic
            Infiltrations or neoplasms
        Polyneuropathy
            Metabolic
            Toxic
            Deficiency
            Infectious/inflammatory
            Malignancy-associated
            Idiopathic

(continued)

Table 15–3. *Continued*

Hereditary forms
  Mixed sensorimotor neuropathy
    Metabolic
    Idiopathic
  Sensory/automatic neuropathy

Syndromic classification
  Acute sensory motor polyneuropathy
  Subacute sensorimotor polyneuropathy
  Chronic sensorimotor polyneuropathy
    Acquired forms
    Genetically determined forms
  Recurrent or relapsing polyneuropathy
  Mononeuropathy or multiple mononeuropathy

Inherited Versus Acquired Neuropathies

As simple as the peripheral nervous system may appear, disorders of this system are numerous and diverse. Many factors, both acquired and inherited, are known to adversely affect its function.[3–5,35,36,39] Moreover, these factors may exert their deleterious effects at varying sites along the peripheral nerve, on different types of nerve fibers, and with varying severity.

Inherited Neuropathies[1–5,35,36,38–40]

Most of the *genetically determined* neuropathies are polyneuropathies, although hereditary factors may predispose certain specific nerve trunks to injury. Typically, a patient with a genetically determined polyneuropathy has a history of a chronic disorder, frequently beginning in childhood. With few exceptions, the onset has been insidious and progression has been slow, occurring over years or decades. These patients often have musculoskeletal deformity in the form of pes cavus and muscle wasting, and the neuropathy tends to be progressive, symmetric, and more distal than proximal. Some display both motor and sensory involvement. Among these are the hereditary motor and sensory neuropathies (HMSNs) which may be subdivided into types I, II, and III.[38–40] Although these genetic disorders are relatively uncommon, HMSN type I is the most common among them (Fig. 15–12). The neuropathies in which the primary manifestations are either sensory or autonomic or both have been linked together as the hereditary sensory and autonomic neuropathies (HSANs), which may also be divided into several subtypes.

The inherited neuropathies may also be categorized as those without a known biochemical cause (i.e., idiopathic) and those associated with a distinct biochemical abnormality (e.g., uremic polyneuropathy). Various modes of genetic transmission occur. Most of these disorders are rare, with the exception of the dominantly inherited peroneal muscular atrophies (see Fig. 15–12).

Acquired Neuropathies[1–5,35,36,38,41–43]

Most acquired neuropathies are also polyneuropathies, which, like the hereditary polyneuropathies, are characterized by widespread symmetric involvement, usually distal and graded. These disorders have a great diversity in both their etiology and their clinical manifestations. They are extremely variable in tempo, severity, and the mix of sensory and motor features. Most of the mononeuropathies and multiple mononeuropathies are also acquired, whether caused by trauma or disease.

The clinical course of the acquired disorders ranges from abrupt onset and rapid progression to insidious progression over many years.[35] The course followed by a particular neuropathy is determined by its underlying pathology. Acute generalized polyneuropathy

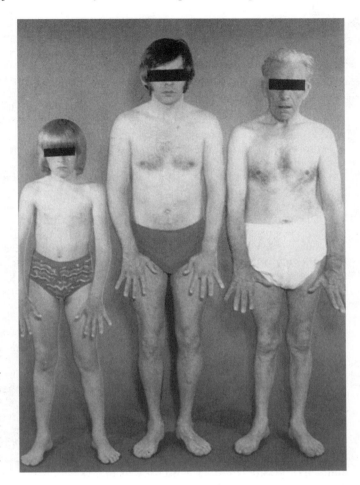

Figure 15–12. *Familial Motor and Sensory Neuropathy (Charcot-Marie-Tooth Disease).* Three generations of this family demonstrated the distal weakness and wasting characteristic of this inherited polyneuropathy. (From Atlas of Clinical Neurology, ed 2, by Perkins, GD, Hochberg, FH, and Miller, DC, Mosby-Wolfe, an imprint of Times Mirror International Publishers Ltd, London, UK, 1993.)

with a rapid and full recovery, such as Guillain-Barré syndrome, reflects a widespread but temporary conduction block related to demyelination. Recovery is associated with remyelination, which can occur quickly. In contrast, acquired neuropathies associated with extensive axonal degeneration have a slow recovery associated with time-consuming axonal regeneration or collateral sprouting from surviving axons.

The Most Common Neuropathies

In the United States, the most common hereditary neuropathy is dominant peroneal muscular atrophy (Charcot-Marie-Tooth; HSMN type I).[38–40] The most common acquired neuropathies are the Guillain-Barré syndrome[43–45] and those associated with diabetes[54,55] and alcoholism.[51,52]

Diabetic Polyneuropathy[4,41,54,55]

Diabetes mellitus is the most common human metabolic disease. In the United States alone, more than 5 million people are thought to have this disorder. Diabetic neuropathy is the most common complication of diabetes, and **diabetes may be the most common cause of peripheral neuropathy.** The most common form of diabetic neuropathy (75% of all cases) is distal, symmetric polyneuropathy. Diabetic polyneuropathy probably develops in 50% of all patients with long-term diabetes, especially those with poor control of blood sugar levels. **Distal sensory disturbances predominate in most cases.** The most common form of polyneuropathy is one in which large nerve fibers are primarily involved and manifests as painless paresthesias beginning in the feet and lower legs, distal impairment of vibratory and joint position sense, and diminished muscle stretch reflexes (ankle jerks). A less common small fiber form is manifested by deep aching pain in the legs and burning feelings in the feet. Touch, pain, and temperature sensations are impaired, whereas joint position sense and tendon reflexes are preserved. Infrequent forms of polyneuropathy also exist in which motor or autonomic disturbances predominate. The precise nature of the underlying primary pathologic process in the distal polyneuropathy remains to be determined, but most studies have revealed a mixture of axonal degeneration and segmental demyelination. The demyelination may be secondary to primary axonal dysfunction. Although the pathogenesis of this dysfunction is poorly understood, it may be due to metabolic abnormalities in the neuron.

Diabetes is also associated with a variety of vascular disorders, so that disease of the small intraneural blood vessels may also be involved. In general, the course of this distal polyneuropathy is improved by careful control of the diabetes. Symptomatic relief of painful diabetic neuropathy and treatment of autonomic dysfunction is difficult. Patients with cutaneous sensory loss and vascular disease are particularly susceptible to trophic ulcers and cutaneous infections in the feet; therefore, skin care is of utmost importance. Ulcers may also respond favorably to reduced weight bearing, local débridement, and antibiotics.[54] Distal weakness may create a need for orthoses and rehabilitative services.

Alcoholic Polyneuropathy[4,41,51,52]

Neuropathy is one of a number of neurologic complications of alcoholism, and **alcoholic neuropathy is one of the most common peripheral neuropathies.** This distal polyneuropathy usually begins insidiously and progresses slowly, but acute exacerbations may occur. A mixture of sensory and motor findings is typical, with sensory signs and symptoms often preceding muscle weakness. In mild cases, symptoms may consist of only mild aching in the calf muscles and discomfort on the soles of the feet. In more severe cases, **distal muscle weakness and wasting, loss of muscle stretch reflexes, and sensory abnormalities are common,** with the legs more severely involved than the arms. Pain (which may be severe) and paresthesias in distal parts of the legs, particularly in the soles of the feet, are characteristic sensory features. The entire plantar surface of the foot may become extremely sensitive to touch, to the extent that shoes or even socks cannot be tolerated. Distal sensory loss may also be severe and sensory ataxia may develop as a result of a loss of proprioceptive feedback. Footdrop, and later wrist drop may result from muscle weakness and when accompanied by atrophy, may evolve into disabling contractures. In chronic cases, trophic changes often develop in the feet, with decubiti, edema, and foot deformity.

Alcoholic neuropathy seems to be primarily a distal axonopathy, although some secondary demyelination may occur. The exact cause of this axonopathy is not known, with debate focused on the relative importance of the neurotoxic effects of alcohol itself and the deleterious effects of the poor nutritional status of most alcoholics. The deficiency of thiamine and other B vitamins, which is often associated with alcoholism, has been specifically implicated. With abstinence and improved nutrition, a slow, incomplete recovery may occur over many months, although considerable discomfort may remain.

Guillain-Barré Syndrome[3,4,43-45]

Guillain-Barré syndrome, like the diabetic and alcoholic disorders, is an acquired polyneuropathy. It differs, however, in lacking any apparent causal relationship with a known disease entity and in revolving around severe motor dysfunction. **Guillain-Barré syndrome is a rapidly evolving paralytic disorder,** which is probably the most common acute paralytic disease seen in developed countries. Its primary clinical manifestation is rapidly progressive muscle weakness. **This weakness is typically symmetric, beginning in the distal muscles of the lower limbs and ascending rapidly over the entire body.** Difficulty in walking is a common early complaint. Most patients reach their maximal deficit in less than 2 weeks, many in a few days. The eventual degree of weakness is highly variable, ranging from mild distal weakness (i.e., bilateral footdrop) to complete, flaccid quadriplegia with an inability to breathe, swallow, or speak. Facial weakness is a common feature, but involvement of the extraocular muscle or muscles of the lower cranial nerves is less common. The tendon reflexes are usually absent. Transient paresthesias (tingling, burning, and numbness) are present in most cases, but, aside from mild impairment of distal vibratory and position sense, are generally not accompanied by significant, objective sensory loss. Patients often complain of pain (especially in muscle) and dyesthesias, which may interfere with rehabilitation. Disturbances of autonomic function are also common and may be difficult to manage. These include tachycardia, facial flushing, fluctuating hypertension and hypotension, and abnormal sweating.

Recovery in Guillain-Barré typically begins within 2 to 4 weeks after progression ceases and may be rapid. Although the pattern of recovery is variable, it normally proceeds at a steady pace, and within 6 months 85% of cases are ambulatory.[45] Although most individuals experience an excellent functional recovery, the overall mortality rate is 5%, and perhaps 20% of all patients remain significantly handicapped by weakness.[45] Pathologic studies reveal inflammation and segmental demyelination throughout the peripheral nervous system. Although peripheral nerves may be affected at any level from the roots to the most distal intramuscular nerve endings, most lesions develop in the ventral roots, limb-girdle plexuses, and proximal nerve trunks. Deleterious changes may also occur in dorsal (sensory) roots, autonomic ganglia, and distal peripheral nerves. Guillain-Barré syndrome is generally considered an autoimmune disorder, although the conditions that trigger this reaction are not known. In about 60% of cases, the symptomatic onset of the disorder is preceded within 1 month by an upper respiratory or gastrointestinal tract infection. This suggests that a virus may be involved; however, all attempts to isolate such a virus or other microbial agents, have failed. Management includes thorough respiratory care and prevention of the complications of autonomic dysfunction. Physical and occupational therapy directed at the prevention of contractures, maintenance of range of motion, and restoration of musculoskeletal function should begin immediately and will hasten recovery.

Hereditary Motor and Sensory Neuropathy Type I[3,4,38–40]

As previously mentioned, the hereditary neuropathies are a heterogeneous group of genetically determined disorders in which the underlying cause of neuronal deterioration is usually unknown. Most of these disorders are rare, with the exception of HMSNs. The most common disorder within this group is HMSN type I, which includes most individuals previously labeled as having peroneal muscular atrophy, Charcot-Marie-Tooth disease, or Roussy-Lévy syndrome. **HMSN type I is a slowly progressive, relatively benign polyneuropathy characterized by weakness and wasting of distal limb muscles.** Common initial complaints are foot deformity (pes cavus) and difficulty in walking or running, which begin in late childhood or adolescence. **Symmetric weakness and wasting are found in intrinsic foot, peroneal, and anterior tibial muscles.** After a period of years, the muscles of the hand and forearm may be similarly involved. Occasionally, the intrinsic muscles of the hand atrophy to produce a clawhand deformity, analogous to pes cavus. Wasting seldom extends beyond midthigh or above the elbow. Tendon reflexes in the involved extremities are usually absent. Paresthesias are common, and some degree of objective distal sensory impairment is usually found by examination. The sensory impairment is rarely symptomatic and typically consists of diminished vibratory sense and light touch in the feet and hands.

HMSN type I progresses very slowly and may stabilize for long periods of time. The principal functional difficulty is in walking, which is caused by a combination of weakness and sensory ataxia, compounded by footdrop and ankle instability. Pathology studies reveal depletion of large myelinated motor and sensory fibers. Axonal degeneration is probably the primary underlying pathology, leading to secondary segmental demyelination. The precise cause of the axonal deterioration is unknown, but it may reflect some inherited abnormality of neuronal or axonal metabolism. There is no known treatment, but the condition is often benign, creating little significant functional impairment. Preservation of proximal strength often enables even seriously involved patients to remain ambulatory, when aided by braces and other orthotic devices and surgery to correct deformity and reduce footdrop and ankle instability.

Syndromic Classification of Neuropathies

One approach to the classification of a neuropathy, particularly when the cause is unclear, is to define it in terms of the signs and symptoms it manifests (i.e., as a syndrome). In this context, emphasis is often placed on the time course of the disease.

Acute neuropathies are those that evolve over hours or days.[5,34,35] These are usually **polyneuropathies, which may be postinfectious, metabolic, or toxic. Guillain-Barré syndrome**, which is typically a postinfectious (viral) inflammatory phenomenon **is the most common.**[43-45] Although most toxins tend to cause relatively chronic neuropathies, thallium and certain other chemicals can produce a polyneuropathy that can be rapidly progressive and resemble Guillain-Barré syndrome. The typical clinical picture is one of symmetric weakness beginning in the feet. This weakness usually evolves over days but may progress rapidly over hours. As it develops, it may be accompanied by sensory disturbances, including pain and paresthesias, and occasionally significant autonomic involvement. **Acute focal damage to peripheral nerves may be caused by physical injury (e.g., laceration, compression, traction, or ischemia) and result in acute onset mononeuropathies.**[46-50] Although rare in Western medical practice, diphtheria (a bacterial infection) can also cause an acute focal neuropathy.

Subacute neuropathies are those that evolve over a period of weeks to months. This group of disorders is heterogenous, although all are acquired. **Most are polyneuropathies due to nutritional deficiency (e.g., alcoholism),**[51,52] **sustained exposure to toxic agents (e.g., heavy metals, such as arsenic and solvents),**[53] **drug intoxications,**[53] **metabolic disturbances (e.g., diabetes),**[54,55] **or inflammatory conditions.**[43-45] In general, symptoms begin with pain, paresthesias, or numbness in the feet, gradually spreading upward to the knees and then involving the fingers and hands (glove-and-stocking distribution). Weakness and wasting of the peripheral muscles may develop.

Chronic polyneuropathies arise over months or years and cause signs and symptoms similar to those in more acute neuropathies.[51-55] **Although many of these disorders can be linked to metabolic disturbances (e.g., diabetes), chronic intoxication (e.g., alcoholism), or malignant disease**, in a significant proportion no cause is ever firmly established.

Difficulties with Classification

Although the distinction made previously in this chapter between neuropathies in which the underlying pathology involves primarily the axon (axonopathies) and those in which it primarily involves the myelin (myelinopathies) is a useful theoretical construct, it cannot always be neatly applied to the specific diseases defined etiologically or syndromically in the clinic. Some neuropathic conditions conform to one of these two pathologic categories (Table 15–4); many more are difficult to classify. In many neuropathies (e.g., diabetic and uremic polyneuropathy; HSMN type I), significant pathology of both axon and myelin exists. In some, this involvement is concurrent; in others, one is a consequence of the other. It is not always clear which is which. In addition, a single cause (e.g., HIV infection, malignancy) may result in several different forms of neuropathy, with varying degrees of axonal or myelin involvement. Finally, in many human neuropathies the underlying pathologic changes are only poorly understood, with conclusions about pathogenesis drawn

Table 15–4. Polyneuropathies with Known Primary Pathology

Pathologic Classification	Origin
Axonopathy (Usually Distal)	
Toxic	Drugs, industrial agents, and environmental contaminants
Metabolic	Diabetes, alcoholism, nutritional deficiency (especially thiamine), uremia (renal insufficiency); porphyria (heme defect)
Infectious	HIV-related, Lyme disease
Inherited	HMSN type II
Malignancy-associated	Lung
Myelinopathy	
Immunologic	Acute inflammatory polyradiculoneuropathy (Guillain-Barré syndrome)
Toxic	Lead; diphtheria toxin (uncommon)

HMSN = hereditary motor and sensory neuropathy.

indirectly from clinical manifestations, electrophysiologic studies, and animal models. As more is learned about the morphologic changes accompanying these disorders, their classification will become easier.

Disorders of Cranial Nerves

Although the emphasis in this chapter has been on the spinal nerves, it should be noted that many of the same types of disorders and injuries can also adversely affect the cranial nerves. **Cranial nerve involvement is an important component of a number of peripheral neuropathies** (e.g., Guillain-Barré syndrome, Lyme disease, and diabetic neuropathy) and in some of these disorders may predominate.[11,12,56,57] In general, the cranial nerves tend to be involved late in the progression of polyneuropathy, well after symptoms in the distal extremities. **Cranial nerves are subject to the same basic pathologic reactions of axon or myelin as spinal nerves,** but share some etiologies rarely affecting the spinal cord.[56,57] Cranial nerves, for example, are more often injured by vascular insults or tumors of the central nervous system from which they emerge (e.g., the brainstem) than their spinal counterparts. Cranial nerves also subserve motor and sensory functions not associated with spinal nerves. Accordingly, their dysfunction may create abnormalities of olfaction, vision, taste, hearing, balance, and craniofacial pain in addition to somatic and autonomic disturbances analogous to those accompanying spinal nerve dysfunction. Disorders of cranial nerves are important clinical entities that can cause considerable discomfort and functional impairment.

Disorders of Spinal Roots (Radiculopathies)

The spinal roots are susceptible to many of the same disorders that affect the other components of the peripheral nervous system.[18,19,22] In fact, the radiculopathies (as these disorders are called) probably represent one of the most common problems brought to the neurologist. **Certain aspects of the anatomy of the spinal roots make them particularly vulnerable to specific types of disturbance.**[18,19] The spinal roots are delicate structures that exit the spinal vertebrae through a narrow, rigid bony canal (foramen). Narrowing of this canal or shifting of these bony structures can easily damage this tissue. The roots also contain much less endoneurial collagen than peripheral nerves and lack the substantial epineurial and perineurial sheaths found in the periphery.[18,19] Because of this, they have much less tensile strength than peripheral nerves and are more susceptible to injury by compression or excessive stretch. In the periphery, the actual nerve fibers of a nerve trunk are effectively isolated from the blood by a barrier formed by the perineurium and capillary wall. Nerve roots and the dorsal root ganglia, however, are covered with only a thin layer of perineurial cells, which does not provide a very effective blood–nerve barrier.[18] This may explain their vulnerability to certain circulating toxic, infectious (e.g., diphtheria and syphilis) or inflammatory (e.g., Guillain-Barré syndrome) factors. There is also some evidence that the blood supply of the spinal roots may be less than that of peripheral nerves. This may account for the susceptibility of nerve roots to ischemic damage, as might occur in diabetes or compression. Finally, because of their proximity to the leptomeninges of the spinal cord (i.e., pia mater and arachnoid), the nerve roots are susceptible to damage by infectious, inflammatory, and neoplastic processes that involve these protective membranes.[19]

Nerve roots, like all peripheral nerves, have a limited number of pathologic responses to injury or disease.[18,19] **Some types of injury produce segmental demyelination as the predominant reaction, whereas others produce primarily axonal atrophy or wallerian degeneration.** In most of the nerve root disorders, there is some combination of the two. Compressive radiculopathies are characterized primarily by axonal degeneration, but some secondary demyelination also occurs. Conversely, in inflammatory radiculoneuropathies such as Guillain-Barré syndrome, the predominant pathology is demyelination, but some degree of axonal degeneration may also occur. When the predominant pathology is demyelination, recovery by remyelination is generally rapid and complete. When axonal degeneration predominates, recovery is slow and incomplete. Moreover, in the centrally directed processes of the dorsal root ganglion cells, the glial scar that forms in the dorsal spinal cord prevents axons that begin to regenerate from reaching their central targets.[23]

The clinical picture presented by a lesion of a single spinal root is one of radicular pain accompanied by sensory loss, weakness, and hyporeflexia.[19] These signs and symptoms are readily distinguishable from those of focal neuropathy. When many roots are involved, the resulting clinical syndrome is difficult to distinguish from that of polyneuropathy.[19] Polyradiculopathies are characterized by generalized weakness, sensory loss, and areflexia. **In most nerve root disorders, dorsal (sensory) and ventral (motor) components are equally affected.** In some conditions, one component may be preferentially involved. In some cases of inflammatory polyradiculopathy, for example, the ventral roots are selectively affected, whereas the dorsal roots are spared, creating a syndrome resembling an anterior horn cell disorder.

RECOMMENDED READINGS

Adams, RD and Victor, M: Principles of Neurology, ed 5. Chapter 46. Diseases of the Peripheral Nerves. McGraw-Hill, New York, 1993.

Bosch, EP and Mitsumoto, H: Disorders of Peripheral Nerves. Chapter 81A. In Bradley, WG, et al (eds): Neurology in Clinical Practice, vol II. Butterworth-Heinemann, Boston, 1990.

Brown, MJ (ed): Neuropathy. Semin Neurol 7(1):1, 1987.

Chadwick, D, Cartlidge, N, and Bates, D: Medical Neurology. Chapter 10. Diseases of the Peripheral Nerves and Muscle. Churchill Livingstone, Edinburgh, 1989.

Dyck, PJ: Diseases of Peripheral Nerves. Chapter 72. In Engel, AG and Franzini-Armstrong, C (eds): Myology: Basic and Clinical, ed 2. McGraw-Hill, New York, 1994.

Dyck, PJ and Thomas, PK (eds): Peripheral Neuropathy, ed 3. WB Saunders, Philadelphia, 1993.

Johnson, PC: Peripheral Nerve. Chapter 18. In Davis, RL and Robertson, DM (eds): Textbook of Neuropathology, ed 2. Williams & Wilkins, Baltimore, 1991.

Schaumburg, HH, Berger, AR, and Thomas, PK: Disorders of Peripheral Nerves, ed 2. FA Davis, Philadelphia, 1992.

Stewart, JD: Focal Peripheral Neuropathies, ed 2. Raven Press, New York, 1993.

Sunderland, Sir S: Nerve Injuries and Their Repair: A Critical Appraisal. Churchill Livingstone, Edinburgh, 1991.

Swash, M and Schwartz, MS: Neuromuscular Diseases, ed 2. Chapter 7. A Clinical Approach to the Neuropathies. Springer-Verlag, London, 1988.

Terzis, JK and Smith, KL: The Peripheral Nerve: Structure, Function, and Reconstruction. Raven Press, New York, 1990.

Thomas, PK, Landon, DN, and King, RHM: Diseases of Peripheral Nerves. Chapter 18. In Adams, JH and Duchen, LW (eds): Greenfield's Neuropathology, ed 5. Oxford University Press, New York, 1992.

REFERENCES

1. Dyck, PJ and Thomas, PK (eds): Peripheral Neuropathy, ed 3. WB Saunders, Philadelphia, 1993.
2. Schaumburg, HH, Berger, AR, and Thomas, PK: Disorders of Peripheral Nerves, ed 2. FA Davis, Philadelphia, 1992.
3. Adams, RD and Victor, M: Principles of Neurology, ed 5. Chapter 46. Diseases of the Peripheral Nerves. McGraw-Hill, New York, 1993.
4. Bosch, EP and Mitsumoto, H: Disorders of Peripheral Nerves. Chapter 81A. In Bradley, WG, et al (eds): Neurology in Clinical Practice, vol II. Butterworth-Heinemann, Boston, 1990.
5. Chadwick, D, Cartlidge, N, and Bates, D: Medical Neurology. Chapter 10. Diseases of the Peripheral Nerves and Muscle. Churchill Livingstone, Edinburgh, 1989.
6. Dyck, PJ: Diseases of Peripheral Nerves. Chapter 72. In Engel, AG and Franzini-Armstrong, C (eds): Myology: Basic and Clinical, ed 2. McGraw-Hill, New York, 1994.
7. Schaumburg, HH, Berger, AR, and Thomas, PK: Disorders of Peripheral Nerves, ed 2. Chapter 1. Basic Concepts and Terminology. FA Davis, Philadelphia, 1992.
8. Gardner, E and Bunge, RP: Gross Anatomy of the Peripheral Nervous System. Chapter 2. In Dyck, PJ and Thomas, PK (ed): Peripheral Neuropathy, ed 3. WB Saunders, Philadelphia, 1993.
9. Thomas, PK, et al: Microscopic Anatomy of the Peripheral Nervous System. Chapter 3. In Dyck, PJ and Thomas, PK (eds): Peripheral Neuropathy, ed 3. WB Saunders, Philadelphia, 1993.
10. Stewart, JD: Focal Peripheral Neuropathies, ed 2. Chapter 1. The Structure of the Peripheral Nervous System. Raven Press, New York, 1993.
11. Role, LW and Kelly, JP: The Brainstem: Cranial Nerve Nuclei and the Monoaminergic Systems. Chapter 44. In Kandel, ER, Schwartz, JH, and Jessell, TM: Principles of Neural Science, ed 3. Appleton & Lange, Norwalk, CT, 1991.
12. Wilson-Paulwels, L, Akesson, EJ, and Stewart, PA: Cranial Nerves: Anatomy and Clinical Comments. BC Decker, Toronto, 1988.
13. Terzis, JK and Smith, KL: The Peripheral Nerve. Structure, Function, and Reconstruction. Chapter 1. Composition of the Peripheral Nerve. Raven Press, New York, 1990.
14. Thomas, PK, Landon, DN, and King, RHM: Diseases of Peripheral Nerves. Chapter 18. In Adams, JH and Duchen, LW (eds): Greenfield's Neuropathology, ed 5. Oxford University Press, New York, 1992.
15. Johnson, PC: Peripheral Nerve. Chapter 18. In Davis, RL and Robertson, DM (eds): Textbook of Neuropathology, ed 2. Williams & Wilkins, Baltimore, 1991.
16. Sunderland, Sir S: Nerve Injuries and Their Repair: A Critical Appraisal. Chapter 9. Connective Tissues of Nerve Trunks. Churchill Livingstone, Edinburgh, 1991.
17. Sunderland, Sir S: Nerve Injuries and Their Repair: A Critical Appraisal. Chapter 10. Blood Supply of Nerves. Churchill Livingstone, Edinburgh, 1991.
18. Parry, GJ: Diseases of Spinal Roots. Chapter 47. In Dyck, PJ and Thomas, PK (eds): Peripheral Neuropathy, ed 3. WB Saunders, Philadelphia, 1993.
19. Chad, DA: Disorders of Roots and Plexuses. Chapter 81B. In Bradley, WG, et al (eds): Neurology in Clinical Practice, vol II. Butterworth-Heinemann, Boston, 1990.
20. Ochs, S and Brimijoin, WS: Axonal Transport. Chapter 21. In Dyck, PJ and Thomas, PK (eds): Peripheral Neuropathy, ed 3. WB Saunders, Philadelphia, 1993.
21. Griffin, JW, Hoffman, PN, and Crawford, TO: Pathophysiology of Neuronal and Axonal Degenerations. Chapter 17. In Asbury, AK, McKhann, GM, and McDonald, WI (eds): Diseases of the Nervous System: Clinical Neurobiology, ed 2. WB Saunders, Philadelphia, 1992.
22. Said, G and Thomas, PK: Pathophysiology of Nerve and Root Disorders. Chapter 18. In Asbury, AK, McKhann, GM, and McDonald, WI (eds): Diseases of the Nervous System: Clinical Neurobiology, ed 2. WB Saunders, Philadelphia, 1992.
23. Jessell, TM: Reactions of Neurons to Injury. Chapter 18. In Kandel, ER, Schwartz, JH, and Jessell, TM: Principles of Neural Science, ed 3. Appleton & Lange, Norwalk, CT, 1991.
24. Griffin, JW and Hoffman, PN: Degeneration and Regeneration in the Peripheral Nervous System. Chapter 22. In Dyck, PJ and Thomas, PK (eds): Peripheral Neuropathy, ed 3. WB Saunders, Philadelphia, 1993.
25. Schaumburg, HH, Berger, AR, and Thomas, PK: Disorders of Peripheral Nerve, ed 2. Chapter 2. Anatomical Classification of Peripheral Nervous System Disorders. FA Davis, Philadelphia, 1992.
26. Terzis, JK and Smith, KL: The Peripheral Nerve. Structure, Function, and Reconstruction. Chapter 3. Peripheral Nerve Regeneration. Raven Press, New York, 1990.
27. Selzer, ME: Nerve Regeneration. Semin Neurol 7(1):88, 1987.
28. Rasminsky, M and Bray, GM: Pathophysiology of Nerve and Root Disorders. Chapter 23. In Asbury, AK, McKhann, GM, and McDonald, WI (eds): Diseases of the Nervous System: Clinical Neurobiology. WB Saunders, Philadelphia, 1988.
29. Jennekens, FGI: Neurogenic Disorders of Muscle. Chapter 16. In Mastaglia, FL and Detchant, Lord Walton (eds): Skeletal Muscle Pathology, ed 2. Churchill Livingstone, Edinburgh, 1992.
30. Bowden, REM and Gutmann, E: Denervation and Reinnervation of Human Voluntary Muscle. Brain 67:273, 1944.
31. Oaklander, AL, Miller, MS, and Spencer, PS: Early Biochemical Changes in Degenerating Mouse Sciatic Nerve Are Associated with Endothelial Cells. Brain Res 419:39, 1987.
32. McDonald, WI: Physiological Consequences of Demyelination. Chapter 8. In Sumner, AJ (ed): The Physiology of Peripheral Nerve Disease. WB Saunders, Philadelphia, 1980.
33. Rowland, LP: Diseases of the Motor Unit. Chapter 17. In Kandel, ER, Schwartz, JH, and Jessell, TM: Principles of Neural Science, ed 3. Appleton & Lange, Norwalk, CT, 1991.
34. Thomas, PK and Ochoa, J: Clinical Features and Differential Diagnosis. Chapter 39. In Dyck, PJ and

Thomas, PK (eds): Peripheral Neuropathy, ed 3. WB Saunders, Philadelphia, 1993.

35. Asbury, AK and Bird, SJ: Disorders of Peripheral Nerve. Chapter 19. In Asbury, AK, McKhann, GM, and McDonald, WI (eds): Diseases of the Nervous System: Clinical Neurobiology. WB Saunders, Philadelphia, 1992.

36. Brown, MJ: Evaluating the Perplexing Neuropathic Patient. Semin Neurol 7(1):1, 1987.

37. Swash, M and Schwartz, MS: Neuromuscular Diseases, ed 2. Chapter 7. A Clinical Approach to the Neuropathies. Springer-Verlag, London, 1988.

38. Dyck, PJ and Thomas, PK (eds): Peripheral Neuropathy, ed 3. Part E. Inherited Peripheral Neuropathies. WB Saunders, Philadelphia, 1993.

39. Schaumburg, HH, Berger, AR, and Thomas, PK: Disorders of Peripheral Nerves, ed 2. Part IV. Inherited Peripheral Neuropathy. FA Davis, Philadelphia, 1992.

40. Swash, M and Schwartz, MS: Neuromuscular Diseases, ed 2. Chapter 10. Genetically Determined Neuropathies. Springer-Verlag, London, 1988.

41. Swash, M and Schwartz, MS: Neuromuscular Diseases, ed 2. Chapter 11. Acquired Polyneuropathies. Springer-Verlag, London, 1988.

42. Pleasure, DE and Schotland, DL: Acquired Neuropathies. Chapter 108. In Rowland, LP (ed): Merritt's Textbook of Neurology, ed 8. Lea & Febiger, Philadelphia, 1989.

43. Lisak, RP and Brown, MJ: Acquired Demyelinating Polyneuropathies. Semin Neurol 7:40, 1987.

44. Arnason, BGW and Soliven, B: Acute Inflammatory Demyelinating Polyradiculoneuropathy. Chapter 80. In Dyck, PJ and Thomas, PK (eds): Peripheral Neuropathy, ed 3. WB Saunders, 1993.

45. Schaumburg, HH, Berger, AR, and Thomas, PK: Disorders of Peripheral Nerves, ed 2. Chapter 5. Inflammatory Demyelinating Neuropathy. FA Davis, Philadelphia, 1992.

46. Schaumburg, HH, Berger, AR, and Thomas, PK: Disorders of Peripheral Nerves, ed 2. Part V. Trauma. FA Davis, Philadelphia, 1992.

47. Terzis, JK and Smith, KL: The Peripheral Nerve: Structure, Function and Reconstruction. Chapter 2. Peripheral Nerve Injury. Raven Press, New York, 1990.

48. Stewart, JD: Focal Peripheral Neuropathies, ed 2. Chapter 2. Pathological Processes Producing Focal Peripheral Neuropathies. Elsevier, New York, 1993.

49. Sunderland, Sir S: Nerve Injuries and Their Repair: A Critical Appraisal. Churchill Livingstone, Edinburgh, 1991.

50. Dyck, PJ and Thomas, PK (eds): Peripheral Neuropathy, ed 3. Part D. Neuropathy Due to Ischemia and Physical Agents. WB Saunders, Philadelphia, 1993.

51. Schaumburg, HH, Berger, AR, and Thomas, PK: Disorders of Peripheral Nerves, ed 2. Chapter 9. Neuropathy Associated with Alcoholism, Nutritional Deficiencies, and Malabsorption. FA Davis, Philadelphia, 1992.

52. Windebank, AJ: Polyneuropathy Due to Nutritional Deficiency and Alcoholism. Chapter 70. In Dyck, PJ and Thomas, PK: Peripheral Neuropathy, ed 3. WB Saunders, Philadelphia, 1993.

53. Dyck, PJ and Thomas, PK (eds): Peripheral Neuropathy, ed 3. Part H. Neuropathy Associated with Industrial Agents, Metals, and Drugs. WB Saunders, Philadelphia, 1993.

54. Schaumburg, HH, Berger, AR, and Thomas, PK: Disorders of Peripheral Nerves, ed 2. Chapter 7. Diabetic Neuropathy. FA Davis, 1992.

55. Thomas, PK and Tomlinson, DR: Diabetic and Hypoglycemic Neuropathy. Chapter 64. In Dyck, PJ and Thomas, PK (eds): Peripheral Neuropathy, ed 3. WB Saunders, Philadelphia, 1993.

56. Chadwick, D, Cartlidge, N, and Bates, D: Medical Neurology. Chapter 3. Disorders of Special Sensation and Cranial Nerves. Churchill Livingstone, Edinburgh, 1989.

57. Adams, RD and Victor, M: Principles of Neurology, ed 5. Chapter 47. Diseases of the Cranial Nerves. McGraw-Hill, New York, 1993.

CHAPTER 16

■

Disorders of Anterior Horn Cells: The Neuronopathies

Christopher M. Fredericks, PhD

- *Clinical Features of Neuronopathies*
- *Injury Due to Physical or Chemical Agents*
- *Conditions Characterized by Motor Neuron and Muscle Hyperactivity*

Motor activity is dependent on the functional integrity of the lower motor neurons that innervate skeletal muscle. These neurons span the blood-brain barrier, with portions of each neuron found within the central and peripheral nervous systems. Although the bulk of these cells, namely their axons and axon terminals, reside within the peripheral nervous system, the cell body of each neuron resides within the protective confines of the central nervous system (i.e., the anterior gray matter of the spinal cord or the cranial motor nuclei of the brainstem). In Chapter 15, a distinction was made between disorders of the central and peripheral components of these neurons. Disorders were discussed that primarily affect the peripheral component of motor neurons and their associated sensory fibers. These are the so-called peripheral neuropathies. **This chapter will focus on the disorders in which the primary pathologic defect is in the region of the motor neuron cell body itself.**[1-4] **These are the** *neuronopathies.*

Although the distinction between the peripheral neuropathies and the neuronopathies provides a convenient way to organize discussion of these disorders, this distinction is something of an oversimplification and may not be possible or appropriate in many disorders. Although a number of disorders have been identified in which the primary pathology is clearly localized in the anterior horn cell, or in the distal axon, in many disorders there is considerable overlap between the two.[1-4] In some cases, it is evident that cell body degeneration is accompanied from the beginning by pathologic alterations in the axon. In other cases, however, the primary disease involves the cell body *or* axon, but leads to secondary effects in other parts of the neuron. In most peripheral neuropathies, for example, there is some proximal spread of dysfunction from the primary site of injury. If the site is close to the cell body, this spread may result in cell body disruption and neuron death.

Although the distinction between central and peripheral disorders of the lower motor neuron is often blurred, the isolation of the anterior horn cell within the central nervous system does have some interesting functional implications. Compared with the cell body, which is situated in the protected milieu behind the blood-brain barrier, the axons and axon terminals are more exposed to toxic and infective agents in the overall extracellular fluid.[4] Some of these offending agents may be carried to the cell body by retrograde axonal transport (see Chapters 1 and 15), but the protective blood-brain barrier surely influences the susceptibility of the central portion of the neuron to injury. In addition, differences in the regenerative capabilities of the central and peripheral nervous systems are reflected in the greater recuperative potential in peripheral neuropathies compared with that in central neuronopathies.

Neuronopathy may occur as one aspect of disorders producing widespread damage to the central nervous system, or within the context of systemic disorders producing disturbance of function throughout the entire nervous system. In this regard, motor neurons, like other kinds of cells, are affected by generalized infections, nutritional deficiencies, metabolic and endocrine disorders, immune disturbances, and various toxic states. This chapter will focus on disorders with a specific predilection for the lower motor neuron cell body.

Discussion of disorders involving more generalized spinal cord dysfunction (e.g., syringomelia, spinal cord tumors, inflammatory myelopathies, and trauma) and more diverse white matter lesions will be found in the chapters concerned with spinal cord disorders (see Chapter 17) and multiple sclerosis (see Chapter 22).

Clinical Features of Neuronopathies

The clinical presentation of neuronopathy reflects neuronal degeneration and loss and is primarily one of skeletal muscle weakness and wasting. In most anterior horn cell disorders, neurons of the spinal cord and the motor nuclei of the brainstem may both be involved. Anterior horn cell diseases in adults are often accompanied by prominent fasciculations at rest. When only the lower motor neurons are involved, the tendon reflexes are usually depressed or absent, but in motor neuron diseases with concurrent lower and upper motor neuron lesions, the tendon reflexes are characteristically more brisk than normal, even in wasted muscles. Sensory abnormalities are infrequent, although some patients complain of paresthesias.

Diseases affecting the anterior horn cell may manifest any time, from infancy to old age. Those diseases beginning in infancy, childhood, or adolescence are usually limited to the lower motor neuron; in adults other parts of the motor system (i.e., upper motor neurons) may be involved.

Motor Neuron Disease: Amyotrophic Lateral Sclerosis

Although there is some debate about exactly what constitutes a motor neuron disease, this term is generally used clinically to refer to a group of disorders characterized by progressively disordered function of both upper and lower motor neurons.[1-5] Patients with motor neuron disease present with progressive muscle wasting, weakness, and fasciculations, accompanied by spasticity, hyperreflexia, and extensor plantar responses.[4-11] These features represent the consequences of a combination of both lower and upper motor neuron lesions. Although most patients with motor neuron disease show features of both upper and lower motor neuron dysfunction, forms of the disease exist in which either upper or lower motor neuron signs predominate, especially early in its progression. Upper motor neuron signs ultimately arise in almost all cases, but they may be initially masked by severe lower motor neuron involvement.

Three clinical forms of motor neuron disease may be described, but probably reflect the same underlying pathology.[4-11] The most common form (about 80% of cases) is classic amyotrophic lateral sclerosis (ALS) in which both upper and lower motor neurons are involved early on. In progressive bulbar palsy, on the other hand, the bulbar neurons and musculature are primarily involved, and in progressive muscular atrophy, the disease is limited to spinal motor neurons. Although these three designations are useful, these are clinical entities only and the longer a patient survives, the greater is the tendency for these entities to overlap. In North America, the term "amyotrophic lateral sclerosis" is used to described all three.

Classic Amyotrophic Lateral Sclerosis

The classic form of ALS is by far the most common form of motor neuron disease.[4–11] This is an important disease, accounting for about 0.1% of adult deaths. ALS is a disease of late middle life and is rarely seen prior to age 40. Its incidence increases linearly from the third decade of life onward. Ninety percent of all cases begin between the ages of 40 and 70 years, with some predominance in men (estimated at 2 to 1.5:1). About 5% to 10% of all cases of ALS are familial,[4, 8,10,23,24] and clustering of cases has been observed in certain small geographic areas (e.g., Guam).

ALS is characterized from the onset by a mixture of upper and lower motor neuron signs and symptoms.[4–11] The first symptom is most often asymmetric weakness, as might be manifested by difficulty in manipulating objects with the fingers or dragging one leg during walking. Muscle cramps are also a common early complaint and are most often found in muscles that are already weak or will become weak early in the course of the disease. Although uncommon as presenting symptoms, fasciculations and muscle wasting are frequently discovered on physical examination early in the progression of the disease. Weakness and wasting are focal at the beginning, but as the disease progresses, signs of lower motor neuron destruction spread to other parts of the body and become more generalized (Fig. 16–1). In addition, manifestations of upper motor neuron (pyramidal tracts) involvement such as spasticity, hyperreflexia, and Babinski's reflexes become a feature of almost all cases at some stage of the disease. **The overall clinical picture of ALS becomes a balance between the two.** It is common to find brisk tendon reflexes superimposed on muscle weakness. On the other hand, depressed tendon reflexes may be found in regions where lower motor neurons are exclusively involved or where muscle weakness and atrophy is so advanced that upper motor neuron signs cannot be elicited.

Progressive Bulbar Palsy

In progressive bulbar palsy, the bulbar motor neurons and musculature are primarily affected, and this form of motor neuron disease is dominated from the outset by dysarthria and dysphagia with difficulty in chewing.[4–11] The tongue is weak, and atrophy and fasciculations may be prominent. There is evidence of combined upper and lower motor neuron involvement of the bulbar musculature. Similar abnormalities develop in the limbs later in the course of the disease.

Progressive Muscular Atrophy

In progressive muscular atrophy, there is primarily lower motor neuron involvement of limb muscles, with less prominent impairment of cranial muscle function, without definite evidence of upper motor neuron affliction.[4–11] Patients fail to develop the usual manifestations (hyperreflexia, Babinski's sign, and spasticity) of corticospinal involvement.

General Clinical and Pathologic Features

Although the length and severity of motor neuron disease are highly variable, the clinical course is almost inevitably progressive, with eventual involvement of all striated muscles, other than the extraocular muscles, which are seldom symptomatically involved.[4–11] Patients often reach a stage at which they have almost no muscle function and,

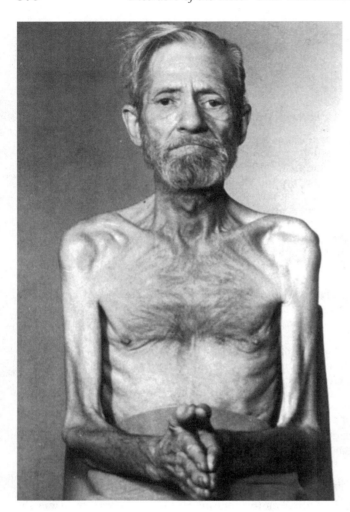

Figure 16–1. *Muscle Wasting in an Amyotrophic Lateral Sclerosis Patient.* Complete atrophy of the deltoid muscle exposes the corocoid process. Other muscles, including the pectoralis major, biceps, triceps, trapezius, rhomboid, supraspinatus, and infraspinatus, are similarly depleted. This patient was ambulatory with no bulbar features at this stage of his illness. (From Hudson,[4] with permission.)

although remaining alert and conscious, have little ability to express themselves by either speech or gesture. Death is usually secondary to involvement of the respiratory muscles. Although the life expectancy of a patient with ALS can vary from less than 1 year to more than a decade with ventilatory support, the average survival rate without ventilatory support is 3 to 4 years. About 20% of patients survive for more than 5 years. A few survive for as long as 20 years. Patients who present with predominantly bulbar paralysis, about 25% of the total, are the most difficult to manage and have the poorest prognosis. The best prognosis is associated with weakness limited to the lower motor neurons of the limbs. Precise determination of the duration of ALS is made difficult by the fact that the exact onset of the illness is impossible to determine.[7] Many patients are uncertain about the date of symptom onset, which may have occurred months or years before their examination. Frequently, the onset is so insidious that it is impossible to define. Although ALS is generally considered a progressive disorder, in some patients the disease seems to stabilize or to progress in a stepwise fashion. These patients usually have a longer clinical course.[7] This apparent stabilization may be related to the patient's ability to compensate temporarily with unaffected sets of muscles, while the disease continues to progress in the affected muscles.

In all the various forms of motor neuron disease, control of bladder, bowel, and autonomic function is largely unimpaired. Although sensory symptoms such as pain and

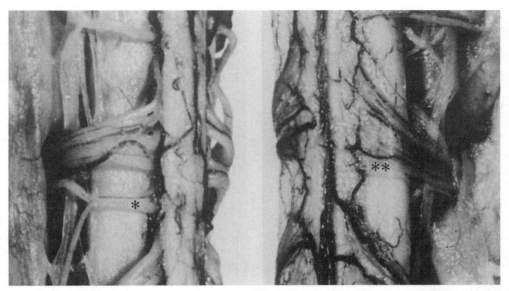

Figure 16–2. *Anterior and Posterior Nerve Roots from the Cervical Cord of a Patient with Amyotrophic Lateral Sclerosis.* There is marked discrepancy in size between the normal posterior roots(*) and the atrophic anterior roots (**). (From Atlas of Clinical Neurology, ed 2, by GD Perkins, FH Hechberg & DC Miller, Mosby-Wolfe, an imprint of Times Mirror International Publishers, Ltd, London, UK, 1993.)

paresthesias are frequently reported, objective impairment of either peripheral sensory systems or of the special senses are rarely a feature of the disease. The intellect is intact and dementia is uncommon.

The essential pathologic feature of all the motor neuron disorders is the loss and atrophy of both upper and lower motor neurons.[1,4–14] There is extensive loss and degeneration of anterior horn cells in the spinal cord and motor cells in the brainstem motor nuclei, as well as of pyramidal cells in the primary motor cortex and of myelinated fibers in the corticospinal tracts.[1,4–6,11–14] The largest and most heavily myelinated neurons seem to be most severely affected. In the brainstem, the hypoglossal, facial, and trigeminal nuclei are most severely involved, whereas the nuclei controlling the extraocular muscles are spared. In myelin-stained cross sections of the spinal cord, the loss of upper and lower motor neurons is evident in the prominent shrinkage of the anterior horns, atrophy of the anterior roots, and pallor of corticospinal tracts in the lateral and anterior columns (Fig. 16–2). This is in contrast to the well-preserved (unaffected) tracts of the posterior columns and spinocerebellar tracts that are usually spared (Fig. 16–3).[11–14]

Involvement of the pyramidal tracts extends throughout the neural axis, but appears to be more pronounced below the medulla than in the upper brainstem or internal capsule.[4–14] In general, spinal cord lower motor neuron involvement is more pronounced in cervical than in lumbar segments. In individual cases, the pattern of motor neuron loss in the spinal cord and brainstem corresponds closely with the clinical pattern of involvement (i.e., wasted skeletal muscles). Although both the cell body and the axon are ultimately affected, cytologic studies suggest that lesions at or near the cell body predominate in the early stages of motor neuron disease and probably represent the primary pathology (hence their inclusion in the broader category of neuronopathy).[8,13]

Because of the loss of lower motor neurons, skeletal muscle undergoes degenerative changes similar to those associated with the denervation produced by peripheral neuropathy (see Chapter 15).[8,10,14,15] The involved skeletal muscles contain large numbers of atrophic muscle fibers (Fig. 16–4). The atrophy of muscle fibers occurs in a motor unit distribution, reflecting the loss of individual motor neurons. In contrast, the denervation atrophy

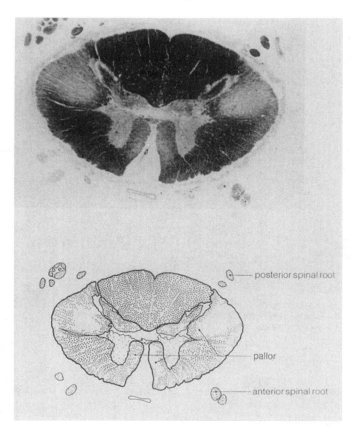

Figure 16–3. *Degeneration of Motor Neurons in the Spinal Cord of Amyotrophic Lateral Sclerosis.* This section of thoracic spinal cord shows poor (*pale*) myelin staining in the degenerating neurons of the lateral and anterior corticospinal tracts; this is in contrast to the heavily staining (*dark*) preserved tracts elsewhere. The anterior roots are less darkly stained than the posterior roots. (From Atlas of Clinical Neurology, ed 2, by GD Perkins, FH Hochberg & DC Miller, Mosby-Wolfe, an imprint of Times Mirror Internationall Publishers, Ltd, London, UK, 1993.)

of most peripheral neuropathies involves much larger areas of muscle, reflecting the large number of motor units supplied by a single peripheral nerve. In any given whole muscle, some fiber bundles are more involved than others and fibers are found in varying stages of atrophy, attesting to the progressive course of denervation. Many unaffected muscle fibers enlarge in compensatory hypertrophy. Over a period of time, denervation followed by reinnervation and the formation of enlarged motor units creates a reorganization of fiber types in which groupings of like fiber types replace the usual checkerboard pattern. This reorganization becomes more evident the longer the cycle of denervation and reinnervation continues.

Few clues to the cause of the motor neuron diseases are found in patient laboratory results, as only minor biochemical abnormalities are present. **Although many factors have been investigated as possible instigators, the cause of the motor neuron deterioration seen in ALS is unknown.**[3–11] Premature aging (abiotrophy),[16] exogenous toxins (e.g., heavy metals),[17] viral diseases, immunologic disturbances,[18,19] and heredity all have been implicated but not proved. Similarities between ALS and poliomyelitis have suggested possible viral origins, but little evidence has been gathered to support this. The association between motor neuron disease and certain autoimmune disorders, the occurrence of unusual antibodies in the blood or nervous system of patients with ALS, and studies of animal models all point toward the possibility of an immune-mediated process underlying ALS. Another interesting hypothesis proposes that some of the central nervous system neurotransmitters themselves may contribute to motor neuron degeneration and death. Glutamate, for example, which is the primary excitatory transmitter in the brain, has been specifically implicated in ALS as well as in a number of other neurologic disorders.[20–22] Glutamate, and

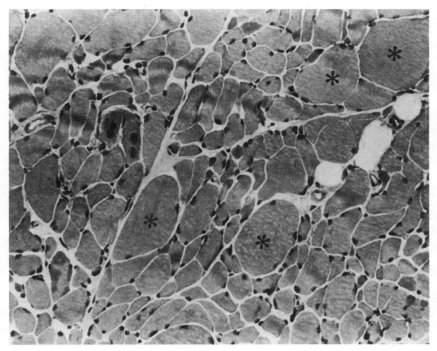

Figure 16–4. *Skeletal Muscle in Amyotrophic Lateral Sclerosis.* Most of the muscle fibers are denervated and have become atrophic and angulated or elongated. Fibers of normal size and hypertrophic fibers (*) are scattered singly or in small groups among the smaller atrophic fibers (×210). (From Mastaglia, FL and Walton, Lord of Detchant (eds): Skeletal Muscle Pathology. Churchill Livingstone, Edinburgh, 1992, p 576, with permission.)

certain related neuropeptides, are elevated in the cerebrospinal fluid and blood in ALS patients to concentrations that could be neurotoxic.[20–22] The implication is that overexcitation of glutamate-sensitive cells in the nervous system may result in their premature degeneration and death.

No specific treatments are available for ALS. General care revolves around the relief of discomfort and measures designed to minimize the musculoskeletal, integumentary, and systemic effects of immobilization.[25–27] Problems with swallowing, speech, postural control, and respiration are common. Despite the lack of any treatment that alters the progression of the disease, patients benefit from active physical, occupational, and speech therapy. Therapy is directed at preventing contractures, skeletal deformity, and respiratory complications. The benefits derived from exercise in ALS patients are similar to those in healthy individuals. ALS is characterized by reinnervation of muscle. Exercise maximizes the effectiveness of the remaining innervated or reinnervated muscle fibers and prevents disuse atrophy that would otherwise develop in disabled patients prone to inactivity.

Spinal Muscular Atrophies

The term *spinal muscular atrophy* is used to denote a group of inherited disorders characterized by the loss and degeneration of lower motor neurons in both the anterior horns of the spinal cord and the motor nuclei of the brainstem.[4,8–10,28,30] Other components of the nervous system, such as peripheral nerves, upper motor neurons, or sensory tracts, are not directly affected. In view of the presence of prominent bulbar involvement, the term spinal muscular atrophy is something of a misnomer.[4,30] A more accurate descriptor might be bulbospinal muscular atrophy or inherited motor neuropathy. Nevertheless, the term spinal muscular atrophy persists.

The spinal muscular atrophies as a group are not particularly common, and some are very rare. Nonetheless, they are important clinically because among children they represent the most common disorder of lower motor neurons.

The spinal muscular atrophies are a heterogeneous group of disorders, but they all are characterized by muscle weakness and atrophy because of the loss of lower motor neurons (Fig. 16–5).[4,8–10,28–31] The presenting symptoms are related to impaired motor function and range from decreased fetal movements *in utero* and an incapacitated floppy infant to deterioration of athletic ability late in life. These disorders usually present as symmetric proximal weakness, with relative sparing of the muscles that move the eye, the anal sphincter, and the diaphragm. In some less common forms, weakness is predominantly distal, bulbar, or focal. In most cases, with progression of the disease, bulbar involvement becomes more evident. Muscle weakness is usually accompanied by wasting, although this may not be obvious initially. The tendon reflexes are nearly always depressed or absent. Sensory systems and the intellect are not affected. The development of skeletal deformities such as scoliosis, lordosis, pes cavus, and joint contracture is related to the age of onset, with the most marked deformities encountered in severe early childhood disease (Fig. 16–6).[30] The age of onset varies from *in utero* to late in life, with most of these disorders evident in infancy or early childhood. The spinal muscular atrophies are most often inherited as autosomal-recessive traits, but autosomal-dominant and sex-linked recessive forms also occur.

Many different schemes have been proposed and considerable debate continues over how to best organize these disorders (Table 16–1).[4,8–10,28,31] In the absence of knowledge of the fundamental pathogenesis of the spinal muscular atrophies, these schemes are

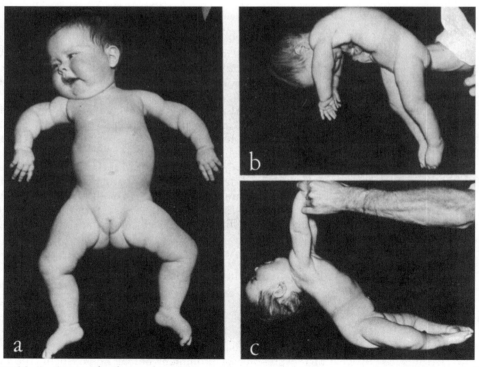

Figure 16–5. *Severe Infantile Spinal Muscular Atrophy.* Six-week-old infant with weakness and hypotonia from birth, showing (A) frog-posture in the supine position, (B) marked flaccid weakness of limbs and trunk in ventral suspension, and (C) head lag in the supine position. Note (A) normal facial expression. (Adapted from Dubowitz, V: Muscle Disorders in Childhood. WB Saunders, London, 1978, p 150, with permission.)

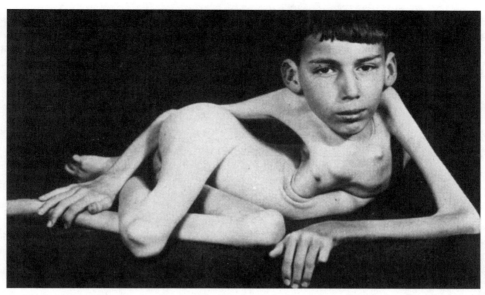

Figure 16–6. *Spinal Muscular Atrophy Patient.* This young patient has marked weakness and atrophy of all muscles except those of the face, and severe scoliosis and lordosis. This individual survived until 8 years of age. (From Dubowitz, V: Muscle Disorders in Childhood. WB Saunders, London, 1978, p 158, with permission.)

essentially descriptive only of the most obvious features of these syndromes, emphasizing primarily the age of onset, the distribution of weakness, and the pattern of inheritance. The boundaries between these individual clinical entities may become obscured by overlap in the infantile, juvenile, and adult ages of onset and, as the disease progresses and weakness becomes more generalized, in the pattern of muscle involvement. Our ability to accurately categorize these disorders will improve as our understanding of their genetic basis advances. These categorizations are important for the accurate prognosis and genetic counseling central to the management of spinal muscular atrophies.

Based on age of onset and rate of progression, essentially three primary clinical variants have been described: (1) acute, infantile spinal muscular atrophy (SMA type I or Werdnig-Hoffman disease), in which onset is noted between birth and 5 months of age and the developmental milestones of rolling, sitting, and walking are never achieved; (2) a more chronic, childhood spinal muscular atrophy (intermediate SMA or SMA type II) with onset at up to 3 years of age and variable impairment of sitting, standing, and walking; and (3) various chronic forms (including SMA type III and Kugelberg-Welander syndrome) in which the age of onset is variable and progression is slower, although motor milestones are delayed and there is difficulty in walking, running, and climbing. SMA type I is rapidly progressive with death occurring within the first 2 years of life, usually from a respiratory complication. In SMA types II and III, most patients survive for at least 10 years after onset, many for much longer.

The pathologic changes observed in spinal muscular atrophies are consistent with the functional deficits observed clinically and **reveal widespread loss of anterior horn cells at all levels of the spinal cord and similar changes in the motor nuclei of the cranial nerves.**[4,8–10,28,31] The lumbar cord is especially severely affected. Although **the histopathologic changes observed in the affected muscles** vary somewhat with the time course and age of onset of the particular form of the disorder, **all are reflective of widespread denervation** (Fig. 16–7).[14,15,33] Large groups of small atrophic muscle fibers are mixed with small numbers of hypertrophied (unaffected) fibers. In more chronic forms of spinal muscular atrophy the reorganization of fiber types that accompanies reinnervation becomes apparent. In SMA type I, in which muscle is affected in the fetal and early neonatal period, evidence of

Table 16–1. *Major Spinal Muscular Atrophies*

Type	Inheritance	Age of Onset	Primary Clinical Features
Proximal			
Acute infantile forms (Werdnig-Hoffmann disease; SMA type I)	Autosomal recessive	In utero to 5 months	Severe generalized muscle weakness and hypotonia; proximal weakness particularly severe; bulbar involvement with progression of disease; external ocular muscles and sphincters spared; tendon reflexes absent; death by 18 months usually due to pulmonary infection
Chronic childhood forms (intermediate form; SMA type II)	Autosomal recessive	3–36 months (most <12 months)	Severe generalized muscle weakness most prominent proximally and in lower limbs; delayed motor milestones; respiratory and bulbar muscles less involved; external ocular muscles and sphincters spared; tendon reflexes depressed or absent; many die in childhood; some survive into adult life, but often with severe disability and skeletal deformity
Juvenile forms (Kugelberg-Welander disease; SMA type III or IV)	Autosomal recessive (also a rare autosomal dominant form)	2–10 years (most <5 years)	Slowly progressive proximal muscle weakness beginning in lower limbs and pelvic girdle extending later to shoulder girdle and upper arms; mild bulbar involvement; external ocular muscles spared; tendon reflexes depressed or absent; variable levels of disability; normal life expectancy
Adult forms (SMA type III or IV)	Various (autosomal recessive; autosomal dominant; x-linked)	15–60 years	Slowly progressive proximal weakness; dominant form more severe with more rapid progression; normal life expectancy
Distal			
Juvenile and adult forms (spinal form of Charcot-Marie disease)	Autosomal recessive and autosomal dominant	2–20 years (juvenile) 20–40 years (adult)	Begins with weakness of distal legs, particularly anterior tibial and peroneal compartments; pes cavus deformity may be prominent early; generally slowly progressive, but tempo varies; tendon reflexes depressed or absent
Other			
Various	Various	Most adult; some in childhood and adolescence (bulbar, scapuloperoneal)	Rare forms of spinal muscular atrophy with various limited presentations, including scapuloperoneal, fascioscapulohumeral, oculopharyngeal, bulbar, and monomelic distributions; slow, relatively benign progression

SMA = spinal muscular atrophies.

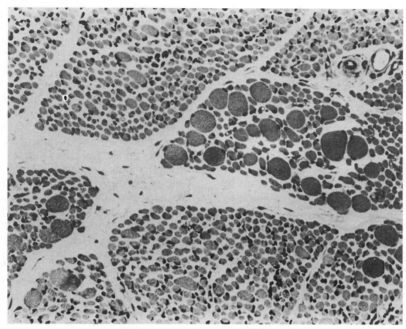

Figure 16–7. *Skeletal Muscle in Werdnig-Hoffmann Disease (SMA Type I).* Large numbers of small muscle fibers are interspersed with a few large fibers occurring either singly or in small groups. The large fibers are innervated or reinnervated, their hypertrophy being a compensatory phenomenon (×210). (From Mastaglia, FL and Walton, Lord of Detchant (eds): Skeletal Muscle Pathology. Churchill Livingstone, Edinburgh, 1992, p 588, with permission.)

retarded muscle maturation (fetal-like muscle fibers) is found, which is not seen in children and adults.

Although considerable progress has been made recently in our understanding of the genetics of spinal muscular disorders, **little is known about the actual genetically determined biochemical or structural defects that cause the neuronal loss characteristic of these diseases.**[32,34]

Treatment of spinal muscular atrophies is symptomatic and supportive.[8–10,29,31] In the severe infantile forms (SMA type I), little specific treatment is possible. In the disorders of later onset and slower progression, treatment is directed toward maintaining joint mobility and preventing contractures, minimizing skeletal deformity, and promoting active exercise to maintain strength in still functioning muscles. In SMA types II and III, prevention of contractures and maintenance of the sitting posture are important goals.[8] These goals are accomplished by regular active exercise, range-of-motion and passive exercise, and the use of splinting, bracing, spinal orthosis, and tendon transfer. Aggressive surgery and bracing are most important in SMA types II and III, in which longer survival or prolonged stabilization may occur. Scoliosis is a common problem, and spinal bracing or fusion may be necessary to prevent respiratory compromise when thoracic scoliotic curvature becomes too great. With immobilization, attention must be directed toward assistance in feeding and prevention of deleterious changes in the respiratory and integumentary systems.

Viral Disorders

The function of the lower motor neuron can be adversely affected by a number of viruses, both as a consequence of selective attack and as one component of more widespread damage to the central nervous system.[4,8,10] The discussion here is about the viral disorders in which the anterior horn cells and the motor nuclei of the brainstem bear the brunt of the viral attack. Three viruses in particular affect lower motor neurons: poliomyelitis, herpes zoster, and rabies.

Poliomyelitis and the Postpolio Syndrome

Although poliomyelitis has almost disappeared in immunized populations, it remains endemic in some underdeveloped regions of the world and is perhaps the most completely studied example of acute anterior horn cell loss in humans. In the United States, in the years immediately preceding the introduction of vaccines, an average of more than 16,000 cases of paralytic poliomyelitis were reported annually. With the widespread application of the polio vaccines, that number fell rapidly to only a few cases per year.[4,8,10,34-36]

Poliomyelitis is an acute disorder caused by any one of three strains of enteroviruses (so named because of their natural habitat within the gastrointestinal tract).[34-36] In most cases, the poliovirus produces only minor nonspecific systemic illness (e.g., headache, malaise, vomiting, diarrhea, sore throat, or fever) or is asymptomatic. **Less than 1% of patients develop paralysis.** Among paralytic patients, the extent of weakness varies markedly from one individual to another. In some patients, only an isolated muscle group in one limb may be involved; in others, all the limbs may be paralyzed.

The poliovirus invades and damages large motor neurons, with a tendency to involve those of the spinal cord more than the brainstem, and a predilection for those of the lumbosacral and cervical regions of the cord.[4,8,10,34-36] The neuronal damage and consequent paralysis are usually asymmetric, more severe proximally than distally, and affect the leg more than the arm. The asymmetry of involvement may be to such a degree that one limb is totally paralyzed, whereas the contralateral limb is spared entirely. In 10% to 15% of those with paralysis, the motor nuclei of the brainstem are affected, causing laryngeal and pharyngeal weakness leading to difficulties in swallowing and speaking. The muscles of the face, tongue, and jaw are less frequently involved, and the extraocular muscles are usually spared. Polio seldom causes permanent paralysis of the bulbar muscles. Whether spinal or bulbar, the affected muscles are flaccid, and the tendon reflexes may be diminished or absent. Muscle atrophy develops rapidly, usually beginning within 1 week of paralysis. The degree of atrophy depends on the number of motor neurons and thus the number of motor units that are affected.

In the areas of the spinal cord or brainstem invaded by the virus, an inflammatory response is evident, with an infiltration of large numbers of leukocytes and other inflammatory cells.[34-36] **The motor cell bodies irreversibly damaged and killed by the virus are ultimately removed by phagocytosis.** With destruction of the cell body, the motor axons undergo wallerian degeneration, whereas **the afflicted muscles undergo rapid denervation atrophy.** Some reinnervation occurs through the sprouting of collateral terminal branches in the preserved motor neurons, forming enlarged motor units. The muscle fibers that are spared undergo compensatory hypertrophy. Certain areas of the brain are also susceptible, including the reticular formation and other nuclei of the medulla, the midbrain, thalamus, hypothalamus, and motor cortex. How the virus gains access to the central nervous system and why certain neurons are more vulnerable than others are not completely understood.

Death in poliomyelitis is usually the result of bulbar involvement and is due to respiratory, cardiac, or autonomic dysfunction. Patients who survive an episode of acute paralysis usually recover considerable muscle function. Recovery of function may begin within 1 to 3 weeks after the peak of paralysis and may continue for several years. Recovery is due to both restoration of function in neurons that are not irreversibly damaged and to reinnervation of denervated muscle fibers by collateral sprouting from surviving axons.

The most important form of treatment for poliomyelitis is prevention. Once the disease is established, only symptomatic and supportive treatment is possible. As with other paralytic disorders, physical and occupational therapy focuses initially on the prevention of contractures, deterioration and deformation of the skeleton, and bed sores, and ultimately on the recovery of function. When there are respiratory and bulbar symptoms, an airway must be maintained, and artificial ventilation and tracheotomy may be required.

The greatest clinical significance of poliomyelitis now resides in the fact that up to two thirds of all persons who have had paralytic polio may experience additional polio-related health problems decades after their initial attack.[4,8,15,37-42] These problems typically arise 30 to 40 years after the original acute attack and constitute a condition called the **postpolio syndrome.** The manifestations of this syndrome include generalized fatigability and lack of endurance (the most common complaint), musculoskeletal pain, slowly progressive muscle weakness, and atrophy (Table 16–2).[37-42] Joint pain is the primary musculoskeletal problem and can occur without any new weakness. This pain reflects joint deterioration, which has been caused by long-term overstress of joints due to chronic muscle weakness and the abnormal movement mechanics accompanying skeletal deformity.[38] Pain may also arise from tendons that have been overstressed because of joint deformities and muscle weakness. These joint problems and the associated muscle weakness frequently lead to loss of mobility and a return to using assistive devices. Difficulty may develop in daily activities such as standing, walking, climbing stairs, and dressing.

The people most likely to develop postpolio problems are those who had the most severe original attack, but (ironically) experienced enough recovery to lead a physically active life.[43] Those who were older at the time of contracting polio are also more vulnerable. The muscles affected are usually at the same segmental level as those affected by the original attack, and may include muscles with long-standing residual atrophy, as well as those that seem fully recovered or even unaffected by the original disease.

Although the cause of postpolio syndrome is not known with certainty, the best explanation is that it reflects a decline in the enlarged motor units that were created by collateral sprouting during the reinnervation period following the original attack (Fig. 16–8). During the decades following their formation, these giant motor units were overworked, placing excessive metabolic demands on the axonal sprouts of the remaining motor neurons, which ultimately caused their premature exhaustion.[37-50] In addition, the original viral attack on the anterior horn cells may have left some motor neurons functional, but with subtle defects making them more vulnerable to later deterioration. **With more than 1.5 million survivors of acute polio remaining in the United States, particularly from the large epidemics of the 1940s and 1950s, the postpolio syndrome represents a significant potential source of motor disability and demand for rehabilitative services.**[37-40]

The general goals of the management of postpolio patients are alleviation of pain, energy conservation, reduction of the mechanical stresses imposed on affected joints and muscles (e.g., through changes in physical activity and the use of assistive devices),

---

Table 16–2. *Principal Clinical Manifestations of Postpolio Syndrome*

- Lack of endurance and excessive fatigue, following even minimal physical activity

- Joint and muscle pain

- Slowly progressive muscle weakness, with or without muscle atrophy and pain; most often in previously affected muscles

- Progressive increase in skeletal deformity, further impeding function

- Progressive respiratory difficulties, particularly in patients with significant residual respiratory impairment

- Progressive weakness in bulbar muscles, especially in larynx and pharynx leading to dysphagia; most often in patients with residual bulbar impairment

- Intolerance to cold, which may exacerbate other symptoms

- Sleep apnea

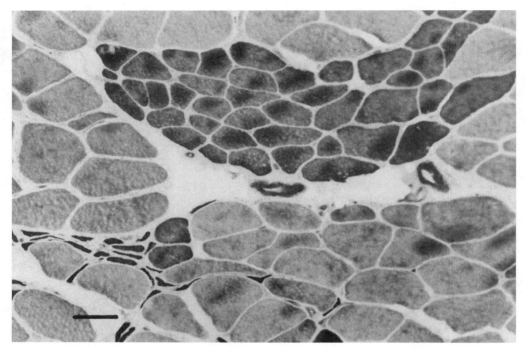

Figure 16–8. *Skeletal Muscle from a Patient with the Postpolio Syndrome.* In this biopsy specimen, fiber type grouping (*Dark Fibers Just Above Center*) confirms prior denervation and reinnervation. There is also a group of angulated, atrophic fibers (*Lower Left*) indicating active denervation. (From Tandan,[9] p 1706, with permission.)

correction of postural and gait deviations, and supportive psychological counseling.[37–40] In the context of maximizing muscle strength and function, considerable controversy exists over the effectiveness and efficacy of exercise in these patients. Although there is general agreement that some kind of formal exercise program benefits almost all postpolio patients by improving muscle strength, endurance, and cardiorespiratory fitness, debate focuses on the form and intensity of this exercise. In particular, the long-term effects of strength training in these patients are unknown, and it is important to determine whether this type of exercise causes further deterioration of already abnormal motor units.

Herpes Zoster

Herpes zoster (shingles) is a common viral infection of the nervous system, which affects primarily the sensory ganglia of the spinal cord or cranial nerves. [44,45] This inflammation may spread to involve contiguous spinal roots and peripheral nerves, as well as the posterior and anterior horns, which **may result in destruction of some anterior horn cells and muscle paralysis.** Lower motor neuron damage may also arise from damage to the anterior root where it joins the dorsal root ganglion.

Herpes zoster is characterized by both skin and, less often, motor involvement.[44,45] Pain or tingling often appears first in the affected dermatome or dermatomes and is usually followed in a few days by a rash, which quickly progresses from redness to vesicular eruptions. Thoracic and cranial dermatomes are most often involved. A motor deficit is reported in about 1% to 2% of patients (Fig. 16–9). The true incidence of motor involvement, however, is probably greater than this, since weakness of a few muscles may easily go unnoticed. The muscles involved are usually those innervated by the same nerve roots that supply the affected dermatomes. For example, cervical herpes zoster may be followed by weakness and wasting of muscles in the hand or arm; thoracic herpes zoster, by

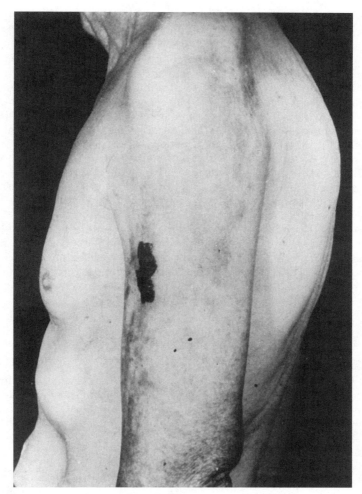

Figure 16–9. *Motor Zoster.* Paralysis of the deltoid muscle occurred after herpes zoster, affecting the C-5 dermatome. Some crusting and staining of the skin are visible at the site of the skin lesions. (From Wood and Anderson,[34] p 605, with permission.)

weakness of intercostal or abdominal muscles. Generally, the prognosis for the motor complications of herpes zoster is good.

The pathogenesis of herpes zoster is not fully understood. It is caused by the same virus that causes chickenpox and may represent spontaneous reactivation of a viral infection that has lain dormant in the dorsal root ganglion neurons since a childhood infection with chickenpox.[44,45] Although herpes zoster can occur at any age, a dramatic increase in incidence occurs after age 50. It is estimated that 50% of those who live to 85 years of age will have at least one attack of shingles.

Rabies

Rabies is a viral infection of the central nervous system transmitted from animals to humans.[46–49] Infection is usually associated with introduction of infected saliva into a victim's subcutaneous or muscle tissue by the bite of a rabid animal. Inoculation may also result from contact of the saliva with abrasions or through the mucous membranes. In rare instances, airborne infection has resulted from exposure in bat-infested caves or from inadvertent exposure to highly contaminated material by laboratory workers. The incubation period of rabies has been reported to vary from as little as 10 days to 1 full year, but most cases are evident within 20 to 90 days following exposure.

After incubating and replicating in the peripheral tissues, the rabies virus travels by axoplasmic transport in peripheral neurons to the central nervous system, first gaining access to the spinal cord and then rapidly spreading throughout the brain.[46–49] Distinct neurologic signs and symptoms are preceded by a 2- to 10-day period of generalized illness (e.g., malaise, headache, and fever) and vague emotional changes (e.g., anxiety or depression). **The more common form of the disease,** *furious rabies,* **is a fulminating, disseminated encephalitis** manifested by fasciculations, agitation, hyperactivity, cerebellar signs, and convulsions, progressing to death in 3 to 5 days. Attacks of furious hyperactivity and apprehension (with hallucinations, muscle spasms, excessive autonomic activity, and occasional seizures), which last a few minutes, alternate with periods of relative stability and mental lucidity. With time, the attacks become more frequent and are increasingly convulsive and asphyxial.

About 20% of patients with rabies have a paralytic form of the disease, termed *dumb rabies,* **which is characterized by lower motor neuron paralysis of a limb or multiple limbs.**[46–49] In these cases, the most striking pathologic findings are seen in the spinal cord, **with degeneration of anterior horn cells** and infiltration by inflammatory cells. Dorsal root ganglia may be similarly affected, as well as the brainstem and cerebrum.

In either type of rabies, death is almost inevitable, resulting from cardiac or respiratory dysfunction.

Injury Due to Physical or Chemical Agents

In the modern world, a variety of physical and chemical agents have the potential for disrupting motor neuron function. Pathologic evidence of **motor neuron destruction and signs and symptoms of motor impairment have been associated with intoxication by various chemical agents, as well as with the physical injury induced by irradiation or electrocution.**[4–6,50–58]

Environmental Contaminants

Among the toxic chemical agents to which we are exposed, the heavy metals and assorted hydrocarbons are of particular concern. Although exposure to **heavy metals,** such as lead, arsenic, manganese, and mercury is not as common as in the past, these elements remain present in the environment and are poisonous when absorbed. **All are toxic to the nervous system, often producing evidence of generalized encephalopathy.**[4–6,57] **In some cases, however, clinical and pathologic observations indicate a more selective involvement of anterior horn cells.** For example, lead poisoning, although typically producing encephalopathy in children, may produce a syndrome in adults involving both upper and lower motor neurons or lower motor neurons alone.[4–6,51] In the latter case, clinical, pathologic, and electrophysiologic evidence suggest that the neuropathy is not a peripheral neuropathy but reflects damage to the central components of the motor neuron. Mercury intoxication may interfere with similar systems. In the case of either lead or mercury intoxication, muscle weakness, wasting, fasciculations, and abnormal deep tendon reflexes may develop. Although the clinical similarities between lead intoxication and ALS were noted by the early 1900s and although heavy metal poisoning may well exacerbate motor neuron disease, it is unlikely that such intoxication accounts for a substantial number of patients with ALS. Other metals such as iron, antimony, barium, bismuth, copper, silver, gold, platinum, and lithium may also produce serious intoxications and resultant evidence of encephalopathy or polyneuropathy.[51]

It is also likely that motor neuron disease can be caused by or at least exacerbated by various industrial hydrocarbons present in the environment.[4] These chemicals include pesticides, herbicides, and various liquid petrochemicals used as solvents, fuels, and lubricants. Both acute and chronic exposure to such agents have been shown to be associated with development of motor neuron disease, in some cases closely resembling ALS.

New types of contaminations will undoubtedly appear in the environment and hence new types of intoxication will continue to occur in the peoples of the industrialized world, some of which will involve primarily motor neuron dysfunction.

Radiation and Electricity

Damage to the motor neuron, both within the anterior horn and within the nerve roots, **may also be induced by various physical agents, such as ionizing radiation and electricity.**[4-6,9,50] Although the adult central nervous system is relatively resistant to the effects of x-radiation, **the anterior horn cells seem especially susceptible to ionizing radiation,** and heavy x-ray exposure may produce irreversible damage to the spinal cord and roots.[9,52-54] This type of exposure is usually coincidental with radiation therapy of intraspinal or paraspinal neoplasms. Irradiation of cervical or thoracic structures (e.g., for carcinoma of mouth, pharynx, esophagus, lung, or paraspinal regions) may lead to delayed spinal cord damage with sensory and motor signs resembling a partial cord transection. On the other hand, excessive irradiation of the lumbar/sacral cord or cauda equina (as in the treatment of lymphoma or metastasized testicular cancer) more often gives rise to evidence of a purely lower motor neuron lesion, with muscle weakness, atrophy, flaccidity, and absent deep tendon reflexes confined to the lower extremities.[4] Evidence is found of specific damage to anterior horn cells or possibly the anterior roots.[4,53] Regardless of the site, these postirradiation syndromes demonstrate neuronal damage, degeneration, and infarction, the extent of which is dose-dependent.

Damage to the nervous system may also occur when an individual is struck by lightning or otherwise electrocuted.[55-58] Cerebral damage is frequently the most obvious result, but damage to the spinal cord is not uncommon. This is particularly so when electricity is conducted along the entire length of the body. Although immediate paralysis, sensory loss, and bladder dysfunction may result, **some patients may develop months later a syndrome of lower motor neuron paralysis due to degeneration of anterior horn cells in the area of the electrical injury.**[55-58] This delayed onset myelopathy may be analogous to that created by irradiation.

Conditions Characterized by Motor Neuron and Muscle Hyperactivity

Although most diseases of the motor neuron are associated with muscle hypoactivity, **some conditions cause hyperactivity of motor neurons and hence excessive muscle activity,** manifested by fasciculations, myokymia, cramps, or even powerful spasms and convulsions. In tetanus or strychnine poisoning, for example, muscle spasms may be violent enough to fracture large bones and to cause asphyxia.

Tetanus

Tetanus is a disease of the nervous system caused by the neurotoxin of an anaerobic bacterium, *Clostridium tetani,* which contaminates soil worldwide.[45,59-62] Human infection occurs as the result of wound infection. *Tetanospasmin,* **the toxin produced by this bacterium,** is carried by retrograde axonal transport in motor axons to the anterior horn cells of the spinal cord. Here the toxin crosses the synaptic cleft to accumulate in the terminals of spinal inhibitory neurons (e.g., Renshaw cells) where it **prevents the release of**

inhibitory transmitters, such as glycine or γ-aminobutyric acid. This results in uncontrolled activation of both alpha and gamma motor neurons, causing muscle rigidity and spasm.[45,59-62] Tetanospasmin may also produce an analogous disinhibition of sympathetic autonomic pathways creating autonomic hyperactivity. Autonomic hyperactivity includes labile hypertension, tachycardia, peripheral vasoconstriction, and sweating. The onset of symptoms from the time of injury is variable, but is usually between 5 and 10 days. Muscle spasms are usually widespread and severe and may involve limb, trunk, and bulbar muscles in various combinations.[45] The most common, and most often the initial presentation, is lockjaw, explaining why tetanus is often diagnosed first by dentists. After the acute spasmodic phase, muscle rigidity may persist for weeks and then gradually subside.

Tetanus requires intensive medical care directed at controlling spasms and maintaining ventilation. The complications of tetanus are those of respiratory and cardiovascular impairment and orthopedic problems from broken bones. Although the course of recovery is variable, intensive care may be necessary for several weeks. With adequate treatment, recovery is usually complete with no residual neurologic deficits.

Because it can be readily prevented by immunization, tetanus has become a rare disease in developed countries. However, as the population of immunocompromised hosts (e.g., HIV-infected) grows, an increasing percentage of patients may not respond to standard immunizations, and a substantial increase in the incidence of this disorder may occur.[60] Tetanus is also of current interest as a model of disordered motor control, which may provide information of value in the treatment of more common causes of neurogenic muscle rigidity.[60]

Strychnine Poisoning

Strychnine poisoning produces a condition similar to that of tetanus with extreme neuronal and skeletal muscle hyperactivity, which may also be lethal unless aggressively treated.[63] Strychnine is a substance that is used as a poison for animal pests such as rats, and although it has no proven therapeutic value, it is widely used in home remedies as a cathartic or tonic and as an adulterant of illicit drugs. **Like tetanospasmin, strychnine produces neuronal hyperexcitability by blocking neuronal inhibition, rather than by direct neuronal stimulation.**[63] Strychnine acts as a selective, competitive antagonist of the inhibitory effects exerted by glycine at glycine receptors wherever they exist in the central nervous system. These receptors are particularly numerous in the gray matter of the spinal cord and brainstem. Strychnine is thus a powerful convulsant. Since strychnine reduces inhibition, including the inhibitory influences existing between the motor neurons of antagonistic muscle groups, the pattern of convulsion is determined by the most powerful muscles acting at a given joint.[63] The treatment for strychnine poisoning is similar to that for tetanus.

RECOMMENDED READINGS

Banker, BQ: The Pathology of the Motor Neuron Disorders. Chapter 71. In Engel, AG and Banker, BQ (eds): Myology: Basic and Clinical. McGraw-Hill, New York, 1986.

Brooks, BR (ed): Amytrophic Lateral Sclerosis. Neurol Clin 5(1):1, 1987.

Dubowitz, V: Muscle Disorders in Childhood. WB Saunders, London, 1978.

Gomez, MR: Motor Neuron Diseases in Children. Chapter 70. In Engel, AG and Franzini-Armstrong, C (eds): Myology: Basic and Clinical, ed 2. McGraw-Hill, New York, 1994.

Harding, AE: Inherited Neuronal Atrophy and Degeneration Predominantly of Lower Motor Neurons. Chapter

55. In Dyck, PJ and Thomas, PK (eds): Peripheral Neuropathy, ed 3. WB Saunders, Philadelphia, 1993.

Hudson, AJ (ed): Amyotrophic Lateral Sclerosis: Concepts in Etiology and Pathogenesis. University of Toronto Press, Toronto, 1990.

Hudson, AJ: The Motor Neuron Diseases and Related Disorders. Chapter 53A. In Joynt, RJ (ed): Clinical Neurology, vol 4. JB Lippincott, Philadelphia, 1991.

Jennekens, FGI: Neurogenic Disorders of Muscle. Chapter 16. In Mastaglia, FL and Detchant, Lord Walton (eds): Skeletal Muscle Pathology, ed 2. Churchill Livingstone, Edinburgh, 1992.

Jubelt, B and Drucker, J: Post-polio Syndrome: An Update. Semin Neurol 13(3):283, 1993.

Kuncl, RW, et al: Motor Neuron Diseases. Chapter 89. In Asbury, AK, McKhann, GM, and McDonald, WI (eds): Diseases of the Nervous System: Clinical Neurobiology, vol 1, ed 2. WB Saunders, Philadelphia, 1992.

Menkes, JH: Textbook of Child Neurology, ed 4. Chapter 13. Diseases of the Motor Unit. Lea & Febiger, Philadelphia, 1990.

Parry, GJ: Myelopathies Affecting Anterior Horn Cells. Chapter 46. In Dyck, PJ and Thomas, PK (eds): Peripheral Neuropathy, ed 3. WB Saunders, Philadelphia, 1993.

Rowland, LP (ed): Amyotrophic Lateral Sclerosis and Other Motor Neuron Diseases. Adv Neurol 56:1, 1991.

Swash, M and Schwartz, MS: Neuromuscular Diseases, ed 2. Chapter 6. Diseases of Anterior Horn Cells. Springer-Verlag, London, 1988.

Tandan, R: Disorders of the Upper and Lower Motor Neurons. Chapter 80. In Bradley, WG, et al (eds): Neurology in Clinical Practice, vol II. Butterworth-Heinemann, Boston, 1990.

Williams, DB and Windebank, AJ: Motor Neuron Disease (Amyotrophic Lateral Sclerosis). Mayo Clin Proc 66:54, 1991.

Williams, DB and Windebank, AJ: Motor Neuron Disease. Chapter 54. In Dyck, PJ and Thomas, PK (eds): Peripheral Neuropathy, ed 3. WB Saunders, Philadelphia, 1993.

Windebank, AJ and Mulder, DW: Motor Neuron Disease in Adults. Chapter 71. In Engel, AG and Franzini-Armstrong, C (eds): Myology: Basic and Clinical, ed 2. McGraw-Hill, New York, 1994.

Wood, M, and Anderson, M: Neurological Infections. WB Saunders, London, 1988.

REFERENCES

1. Hays, AP: Separation of Motor Neuron Diseases from Pure Motor Neuropathies: Pathology. Adv Neurol 56:385, 1991.
2. Thomas, PK: Separating Motor Neuron Diseases from Pure Motor Neuropathies: Clinical Clues and Definitions. Adv Neurol 56:381, 1991.
3. Rowland, LP: Ten Central Themes in a Decade of ALS Research. Adv Neurol 56:3, 1991.
4. Hudson, AJ: The Motor Neuron Diseases and Related Disorders. Chapter 53A. In Joynt, RJ (ed): Clinical Neurology, vol 4. JB Lippincott, Philadelphia, 1991.
5. Williams, DB and Windebank, AJ: Motor Neuron Disease (Amyotrophic Lateral Sclerosis). Mayo Clin Proc 66:54, 1991.
6. Williams, DB and Windebank, AJ: Motor Neuron Disease. Chapter 54. In Dyck, PJ and Thomas, PK (eds): Peripheral Neuropathy, ed 3. WB Saunders, Philadelphia, 1993.
7. Windebank, AJ and Mulder, DW: Motor Neuron Disease in Adults. Chapter 71. In Engel, AG and Franzini-Armstrong, C (eds): Myology: Basic and Clinical, ed 2. McGraw-Hill, New York, 1994.
8. Kuncl, RW, et al: Motor Neuron Diseases. Chapter 89. In Asbury, AK, McKhann, GM, and McDonald, WI (eds): Diseases of the Nervous System: Clinical Neurobiology, vol 1, ed 2. WB Saunders, Philadelphia, 1992.
9. Tandan, R: Disorders of the Upper and Lower Motor Neurons. Chapter 80. In Bradley, WG, et al (eds): Neurology in Clinical Practice, vol II. Butterworth-Heinemann, Boston, 1990.
10. Swash, M and Schwartz, MS: Neuromuscular Diseases, ed 2. Chapter 6. Diseases of Anterior Horn Cells. Springer-Verlag, London, 1988.
11. Swash, M and Schwartz, MS: What Do We Really Know About Amyotrophic Lateral Sclerosis? J Neurol Sci 113:4, 1992.
12. Oppenheimer, DR and Esiri, MM: Diseases of the Basal Ganglia, Cerebellum, and Motor Neurons. Chapter 15. In Adams, JH and Duchen, LW (eds): Greenfield's Neuropathology ed 5. Oxford University Press, New York, 1992.
13. Hirano, A: Cytopathology of Amytrophic Lateral Sclerosis. Adv Neurol 56:91, 1991.
14. Banker, BQ: The Pathology of the Motor Neuron Disorders. Chapter 71. In Engel, AG and Banker, BQ (eds): Myology: Basic and Clinical. McGraw-Hill, New York, 1986.
15. Jennekens, FGI: Neurogenic Disorders of Muscle. Chapter 16. In Mastaglia, FL and Detchant, Lord Walton (eds): Skeletal Muscle Pathology, ed 2. Churchill Livingstone, Edinburgh, 1992.
16. Eisen, AA and Calne, DB: Latent Neuro-Abiotrophies: A Clue to Amyotrophic Lateral Sclerosis: Concepts in Pathogenesis and Etiology. University of Toronto Press, Toronto, 1990, pp. 296–316.
17. Brooks, BR (ed): Amyotrophy Lateral Sclerosis. Neurol Clin 5:1, 1987.
18. Drachman, DB and Kuncl, RW: ALS: An Unconventional Autoimmune Disease? Ann Neurol 26:269, 1989.
19. Engelhardt, JI and Appel, SH: IgG Reactivity in the Spinal Cord and Motor Cortex in Amyotrophic Lateral Sclerosis. Arch Neurol 47:1210, 1990.
20. Plaitakis, A: Altered Glutamatergic Mechanisms and Selective Motor Neuron Degeneration in Amyotrophic Lateral Sclerosis: Possible Role of Glycine. Adv Neurol 56:319, 1991.
21. Rothstein, JD, et al: Excitatory Amino Acids in Amyotrophic Lateral Sclerosis: An Update. Ann Neurol 30:224, 1991.
22. Perry, TL, et al: ALS: Amino Acid Levels in Plasma and Cerebrospinal Fluid. Ann Neurol 28:12, 1990.
23. Strong, MJ, Hudson, AJ, and Alvord, WG: Familial Amyotrophic Lateral Sclerosis, 1850–1989. A Statistical Analysis of the World Literature. Can J Neurol Sci 18:45, 1991.
24. Hirano, A, Hirano, M, and Dembitzer, HM: Pathological Variations and the Extent of the Disease Process in Amyotrophic Lateral Sclerosis. In Hudson, AJ (ed): Amytrophic Lateral Sclerosis: Concepts in Etiology and Pathogenesis. University of Toronto, Toronto, 1990, pp. 166–192.
25. Kuncl, RW and Clawson, LL: Amyotrophic Lateral Sclerosis. In Johnson, RT (ed): Current Therapy in Neurological Diseases, ed 3. BC Decker, Philadelphia, 1990.

26. Sanjak, M, Reddan, W, and Brooks, BR: Role of Muscular Exercise in Amyotrophic Lateral Sclerosis. Neurol Clin 5:251, 1987.

27. Hudson, AJ, Jr: Outpatient Management of Amyotrophic Lateral Sclerosis. Semin Neurol 7:344, 1987.

28. Hausmanowa-Petrusewicz, I: Spinal Muscular Atrophies: How Many Types. Adv Neurol 56:157, 1991.

29. Menkes, JH: Textbook of Child Neurology, ed 4. Chapter 13. Diseases of the Motor Unit. Lea & Febiger, Philadelphia, 1990.

30. Harding, AE: Inherited Neuronal Atrophy and Degeneration Predominantly of Lower Motor Neurons. Chapter 55. In Dyck, PJ and Thomas, PK (eds): Peripheral Neuropathy, ed 3. WB Saunders, Philadelphia, 1993.

31. Gomez, MR: Motor Neuron Diseases in Children. Chapter 70. In Engel, AG and Franzini-Armstrong, C (eds): Myology: Basic and Clinical, ed 2. McGraw-Hill, New York, 1994.

32. Gilliam, TC and Brzustowicz, LM: The Molecular and Genetic Basis of the Spinal Muscular Atrophies. Chapter 59. In Rosenberg, RN, et al (eds): The Molecular and Genetic Basis of Neurological Disease. Butterworth-Heinemann, Boston, 1993.

33. Harriman, DGF: Diseases of Muscle. Chapter 21. In Adams, JH and Duchen, LW (eds): Greenfield's Neuropathology, ed 5. Oxford University Press, New York, 1992.

34. Wood, M, and Anderson, M: Neurological Infections. Chapter 7. Poliomyelitis and Allied Infections. WB Saunders, London, 1988.

35. Krugman, S, et al: Infectious Diseases in Children, ed 9. Chapter 5. Enteroviral Infections. Mosby-Year Book, St. Louis, 1992.

36. Cherry, JD: Enteroviruses: Polioviruses (Poliomyelitis), Coxsackieviruses, Echoviruses, and Enteroviruses. Chapter 157. In Feigin, RD and Cherry, JD (eds): Textbook of Pediatric Infectious Diseases, ed 3. WB Saunders, Philadelphia, 1992.

37. Halstead, LS: Late Complications of Poliomyelitis. Chapter 24. In Goodgold, J (ed): Rehabilitation Medicine. CV Mosby, St. Louis, 1988.

38. Jubelt, B and Drucker, J: Post-polio Syndrome: An Update. Semin Neurol 13(3):283, 1993.

39. Bruno, RL: Post-polio Sequelae: Research and Treatment in the Second Decade. Orthopedics 14:1169, 1991.

40. Agre, JC, Rodriquez, AA, and Tafel, JA: Late Effects of Polio: Critical Review of Literature on Neuromuscular Function. Arch Phys Med Rehabil 72:929, 1991.

41. Agre, JC, And Rodriquez, AA: Intermittent Isometric Activity: Its Effects on Muscle Fatigue in Postpolio Subjects, Arch Phys Med Rehabil 72:971, 1991.

42. Dalakas, M and Illa, I: Post-Polio Syndrome: Concepts in Clinical Diagnosis, Pathogenesis, and Etiology. Adv Neurol 56:495, 1991.

43. Klingman, J, et al: Functional Recovery: A Major Risk Factor for the Development of Postpoliomyelitis Muscular Atrophy. Arch Neurol 45:645, 1988.

44. Hope-Simpson, RE: The Nature of Herpes Zoster: A Long-Term Study and New Hypothesis. Proc R Soc Med 58:9, 1965.

45. Wood, M and Anderson, M: Neurological Infections. Chapter 12. Infections Affecting Peripheral Nerves and the Motor End-Plate. WB Saunders, London, 1988.

46. Plotkin, SA and Clark, HF: Rabies. Chapter 153. In Feigin, RD and Cherry, JD (eds): Textbook of Pediatric Infectious Diseases, ed 3. WB Saunders, Philadelphia, 1992.

47. Esiri, MM and Kennedy, PGE: Virus Diseases. Chapter 7. In Adams, JH and Duchen, LW (eds): Greenfield's Neuropathology, ed 5. Oxford University Press, New York, 1992.

48. Bharucha, NE, Bhabha, SK, and Bharaucha, EP: Viral Infections. Chapter 60B. In Bradley, WG, et al (eds): Neurology in Clinical Practice: The Neurological Disorders. Butterworth-Heinemann, Boston, 1990.

49. Wood, M and Anderson, M: Rabies. Chapter 8. Infections Affecting Peripheral Nerves and the Motor End-Plate. WB Saunders, London, 1988.

50. Parry, GJ: Myelopathies Affecting Anterior Horn Cells. Chapter 46. In Dyck, PJ and Thomas, PK (eds): Peripheral Neuropathy, ed 3. WB Saunders, Philadelphia, 1993.

51. Windebank, AJ: Metal Neuropathy. Chapter 85. In Dyck, PJ and Thomas, PK (eds): Peripheral Neuropathy, ed 3. WB Saunders, Philadelphia, 1993.

52. Goldwein, JW: Radiation Myelopathy. Med Pediatr Oncol 15:89, 1987.

53. Bradley, WG, et al: Post-Radiation Motor Neuron Syndromes. Adv Neurol 56:341, 1991.

54. deCarolis, P, et al: Isolated Lower Motor Neuron Involvement Following Radiotherapy. J Neurol Neurosurg Psychiatry 49:718, 1986.

55. Panse, F: Electrical Lesions of the Nervous System. Chapter 13. In Vinken, PJ and Bruyn, GW (eds): Handbook of Clinical Neurology, vol 7. North-Holland Publishing Company, Amsterdam, 1979.

56. Sirdofsky, MD, Hawley, RJ, and Manz, H: Progressive Motor Neuron Disease Associated with Electrical Injury. Nerve Muscle 14:977, 1991.

57. Farrell, DF and Starr, A: Delayed Neurological Sequelae of Electrical Injuries. Neurology 18:601, 1968.

58. Holbrook, LA, Beach, FXM, and Silver, JR: Delayed Myelopathy: A Rare Complication of Severe Electrical Burns. Br Med J 4:659, 1970.

59. Bharucha, NE, Bhabha, SK, and Bharucha, EP: Bacterial Infections. Chapter 60A. In Bradley, WG, et al (eds): Neurology in Clinical Practice, vol II. Butterworth-Heinemann, Boston, 1990.

60. Bleck, TP: Tetanus: Pathophysiology, Management, and Prophylaxis. Dis Mon 37:545, 1991.

61. Facchiano, F, et al: The Transglutaminase Hypothesis for the Action of Tetanus Toxin. Trends Biochem Sci 18:327, 1993.

62. Roos, KL: Tetanus. Semin Neurol 11:206, 1991.

63. Franz, DN: Central Nervous System Stimulants. Chapter 24. In Gilman, AG, et al (eds): Goodman and Gilman's: The Pharmacological Basis of Therapeutics, ed 7. Macmillan, New York, 1985.

SECTION

DISORDERS OF CENTRAL MOTOR CONTROL

Overview

Ultimately, all motor commands exert an effect through activation of the motor unit. This is true of the simplest reflex motor responses, as well as the most complex motor behaviors of volition. Accordingly, all normal motor activity requires the functional integrity of both the central motor control systems that give rise to these commands, as well as the peripheral motor unit through which these commands are expressed. In Section IV, various pathologic conditions were discussed in which the motor unit itself was dysfunctional. These "neuromuscular diseases" are manifested by a characteristic array of signs and symptoms that reflect the inability of motor units to respond to the motor commands impinging on them. Some form of depressed motor activity, such as muscle weakness, fatigability, hypotonia, or hyporeflexia, is most common. In central motor disorders, on the other hand, the motor effector unit is usually intact, whereas control of this unit is impaired. In these disorders, the loss or distortion of motor directives sent to the motor unit may result in a wide variety of functional deficits and clinical findings. These presentations include various forms and combinations of unrestrained (e.g., spasticity, rigidity, hyperreflexia, or involuntary movements), depressed (e.g., paresis, paralysis, or hypokinesia), or disordered (e.g., ataxia or unusual activation patterns) motor activity. The purpose of this section is to discuss the fundamental pathophysiologic and clinical features of the central motor disorders.

The conditions described in Chapters 17, 18, and 19 involve damage that is largely limited to one specific functional component of central motor control (e.g., spinal cord, basal ganglia, or cerebellum). Accordingly, the clinical presentations characteristic of these disorders are relatively limited and predictable, reflecting the particular contribution that the involved system makes to motor control. In Chapters 20, 21, and 22, conditions are discussed in which more generalized damage to the central nervous system is usually involved (e.g., traumatic brain injury, stroke, or multiple sclerosis). These disorders may disrupt the integrity of many regions involved in motor function and their interconnections. Because so many different patterns of involvement and levels of severity are possible, the clinical presentations of these disorders are extremely varied and may be catastrophic.

CHAPTER 17

■

Disorders of the Spinal Cord

Christopher M. Fredericks, PhD

- ■ *Review of the Overall Organization of the Spinal Cord*
- ■ *The Somatotopy of the Spinal Cord*
- ■ *Functional Deficits Caused by Spinal Cord Lesions: General Principles*
- ■ *Signs and Symptoms Caused by Spinal Cord Lesions*
- ■ *Classification of Spinal Cord Lesions*
- ■ *Etiology of Spinal Cord Lesions*

*T*he integrity of the spinal cord is necessary for much of our normal motor and sensory function. Unfortunately, a variety of pathologic conditions can adversely affect both the structure and function of the spinal cord. These conditions range from slowly evolving chronic disorders to acute insults wrought by physical trauma or vascular accident. Such pathologies may be focal or diffuse, may involve primarily the spinal cord or the vertebral column, and may reflect many disparate etiologies. The functional impairments caused by these pathologies may be severe, resulting in permanent disability and a lifelong need for care.

The purpose of this chapter is to discuss the principal pathologic conditions that affect the spinal cord. Several important disorders that extensively involve the spinal cord are also discussed in a slightly different context in other chapters. These are disorders of the anterior horn cell, such as amyotrophic lateral sclerosis and spinal muscular atrophy (see Chapter 16), and demyelinating disorders, such as multiple sclerosis (see Chapter 22).

The spinal cord is a complex neural structure composed of many different types of long ascending and descending fibers, as well as many interneurons and other short interconnecting fibers. The pathways of the spinal cord are arranged in a consistent pattern at each spinal level. A familiarity with the anatomic and functional organization of the cord provides a basis for understanding the functional deficits that arise from injury or disease of this structure. Accordingly, the first two sections of this chapter are devoted to a review of the structure of the spinal cord. The remainder of the chapter considers various spinal cord pathologies and the functional deficits that they produce.

394

Review of the Overall Organization
of the Spinal Cord

As described in Chapter 5, the spinal cord is composed of an outer layer of white matter and an inner core of gray matter (Fig. 17–1).[1–3] The white matter is divided into three longitudinally aligned funiculi (columns), each containing ascending and descending fibers. These fibers are generally organized into bundles. Fiber bundles that follow essentially the same course and have similar terminations are known as **fasciculi** or **tracts**. Although the location of various spinal cord tracts has been approximated from clinical and pathologic studies in humans and through experimental studies in animals, the precise position of some tracts remains unknown. There may also be considerable overlap between tracts and variations among individuals.

Descending tracts are found primarily in the lateral and anterior funiculi. Ascending tracts are found in all funiculi. Most descending fibers convey motor control signals to the motor neurons and interneurons of the spinal cord, whereas ascending fibers are either first-order or second-order sensory fibers conveying somatosensory information to integrative structures in the brain. In general, the longest tracts are found in the periphery of the white matter, whereas shorter tracts are found nearer the gray matter. Propriospinal fibers are largely confined to a thin shell surrounding the gray matter, called the **propriospinal tract** or **fasciculus proprius**.

The gray matter is composed of the complex, compact spinal circuitry responsible for the integration of motor and sensory information and the programming of certain motor behaviors (see Chapter 5). The most abundant cell within the gray matter is the interneuron, which seldom sends branches over more than several segments and seldom reaches supraspinal structures.

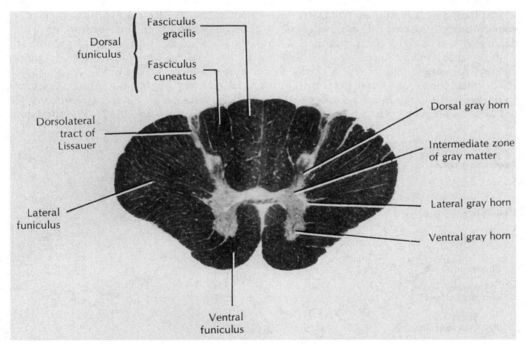

Figure 17–1. Transverse section of the spinal cord (T-2 segment). (From Barr and Kiernan,[3] p 71, with permission.)

Descending Spinal Tracts[1-5]

The descending spinal tracts provide a mechanism by which higher centers can directly regulate somatic motor activity, exert important influences on reflex pathways and afferent inputs to the spinal cord, and control certain visceral activities (Fig. 17–2).

The longest and most clinically significant of the descending spinal tracts are the corticospinal or the so-called *pyramidal* **tracts. All the fibers of these tracts arise in the cerebral cortex** (see Chapter 7). On leaving the cortex, the corticospinal tract fibers descend through a small compact region of the posterior limb of the internal capsule, pass through the medullary pyramids (hence the name), and descend into the spinal cord. At the junction of the medulla and spinal cord, most of the corticospinal tract fibers decussate to descend in the posterior portion of the lateral funiculus of the opposite side of the spinal cord. This large *lateral* **corticospinal tract** gives off branches to the spinal gray matter as it travels down the cord. Most of these branches enter the intermediate gray matter. About 15% of the fibers in each pyramid do not cross but continue into the ipsilateral cord as the *anterior* **(ventral) corticospinal tract.** This tract occupies a small oval area of the anterior funiculus adjacent to the anterior median fissure. These fibers terminate in the anterior horn or intermediate gray matter, mainly in cervical and thoracic segments. Finally, a few uncrossed fibers descend as a small tract in a portion of the lateral funiculus more ventral than that occupied by the lateral corticospinal tract.

As the corticospinal fibers travel down the cord, they give off many collateral branches to different spinal segments. These branches terminate on alpha and gamma motorneurons, as well as on spinal interneurons, such as Ia interneurons and Renshaw cells.[1,2,4] Throughout most of their course, the corticospinal fibers are thought to maintain a somatotopic organization, with fibers to the leg found lateral to those of the arm and trunk. This arrangement is maintained in their terminations on specific neurons of the spinal gray matter.

Three distinct descending spinal cord tracts arise from the midbrain: the rubrospinal, tectospinal, and interstitiospinal tracts (see Chapter 6).[2,4,5] **The rubrospinal tract arises somatotopically from the red nucleus,** crosses completely in the ventral segmental decussation, and descends to the spinal cord. This tract travels in the cord ventral and slightly lateral to the lateral corticospinal tract in the lateral funiculus. The red nucleus receives important input from both the motor cortex and cerebellum. The corticorubral-rubrospinal connections constitute a nonpyramidal pathway linking the motor cortex and spinal cord. Although opinions differ regarding the importance of this tract in humans, the red nucleus seems to play a role in the control of muscle tone, particularly in contralateral

Descending Tracts

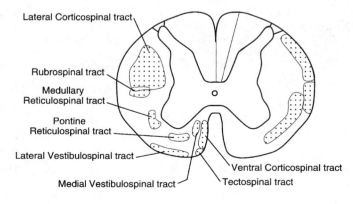

Figure 17–2. Schematic diagram of the location of the principal descending (motor) tracts of the human spinal cord.

flexor muscle groups. The rubrospinal tract may also be clinically important because it may subserve some residual motor function after damage to the lateral corticospinal tract.

The tectospinal tract originates primarily from cells of the deeper layers of the superior colliculus, crosses in the dorsal tegmental decussation, and descends to the spinal cord. This tract travels in the medial part of the anterior funiculus near the anterior median fissure and descends only as far as the cervical segments. Most fibers terminate in high cervical segments. Although little is known of the function of the tectospinal tract in humans, it is believed to participate in the control of neck, shoulder, and upper trunk muscles and may take part in head and neck orienting reactions to visual and possibly auditory stimuli.[4]

The interstitiospinal tract is a small uncrossed tract that arises from the interstitial nucleus of Cajal and descends in the medial portion of the anterior funiculus. This tract is well defined only in cervical segments, although some fibers descend all the way to the sacral cord. The tract's fibers terminate in areas overlapping termination of vestibulospinal fibers.

Four distinct tracts descend from the pons and medulla: the vestibulospinal and the pontine and medullary reticulospinal tracts (see Chapter 6).[1,2,4,5] The vestibular nuclei form a complex extending into both the pons and medulla. **A large lateral vestibulospinal pathway arises somatotopically from cells of the lateral vestibular nucleus** and descends the length of the ipsilateral cord in the anterior funiculus. A few fibers from the medial vestibular nucleus form a small separate medial vestibulospinal tract, descending only to cervical segments. The lateral vestibulospinal tract is thought to exert an excitatory influence on extensor motor neurons and an inhibitory influence on flexor motor neurons at many levels of the spinal cord. The medial vestibulospinal tract, with its limited distribution, may influence neck and upper back muscles and play a role in controlling head position. **The** *pontine* **reticulospinal tract arises in cells of the pontine reticular formation** to descend uncrossed in the medial part of the anterior funiculus. These fibers traverse the entire length of the cord. **The** *medullary* **reticulospinal spinal tract arises in cells of the medullary reticular formation** and projects bilaterally (crossed and uncrossed) to the anterior part of the lateral funiculi. The reticular formation has many inputs, among them many direct projections from the cerebral cortex. As with the red nucleus, these corticoreticular-reticulospinal connections constitute a nonpyramidal pathway linking the cortex and the spinal cord. The reticulospinal tracts exert both facilatory and inhibitory influences on voluntary movements, reflex activities, and muscle tone.

Ascending Spinal Tracts[1-4,7,8]

Motor control is dependent on a continual flow of sensory information to supraspinal centers (see Chapter 4). The ascending tracts of the spinal cord provide most of this input, transmitting sensory information to the cerebellum and to the thalamus, from which it is distributed to the cerebral cortex (Fig. 17–3). Although both the cerebral cortex and the cerebellum contribute to the control of motor function, it is only the information that reaches the cerebral cortex that is consciously perceived.

Two major tracts of great clinical significance carry sensory information to the thalamus: the dorsal (posterior) column–medial lemniscal pathway and the anterolateral (spinothalamic) pathway (see Chapter 4).[1-4,7,8,11] The dorsal columns are made up primarily of large myelinated dorsal root fibers carrying impulses from a variety of mechanoreceptors. Most of these first-order neurons ascend immediately on entering the spinal cord and terminate without crossing the spinal midline in ipsilateral dorsal column nuclei in the medulla (see Fig. 4–9). Here, they terminate on second-order neurons that cross over the neural axis and form a compact bundle called the **medial lemniscus.** The medial lemniscus ascends through the contralateral half of the brainstem and ultimately terminates in the thalamus. From there, third-order fibers project to the cerebral cortex. The manner in which the dorsal root fibers enter the dorsal column as it ascends through the spinal cord creates a distinct somatotopic arrangement.[1,2,7] Specifically, new fibers entering

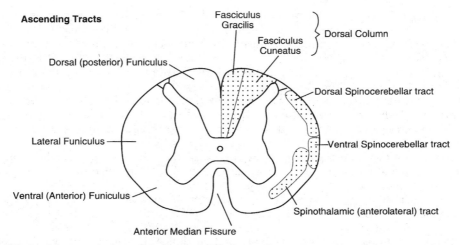

Ascending Tracts

Figure 17-3. Schematic diagram of the location of the principal ascending (sensory) tracts of the human spinal cord.

the dorsal column occupy the most lateral position, displacing medially those already present (Fig. 17–4). The result is a laminar arrangement in which layers of fibers from the most caudal levels (the leg) are most medial, whereas fibers from more rostral levels (neck and back of the head) are most lateral. This basic arrangement is maintained in the medullary nuclei, medial lemniscus, and thalamus and in the final cortical projections. **The dorsal columns convey information related to touch (including the vibratory sense), pressure, and joint position and movement,** much of which reaches conscious perception. This tract also contains group Ib afferents from Golgi tendon organs. These afferents contribute to our kinesthetic or proprioceptive sense, but it is a matter of debate as to how much of this information reaches conscious awareness. In addition to first-order afferent fibers, the dorsal column contains many axons of second-order neurons, propriospinal neurons, and descending branches from afferent fibers and descending fibers arising from

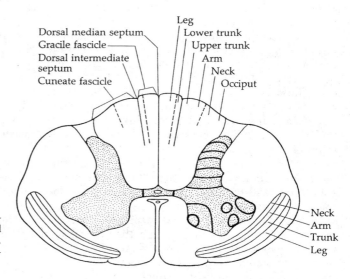

Figure 17-4. The somatotopic organization of the dorsal columns and anterolateral (spinothalamic) tracts. (From Martin,[7] p 116, with permission.)

the medullary dorsal column nuclei.[2,4] Lesions of the dorsal columns characteristically impair tactile and kinesthetic sense. However, since input from touch and pressure receptors also reaches the cortex by other routes, damage to the dorsal columns causes impairment but not abolition of tactile sensibility.[1]

Primary thermoreceptive and nociceptive fibers, as well as some collateral branches from first-order touch and pressure afferent fibers, instead of ascending within the dorsal column upon entry into the cord, synapse within the dorsal horn on second-order neurons. These second-order fibers then project across the spinal cord midline to form the ascending spinothalamic tract. This tract occupies most of the anterior half of the lateral funiculus. The spinothalamic tract ascends through the medulla and pons in a more dorsal position than the medial lemniscus and terminates on third-order neurons in the thalamus. Like the dorsal column, the spinothalamic tract is somatotopically arranged (see Fig. 17–4).[2–4,7] In this case, fibers with the more caudal origins (sacral and lumbar) occupy the more lateral positions, whereas the most rostral (thoracic and cervical) are most medially situated. The spinothalamic somatotopy is not as precise as that of the dorsal columns. **The spinothalamic tracts have been traditionally divided into lateral and anterior spinothalamic tracts, the former subserving pain and temperature sensation and the latter some aspects of tactile sensation.** It has been argued that since all these fibers are extensively intermingled in the spinal cord, it may be more appropriate to refer to the whole complex as a single spinothalamic tract.[1] **A commonly used alternate term for this group of tracts is the *anterolateral pathway*.** Although the spinothalamic tract represents an alternate route by which some tactile information reaches the cerebral cortex, it is most important clinically as the primary pathway for pain and temperature sensation. In addition to light touch, pain, and temperature, several other types of sensation are also subserved by the spinothalamic tracts. These include itch, pressure sensations from the bladder and bowel, and sexual sensations.[1] However, with the exception of itch, this sensory information is carried bilaterally, so that unilateral damage causes little impairment.

Considerable sensory information is conveyed through the spinal cord to the cerebellum, where it is used in the coordination of movement (see Chapter 8). Somatosensory fibers synapse on neurons of the ipsilateral Clarke's column, which ascend in the posterolateral part of the lateral funiculus as the dorsal spinocerebellar tract.[1,2] In the medulla, the fibers of this tract enter the ipsilateral cerebellum through the inferior cerebellar peduncle. Since Clarke's column does not extend lower than L-2 or L-3, afferent fibers from segments below this level ascend in the dorsal column to join the tract. Many of the most rostral (i.e., cervical and upper thoracic) spinocerebellar afferents do not travel in the dorsal spinocerebellar tract but form the separate cuneocerebellar tract. This tract projects to the ipsilateral cerebellum via the inferior peduncle. Sensory fibers from coccygeal, sacral, and lumbar segments form an additional tract, the anterior spinocerebellar tract, which ascends in the lateral aspect of the cord just anterior to the posterior spinocerebellar tract. Unlike the posterior tract, this tract is crossed and enters the cerebellum via the superior peduncle. There, most of its fibers recross the midline before terminating in the cerebellar cortex. In this way, the cerebellar terminations of this tract ultimately end up on the same side as their origins. **The spinocerebellar tracts receive input from a variety of muscle, joint, and cutaneous proprioceptors and convey information about the position of the body in space and the relative position of body segments.** Clinically detectable deficits due to damage to the spinocerebellar tracts are rare, because when these tracts are affected other areas of the cord are almost always affected as well. Early indicators of damage to the spinocerebellar tracts include various forms of ataxia, but, as might be expected, no conscious loss of sensation.

Additional ascending spinal tracts have been identified, but little is known of their function or clinical significance in humans. Spinoreticular fibers may provide substantial input to the reticular formation, spino-olivary fibers project to the accessory olivary nuclei that project to the cerebellum, and spinotectal fibers project to the superior colliculus and other parts of the tectum of the midbrain.

The Somatotopy of the Spinal Cord

As alluded to in the other chapters of this textbook, **many of the tracts and control centers of the central nervous system are somatotopically organized.**[1-5,7] In other words, they are arranged in such a way that particular portions of the body are represented in a particular anatomic location. **This is true of both the motor and sensory systems of the spinal cord.**

Descending Motor Control Systems[4,5,9,10]

The **motor pathways** descend in the ventral and lateral regions of the spinal cord white matter and ultimately synapse on motor neurons in the ventral horn and on interneurons and propriospinal neurons in the intermediate zone. For the sake of discussion, these pathways **can be divided into the medial descending pathways** (the ventral corticospinal, reticulospinal, vestibulospinal, and tectospinal tracts) **and the lateral descending pathways** (the lateral corticospinal and rubrospinal tracts).[4,5,10] The medial pathways terminate in the medial regions of the intermediate zone and ventral horn where the neurons controlling girdle and axial muscles are located. In contrast, the lateral descending pathways terminate in the lateral parts of the intermediate zone and ventral horn where the neuronal pools controlling the distal muscles of the extremities are located. In addition, flexor muscles are specifically innervated by motor neurons that are located dorsal to the extensor muscle motor neurons. This mediolateral and dorsoventral localization of proximal-distal and flexor-extensor functions can be graphically represented by a partial homunculus superimposed on the ventral gray matter (Fig. 17–5).

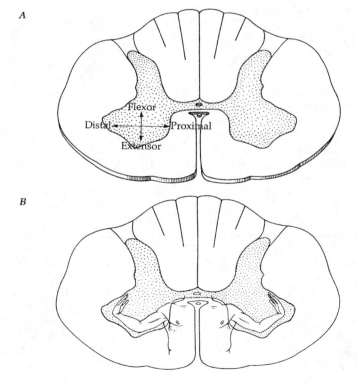

A

B

Figure 17–5. *The Somatotopic Organization of the Ventral Horn.* (*A*) Schematic diagram of the spinal cord indicating the general locations of motor neurons innervating limb and axial muscles and flexor and extensor muscles. (*B*) A partial "homunculus" superimposed on the ventral horns. (From Martin,[5] [Adapted with the permission of Macmillan College Publishing Company from CORRELATIVE ANATOMY OF THE NERVOUS SYSTEM by E. Crosby, T. Humphrey, E. Lauer. Copyright © 1962 Macmillan College Publishing Company.] p 211, with permission.)

Ascending Sensory Tracts[1,2,4,11]

The fibers of the major ascending sensory tracts are also somatotopically arranged. Recall that as the dorsal column reaches successively more rostral spinal levels, new fibers are added to the lateral margin of the tract, displacing fibers of more caudal origins toward the spinal midline. The result is a somatotopic arrangement in which input from the leg is carried by fibers in the most medial portion of the dorsal column, whereas input from the neck and the back of the head is conveyed in the most lateral portions of the column (see Fig. 17–4). New fibers are also added to the ascending anterolateral pathway in an orderly fashion. In this tract, however, the most rostral fibers accrue to the dorsomedial portions of the tract, displacing the fibers already present to a more ventrolateral position. This results in a somatotopy in which input from the leg is dorsomedial and from the neck is ventrolateral.

The dorsal horn itself displays several types of spatial organization in the terminations of primary afferent (dorsal root) fibers.[9,10] First, there is a mediolateral somatotopic organization of incoming fibers. Distal parts of limbs are represented medially, and proximal parts are represented laterally. This is essentially the opposite of that found in the origins of the efferent fibers of the ventral horn. In the thoracic region of the body, ventral parts are represented medially and dorsal parts laterally. Second, there is a ventral-dorsal segregation of afferent fiber types (and hence modality), which is superimposed on the somatotopic pattern. The specific site at which sensory fibers terminate within the dorsal horn is related to the diameter of the fiber.[4,9] The smallest-diameter afferent fibers (mediating pain and temperature) terminate predominantly in the most posterior aspects of the dorsal horn, whereas large-diameter myelinated fibers from touch receptors and proprioceptors terminate in more ventral layers of the gray matter.

Gray Matter

As discussed in Chapter 5, the spinal gray matter is a mass of nerve cell bodies, dendrites, myelinated and unmyelinated axons, and glial cells, which extends the length of the spinal cord. The gray matter on each side consists of dorsal and ventral horns and an intermediate zone (see Fig. 17–1). A small lateral horn is apparent in thoracic and upper lumbar segments. **Within the gray matter, neurons of the same type tend to be grouped together.** When viewed in transverse section, these histologic groupings of cells appear as layers, especially within the dorsal horn. **The layers of neurons are known as the *Rexed's laminae*.**[1,3,5,11,12] These laminae are numbered consecutively with Roman numerals, starting at the top of the dorsal horn and moving ventrally into the ventral horn (Fig. 17–6). The dorsal horn is formed by laminae I through VI, the intermediate zone and Clarke's column corresponds to lamina VII, and the ventral horn is composed of laminae VIII and IX.[5] Lamina X is the gray matter surrounding the central canal. This scheme is just one way of categorizing the location of spinal cord neurons, but it has proved useful because the **histologic differences among laminae correspond well to functions being undertaken within the laminae** (Table 17–1). For example, although dorsal root afferent fibers terminate in all laminae, they predominate in those of the dorsal horn (i.e., I through VI). Moreover, because the small-diameter afferent fibers predominate in the more superficial laminae, whereas large-diameter fibers predominate in deeper layers, terminations of pain (nociceptive) and temperature are prominent in laminae I and II, whereas proprioceptive (i.e., muscle spindle and Golgi tendon organ) and tactile afferents are prominent in laminae V, VI, VII, and IX. Lamina IX contains large numbers of alpha and gamma motor neurons.

Laminae of Rexed

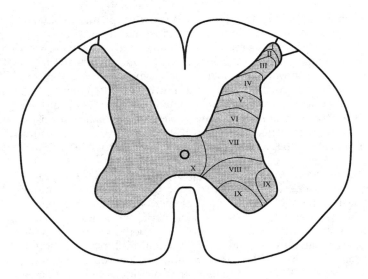

Figure 17–6. Schematic diagram of the general arrangement of the laminae of the gray matter of the human spinal cord.

Functional Deficits Caused by Spinal Cord Lesions: General Principles

A familiarity with the topography and somatotopy of the spinal cord provides a basis for understanding the functional deficits that arise from spinal cord injury or disease.[13-15] Clearly, if the regions of the cord in which motor tracts predominate are damaged, motor deficits will develop. For example, disruption of the corticospinal tracts impairs volitional motor activity, resulting in selective muscle weakness or paralysis. On the other hand,

Table 17–1. Projections to and from the Laminae of Rexed

Projections	Laminae
To Lamina	
Nociceptors	I, II, V
Mechanoreceptors	II–VI
Group Ia (primary endings in muscle spindles)	VI, VII, IX
Group II (secondary endings in muscle spindles)	IV–VII, IX
Group Ib (Golgi tendon organs)	V–VII
Nonmyelinated C fibers	II
Corticospinal tract	III–VII
Reticulospinal tract	I, II, V–VIII
Propriospinal fibers	I, II
From Lamina	
Ventrospinocerebellar	V–VII
Spinothalamic	IV–VI
Postsynaptic dorsal column neurons	III–V
Preganglionic sympathetic neurons	VII
Alpha, gamma motor neurons	IX

Adapted from Daube et al.[12]

disruption of the motor control tracts descending from the brainstem results in more subtle alterations in somatic reflex activity and muscle tone. By the same token, if the regions of the spinal cord in which sensory tracts predominate are damaged, sensory deficits will arise. The specific modality involved is determined by the particular tract disturbed. Disruption of the dorsal columns, for example, results in an impaired sense of fine touch, vibration, and joint position. Disturbance of the anterolateral (spinothalamic) tracts impairs perception of pain, temperature, and crude touch. Although no loss of conscious sensation occurs with disruption of the spinocerebellar tracts, the proprioceptive input that they transmit is important in motor control (though subconscious) and its loss results in a type of incoordination called **sensory ataxia.**

Beyond this simple differentiation between motor and sensory deficits, the specific signs and symptoms that accompany lesions of the spinal cord predictably reflect the anatomic level at which the lesions occur, the somatotopy of the tracts involved, and whether the tracts are crossed or uncrossed.

Anatomic Level of the Lesion

Lesions of the spinal cord often give rise to motor and sensory deficits that are specifically related to the involvement of particular spinal segments.[12,13] In this regard, these deficits may be limited to a small number of involved segments or may extend to all segments below the level of involvement. When the white matter of the spinal cord is damaged at a given level, the long sensory and motor tracts passing through that level may be interrupted. This results in a loss of function in those parts of the body innervated from that level and below. In the case of a complete transverse sectioning of the cord, all motor and sensory function is lost below the level of the injury. On the other hand, when the gray matter is selectively damaged in a given region of the cord, functional loss is limited to those parts of the body innervated by the specific spinal segments involved. This may include both sensory loss and lower motor neuron motor deficits. When substantial injury is done to both white and gray matter in a specific region of the cord, a mixture of deficits results, reflecting disruption of both long pathways passing through the region and disruption of local (segmental) pathways. A good example of such mixed findings is the Brown-Séquard syndrome, which is described later in this chapter.

In the case of either white matter of gray matter damage, the particular deficits that develop provide evidence of the level or region of the spinal cord that is injured. **Muscle weakness, atrophy, and abnormal deep tendon reflexes may provide a good indication of the level at which the cord is affected** (Table 17–2). This is particularly true of the segments involved in the control of the muscles of the extremities. Because it is difficult to relate the innervation of muscles of the trunk and thorax to specific segments, the lesion level may not be as obvious in these segments. **Often the pattern of sensory loss provides an even better indication of the site of a spinal cord lesion.**

Tract Somatotopy

Most of the major motor and sensory tracts are somatotopically organized, which implies that damage occurring within this somatotopy will cause predictable involvement of specific body parts.[7,13,14] The fibers of the corticospinal, dorsal column, and spinothalamic tracts all are somatotopically arranged. The clinical importance of this arrangement is clearly illustrated by two clinical situations affecting the spinothalamic tracts.[7,13,14] First, when a lesion such as a tumor arises in the innermost portion of the thoracic or cervical cord, it first compresses the most medial fibers of the spinothalamic tract, which are those with origins in the more rostral segments of the cord. It may not affect the most lateral fibers, which originate in more caudal segments. In such a case, pain and temperature sensation

***Table 17-2.** Functional Indicators of Lesion Level*

MOTOR

Root	Major Muscles Affected	Reflex Loss
C-3-5	Diaphragm	
C-5	Deltoids, elbow flexors	Biceps, brachioradialis
C-6	Wrist extensors	
C-7	Elbow extensors	Triceps
C-8	Finger flexors	Finger flexor
T-1	Hand intrinsics	
L-2-4	Hip flexors, knee extensors, ankle dorsiflexors	Knee jerk, cremasteric
L-5	Long extensor of great toe	
S-1-2	Ankle plantar flexors	Ankle jerk
S-3-5	Bladder and anal sphincters	

SENSORY

Root	Major Sensory Areas Affected
C-4	Clavicle
C-8	Fifth finger
T-4	Nipples
T-10	Umbilicus
L-1	Inguinal ligament
L-3	Anterior surface of the thigh
L-5	Great toe
S-1	Lateral aspect of the foot
S-3-5	Perineum

will be lost below the level of the lesion, with the exception of the most caudal areas (e.g., perineum, scrotum, and saddle area), the fibers from which are most lateral and thus spared. Second, clinical advantage may be taken from the somatotopic arrangement of these fibers in an operation called an **anterolateral cordotomy**. In this procedure, the spinothalamic tracts are selectively sectioned in an effort to relieve certain types of intractable pain in the pelvis or legs. As an incision is made into the anterolateral cord, the lateral fibers of the spinothalamic tract will be the first to be transected, producing contralateral analgesia in the most caudal regions. As deeper fibers of more rostral origins are cut, the level of anesthesia rises. Because pain is not experienced in the cord itself, it is possible to perform this procedure in an awake patient under local anesthesia. In this way, the extent of sensory loss can be continually ascertained from the patient during the procedure so that only the desired level of anesthesia is obtained.

Crossed or Uncrossed Tracts

Whether a particular tract crosses the neural axis in its descent or ascent and, if crossed, where it crosses in relation to a specific lesion, will determine the distribution of the deficits created by its disruption. For example, unilateral lesions that disrupt the corticospinal tracts above the level of their medullary decussation produce primarily contralateral muscle weakness. If, however, these tracts are disrupted below the decussation (in the spinal cord), the resultant muscle weakness will be ipsilateral to the lesion. The

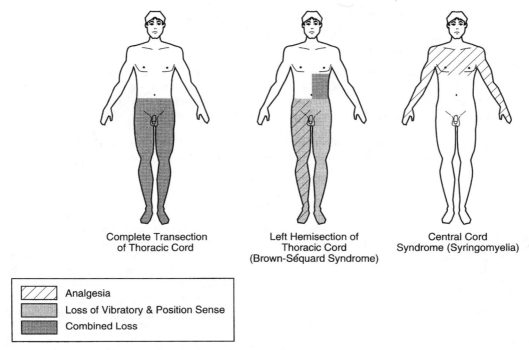

Complete Transection of Thoracic Cord	Left Hemisection of Thoracic Cord (Brown-Séquard Syndrome)	Central Cord Syndrome (Syringomyelia)

[///] Analgesia

[ ] Loss of Vibratory & Position Sense

[■] Combined Loss

Figure 17–7. The pattern of sensory impairment associated with several types of spinal cord injury.

effects of decussation are perhaps most dramatically illustrated by the motor and sensory deficits accompanying spinal cord hemisection in the so-called Brown-Séquard syndrome (Fig. 17–7).[7,13] Because the fibers of the dorsal columns do not cross within the spinal cord, the Brown-Séquard deficits in tactile, vibratory, and position sense are unilateral and ipsilateral. On the other hand, because the spinothalamic fibers cross upon entry into the spinal cord, deficits in pain and temperature perception are unilateral and *contralateral* to the site of injury. A somewhat different situation arises in syringomyelia, in which a cavity forms in the central portions of the spinal cord. This lesion selectively damages the spinothalamic fibers crossing from both sides of the body, creating a bilateral loss of pain and temperature.

At first glance, it would seem that the functional deficits caused by spinal cord lesions can be reliably predicted from a knowledge of the location, arrangement, and course followed by the major motor and sensory tracts. It is not this simple, however, because anatomic variations among individuals, collateral connections between tracts, overlap of somatotopic areas, and redundant innervation all tend to blur these distinctions. Transection of the dorsal column, for example, produces only a partial loss of touch and position sense rather than abolition (as one might expect), because some crude touch and pressure sensation reach the cerebral cortex by other routes (probably the anterolateral pathways). The recurrence of pain following sectioning of spinothalamic tracts may reflect a small proportion of uncrossed fibers, the presence of some spinothalamic fibers in more dorsal areas of the cord, and the presence of pain fibers in other pathways (e.g., propriospinal).[1,14] Unilateral lesioning of the corticospinal tracts innervating axial muscles produces much less of an effect than might be expected because of the redundancy inherent in their bilateral innervation. Similarly, because certain types of sensations (e.g., pressure sensations from bladder and bowel and sexual sensations) are carried bilaterally in the spinothalamic tracts, unilateral damage usually results in little impairment.[1]

Signs and Symptoms Caused by Spinal Cord Lesions[13,15–19]

The neurologic abnormalities associated with spinal cord disease or injury are relatively few. In most cases, a careful exploration of a patient's signs and symptoms by means of a thorough history and physical examination can indicate which tracts are involved and at what level. Confirmation can be provided by electrophysiologic studies (e.g., evoked potentials) and various imaging techniques. Patients with spinal cord lesions typically present with varying combinations of pain, paresthesias and numbness, muscle weakness, abnormal somatic reflexes and muscle tone, and autonomic dysfunction.

Pain

Three main types of pain are seen in patients with spinal cord disease.[15,16,20] The most common is that associated with the site of the spinal cord lesion itself. This **local pain** arises from damage to the bony and ligamentous structures surrounding the cord. Local pain may develop rapidly in conditions such as spinal fracture, spinal infarction, or disk herniation, or more slowly in conditions such as transverse myelitis, syringomyelia, or tumor. Local pain is most severe over the vertebral column at the level of the spinal involvement but may spread to more distant areas. **Radicular pain** is created by damage to sensory nerve roots. This pain, which may be excruciating, is often associated with local pain. Radicular pain usually radiates in a pattern restricted to the affected dermatomes. A **diffuse aching or burning pain** is occasionally seen in spinal cord–injured patients, which is attributed to dysfunction of spinal cord pain pathways. Most frequently seen in patients with traumatic spinal cord injury, this type of pain usually develops relatively late, often occurring months after other spinal cord symptoms. It is not localized to the segment of injury but is usually referred to areas well below the level of the lesion (e.g., to the feet, legs, and buttocks).

Sensory Abnormalities

A variety of sensory disturbances also accompany spinal cord disease.[15,16] **Paresthesias** manifest as an assortment of abnormal sensations and reflect aberrant activity in sensory root or spinal cord sensory fibers. The most common (e.g., "pins and needles," tingling) seem to be due to abnormal activity in dorsal root and dorsal column pathways that convey touch. Patients may also experience a **loss of sensation** in some part of the body. All sensory modalities may be affected (e.g., touch, position sense, vibration, pain, and temperature), or some may be lost and others preserved. A difference seems to exist between the analgesia produced by sectioning of spinothalamic pathways (such as during anterolateral cordotomy) and the numbness or "deadness" reported by patients which arises from dorsal column involvement.[15] As mentioned earlier, a careful mapping of any sensory impairment provides valuable information regarding the level of the lesion.

Muscle Weakness

Muscle weakness is present to some extent in most disorders of the spinal cord. Upper motor neuron weakness is produced when the corticospinal tracts are disrupted. Involvement of the lateral corticospinal tracts innervating the distal extremities produces a more profound deficit than involvement of the medial tracts because of extensive bilateral input to the axial muscles. Lower motor neuron weakness is produced when the gray matter is damaged, disrupting the function of alpha motor neurons. **Upper motor neuron** weakness is typically combined with hyperreflexia, spasticity, and abnormal reflex responses such as Babinski's sign. **Lower motor neuron** weakness is characterized by atrophy, hypotonia, hyporeflexia or areflexia, and fasciculations in the involved muscle.

Abnormal Reflexes and Muscle Tone

Extensive spinal cord lesions, such as trauma, infarction or hemorrhage, and transverse myelitis, **usually produce a condition termed** *spinal shock.* Spinal shock is a transient state of markedly depressed spinal cord activity, which manifests as anesthesia, somatic and visceral areflexia, paralysis, and atonia below the level of the lesion. This depression of neural activity probably reflects the sudden withdrawal of facilitatory influences descending from cerebral and brainstem structures to spinal interneuron and motor neuron pools. **Spinal shock usually resolves within several weeks and is supplanted by an evolving state of hyperreflexia and spasticity.**

More slowly developing conditions may be associated with increased muscle tone and heightened reflexes from their onset, rather than spinal shock. Hyperreflexia, particularly in the extremities, is eventually present in all spinal cord disorders. This clinical picture can become somewhat confusing in disorders in which the upper motor neuron dysfunction producing the hyperreflexia and spasticity is accompanied by significant destruction of lower motor neurons (e.g., in amyotrophic lateral sclerosis). As increasing numbers of lower motor neurons are destroyed, areflexia and hypotonia may predominate. Somatic reflexes may also be abnormal in form. The extensor plantar response (Babinski's response), which is a distorted form of a primitive withdrawal response, is often an early sign of upper motor neuron disease. Other superficial reflexes (e.g., the cremasteric reflex) may be disturbed as well. As with the other functional deficits produced by spinal cord disease, the level at which the abnormal reflexes occur provides a useful indication of the site of the spinal cord lesion. For example, hyperactive reflexes in the legs with normal reflexes in the arms usually indicate a lesion of the thoracic or upper lumbar spinal cord.

Urinary Incontinence and Other Forms of Visceral Dysfunction

The spinal cord contains pathways mediating both the volitional and reflex control of a variety of visceral functions. Any or all of these pathways can be interrupted by spinal cord injury or disease, and the resultant visceral dysfunction may make a significant contribution to patient morbidity and mortality (see Chapter 24). **The corticospinal tracts mediate the volitional control of breathing. The pathways for the volitional control of micturition and for the automatic control of breathing, micturition, sweating, and blood pressure are located in the ventral half of the lateral column,** ventral to the corticospinal tracts.

Some of the most common and difficult to manage visceral problems relate to urinary bladder dysfunction.[21-24] The lower urinary tract is particularly vulnerable because many of the responses of this system require the coordination of autonomic and somatic mechanisms at various levels of the lumbosacral spinal cord, as well as input from higher centers in the brain. The innervation of the lower urinary tract involves three sets of peripheral motor nerves, namely, parasympathetic, sympathetic, and somatic. Most of the reflex mechanisms involved in urinary function are in lumbar and sacral segments. Sensory impulses arising in the bladder, urethra, sphincters, and related pelvic muscles are conveyed to the spinal cord within each of the three types of motor nerves. Segmental parasympathetic, sympathetic, and somatic mechanisms all are subject to a variety of inhibitory and facilitatory influences descending from higher centers. Most of the descending fibers involved in micturition lie in the lateral column just about level with the central canal.[16] This places these tracts just ventral to the corticospinal tracts, which occupy the dorsal half of the lateral columns. The bladder pathways are slightly dorsolateral to the descending fibers mediating reflex breathing and slightly medial to spinothalamic pain and temperature tracts from the sacral regions.

Spinal cord disease can cause a variety of lower urinary tract problems, depending on the level and severity of the lesion.[21-24] If spinal shock develops, such as with acute spinal cord injury, the bladder becomes areflexic and acute urinary retention develops. In the absence of spinal shock or after it has resolved, lesions of the cauda equina or the S-2 through S-4 segments disrupt the spinal reflex arcs necessary for micturition, so that the bladder remains **areflexic or "paralytic"** (see Chapter 24). Areflexia can result from destruction of sacral lower motor neurons (parasympathetic fibers), afferent pathways, or both. In patients with spinal cord lesions above the level of the sacral micturition reflexes, a **hyperreflexic or "spastic" bladder** usually develops. With disruption of neural connections to higher control centers, conscious awareness of bladder fullness and volitional control over micturition are lost. Reflex pathways below the level of the lesions usually become disinhibited and hyperirritable, resulting in hyperactivity of the detrusor and urethral sphincters. As a consequence, bladder capacity is diminished, high intravesical pressures develop, emptying is incomplete, and large residual urine volumes are retained. The so-called neurogenic bladders accompanying spinal cord disease predispose patients to urinary tract infection, stone formation, and upper urinary tract deterioration. Spinal cord lesions adversely affecting urinary tract function are common, not only following acute injury but also in association with conditions such as multiple sclerosis, tumor, and tabes dorsalis due to syphilis.

The lower urinary tract also subserves certain sexual functions, particularly in men, so that it is not surprising that **urinary dysfunction is often accompanied by genital dysfunction.**[25,26] Sexual function relies on spinal lower motor neurons and first-order sensory fibers, as well as on ascending and descending pathways. Most fibers carrying sensory information from sexual organs seem to lie primarily within the anterolateral tracts of the spinal cord. Many of the structures are bilaterally innervated. Most of the reflex mechanisms involved in sexual function are located in sacral and lower lumbar segments. Lesions in these areas disrupt both erection and ejaculation. In patients with lesions above the T-12 level, psychogenic erections are abolished, but reflexive responses may persist as long as lower motor neurons are intact. Ejaculation, however, occurs in a relatively small percentage of patients with significant lesions.

Breathing is also dependent on an intact spinal cord but is significantly impaired only by lesions involving the most rostral spinal segments.[27,28] Three major muscle groups are involved in respiration: the diaphragm (innervated from C-3 through C-5), the intercostal muscles (innervated from T-1 through T-12), and the abdominal muscles (innervated from T-6 through T-12). Although the diaphragm is the primary muscle of quiet breathing, the intercostal muscles assist normal inspiration by elevating the rib cage and in expiration at high ventilatory volumes. The abdominal muscles assist in forced expiration and coughing. In addition, a number of secondary or accessory muscles may assist in particularly forceful breathing or assume functional importance when the primary respiratory muscles are impaired. These include the sternocleidomastoids (innervated from C-1 through C-3), the scalenes (innervated from C-4 through C-11), and the trapezius (innervated from C-1 through C-4 and by cranial nerve XI). The muscles of the mouth and throat represent an additional group of muscles whose impairment may interfere with respiration.

The degree to which spinal cord disease or injury impairs respiration depends on the level of the lesion and how complete it is.[27,28] Lesions of the lumbar cord have little or no effect on ventilation or cough. Lesions of the thoracic cord can impair cough but have little effect on normal breathing. Lesions of the lower cervical cord are associated with increasing effects on breathing. Lesions at C-5 or higher can affect diaphragmatic function, with complete lesions at C-3 or higher producing bilateral diaphragmatic paralysis, which necessitates artificial ventilation.

Because separate pathways control voluntary breathing and automatic (involuntary) breathing, relatively circumscribed lesions in the spinal cord may adversely affect one without the other.[16] **Corticospinal tracts mediate the voluntary control of breathing. Their interruption eliminates voluntary respiration.** Such a patient may breathe adequately whether awake or asleep, because automatic breathing pathways remain intact. **Bilateral interruption of the ventrolateral white matter (sparing the more dorsally situated corticospinal tracts) disrupts the pathways from the medulla that mediate automatic breathing.** Such a patient may breathe adequately while awake, using the volitional pathways and the extra drive to breathe provided by the waking state. However, when asleep and dependent on automatic pathways, the patient may stop breathing. The clinician must be attentive to the possibility of death from sleep apnea in any patient who has a high cervical cord lesion affecting the ventrolateral quadrants.[16]

A variety of sensory stimuli from the periphery influence breathing, including input from pain, lung receptors, chemoreceptors, and possibly proprioceptors. It is likely that some of the adverse effects of spinal cord lesions on ventilation reflect the interruption of **ascending** rather than solely descending pathways. Some patients, for example, experience respiratory insufficiency, not due to weakness of the diaphragm or of the muscles of the chest wall, but to a reduced responsiveness to carbon dioxide.[16]

In addition to urinary incontinence and respiratory insufficiency (in the case of high lesions), spinal cord–injured patients may present with a variety of disturbances of gastrointestinal tract function, thermoregulation, and blood pressure control.

Classification of Spinal Cord Lesions[13,17–19]

Among the various tracts that course through the spinal cord, only four have major clinical importance.[13] Clinically significant signs and symptoms are produced by lesions of the descending lateral corticospinal tracts and the ascending dorsal column, spinothalamic, and spinocerebellar tracts. The greater the involvement of these pathways, the more extensive will be the resultant functional deficits.

Spinal cord lesions may be classified according to their etiology, the deficits that they produce, or **their anatomic criteria.**[13,17–19] The latter approach is a common one and is described in the following text (Fig. 17–8). Using this approach, in combination with a knowledge of the function of the major spinal cord pathways, one can readily predict the clinical presentations produced by various spinal cord lesions.

Complete Spinal Cord Transection

With complete spinal cord transection, all tracts ascending from below the level of the lesion and all tracts descending from above the level of the lesion are interrupted.[17,18,30] As a result, **both motor and sensory function below the level of spinal cord damage are profoundly disturbed.** All sensory modalities below the lesion level are lost. Radicular pain, segmental paresthesias, and localized vertebral pain all may occur at the level of injury, particularly in the case of destructive lesions such as trauma. Depending on the level of the lesion, paraplegia or tetraplegia will develop as a result of interruption of the corticospinal tracts (Table 17–3). If spinal shock has developed (i.e., with an acute lesion), this paralysis is initially flaccid and areflexic. Eventually, the hypertonia, hyperreflexia, spasticity, and plantar extensor signs characteristic of upper motor neuron lesions develop. At the level of the lesion itself, lower motor neuron signs (paresis, atrophy, fasciculations, and areflexia) may occur in a segmental distribution because of damage to anterior horn cells or their ventral roots. Bladder and bowel deficits develop as a result of the disruption of autonomic pathways. A spastic bladder with urgency of micturition is the most common bladder

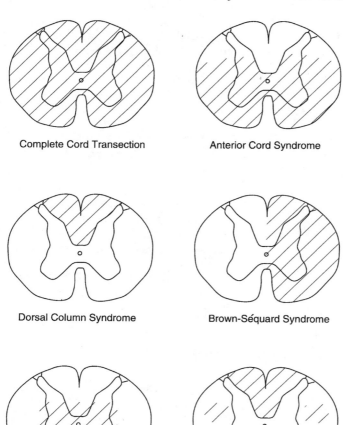

Complete Cord Transection   Anterior Cord Syndrome

Dorsal Column Syndrome   Brown-Séquard Syndrome

Central Cord Syndrome   Posterolateral Syndrome

Figure 17–8. Schematic representations of various forms ("syndromes") of spinal cord injury.

symptom. Constipation is the most common bowel symptom. Anhidrosis (diminished sweating), trophic skin changes, impaired temperature control, and vasomotor instability all are seen below the level of the lesion (see Chapter 24).

Complete transverse myelopathy is most often caused by trauma, tumor, multiple sclerosis, or vascular disorders.[18] Other causes are spinal epidural hematoma or absess, herniated intervertebral disk, and parainfectious or postvaccinal syndromes.

Incomplete Lesions[13,17–19]

Usually lesioning of the spinal cord is incomplete, with the associated clinical findings reflecting the specific damage done to the tracts of the spinal cord. Incomplete lesions may be classified according to the specific portions of the cord involved, creating an assortment of fairly standardized syndromes (Fig. 17–8). It should be remembered that spinal cord lesions show great variability, and these syndromes are rarely seen in pure form (i.e., exactly as described).

Table 17–3. *Functional Deficits Associated with Lesions at Specific Spinal Cord Segments*

Segment	Deficit
C-4, C-5, C-6, C-7	Tetraplegia Impaired respiration Reflex bladder
C-8, T-1	Impaired respiration Reflex bladder Paraplegia Hand weakness
T-2, T-3	Impaired respiration Reflex bladder Paraplegia
T-12, L-1	Paraplegia Reflex bladder
L-4, L-5	Paraplegia Reflex bladder
S-2, S-3	Areflexic bladder

Adapted from Daube et al.[12]

Anterior Cord Syndrome[17–19]

Anterior cord syndrome reflects destruction of the anterior two thirds of the spinal cord. Damage thus includes the anterior gray matter containing alpha motor neurons, as well as the corticospinal and spinothalamic tracts of the anterior and lateral white matter. The posterior gray matter and dorsal columns are preserved. **In a patient so affected, fine touch, vibratory sense, and joint position sense are intact, but motor control and pain and temperature sense are lost below the level of the lesion.** The most common causes of anterior cord syndrome are ischemia, infarction, and trauma. This type of injury is usually seen with flexion type injury, but it may also be associated with acute traumatic herniation of an intervertebral disk. The portion of the spinal cord involved in this syndrome corresponds to the anterior part of the spinal cord that is supplied by the anterior spinal artery. Perhaps the most important vascular (ischemic) syndrome of the spinal cord results when this artery is compromised.[17]

Posterior Cord (Dorsal Column) Syndrome[17–19]

The posterior cord syndrome involves damage restricted to the dorsal columns. Patients with this syndrome present with impaired fine touch, vibratory sense, and joint position sense but have intact senses of pain and temperature and intact motor function. The dorsal columns and their roots may be selectively destroyed by tabes dorsalis, a central nervous system form of syphilis. This syndrome is characterized by marked sensory ataxia caused by the loss of the dorsal proprioceptive pathways. Selective dorsal column injury is seldom caused by trauma, but when it is, it is usually associated with a hyperextension type of injury.

Lateral Cord Syndrome (Brown-Séquard Syndrome)[17–19,29,31,32]

Brown-Séquard syndrome is caused by lateral hemisection of the spinal cord. It is especially interesting because it is so illustrative of the clinical significance of the specific course followed by particular motor and sensory tracts (Fig. 17–9). Because the corticospinal

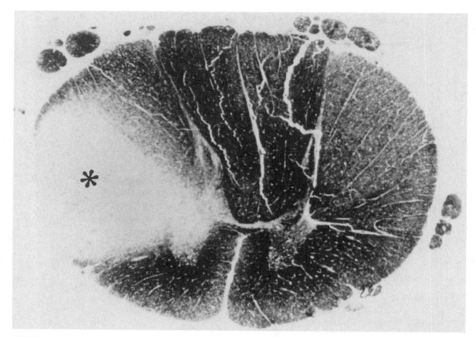

Figure 17–9. *Brown-Séquard Syndrome Resulting from Multiple Sclerosis.* In this transverse section through the spinal cord, the lesion (*) is seen to be incomplete, although the patient had all of the clinical features of a complete hemisection. (From Woolsey and Young,[15] p 573, 1991, with permission.)

tracts and the dorsal column sensory tracts do not decussate within the spinal cord, **affected patients experience ipsilateral loss of fine touch, vibratory sense, and position sense, as well as ipsilateral upper motor neuron deficits.** Because the spinothalamic pathways decussate near their level of entry into the cord, **pain and temperature loss are contralateral to the site of injury.** This creates a memorable clinical scenario in which the patient retains the feeling of pain and temperature on the paralyzed side. Ipsilateral *lower* **motor neuron paralysis** and analgesia or hypalgesia may occur at the segment of injury caused by local damage to sensory and motor fibers. Functional hemisection may result from multiple sclerosis, penetrating injury of the spinal cord (e.g., stab wound), syringomyelia, and tumor. In practice, a pure Brown-Séquard syndrome is seldom seen.

Central Cord Syndrome[17–19,29,31]

The central cord syndrome results when damage is predominantly in the central portion of the spinal cord. Cord damage starts centrally and often spreads to involve more peripheral structures. **Spinothalamic fibers that decussate through the central cord are the first to be involved, producing a bilateral loss of pain and temperature sensation in the presence of normal tactile sense.** The central cord syndrome is probably most often associated with syringomyelia. **Syringomyelia** is a chronic, progressive disorder characterized by cavities that form in the central part of the spinal cord (Fig. 17–10). The precise clinical picture of syringomyelia depends on the extent and shape of the cavity (syrinx) formed. Because the corticospinal fibers to the lower extremities are the most laterally situated in the corticospinal tracts, they are the last to be affected. An acute cervical central spinal cord syndrome also can result from severe hyperextensive injury of the neck. The hallmarks of this syndrome are the dissociated sensory loss and disproportionate weakness of the arms compared with the legs. Central cord damage may also be produced by intramedullary tumor, postirradiation myelopathy, and infarction.

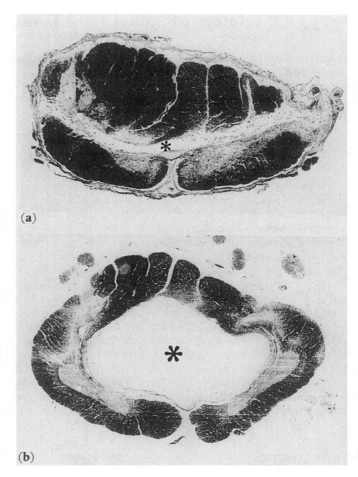

Figure 17-10. *Syringomyelia Evident in Transverse Sections of the Spinal Cord Stained for Myelin.* (A) At the cervical level, the cavity (*) extends into both posterior horns. (B) At the thoracic level, the large cavity (*) merges with the central canal. (From Adam, JH and Duchen, LW: Greenfield's Neuropathy, ed 5. Oxford University Press, New York, 1992, p 551, with permission.)

Posterolateral Cord Syndrome[17]

Bilateral degeneration of the dorsal columns and lateral columns is often evident in a condition called **subacute combined degeneration** of the spinal cord, which is seen in severe vitamin B_{12} deficiency, AIDS, and certain other conditions. **Affected patients complain of paresthesias in the feet and have signs of impaired vibratory sense and proprioception in the legs, which may create a sensory ataxia. Pain and temperature sense remain intact** because of preservation of the spinothalamic tracts. Corticospinal tract disruption results in spastic weakness, hyperreflexia, and bilateral Babinski's signs.

Anterior Horn Cell Syndrome

Certain inherited and acquired disorders selectively damage the anterior horn cells of the spinal cord. These disorders are discussed in Chapter 16.

Combined Anterior Horn Cell and Corticospinal Disease

Certain motor neuron disorders, such as amyotrophic lateral sclerosis, are characterized by degenerative changes in both anterior horn cells and corticospinal tracts of the spinal cord. Diffuse lower motor neuron signs (progressive muscle atrophy, paresis, and fasciculations) are superimposed upon the consequences of upper motor neuron dysfunction (paresis, spasticity, hyperreflexia, and extensor plantar responses).

Etiology of Spinal Cord Lesions[15,29,32-37]

One way of classifying the numerous pathologic conditions adversely affecting the spinal cord is to organize them according to etiology. In the discussion that follows, the main etiologic categories are described, and selected disorders that primarily affect the spinal cord are discussed. Spinal muscular atrophies, amyotrophic lateral sclerosis, and multiple sclerosis, all of which are important disorders, are discussed in other chapters.

Congenital and Developmental Disorders[29,32-39]

A variety of congenital conditions may arise when the spinal cord, vertebral column, or both fail to form properly during embryonic development.[38,39] Failure of the embryonic neural tube to close properly is called dysraphism. Spinal cord dysraphism may be associated with failure to fuse of the overlying meninges, vertebrae, and skin. **The most common of the spinal dysraphisms is *spina bifida,* in which there is incomplete closure of the vertebral canal.** The most common form of this defect is posterior spina bifida, in which the defect occurs in the posterior aspect of the spinal cord, most frequently in the lumbosacral region. The severity of the structural malformations caused by this condition varies markedly. Sometimes only a minor bony defect is evident radiographically, with no cord dysraphism (spina bifida occulta). Spina bifida occulta may be present in as much as 24% of the population.[38] In more severe forms of spina bifida, a sac or cyst protrudes through the vertebral defect and is apparent as an obvious mass in the dorsal midline (Fig. 17–11). This sac may contain both dura and arachnoid (i.e., a meningocele), with the spinal cord remaining in a normal position in the spinal canal, or it may contain both meninges and spinal cord (i.e., meningomyelocele). **The neurologic deficits associated with spina bifida vary considerably, reflecting the severity of the malformation.** For example, patients with spina bifida occulta may be asymptomatic, whereas patients with a large vertebral defect and

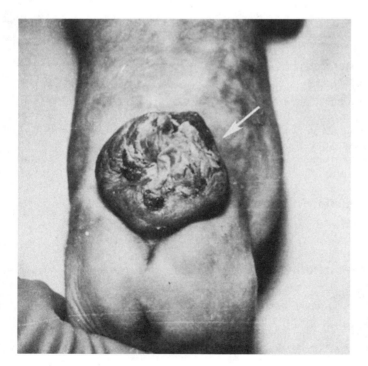

Figure 17–11. Lumbar myelomeningocele in an infant with hydrocephalus and paraplegia. (From Adams, JH and Duchen, LW: Greenfield's Neuropathology, ed 5. Oxford University Press, New York, 1992, p 542, with permission.)

meningomyelocele may be paraplegic and areflexic and often die without treatment. Hydrocephalus occurs in many infants with one of these defects. In some instances, retardation occurs as a result of hydrocephalus or other ill-defined factors. Genetic factors have been suggested in spina bifida because of a predominance in girls and a recurrence in siblings.[37]

In addition to the dysraphic states, other malformations of the spinal cord also occur. Diastematomyelia and diplomyelia are conditions in which the spinal cord forms as two separate hemicords or two duplicate cords, respectively.[35,36,38]

Syringomyelia is a chronic, progressive disorder of the spinal cord, characterized by the presence of large cavities (syringes) within the central portion of the cord.[29,32,35,36,38,40–42] These cavities are most frequently found extending over multiple segments of cervical and upper thoracic regions but may extend upward in some cases into the medulla and pons or downward into thoracic or even lumbar segments. The syrinx first forms in the central gray matter of the cervical cord, where it interrupts decussating pain and temperature fibers at several successive cord segments. Enlargement of the cavity leads to progressive destruction of anterior horn cells in the ventral horns and of ascending and descending tracts in the lateral and posterior funiculi. What causes the formation and extension of this central cavity is not entirely understood.

Usually syringomyelia is associated with certain congenital malformations of the central nervous system. This has led to the theory that formation of the syrinx is linked to these malformations and may specifically reflect abnormal cerebrospinal fluid flow or pressure. In some instances, syringomyelia is not associated with developmental defects and may be acquired as a result of trauma, vascular infarct, or tumor.[17] The associated clinical picture depends not only on the extent of the syrinx but also on any associated malformations. Symptoms usually begin in adulthood with a dissociated sensory loss on one or both sides (i.e., loss of pain and temperature sensitivity with retention of other tactile modalities), then progresses to more widespread motor and sensory signs as the cavity expands. Unless associated with bulbar deficits, this condition rarely causes death directly, but considerable disability may be produced by the weakness of limbs and trunk and by the almost inevitable spinal deformity. Because of the loss of pain and temperature perception, the avoidance of burns and other injuries should be stressed.

Hydromyelia is another condition in which the central canal of the spinal cord is enlarged into a central cavity. Hydromyelia may occur in isolation and may be asymptomatic or may occur in the context of more complex syndromes such as spina bifida or Arnold-Chiari malformations.

Disorders of the Vertebral Column[29,32,35–38]

The vertebral column encases the spinal cord, both protecting and stabilizing this delicate neural structure. **The bony, cartilaginous, and ligamentous components of the spinal column all may be diseased or malformed, threatening the integrity of the spinal cord within.** Alterations in the shape or alignment of the vertebrae or other components of the spine may cause compression of the spinal cord itself or of the blood vessels on which the cord depends. By the same token, deterioration and weakness of the spinal column may make the spinal cord more vulnerable to trauma or even to the mechanical stresses of normal movement and posture.

Intervertebral disk disease and spondylosis (vertebral ankylosis) are probably the most common pathologic conditions affecting the spinal column.[29,32,35–38,43,44] Disk deterioration and accompanying changes in the vertebrae are a common consequence of the normal aging of the spine. By age 50, the intervertebral disks begin a process of degeneration, notable in the dehydration and shrinkage of the soft central portion of the disk called the **nucleus pulposus.** This degeneration is commonly accompanied by the formation of spurlike or rigid bony overgrowths on the margins of the upper and lower surfaces of the vertebral bodies (Fig. 17–12). These bony overgrowths or portions of the intervertebral disk

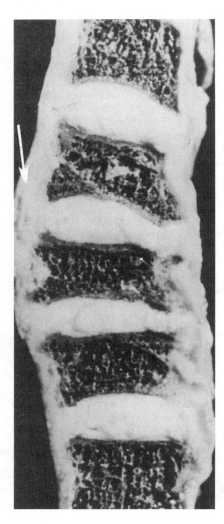

Figure 17–12. *Cervical Spondylosis.* Severe spondylosis affects these cervical disc spaces and has caused a large posterior protrusion (*Arrow*) seen directed to the left of the picture. A corresponding deep indentation was evident in the cord at this level. (From Adams, JH and Duchen, LW: Greenfield's Neuropathology, ed 5. Oxford University Press, New York, 1992, p 1094, with permission.)

may protrude into the spinal canal or intervertebral foramina compressing spinal roots, spinal cord, or both, as well as blood vessels such as radicular arteries. Anterior protrusion or minor posterior protrusion of bone or disk often produces no neurologic symptoms. However, substantial overgrowth of the posterior surface of the vertebrae or posterior protrusion of disk substance can damage the cord, causing both sensory and motor symptoms. Spondylosis is most evident and is most likely to produce neurologic findings when it is present in the mid to lower cervical and lumbar segments—the most mobile parts of the spine. Patients with cervical spondylosis present with a painful stiff neck, spinal root pain in the arms and hands, and upper motor neuron weakness in the legs. Chronic disk degeneration and spondylosis in the lumbar segments cause symptoms of backache and leg pain. Because most protrusions at this level occur between the lower lumbar vertebrae or between the lowest lumbar vertebra and the sacrum, they do not damage the spinal cord per se but their effects result from compression of the roots of the cauda equina.

Herniation of an intervertebral disk may also occur on an acute basis, as a result of physical force applied to a region of the spinal column. For example, acute posterior rupture and protrusion of a disk may be caused by sudden traumatic flexion of the neck, or by heavy compression strain applied to the lumbar spine (e.g., in a fall or in athletic activity). The most common site for acute prolapse is the lumbar region between the fifth lumbar vertebra and the first sacral vertebra.

Rheumatoid arthritis and other joint disorders may affect the vertebrae of the spinal column, producing symptoms that may mimic spondylosis.[29,35,36] Although rheumatoid arthritis of the spine does not itself stimulate the bone formation characteristic of spondylosis, these two disorders may coexist. Rheumatoid spondylosis most commonly affects the cervical spine and may result in cervical dislocations that damage the spinal cord. Other bone disorders, such as osteitis deformans (Paget's disease), may also affect the vertebral column, causing spinal deformity and lesions of the spinal cord or spinal nerve roots.

Inflammatory Disease (Myelitis)[32,33,35,36]

A number of inflammatory disorders of both infective and noninfective origins can involve the spinal cord. Most have a known microbial cause. The spinal cord may be infected by a number of conventional **viruses,** such as rabies, poliomyelitis, and herpes zoster, as well as by certain so-called slow viruses. The list of viral infections has rapidly expanded with the recognition that many other viruses (e.g., herpes simplex, cytomegalovirus, and Epstein-Barr virus) may infect the cord, particularly in immunodeficient states such as HIV infection. Myelitis may also occur as a result of infection by a number of **bacteria,** which may invade the neural tissue itself, as well as the membranes and spaces around the cord. In some diseases, both the spinal cord and the meninges are simultaneously affected; in others, cord lesions predominate. Bacterial infection of the spinal cord or meninges may occur in the context of a generalized infection of the central nervous system or systemic septicemia, or it may be localized (e.g., an absess seeded from an infected vertebra or a penetrating wound). A wide variety of **fungal and parasitic agents** may also involve the spinal cord and its coverings. These disorders are more common in underdeveloped regions of the world and within immunodeficient populations (e.g., those with AIDS).[43]

Inflammatory lesions of the spinal cord also occur, which appear to be due to a disordered immune response rather than to the direct effects of an infectious agent. The fact that some of these lesions occur within 1 or 2 weeks after a viral illness or immunization suggests that an immune response to an antigenic stimulus may be involved.[32,46,47] These disorders usually run a monophasic course, with a single attack followed by a variable degree of recovery and no recurrence. Although in most cases of myelitis the brain is also involved, in some the spinal cord is primarily or exclusively involved. In these cases, which are often described as **transverse myelitis,** weakness and numbness of the feet and legs (less often the hands and arms) and difficulty in emptying the bladder develop over a period of a few days. After their progression, these neurologic symptoms remain stationary for some time and then slowly recede.

Vascular Disorders[29,32,35,47-49]

Although the spinal cord is less susceptible to vascular disease than the brain, ischemia and infarction due to arterial obstruction or hemorrhage occasionally occur and may severely damage the cord. Spinal "stroke" is seldom due to atherosclerosis or another occlusive disease. The segmental and spinal vessels are not susceptible to atherosclerosis and, although atherosclerosis is common in the aorta and may narrow the ostia of the segmental arteries, this usually progresses slowly enough that adequate collateralization develops, sparing the cord. Emboli, whether thrombotic or atheromatous, rarely lodge in the spinal arteries. A dissecting **aortic aneurysm,** however, is a common cause of vascular injury to the spinal cord. Spinal cord ischemia is also an acknowledged complication of vascular surgery, particularly surgery involving the thoracic aorta. In addition to direct manipulation, other medical procedures such as catheterization of thoracic or abdominal vessels or spinal anesthesia can also cause ischemic myelopathy.

Vascular malformations are the most common of the vascular abnormalities of the spinal cord and its meninges.[35,36,50] Arteriovenous malformations appear as a tangled mass of distended, tortuous vessels on the posterior surface of the cord. They most often occur in the thoracolumbar regions. They are occasionally found in association with spina bifida, but more often in isolation. When symptomatic, vascular malformations usually create a syndrome of slowly progressing signs of cord compression or ischemia. Occasionally, a sudden onset or exacerbation of symptoms may be brought on by thrombosis of a vessel within the malformation or hemorrhage into the subarachnoid space or cord itself.

Spinal cord ischemic injury can also occur as a result of conditions causing generalized systemic hypoxia/ischemia or hypotension. The cord can be damaged along with the brain during perinatal asphyxia. Spinal cord necrosis is also known to occur as a result of the severe hypotension following cardiac arrest or hemorrhage. The blood supply to the spinal cord may also be disrupted by trauma and spondylosis, which are discussed elsewhere.

Intraspinal Tumors[29,32,37,51]

Tumors of the spinal cord are considerably less common than tumors of the brain. Moreover, in contrast to brain tumors, most spinal tumors are benign and produce effects mainly by compression of the cord rather than by invasion. Neoplasms of the spine can be divided into those that form within the substance of the spinal cord itself (intramedullary) and those that arise outside the spinal cord (extramedullary). Extramedullary tumors may be further subdivided into those of the vertebral bodies or epidural tissues (extradural) and those arising in the leptomeninges or roots (intradural). Intramedullary tumors represent only about 5% of all spinal cord tumors, with the remaining tumors approximately equally divided among intradural and extradural tumors.[32] **Extramedullary** masses induce neurologic signs and symptoms by compression of both the neural tissue and the blood vessels that supply it. **Intramedullary** growths invade as well as compress the substance of the spinal cord. The most common primary intraspinal tumors are extramedullary (benign neurofibromas and meningiomas). Primary intramedullary tumors have the same cellular origins as those arising in the brain. Secondary intraspinal tumors may also be either intramedullary or extramedullary, the latter being the more common. **Extradural metastases,** such as those from lung, breast, and prostate carcinoma, **are probably the most common of all spinal tumors.** Patients with spinal cord tumors are likely to present with either a sensorimotor spinal tract syndrome due to compression or (less often) invasion of spinal cord tracts, or a painful radicular-spinal cord syndrome in which the signs of spinal cord compression are accompanied (often preceded) by radicular pain in the distribution of the involved sensory roots.[32] The deficits caused by spinal cord compression include asymmetric spastic weakness of the legs with thoracolumbar lesions and of the arms and legs with cervical lesions; dorsal column signs such as paresthesias; impaired pain and thermal sense; and a loss of voluntary bladder and bowel control.

Traumatic Spinal Cord Injury[52-61]

Each year an estimated 8,000 to 10,000 people in the United States sustain a significant traumatic spinal cord injury.[52-54,56,58] Motor vehicle accidents account for about 50% of these injuries, with motorcycle accidents claiming a disproportionate share. Vehicular accidents are followed by falls (about 20%), sports-related accidents (about 14%),[52] and gunshot or stab wounds (about 13%). The incidence and specific cause of spinal cord injury varies with gender, age, and race. About 80% of all injuries are sustained by males between 16 and 30 years of age. This is largely due to risk-taking behaviors within this population. Because of anatomic and biomechanical conditions in the spine, **the cervical region and the thoracolumbar junction are the most common sites of traumatic damage.** Cervical spine injuries are particularly devastating and often cause death (Fig. 17–13).

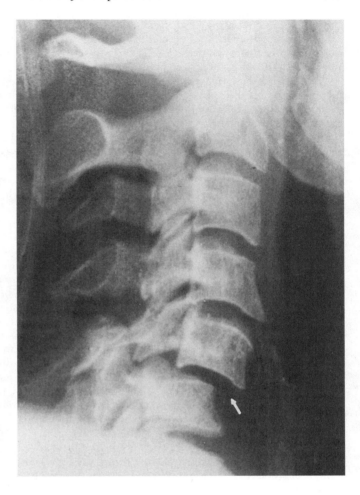

Figure 17–13. *A Dislocation-Fracture Injury of the Cervical Spine.* An accident rendered this patient completely quadriplegic. He died 5 days later from a large pulmonary embolus. (From Errico, TJ et al (eds): Spinal Trauma. JB Lippincott, Philadelphia, 1990, p 110, with permission.)

Mechanism of Injury[35,53–58]

The spinal cord is generally well protected from injury by the bony vertebral column and its muscular elements. Except for the cervical region, a considerable amount of force is required to damage the cord itself. Damage to the cord may be direct, indirect, or both. **The spinal cord may be directly injured,** with or without serious damage to the spine, by stab wounds from knives or other sharp instruments and by small penetrating missiles. The extent and shape of the resultant cord damage depend on the size, velocity, and direction of impact of the penetrating object. In general, with direct injury, the damage to the spine is less severe than that in the cord itself. **The most common cause of cord trauma is indirect injury, with violent force being transmitted to the cord by way of the spinal column.** This may or may not be accompanied by injuries such as fractures, dislocations, or subluxations of the spine. Often there is injury to both the spine and the spinal cord. Spinal cord injury may also be produced by a combination of direct and indirect violence. This is common with high-velocity missiles and in spinal fracture-dislocations in which the cord is directly penetrated or lacerated by small displaced fragments of bone.

As with head injury, a distinction is made between open and closed injury, depending on the integrity of the dura. In general, direct or sharp violence to the cord results in penetrating or open injury, whereas indirect or blunt trauma results in closed or nonpenetrating injury. **Closed injuries constitute the majority of spinal cord injuries.** In fact, the incidence of penetrating cord injuries in which the dura mater and meninges are slit open represents less than 10% of all civilian injuries.[57] Damage due to penetrating injury may be quite circumscribed, whereas closed-cord injury is seldom confined to the point of impact on the spine but may spread over many segments.

The neurologic damage produced by spinal trauma reflects both the nature and magnitude of the force applied to the spine, as well as the particular biomechanical properties and architecture of the region of the spine to which it is applied. Ultimately, the neurologic damage will be determined by the extent to which the vertebrae and associated structures impinge upon the cord, the vascular supply of the cord, or the spinal roots and nerves during and after the trauma. The kinds of forces commonly involved in spinal cord injury include flexion, compression, hyperextension, and flexion-rotation.

CERVICAL SPINE.[54,55,57,59] Because of its exposure, its relatively poor mechanical stability, and the weight of the head to which it is attached, the cervical spine is more vulnerable to trauma than other areas of the vertebral column. About two thirds of all traumatic spinal cord injuries occur in the cervical region. At the C-1–2 level, the spinal canal is the largest of the entire spine. This provides a certain margin of safety for the spinal cord when C-1–2 fractures or subluxations occur. In fact, about 75% of patients with C-1–2 fractures suffer no neurologic injury. Below C-2, the spinal canal rapidly narrows, reaching its most narrow point between C-4 and C-6. Lower cervical spinal cord or nerve root damage is usually due to compression resulting from vertebral body fracture or intervertebral disk herniation or due to stretch resulting from excessive movement between vertebral segments (see Fig. 17–13). The forces most frequently causing injury to the cervical spine are flexion, vertical compression, and hyperextension. Flexion injury (as might be caused in an automobile accident) most consistently results in neurologic injury. Vertical compression is most often the result of striking the head while diving into shallow water. This occurs most frequently at C-4–5 and results in complete quadriplegia.

THORACIC SPINE.[54,55,57,58] The rib cage is attached to the thoracic spine, making this the stiffest and most mechanically stable portion of the spine. As a result, greater force is required to injure this region. Although thoracic spinal cord injuries are less common than cervical, they are more likely to be complete. This may reflect the fact that the thoracic spinal canal is smaller than in the cervical or lumbar spine. Although the stiffness of the thoracic spine protects it somewhat from the effects of perpendicular forces, it is still vulnerable to vertical compression and flexion injury. The thoracic spine may be compressed from above by a falling object or from below when landing on the feet or buttocks after a fall. This region of the spine is also at particular risk for vascular injury because of its dependence on perfusion by vessels from both above and below it. Direct injury by penetrating violence (e.g., stab wounds or gunshot wounds) is not uncommon.

THORACOLUMBAR SPINE.[54,55,57,58] The thoracolumbar spine is second only to the cervical spine in the frequency of injury. The transition that occurs here from an area of rigidity provided by the rib cage to the more mobile lumbar spine makes this a likely site of injury. The shift from terminal spinal cord to cauda equina and the increasing width of the spinal canal between T-11 and L-2, however, mitigates somewhat the neurologic damage produced by trauma to this region of the spine.

LOWER LUMBAR SPINE AND SACRUM.[54,55,57,58] Although the lower lumbar spine lacks the stability afforded by the rib cage, it is supported by strong paraspinal and abdominal muscles. Falls from heights producing vertical compression are the most common injury, followed by flexion injury and penetrating wounds (e.g., gunshots). The neurologic damage resulting from trauma to the lumbar spine is usually incomplete, because of relatively rich vascular supply, a wide spinal canal, and the fact that the spinal cord is not present within the vertebral canal (e.g., the cauda equina).

Pathophysiology of Injury[19,54,57–62]

Compression or shearing of the spinal cord results in destruction of both gray and white matter. Damage is greatest at the level of injury but may extend for several segments above or below this site. In most traumatic lesions, the central part of the cord suffers greater damage than the peripheral parts. **The neurologic damage that results from trauma is only partly due to the initial damage to the cord neurons. Much of the damage is caused by the evolving sequelae of the initial insult.**[60–62] Within hours of the initial trauma, a process of progressive tissue destruction begins within the cord, which can significantly extend the region of neuronal damage. **These secondary reactions,** by mechanisms not entirely understood, **lead to ischemia, edema, demyelination, and necrosis of the spinal cord.** In the hope of developing better therapeutic measures, considerable research has been carried out on both laboratory animals and postmortem human specimens in an effort to define the pathophysiologic mechanisms underlying these secondary effects. Among the factors implicated are hemorrhage, ischemia, local electrolyte derangements, inflammatory reactions, and the local accumulation of various bioreactive substances.[54,55,60–62] With time, the necrotic region of the spinal cord undergoes resorption and is replaced by scar tissue or the formation of cysts or cavities.

Functional Classification of Spinal Cord Injury

Spinal cord injuries are usually divided into two broad functional categories: quadriplegia and paraplegia.[53,54] Quadriplegia is partial or complete paralysis of all four extremities and the trunk, including the respiratory muscles and results from lesions of the cervical cord. Paraplegia is partial or complete paralysis of all or part of the trunk and both lower extremities and results from lesions of the thoracic and lumbar spinal cord or sacral roots. **Patients are further characterized by the level of the lesion, which is usually defined by the most distal uninvolved nerve root segment with normal function. In addition, a spinal lesion is defined as** *complete* **if there is no sensory or voluntary motor function below the level of the neurologic injury and is defined as** *incomplete* **if there is some preservation of sensory or motor function below the level of the lesion.** Thus, a patient who has an intact C-7 nerve root segment with no sensory or motor function below C-7 would be classified as a C-7 complete quadriplegic. If some sensation or motor function were evident below C-7, the patient would be classified as a C-7 incomplete quadriplegic. In reality, injury to the spinal cord often manifests as asymmetric motor or sensory deficits, and it may be necessary to designate the most distal nerve root segment with normal function on each side of the body. Several semiquantitative scales have been developed to more precisely define the neurologic function remaining after spinal cord injury.[63] As described previously spinal cord injury may also be classified according to neuroanatomic criteria.

RECOMMENDED READINGS

Adams, JH and Duchen, LW (eds): Greenfield's Neuropathology, ed 5. Chapters 10 and 17. Oxford University Press, New York, 1992.

Adams, RD and Victor, M: Principles of Neurology, ed 5. Chapter 45. Diseases of the Spinal Cord. McGraw-Hill, New York, 1993.

Barr, ML and Kiernan, JA: The Human Nervous System, ed 6. Chapters 5 and 19. JB Lippincott, Philadelphia, 1993.

Biller, J and Brazis, PW: The Localization of Lesions Affecting the Spinal Cord, ed 2. Chapter 4. In Brazis, PW, Masdeu, JC, and Biller, J: Localization in Clinical Neurology. Little, Brown, & Company, Boston, 1990.

Carpenter, MB. Neuroanatomy, ed 4. Chapter 4. Tracts of the Spinal Cord. Williams & Wilkins, Baltimore, 1991.

Chadwick, D, Cartlidge, N, and Bates, D: Medical Neurology. Chapter 9. Disorders of the Spinal Cord and Cauda Equina. Churchill Livingstone, Edinburgh, 1989.

deGroat, WC and Booth, AM: Autonomic Systems to the Urinary Bladder and Sexual Organs. Chapter 12. In Dyck, PJ and Thomas, PK (eds): Peripheral Neuropathy, ed 3. WB Saunders, Philadelphia, 1993.

deMyer, W: Anatomy and Clinical Neurology of the Spinal Cord. Chapter 43. In Joynt, RJ (ed): Clinical Neurology, vol 3. JB Lippincott, Philadelphia, 1993.

Errico, TJ, et al (eds): Spinal Trauma. JB Lippincott, Philadelphia, 1990.

Martin, JH: Neuroanatomy: Text and Atlas. Chapters 5 and 9. Elsevier, New York, 1991.

Nolte, J: The Human Brain: An Introduction to Its Functional Anatomy, ed 3. Chapter 7. Spinal Cord. Mosby-Year Book, St. Louis, 1993.

Powell, M: Neurological Manifestations of Vertebral Column Disorders. Chapter 114. In Asbury, AK, McKhann, GM, and McDonald, WI (eds): Diseases of the Nervous System: Clinical Neurobiology, ed 2. WB Saunders, Philadelphia, 1992.

Rothman, RH and Simeone, FA (eds): The Spine, ed 3. WB Saunders, Philadelphia, 1991.

Rothwell, JC: Control of Human Voluntary Movement. Chapter 7. Ascending and Descending Pathways of the Spinal Cord. Aspen Publishers, Rockville, MD, 1987.

Rowland, LP: Clinical Syndromes of the Spinal Cord and Brainstem. Chapter 46. In Kandel, ER, Schwartz, JH, and Jessell, TM (eds): Principles of Neural Science, ed 3. Appleton & Lange, Norwalk, CT, 1991.

Schmitz, TJ: Traumatic Spinal Cord Injury. Chapter 26. In O'Sullivan, SB and Schmitz, TJ: Physical Rehabilitation: Assessment and Treatment, ed 3. FA Davis, Philadelphia, 1994.

Somers, MF: Spinal Cord Injury: Functional Rehabilitation. Appleton & Lange, Norwalk, CT, 1991.

Woolsey, RM and Young, RR: Disorders of the Spinal Cord. Neurol Clin 9(3):1, 1991.

REFERENCES

1. Nolte, J: The Human Brain: An Introduction to Its Functional Anatomy, ed 3. Chapter 7. Spinal Cord. Mosby-Year Book, St. Louis, 1993.
2. Carpenter, MB. Neuroanatomy, ed 4. Chapter 4. Tracts of the Spinal Cord. Williams & Wilkins, Baltimore, 1991.
3. Barr, ML and Kiernan, JA: The Human Nervous System: An Anatomical Viewpoint, ed 6. Chapter 5. Spinal Cord. JB Lippincott, Philadelphia, 1993.
4. Rothwell, JC: Control of Human Voluntary Movement. Chapter 7. Ascending and Descending Pathways of the Spinal Cord. Aspen Publishers, Rockville, MD, 1987.
5. Martin, JH: Neuroanatomy: Text and Atlas. Chapter 9. Descending Projection Systems and the Motor Function of the Spinal Cord. Elsevier, New York, 1989.
6. Barr, ML and Kiernan, JA: The Human Nervous System: An Anatomical Viewpoint, ed 6. Chapter 23. Motor Systems. JB Lippincott, Philadelphia, 1993.
7. Martin, JH: Neuroanatomy: Text and Atlas. Chapter 5. The Somatic Sensory System. Appleton & Lange, Norwalk, CT, 1989.
8. Barr, ML and Kiernan, JA: The Human Nervous System: An Anatomical Viewpoint, ed 6. Chapter 19. General Sensory Systems. JB Lippincott, Philadelphia, 1993.
9. Schoenen, J and Gunnar, G: Spinal Cord Connections. Chapter 4. In Paxinos, G (ed): The Human Nervous System. Academic Press, San Diego, 1990.
10. Willis, WD, Jr: The Peripheral Nervous System, ed 3. Chapter 7. In Berne, RM and Levy, MN (eds): Physiology. Mosby-Year Book, St. Louis, 1993.
11. Martin, JH and Jessell, TM: Anatomy of the Somatic Sensory System. Chapter 25. In Kandel, ER, Schwartz, JH, and Jessell, TM (eds): Principles of Neural Science, ed 3. Appleton & Lange, Norwalk, CT, 1991.
12. Daube, JR, et al: Medical Neurosciences, ed 2. Chapter 13. The Spinal Level. Little, Brown & Company, Boston, 1986.
13. Rowland, LP: Clinical Syndromes of the Spinal Cord and Brainstem. Chapter 46. In Kandel, ER, Schwartz, JH, and Jessell, TM (eds): Principles of Neural Science, ed 3. Appleton & Lange, Norwalk, CT, 1991.
14. Schoenen, J: Clinical Anatomy of the Spinal Cord. Neurol Clin 9(3):503, 1991.
15. Woolsey, RM and Young, RR: The Clinical Diagnosis of Disorders of the Spinal Cord. Neurol Clin 9(3):573, 1991.
16. deMyer, W: Anatomy and Clinical Neurology of the Spinal Cord. Chapter 43. In Joynt, RJ (ed): Clinical Neurology, vol 3. JB Lippincott, Philadelphia, 1991.
17. Biller, J and Brazis, DW: The Localization of Lesions Affecting the Spinal Cord. Chapter 4. In Brazis, PW, Masdeu, JC, and Biller, J: Localization in Clinical Neurology, ed 2. Little, Brown & Company, Boston, 1990.
18. Stern, J: Neurologic Evaluation and Neurologic Sequelae of the Spinal Cord Injured Patient. Chapter 9. In Lee, BY, et al (ed): The Spinal Cord Injured Patient: Comprehensive Management. WB Saunders, Philadelphia, 1991.
19. Donovan, WH: Neurologic and Orthopedic Considerations. Chapter 3. In Whiteneck, G (ed): Management of High Quadriplegia. Demos Publishing, New York, 1991.
20. Woolsey, RM: Chronic Pain Following Spinal Cord Injury. J Am Paraplegia Soc 9:39, 1986.
21. Nanninga, JB: Anticipated Urologic-Sexual Dysfunction. Chapter 11. In Meyer, PR, Jr (ed): Surgery of Spine Trauma. Churchill Livingstone, New York, 1989.
22. deGroat, WC and Booth, AM: Autonomic Systems to the Urinary Bladder and Sexual Organs. Chapter 12. In Dyck, PJ and Thomas, PK (eds): Peripheral Neuropathy, ed 3. WB Saunders, Philadelphia, 1993.
23. Krane, RJ and Siroky, MB: Clinical Neuro-Urology, ed 2. Part III. Neurogenic Vesico-urethral Dysfunction. Little, Brown & Company, Boston, 1991.
24. Abdel-Azim, M, Sullivan, M, and Yalla, SV: Disorders of Bladder Function in Spinal Cord Disease. Neurol Clin 9(3):727, 1991.
25. Bors, E and Comarr, AE: Neurologic Disturbances of Sexual Dysfunction with Special Reference to 529 Patients with Spinal Cord Injury. Urol Surv 10:191, 1960.
26. Seftel, RD, Oates, RD, and Krane, RJ: Disturbed Sexual Function in Patients with Spinal Cord Disease. Neurol Clin 9(3):757, 1991.
27. Schmitt, J, Midha, M, and McKenzie, N: Medical Complications of Spinal Cord Disease. Neurol Clin 9:779, 1991.
28. Morgan, MDL, Silver, JR, and Williams, JJ: The Respiratory System of the Spinal Cord Patient. Chapter 3. In Bloch, RF and Basbaum, M (eds): Management of Spinal Cord Injuries. Williams & Wilkins, Baltimore, 1986.

29. Chadwick, D, Cartlidge, N, and Bates, D: Medical Neurology. Chapter 9. Disorders of the Spinal Cord and Cauda Equina. Churchill Livingstone, Edinburgh, 1989.

30. Bastian, HC: On the Symptomatology of Total Transverse Lesions of the Spinal Cord with Special Reference to the Condition of Various Reflexes. Med Clin Trans 73:151, 1980.

31. Koehler, PJ and Endtz, LJ: The Brown-Séquard Syndrome: True or False? Arch Neurol 43:921, 1986.

32. Adams, RD and Victor, M: Principles of Neurology, ed 5. Chapter 45. Diseases of the Spinal Cord. McGraw-Hill, New York, 1993.

33. Elghazawi, AK: Clinical Syndromes and Differential Diagnosis of Spinal Disorders. Radiol Clin North Am 29(4):651, 1991.

34. Berger, JR, Levy, RM, and Snodgrass, S: Medical Myelopathies. Chapter 41. In Rothman, RH and Simeone, FA (eds): The Spine, ed 3. WB Saunders, Philadelphia, 1991.

35. Hughes, JT: Disorders of the Spine and Spinal Cord. Chapter 17. In Adams, JH and Duchen, LW (eds): Greenfield's Neuropathology, ed 5. Oxford University Press, New York, 1992.

36. Hughes, JT: Neuropathology of the Spinal Cord. Neurol Clin 9(3):551, 1991.

37. Adams, RD and Salam-Adams, M: Chronic Nontraumatic Diseases of the Spinal Cord. Neurol Clin 9(3):605, 1991.

38. Harding, BN: Malformations of the Nervous System. Chapter 10. In Adams, JH and Duchen, LW (eds): Greenfield's Neuropathology, ed 5. Oxford University Press, New York, 1992.

39. Sutton, L: Congenital Anomalies of the Spinal Cord. Chapter 11. In Rothman, RH and Simeone, FA (eds): The Spine, ed 3. WB Saunders, Philadelphia, 1991.

40. Finlayson, AI: Syringomyelia and Related Conditions. Chapter 45. In Joynt, RJ (ed): Clinical Neurology, vol 3. JB Lippincott, Philadelphia, 1991.

41. Madsen, PW, Green, BA, and Bowen, BC: Syringomyelia. Chapter 42. In Rothman, RH and Simeone, FA (eds): The Spine, ed 3. WB Saunders, Philadelphia, 1991.

42. Batzdorf, U (ed): Syringomyelia: Current Concepts in Diagnosis and Treatment. Williams & Wilkins, Baltimore, 1991.

43. Bohlman, HH and Emery, SE: The Pathophysiology of Cervical Spondylosis and Myelopathy. Spine 13:843, 1988.

44. Connell, MD and Wiesel, SW: Natural History of Cervical Disk Disease. Orthop Clin North Am 23(3):369, 1992.

45. Herskovitz, S, et al: Spinal Cord Toxoplasmosis in AIDS. Neurology 39:1552, 1989.

46. Berman, M, et al: Acute Transverse Myelitis: Incidence and Etiologic Considerations. Neurology 31:966, 1981.

47. Dawson, DM and Potts, F: Acute Nontraumatic Myelopathies. Neurol Clin 9(3):585, 1991.

48. Satran, R: Spinal Cord Infarction. Stroke 19:529, 1988.

49. Sandson, TA and Friedman, JH: Spinal Cord Infarction: Report of 8 Cases and Review of the Literature. Medicine 68:282, 1989.

50. Stein, BM and Soloman, RA: Arteriovenous Malformations of the Spinal Cord. Chapter 40. In Rothman, RH and Simeone, FA (eds): The Spine, ed 3. WB Saunders, Philadelphia, 1991.

51. Masaryk, TJ: Neoplastic Disease of the Spine. Radiol Clin North Am 29(4):829, 1991.

52. Tall, RL and DeVault, W: Spinal Injury in Sport: Epidemiological Considerations. Clin Sports Med 12(3):441, 1993.

53. Schmitz, TJ: Traumatic Spinal Cord Injury. Chapter 26. In O'Sullivan, SB and Schmitz, TJ: Physical Rehabilitation: Assessment and Treatment, ed 3. FA Davis, Philadelphia, 1994.

54. Somers, MF: Spinal Cord Injury: Functional Rehabilitation. Chapter 2. Spinal Cord Injuries. Appleton & Lange, Norwalk, CT, 1991.

55. Bohlman, HH and Ducker, TB: Spine and Spinal Cord Injuries. Chapter 28. In Rothman, RH and Simeone, FA (eds): The Spine, ed 3. WB Saunders, Philadelphia, 1991.

56. Apple, DF, Jr: Spinal Cord Injury. Chapter 6. In Fletcher, GF, et al (eds): Rehabilitation Medicine: Contemporary Clinical Perspectives. Lea & Febiger, Philadelphia, 1992.

57. Jellinger, K: Pathology of Spinal Cord Trauma. Chapter 18. In Errico, TJ, et al (eds): Spinal Trauma. JB Lippincott, Philadelphia, 1990.

58. Meyer, PR Jr, et al: Spinal Cord Injury. Neurol Clin 9(3):625, 1991.

59. Meyer, PR, Jr: Cervical Spine: Overview and Conservative Management. Chapter 14. In Meyer, PR, Jr. (ed): Surgery of Spine Trauma. Churchill Livingstone, New York. 1989.

60. Anderson, DK and Hall, ED: Pathophysiology of Spinal Cord Trauma. Ann Emerg Med 22(6):987, 1993.

61. Tator, CH and Fehlings, MG: Review of the Secondary Injury Theory of Acute Spinal Cord Trauma with Emphasis on Vascular Mechanisms. J Neurosurg 75(1):15, 1991.

62. Martinez-Arizala, A, Green, BA, and Bunge, RP: Experimental Spinal Cord Injury: Pathophysiology and Treatment. Chapter 32. In Rothman, RH and Simeone, FA (eds): The Spine, ed 3. WB Saunders, Philadelphia, 1991.

63. American Spinal Injury Association. Standards for Neurologic Classification of Spinal Cord Injury Patients. 2020 Peachtree Road, NW, Atlanta, GA 30309.

CHAPTER 18

■

Parkinson's Disease and Other Involuntary Movement Disorders of the Basal Ganglia

James G. Phillips, PhD,
and
George E. Stelmach, EdD

- ■ *General Concepts Related to Normal Movement*
- ■ *Parkinson's Disease*
- ■ *Huntington's Disease*
- ■ *Tourette's Syndrome*
- ■ *Other Movement Disorders*
- ■ *Conclusions*

As outlined in Chapter 9, the basal ganglia consist of a number of subcortical nuclei. The putamen and caudate nucleus are the principal input nuclei, whereas the internal segment of the globus pallidus and the substantia nigra pars reticulata make up the principal output nuclei. Additional nuclei of the basal ganglia, such as the external segment of the globus pallidus, the subthalamic nucleus, the substantia nigra pars compacta, and to a lesser extent, the pedunculopontine nucleus, constitute reentrant loops, which modify the activity of the main input and output nuclei.

The putamen and caudate nucleus receive widespread cortical inputs, whereas the internal globus pallidus and substantia nigra pars reticulata appear to have more circumscribed effects on specific cortical areas via thalamic relay nuclei. This apparent funneling of influences suggests that the basal ganglia have a selective role in the control of movement. Indeed, disturbances of this selective role in basal ganglia disease can cause both problems of voluntary movements and involuntary movements.

Extrinsic and intrinsic connections of the basal ganglia have a topographic organization, which appears to be maintained functionally. The basal ganglia may therefore consist of a number of relatively segregated parallel circuits, centered primarily on the putamen, caudate nucleus, and ventral striatum, which perform motor, cognitive, and limbic functions, respectively (see Chapter 9). Basal ganglia diseases cause disorders of movement, as well as disturbances of cognitive processes and emotion.[1]

This chapter addresses the disorders of voluntary movement, as well as the involuntary movements caused by basal ganglia disease. Since a disease state does not necessarily respect the topographic and anatomic boundaries of the parallel circuits running through the basal ganglia, any basal ganglia disease may cause disturbances in a number of putative basal ganglia functions. Nevertheless, Parkinson's disease is thought to serve as an example of disruption of the motor circuit, whereas Huntington's disease is thought to cause disruption of cognitive circuits and Tourette's syndrome has been proposed to disrupt limbic circuits. More specific disorders such as focal dystonia may illustrate the parallelism inherent within basal ganglia circuits, whereas hemiballismus illustrates a potential axial/proximal organization of the motor circuit. Both Parkinson's disease and Huntington's disease illustrate disturbances of voluntary movement, and Huntington's disease and Tourette's syndrome illustrate involuntary movements.

General Concepts Related to Normal Movement

To understand disordered movement, it is important to have an understanding of normal movement. Normal unskilled movements tend to be jerky and hesitant and use visual feedback and successive corrections to approximate a desired goal. The extent to which feedback guidance is used can be inferred to some degree from the duration of the movement and the jerkiness of the movement and from any prolongation of the period spent decelerating at the termination of a movement.[2] With the development of skill, an internal representation (a motor program) forms, such that the movement is prepared in advance and executed ballistically without the same use of visual feedback. Since it is not feasible to have a program for every unique movement, it has been proposed that programs are more generalized in nature and that parameters are specified for each unique movement. The extent to which a movement is programmed in advance can to some degree be inferred from the response latency, the speed, smoothness, and fluency of the movement, and the proportionately greater periods of time spent in the accelerative phase of movement.[3] **Basal ganglia disorders such as Parkinson's disease and Huntington's disease seem to degrade the programmed control of movement, so that patients rely on feedback guidance to control their movements. In addition, disorders such as Tourette's syndrome and Huntington's disease seem to cause the inappropriate release of fragments of motor programs.**

Parkinson's Disease

Parkinson's disease affects about 1% of the population older than 65 years of age.[4] **The cardinal features of Parkinson's disease are problems of voluntary movement.**[5-8] **The disease causes both akinesia** (difficulty initiating movement) **and bradykinesia** (slowness and difficulty maintaining movement). **Parkinson's disease is also associated with involuntary movement.** The disease causes both **tremor** and muscle **rigidity.** In addition, **it may cause emotional and cognitive disturbances.** Depression has been linked to Parkinson's disease, and up to 33% of patients have been reported to be demented in later stages of the disease.[5]

Parkinson's disease can be caused by toxins, infection, or trauma. There are also inherited variants of the disease.[6-9] The cause of the majority of cases is unknown (idiopathic Parkinson's disease), but the discovery of the neurotoxic effects of the substance, MPTP (1-methyl-4-phenyl-1,2,3,6-tetrahydropyridine) suggests that it may be caused by cumulative exposure to some environmental toxin.[6-9] **The severity of Parkinson's disease correlates well with the extent of degeneration of dopaminergic neurons in the substantia**

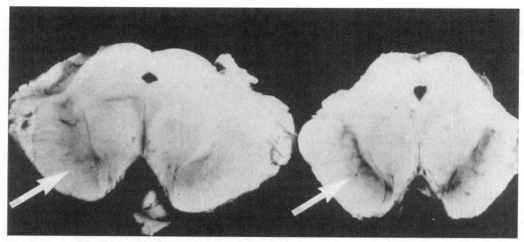

Figure 18–1.   *The Substantia Nigra in Parkinson's Disease.* The upper layer (zona compacta) of the substantia nigra normally has many melanin-containing neurons. In this transverse section through the midbrain (*Left*), the substantia nigra of a patient with Parkinson's disease shows a marked depletion of melanin-containing nerve cells. This produces a characteristic pallor (depigmentation) compared with a normal control (*Right*). (From Rowland, LP (ed): Merritt's Textbook of Neurology, ed 8. Copyright © Lea & Febiger, Philadelphia, 1989, p 659, with permission.)

nigra pars compacta.[6–8,10] Even so, 80% of the cells in the substantia nigra pars compacta may be lost before Parkinson's disease is clinically evident (Fig. 18–1). Subclinical losses of dopaminergic cells appear to be offset by increases in the rate of synthesis and release of dopamine.[11] Since dopamine concentrations are reduced more in the putamen than in the caudate nucleus,[12] and the putamen is a primary component of the motor circuit, there is a preponderance of motor symptoms in Parkinson's disease.

As outlined in Chapter 9, dopaminergic cells in the substantia nigra pars compacta receive inputs from the ventral striatum. These dopaminergic cells appear to modulate the activity of the striatum by means of two types of receptors: D_1 and D_2. D_1 receptors appear to have an excitatory effect on the direct pathway (which has an excitatory role) through the basal ganglia, whereas D_2 receptors appear to have an inhibitory effect on the indirect pathway (which has an inhibitory role) through the basal ganglia. **The loss of dopaminergic neurons from the substantia nigra pars compacta leads to loss of activity in the direct pathway,[6–8,13] and a reduction in spontaneous movement.**

Treatment is primarily palliative and is directed at improving the quality of life by restoring lost dopaminergic function with dopamine precursors or dopamine agonists.[14,15] The decline in dopaminergic influence (linked to akinesia and bradykinesia) may also produce a relative excess of cholinergic activity (linked to tremor and rigidity). Accordingly, anticholinergics are sometimes used to control rigidity and tremor. Unfortunately, after several years of chronic dopaminergic therapy, treatment may become increasingly ineffective for some patients, such that the patient may be mobile at some times and immobile at other times (on-off phenomenon). Higher doses of dopaminergic agents can produce dyskinesias (abnormal, involuntary, choreiform movements) and to a lesser extent cognitive disturbance. Anticholinergic agents in higher doses may also cause cognitive disturbances.[14,15]

Akinesia

Akinesia, which is prominent in patients with Parkinson's disease, is thought to be the result of problems in the preparation of movement. This view is supported by studies of response latency as measured by reaction time and by studies of the electrical potential occurring before movement (the Bereitschaftspotential), which may indicate the preparatory activity of structures such as the supplementary motor area.[16]

Reaction Times and Response Latency

Researchers infer the extent of preparatory processing from the duration of the period before a response is initiated to a stimulus (**reaction time**). Patients are asked to initiate their movements quickly in response to a stimulus. A longer reaction time indicates that more preparation is required for the movement. It is reasoned that the more complex the movement, the more preparation that is required, and thus the longer the reaction time. Therefore, researchers expect that movement complexity and disease states should prolong preparatory processes, leading to longer reaction times. By systematically varying the complexity of the required movements (e.g., movement direction or accuracy), researchers can assess the time to prepare specific movement parameters. In particular, researchers are interested in parameters of movement that cause patients disproportionate problems, in the hope that this will indicate the specific nature of the impairment in preparatory processes.[17]

The classic experiments have compared the performance of Parkinson's disease patients with that of age-matched controls on simple reaction time tasks (one stimulus and one response) and more complex choice reaction time tasks (e.g., two stimuli and two responses). **Patients with Parkinson's disease typically have prolonged simple reaction times, but their choice reaction times are relatively normal** (Fig. 18–2). However, there are two problems with such experiments. First, it is never possible from these studies to determine whether any differences noted are a result of an increase in the number of **stimuli** to attend to or are due to an increase in the number of **responses** to perform. Second, since the emphasis of such research is on disproportionate increases in **difficulty** as indicated by increases in reaction time, it implies that patients are **less** affected by increasing task demands.[17] This is unlikely to be the case, since patients can have problems with more complicated cognitive tasks, particularly in the later stages of the disease. Instead, patients have problems performing simple, automatic tasks. In Parkinson's disease, the simple direct route through the basal ganglia is not functioning properly, and tasks are probably performed using more complicated strategies.

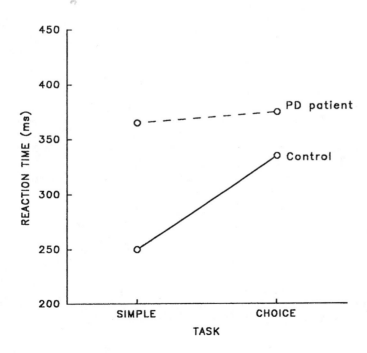

Figure 18–2. *Task Complexity and Parkinson's Disease.* Patients with Parkinson's disease typically have prolonged simple reaction times, but their choice (i.e., more complex) reaction times are relatively normal.

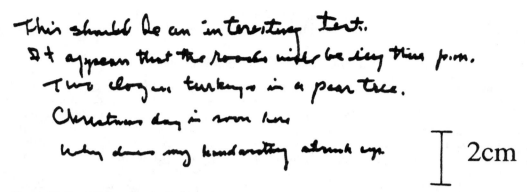

Figure 18–3. *Micrographia in Parkinson's Disease.* Patients with Parkinson's disease may have problems maintaining the scale of their movements. (From Phillips, JG, Stelmach, GE, and Teasdale, N: What can indices of handwriting quality tell us about parkinsonian handwriting? Hum Movt Sci 10:301, 1991, with permission.)

Patients with Parkinson's disease appear to have some problem with the production of simple, relatively automatic movements. Since the shape of movements (e.g., written letters) is intact, but the movements are reduced in size and speed (Fig. 18–3), this might mean that patients have problems specifying parameters such as the size and speed of movement.[18] As one way of studying this possibility, Stelmach and associates[19] looked at the ability of patients with Parkinson's disease to use advance information to specify parameters of their movement. They provided an initial warning stimulus (precue), and then an imperative stimulus signifying movement was required. The precue could be uninformative, or it could specify which arm to move, the direction to move, or the extent of movement (or more complex combinations such as direction and extent). Although patients took longer in movement preparation and were slower in execution, the investigators did not find that any specific parameter was more difficult to prepare than any other. In addition, patients seemed to specify their movement parameters at about the same rate as normal subjects of the same age.

This normal specification of movement parameters is surprising, in view of our previous clinical observations. Perhaps we have focused on the wrong sort of movement parameters. We know from Chapter 9 that the basal ganglia principally affect the supplementary motor area, which has more of a role in the proximal control of movement. Even so, the reaction times for proximal and distal movements do not appear to be differentially affected by Parkinson's disease.[20] However, we know that the basal ganglia consist of relatively segregated parallel circuits. Indeed, Parkinson's disease is very heterogeneous in its effects, initially affecting the left or right side or upper or lower limb. Patients may have problems with a definite movement parameter, but each patient might differ as to which specific parameter is affected (e.g., left versus right side). Alternatively, the basal ganglia may act in a massively parallel fashion, in concert across a number of muscle groups.[21] Although we have been looking for impairment in a specific parameter (e.g., as a voice in a crowd), the basal ganglia may serve to specify many parameters (e.g., as a coordinated choir).

Although patients with Parkinson's disease do not appear to have problems in the specification of movement parameters, they do appear to have problems maintaining readiness for a movement. Patients with Parkinson's disease appear less able to use warning information to prepare their movement,[22,23] and to maintain such a preparatory state during the performance of sequential movements, particularly when the movements involve disparate elements.[13]

More specifically, **patients with Parkinson's disease seem to have a problem with an internal cue that signals when their movements should occur.** However, it must be noted that such an internal cue is specific to simple learned movements, and *not* for any response

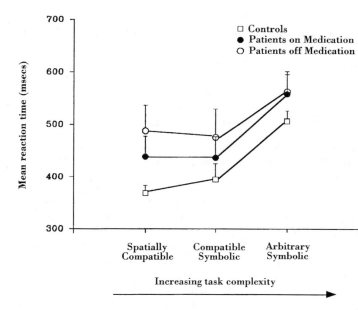

Figure 18–4. *Parkinsonian Medication Improves Performance on Simple Tasks.* Patients with Parkinson's disease usually show more impairment on simple tasks, unless there is a substantial cognitive decline. In this experiment involving tasks of varying complexity, medication promoted the greatest improvement (i.e., shortened reaction time) in the simpler tasks. (Reprinted from Neuropsychologia 31. Brown, VH, et al: Dopamine dependent reaction time deficits in patients with Parkinson's disease are task specific, p 459, 1993, with kind permission from Elsevier Science, Ltd, The Boulevard, Langford Lane, Kidlington OX5 IGb, UK.)

that follows internally generated rules. Brown and colleagues[24] examined the ability of Parkinson's disease patients to follow complex, incompatible, internally generated rules when performing button pressing tasks. In particular, they considered the extent to which these abilities were affected by medication status, reasoning that abilities directly affected by Parkinson's disease would show the most improvement when patients took their medication. Medication caused the greatest improvement in performance of simple tasks and no improvement in performance of the most complex tasks (Fig. 18–4).

Bereitschaftspotential

The Bereitschaftspotential is a surface electroencephalographic potential that occurs before voluntary movement, which may indicate preparatory neural activity.[16] The early component has its peak amplitude over the midline and reflects supplementary motor area activity, whereas late components are greatest in the hemisphere contralateral to movement and reflect activity of other cortical areas. There are reports that the early component of the Bereitschaftspotential is reduced in patients with Parkinson's disease, whereas the late component of the Bereitschaftspotential is greater. This implies impaired or inadequate preparatory activity, which is combined with an increased reliance on alternative mechanisms for controlling movement.[16] Converging evidence from studies of regional cerebral blood flow indicate that activity of the supplementary motor area is indeed impaired in patients with Parkinson's disease and that medication allows the supplementary motor area to function more normally when patients perform motor tasks.[25]

Other Factors Contributing to Akinesia

Thus far, we have limited our discussion to how disturbances in preparatory processes can contribute to akinesia. However, Narabayashi[26] suggested that akinesia may arise in three different ways:

1. Akinesia can be a direct result of impaired preparatory processes, caused by nigrostriatal dopamine deficiency, and thus can be treated by dopamine replacement therapy.

2. Akinesia can be a secondary consequence of rigidity, caused by the release of control of thalamic structures, and thus can be relieved by stereotaxic lesions of the ventrolateral nucleus of the thalamus.

3. Akinesia can be associated with depressive mood and attentional disturbances in later stages of the disease.

Bradykinesia

The movements of **Parkinson's patients are typically slow and hesitant, with an increased reliance on visual feedback.** There is sometimes a tendency to dismiss bradykinesia as the end product of impaired preparatory processes (akinesia). However, it is not that simple. In fact, akinesia and bradykinesia may to some extent reflect different mechanisms. This is suggested by the following: akinesia remains consistently more difficult to demonstrate than bradykinesia; the degree of akinesia does not correlate with bradykinesia; and it is bradykinesia that responds to dopamine therapy.[17]

Hallett and Khoshbin[27] suggest that patients with Parkinson's disease have problems energizing their muscles. This is not a simple problem of muscle strength, but one of coordination and activation.[28] Patients require more cycles of agonist and antagonist muscle activity to perform the same movement as age-matched controls. **Patients simply cannot produce movement forces as quickly, accurately, or smoothly as normal subjects do** (Fig. 18–5)[17]. Such problems in the accuracy of force production lead patients to undershoot their aiming movements and to produce more force when a precision grip is required.

There is reason to believe that problems in the control of movement forces are compounded during production of more complex simultaneous movements or complex movement sequences (particularly those comprising disparate movements).[17] For example,

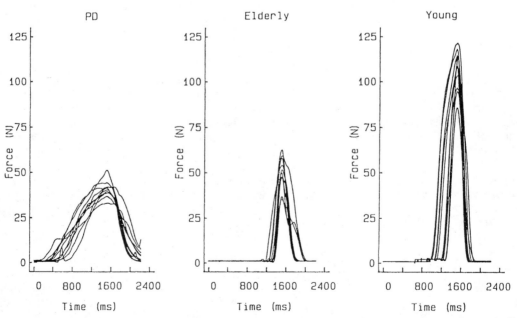

Figure 18–5. *Irregular Force Production in Patients with Parkinson's Disease.* Representative trials in which patients with Parkinson's disease, an elderly subject, and a young subject produced 45% of their maximum force. Patients with Parkinson's disease show slower and less regular force production. (From Stelmach, GE, et al: Force production characteristics in Parkinson's disease. Exp Brain Res 76:165, 1989. Permission by Oxford University Press.)

Bennett and associates [29] examined how a reaching-and-grasping movement was affected in a patient unilaterally affected by Parkinson's disease (Fig. 18–6). Whereas reaching and the opening of the hand for grasping are near-simultaneous movements in healthy adults,

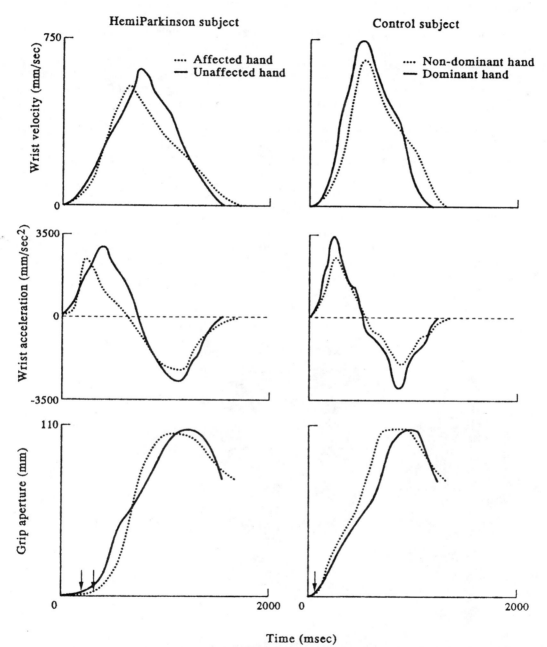

Figure 18–6. *Coordination of Reaching and Grasping Movements in Patients with Parkinson's Disease.* Kinematic profiles obtained from a single reach to grasp a large cylinder at 40 cm distance for a hemiparkinsonian patient (*Left*) and a control subject (*Right*). The vertical arrows indicate the onset of the manipulation component. (Reprinted from Neuropsychologia 31. Bennett, KMB, et al: A kinematic study of the reach to group movement in a study with hemi-Parkinson's disease, p 713, 1993, with kind permission from Elsevier Science, Ltd, The Boulevard, Langford Lane, Kidlington OX5 IGb, UK.)

parkinsonian movements were found to be slower in reaching for objects and, in particular, were delayed in the opening of the hand ready to grip the object. After the hand was open, it reached maximum aperture sooner, indicating less precise control over grip. The patient's affected hand tended to perform like a clumsy nondominant hand. Such observations indicate dysfunction in the performance of near-simultaneous or sequential movement.

Although we have suggested that bradykinesia reflects defective force control, the slowness and jerkiness of movement could also be associated with tremor or depression. Tremor can entrain patients' movements, such that they can have trouble moving at a frequency that differs from that of their tremor.[30] Whereas tremor may contribute to problems in timing movements, parkinsonian tremor occurs at rest and can be alleviated by stereotaxic lesions to the ventralis intermedius nucleus of the thalamus, and so is unlikely to be the sole cause of bradykinesia. Depression can lead to slower movement, and although severity of depression may be related to rate of force production,[28] patients with depressive symptoms do not show the precise problems coordinating simultaneous movements seen in patients with Parkinson's disease.[31]

Rigidity

An increased (but uniform) resistance to passive muscle stretch in patients with Parkinson's disease is known as *muscle rigidity*. Both an increase in muscle tone and an inability to relax contribute to postural abnormalities in these patients (Fig. 18–7). Rigidity is reflexive in origin, although its exact cause is still unclear. It is abolished by dorsal root

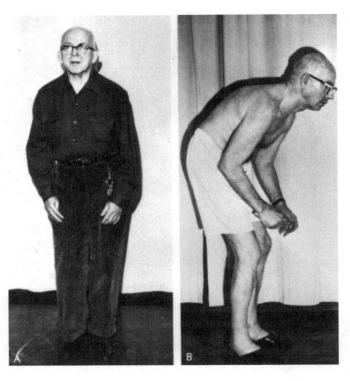

Figure 18–7. Posture and Parkinson's Disease. The body posture of a patient with Parkinson's disease. (*A*) Front view. (*B*) Side view. (From Rowland, LP (ed): Merritt's Textbook of Neurology, ed 7. Copyright © Lea & Febiger, Philadelphia, p 529, with permission.)

section and by intramuscular injection of local anesthetic. Although **peripheral** mechanisms (e.g., H-reflex, tendon jerk, and short-latency stretch reflexes) appear relatively intact, rigidity seems to result from the abnormal responses of **central** mechanisms to stretch.[16] Rigidity appears to be due to exaggerated tonic stretch reflexes such as the shortening reaction (shortening of unloaded muscles), which is enhanced in patients with Parkinson's disease. Rigidity may contribute to akinesia and bradykinesia as well as promote the development of contractures and postural deformities (see Fig. 18–7).[32]

Tremor

About 70% of patients with Parkinson's disease experience involuntary rhythmic movement at rest, which is most noticeable in the distal extremities and most evident following movement. Such tremor is exacerbated by stress and reduced by voluntary movement. This resting tremor occurs at a frequency of 4 to 6 Hz. Tremors are additive and may be worse in specific postures when postural tremor contributes. The tremor disappears when the limb is moved or when the patient is asleep (although getting to sleep may be a problem in patients with severe tremor).

Animal experimentation suggests that resting tremor is driven at a thalamic or cortical level, since tremor is not stopped by the elimination of peripheral mechanisms (whether by deafferentation or by paralysis).[16] Resting tremor can be produced in animals through damage to the nigrostriatal dopaminergic pathway, combined with damage to cerebellar rubrothalamic pathways.[12] Stereotaxic surgery in humans indicates that the ventralis intermedius nucleus of the thalamus has a role in the generation of tremor. However, the basal ganglia do not appear to have connections with this nucleus. Resting tremor appears to be the result of an imbalance in the actions of basal ganglia and cerebellar mechanisms or of the release of control over other structures. Deiber and associates[33] found that suppression of resting tremor in humans by stimulation of the ventralis intermedius nucleus led to decreased cerebellar activity (as indicated by regional cerebral blood flow). On the basis of these observations, Deiber and associates[33] suggest that resting tremor is the result of enhanced cerebellar activity, rather than any cortical mechanism.

Difficulty in Walking

In Parkinson's disease, posture, balance, and gait are impaired. Evidence that the pedunculopontine nucleus is involved in the impairment of walking includes the fact that its stimulation induces locomotion in animals, it has reciprocal connections with the basal ganglia, and it loses neurons in Parkinson's disease. **Functionally, the abnormalities of balance and gait are the result of akinesia, bradykinesia, rigidity, and impairments in postural reflexes.**[16]

Preparatory postural adjustments before voluntary movement are less likely to occur or are diminished in scale (hence less functionally useful) in patients with Parkinson's disease. Steps are reduced in size during walking, patients spend longer in the double-support phase, and there are reductions in the associated arm swings.[34] Increasing rigidity leads to a stooped, flexed posture, with the head projecting forward (see Fig. 18–7). Bradykinesia causes patients to take short shuffling steps and, when combined with the displacement of the center of gravity in the forward direction due to the flexion in the hips and trunk, may cause patients' forefeet to strike the ground before the normal heel strike. Patients take quicker, shorter steps, so that they can keep up with their center of gravity.[16] In addition to the reduction in anticipatory postural adjustments and the tendency to sway forward, corrective mechanisms are also impaired. Patients' corrective postural reflexes are impaired, and voluntary corrective responses are rendered less effective by bradykinesia. This results in delayed and abnormal balance reactions and subsequent risk for falls.

Huntington's Disease

Huntington's disease affects 0.005% to 0.01% of the population. **The disease can lead to cognitive and emotional disturbances as well as problems of voluntary (akinesia, bradykinesia) and involuntary movement.**[6,7,35–38] Among the involuntary movements are the abnormal movements of **chorea.** Choreiform movements are relatively rapid and irregularly timed and may occur in any combination of muscles (Fig. 18–8). *Hypotonia* **(reduced muscle tone) is also common in Huntington's disease patients,** although the young-onset variant causes rigidity.

Huntington's disease has an insidious onset, generally manifesting in the fourth or fifth decade of life. Although it may initially cause depression or cognitive impairments, the appearance of involuntary movements (chorea) and a family history have tended to confirm the diagnosis of Huntington's disease.[35–38] This is a hereditary disorder, with a 50% chance of transmission from affected parent to offspring (autosomal-dominant inheritance). The disease is caused by a mutation of a gene near the tip of the short arm of chromosome 4, involving the excessive repetition of a trinucleotide (CAG). **Huntington's disease is a progressive degenerative disorder,** which is thought to involve a glutamate-dependent excitotoxic process specifically involving one type of glutamate receptor (NMDA subgroup).[39] There are reports of presymptomatic reductions of cerebral blood flow in the striatum, and neuroimaging suggests that cognitive impairments in Huntington's disease are closely related to caudate atrophy (Fig. 18–9). This finding is in contrast to the cognitive impairments seen in Parkinson's disease, which tend to be related more to the disruptions of frontal lobe function occurring in later stages of the disease. The characteristic manifestations of the disease (movement disorder, personality disturbance, and mental deterioration) progress relentlessly, ultimately necessitating extended care in a nursing home or psychiatric hospital. The disease tends to run its course over a period of 15 years and progresses more rapidly in patients with an earlier age of onset.

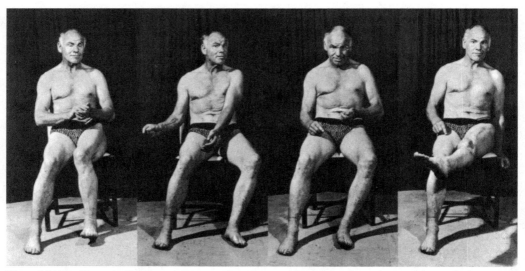

Figure 18–8.   Chorea in Huntington's Disease. This 47-year-old patient with Huntington's disease had a positive family history for four generations. He had a progressive dementia and chorea for 10 years. He was restless, fidgety, and aggressive, and had great difficulty with feeding. Unobserved, there was continuous involuntary movement. When posed before a camera, he was quieter. When engaged in conversation, he exhibited the movements shown in these photographs. (From Spillane, JD: An Atlas of Clinical Neurology. Oxford University Press, New York, 1968, p 219, with permission.)

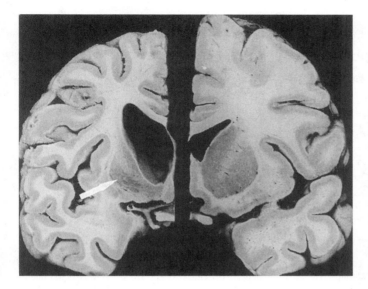

Figure 18–9. *Caudate Degeneration in Huntington's Disease.* The hemisphere on the left is from a female patient aged 49 (brain weight, 1065 g) who had Huntington's disease. The hemisphere on the right is from a normal woman aged 69 (brain weight, 1415 g). The abnormal brain (*Left*) has a dilated lateral ventricle, with atrophy of the caudate and lentiform nuclei (*Arrow*). (From Adams, JH and Duchen, LW (eds): Greenfield's Neuropathology, ed 5. Oxford University Press, New York, 1992, p 1003, with permission.)

Although **degeneration of caudate and putamen are most characteristic of Huntington's disease**, other structures are also affected. Degeneration of the frontal cortex, globus pallidus, and thalamus occurs as the disease progresses.[35–38] Although degeneration is progressive, it may occur at different rates. For example, the striatum may be affected before the globus pallidus, and neurons containing γ-aminobutyric acid (GABA) and enkephalin may be affected before neurons containing GABA and substance P.[35–38]

The striatal degeneration in Huntington's disease affects both cognitive and motor circuits through the basal ganglia. The progression of the disorder leads to changes in symptoms, with an initial increase and then decrease in abnormal movement (chorea), but a steady increase in akinesia and bradykinesia.[40,41]

Progressive striatal degeneration causes an overall reduction in striatal input to the tonic inhibitory output neurons of the basal ganglia, and this probably leads to akinesia and bradykinesia. Although there is a reduction in striatal input, a reduction in striatal activity may also occur. A reduction in the dopaminergic activity of cells from the substantia nigra pars compacta may lead to a further reduction in the ability of a damaged striatum to inhibit tonic inhibitory output neurons.[42]

The situation with chorea is more complex, since it increases and decreases during the course of the disease. In the early stages of the disease, there appears to be a selective loss of those neurons projecting to the external globus pallidus containing GABA and enkephalin.[43] The loss of these neurons disrupts the inhibitory indirect pathway and leads to abnormal movements (chorea). Treatment with dopaminergic antagonists (e.g., neuroleptics such as haloperidol) reduces the chorea, but enhances any akinesia and bradykinesia. In the later stages of Huntington's disease, a further loss of neurons containing GABA and substance P redresses the imbalance between direct and indirect pathways, with a resultant reduction in chorea.[42]

Akinesia and Bradykinesia

An impression of the nature of functional impairments may be gained from a consideration of patients' handwriting (Fig. 18–10).[18] Handwriting is intact in the early stages of the disease, but becomes slow and laborious and may even increase in size as the disease progresses. At first, patients may show difficulty with the shape and slant of letters,

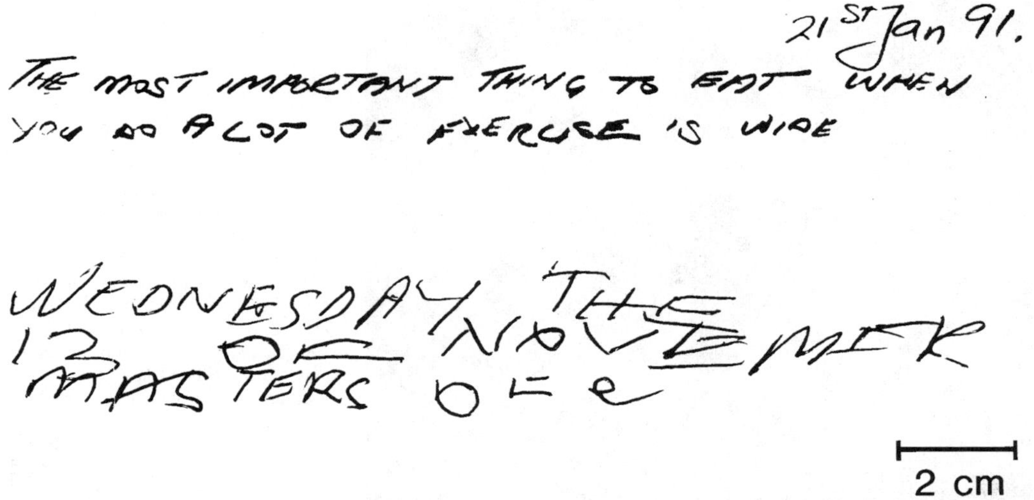

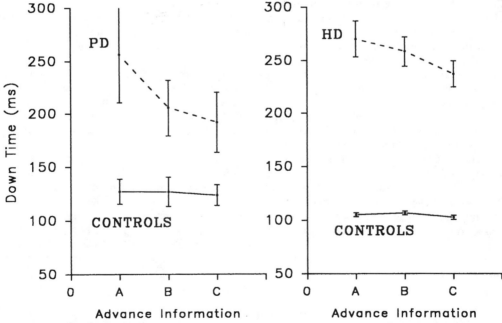

Figure 18–10. *Macrographia in Huntington's Disease.* Patients with Huntington's disease may have problems maintaining the scale of their movements. Handwriting samples are from January 21st and November 13th of the same year. (From Phillips,[18] p 178, with permission.)

Figure 18–11. *Comparison of Preparatory Processes of Patients with Parkinson's and Huntington's Diseases.* In this study requiring a sequential button-pressing task, the period spent holding a button down (i.e., down time) provides a measure of movement preparation time. This measures akinesia. Down time is shown for Parkinson's disease patients (PD) and Huntington's disease (HD) patients and age-matched controls, at three levels of advance information (A=none; B=medium; C=high). Both patient groups have problems using advance information to prepare their movements. (From Phillips,[18] p 177, with permission.)

and then prominent distortions of letter shape occur. There are considerable variations in the amount of force used during writing, reflecting pauses and choreic jerks. These disruptions are unlikely to reflect language impairment, since language function tends to be preserved. Although the overall shape of movements is intact, movement tends to be disrupted by involuntary movements.[44] As dementia progresses, patients show omissions, perseveration (repetition), and substitutions of letters.

Akinesia and bradykinesia steadily increase with the progression of the disease and reflect diminished striatal function. These symptoms appear to be due to problems using advance information to prepare their movements.

Phillips and associates[45] compared the preparatory processes of patients with Parkinson's disease with those of patients with Huntington's disease (Fig. 18–11). The amounts of advance information were varied in a sequential button-pressing task. In condition A, there was no advance information. In condition B, one button was illuminated in advance. In condition C, a button further ahead was illuminated, requiring that two buttons be prepared in advance. The period spent holding a button down (**down time**) provided an index as to the time required to prepare movements and measured akinesia, whereas the time spent moving between buttons (**movement time**) measured bradykinesia. When examining down time, patients with Parkinson's disease and Huntington's disease showed a similar inability to spontaneously initiate movements without cues (condition A). When examining movement time, both groups of patients could use advance information to improve their movements, but they were less able to use the maximal amounts of advance information (condition C) (Fig. 18–12). Although the patterns of impairment are similar for both Parkinson's disease and Huntington's disease patients, patients with Huntington's disease are more impaired,

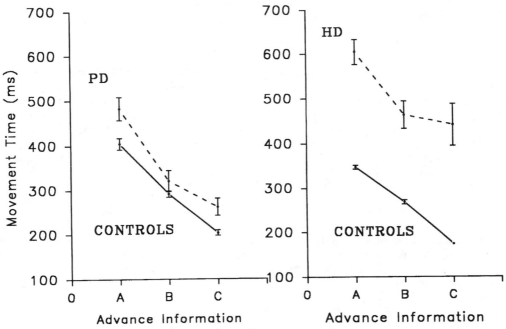

Figure 18–12. *Comparison of Preparatory Processes of Patients with Parkinson's and Huntington's Diseases.* In the same study of button-pressing tasks recorded in Figure 18–11, the time spent moving *between* buttons (i.e., the movement time) measures bradykinesia. Movement time is shown for Parkinson's disease (PD) patients and Huntington's disease (HD) patients and age-matched controls, at three levels of advance information (A=none; B=medium; C=high). Both patient groups have problems using advance information to produce faster movements. (From Phillips,[18] p 177, with permission.)

reflecting the more pervasive striatal damage and the lack of a suitable treatment for akinesia/bradykinesia in these patients.

Bradykinesia is not simply the result of problems in preparatory processes. **Patients with Huntington's disease (like patients with Parkinson's disease) have problems in the development of movement forces and take longer to attain peak force.**[46] **Patients also have problems performing complex simultaneous or sequential movements.**[46] Unlike in Parkinson's disease, however, there is not a progressive slowing during the performance of sequential movements.[47]

Chorea

Choreiform movements are involuntary movements that are difficult to characterize, exhibiting no obvious pattern or purpose (see Fig. 18–8). No obvious rhythmicity or dominant frequency of involuntary movement occurs, as seen in tremor. Muscle activation is not correctly sequenced, and co-contractions can occur that interfere with voluntary movement.[46] **Choreiform movements may show any pattern of activity** (reflexive, ballistic, or tonic) in any muscle at any time. Muscle activation in chorea ranges from brief bursts (50 to 200 milliseconds) to prolonged contractions (2 seconds).[46] Faster contractions could be considered tics, and the more sustained contractions could be considered dystonic. Although the more sustained dystonic contractions show no particular spatial distribution (unlike focal dystonia), dystonic contractions may become more severe in advanced stages of the disease, causing postural abnormalities.[40] Chorea is exacerbated by stress, is reduced by voluntary movement, and ceases during sleep.[40]

Since long-latency stretch reflexes are elicited when a preactivated muscle or a voluntary movement is perturbed, chorea may reflect a failure of the mechanisms controlling long-latency reflexes. However, this does not appear to be the case, because delays or abnormalities in the magnitude of long-latency reflexes do not appear to be related to the severity of chorea.[48]

Hypotonia

Changes in muscle tone in Huntington's disease patients are difficult to characterize. Although most patients have reduced muscle tone (hyptonia), this may change with progression of the disease, with rigidity occurring in advanced stages. There is also a variant of the disease with an early onset and faster progression, which causes akinesia and rigidity rather than chorea. Hypotonia may be related to reduced size of long-latency reflexes. Although short-latency reflex responses to stretch appear normal, the long-latency stretch reflexes are delayed and reduced in amplitude but prolonged in duration. Such reflexes rapidly habituate, but they are less likely to habituate in patients with Huntington's disease.[48]

Difficulty in Walking

Patients with Huntington's disease have a wide-based staggering gait, sometimes with a zigzag progression. Associated arm swings are abnormal, with the arms being held in a fixed posture. Walking speed and stride length decrease and become more variable. Although chorea may cause the occasional sudden knee bend, the wide-based gait, slower walking speed, and impaired balance can occur in patients with minimal choreiform movements.[40]

Tourette's Syndrome

Estimates of the prevalence of Tourette's syndrome vary from 0.0005% to 0.07% of the population. **The syndrome is associated with involuntary movements such as** *tics.*[7,49–51]

Tics are sudden contractions of related muscle groups causing movement or sound. Although these contractions may be repetitive, they are not rhythmic in nature. The movements may involve simple twitches or more complex, seemingly coordinated, but inappropriate movements (e.g., touching, jumping, and speaking). There is also a disturbance of the distinction between voluntary and involuntary movement. In this regard, Tourette's syndrome is associated with impulsions. An *impulsion* is an urge to move or perform a tic, which is relieved by allowing the tic to occur.[52]

Tourette's syndrome may be inherited, but with variations in its mode of expression. It may be linked to attention deficit hyperactivity disorder and obsessive-compulsive disorder.[53] It affects three times as many males as females. Tourette's syndrome tends to affect young males, with tics initially affecting the face and then involving other parts of the body. The severity of symptoms waxes and wanes, but declines (or becomes more manageable) after adolescence.[43]

Tourette's syndrome is thought to involve the limbic circuits of the basal ganglia. This conclusion is drawn in part from the nature of some of the tics, which may contain inappropriate scatologic or sexual reference.[55] For example, patients may exhibit coprolalia (swearing) or a tendency for their tics to incorporate gestures signifying sexual acts. The rostrocaudal evolution of tics as the disease progresses may reflect the topographic organization of the basal ganglia.[56]

Patients with Tourette's syndrome show reduced cerebral blood flow in orbitofrontal cortex, inferior insular cortex, parahippocampal regions, and ventral striatum and, to a lesser extent, putamen.[57] Although metabolic rates of putamen and limbic structures are negatively correlated in normal subjects, these rates are positively correlated in patients with Tourette's syndrome. The limbic system may provide an inhibitory drive (presumably through the striatum) suppressing the substantia nigra pars compacta, which would otherwise excite the direct pathways through the basal ganglia. The decreased activity of the limbic system in Tourette's syndrome would appear to allow excess activity of the substantia nigra pars compacta, which stimulates the direct excitatory pathways of the basal ganglia. Tics may therefore respond to dopamine antagonists (e.g., haloperidol). Other medications may also be effective.[55]

A somewhat different mechanism may explain vocal tics. Brain imaging has indicated reductions in the volume of the left lenticular nucleus (putamen and globus pallidus) and reductions in the left-right asymmetry of this region.[58] As outlined in Chapter 9, the basal ganglia in the dominant hemisphere may have a significant role in the control of language. A reduction in left basal ganglia activity may release excitatory thalamic inputs from the ventral anterior thalamus to the language cortex, producing involuntary vocalizations.

Tics

Tics are difficult to characterize on the basis of muscle activity, since they reveal the normal triphasic agonist, antagonist, agonist pattern expected of normal ballistic movements.[59] However, there are abnormalities in electroencephalographic potentials in these patients. Although a Bereitschaftspotential occurs before voluntary movements, Obeso and associates[60] did not find a Bereitschaftspotential occurring before spontaneous simple tics in patients with Tourette's syndrome. This indicates that tics are not movements that are prepared in the normal manner.

It has been suggested that tics are simply fragments of common motor programs that are spontaneously released.[55] In particular, it was suggested that coprolalia could simply result from the random emission of high-probability phonemes. However, Lang and associates[61] reported a case study indicating that tics do not simply reflect a reduced threshold for high-probability movements. They described a patient with Tourette's syndrome who learned sign language. Tics were suppressed while she was learning sign language. But, as the patient's skill in sign language developed (and became automatic), she began to have tics that signed out obscenities. This occurred in two stages. Tics occurred initially with some conscious thought or urge, but later with little accompanying thought. Lang and associates[61] suggest that an abnormal limbic system provides inputs to both cortical and subcortical structures. The cortical input provides the premonitory urge for a tic, whereas the basal ganglia assumes a greater role in tics when the behavior is made more automatic.

Other Movement Disorders

Our discussion of Parkinson's disease, Huntington's disease, and Tourette's syndrome has illustrated the existence of a number of relatively parallel circuits through the basal ganglia. Each disorder predominantly disturbs a specific circuit: motor circuit (Parkinson's disease), cognitive circuit (Huntington's disease), and limbic circuit (Tourette's syndrome). The fact that these circuits are parallel but contiguous explains how a disorder primarily affecting a specific circuit (e.g., motor) can also cause lesser amounts of disturbance in contiguous circuits (e.g., cognitive, limbic). Two additional disorders are discussed here which illustrate the importance of the topographic organization within each circuit.

Focal Dystonia

Dystonic movements can be produced by a number of diseases (symptomatic dystonia).[62-64] However, we restrict our discussion to a more limited and specific form of idiopathic dystonia (focal dystonia). It is a rare disorder that may illustrate how the topographic organization of the basal ganglia is of direct clinical relevance. *Focal dystonia* involves **sustained muscle contractions that affect related muscles and cause abnormal postures, prolonged twisting movements, and repetitive movements** (Fig. 18–13).[62-64] Different terms are used to describe focal dystonias affecting specific body parts (Table 18–1).

Although the cause of focal dystonia is as yet unclear, the examination of patients with dystonia resulting from obvious lesions indicates that dystonia arises from basal ganglia damage. Computed tomography of 71 patients with symptomatic dystonia indicated that basal ganglia damage (caudate or lentiform nucleus) contributes to dystonic movement.[65] Better resolution is available using magnetic resonance imaging (MRI). MRI revealed abnormalities in the globus pallidus in 15 of 20 cases with a variety of symptomatic dystonic disorders.[66] Although the lesion centered on the globus pallidus in 4 cases, the putamen was involved in 11 of the cases as well. Dystonia may therefore result from the release of the usual inhibitory control of thalamic nuclei (exerted by indirect and direct pathways through the basal ganglia), leading to excess activation of cortical structures.

Focal dystonia may be inherited and may reflect a milder version of generalized dystonia.[64] Generalized dystonia is associated with childhood onset of symptoms (median age 8 years). When the disorder commences in childhood, it is likely to initially affect a leg. The disorder gradually progresses, with symptoms worsening in the affected limb and spreading to other body segments. In contrast to generalized dystonia, focal dystonia is associated with onset in adulthood (median age 45 years). The disorder is milder with adult onset and is more likely to affect the upper body.

Focal dystonia initially occurs during a specific movement (e.g., writing) and seems to involve an overflow and excessive activation of related muscles, with contraction of adjacent muscle groups that are unnecessary for the task. It is exacerbated by movement and improved by rest. The disorder causes co-contraction of muscles and an inability to "turn off" muscles and as such may reflect a failure of the reciprocal inhibition of muscles.[67] Ghez and associates[67] found that patients were relatively accurate in their force production and movement trajectories, but were restricted in the number of ways that they could perform a task. For example, people can normally draw and write in a variety of postures, but a patient with dystonia may be able to perform such tasks only while standing. Symptoms may be relieved by sensory "tricks." For example, a patient with spasmodic torticollis may touch the chin to return the head to the midline.[64]

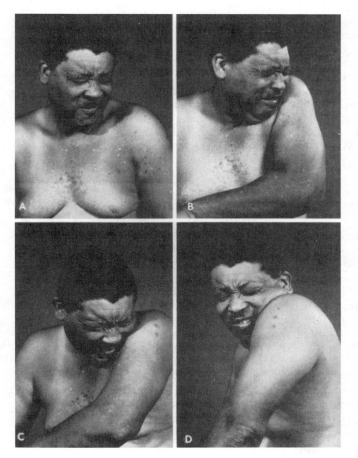

Hemiballismus

Ballismus consists of involuntary, violent, limb movements. When ballismus is unilateral (which is more common), it is called *hemiballismus.* **Hemiballismus affects proximal muscles, leading to wild, rapid flinging of the limbs about the shoulder or hip joint.** The disorder is of interest because it potentially reflects the topographic organization of basal ganglia circuitry. Unlike athetosis, which tends to cause slow, irregular involuntary

Table 18–1. *Focal Dystonias and the Affected Body Part*

Dystonia	Affected Part
Blepharospasm	Eyelids
Oromandibular dystonia	Mouth
Dystonic adductor dysphonia	Larynx
Torticollis	Neck
Writer's cramp	Hand, forearm, arm
Soliosis, lordosis, kyphosis, tortipelvis	Back
Leg dystonia	Foot, leg, thigh

contractions of the **distal** musculature, hemiballismus leads to rapid activation of the **proximal** musculature.[1]

Hemiballismus is most commonly associated with cerebrovascular accidents that have caused lesions to the subthalamic nucleus or its efferent projections to the globus pallidus. Such lesions damage the indirect (inhibitory) pathway through the basal ganglia, leading to excess activity in thalamic nuclei. For this reason, treatment has involved stereotaxic lesions of the thalamus. Hemiballismus may also be treated pharmacologically, since the direct (excitatory) pathway can be controlled by dopamine antagonists. It has been suggested that hemiballismus is the product of impairments in postural mechanisms, such that slight postural disturbances cause wild adjustments at proximal joints.[1]

Conclusions

Basal ganglia disorders disrupt motor coordination, create problems in the execution of voluntary movement, and cause involuntary movements. There may be a slowness initiating (akinesia) and executing (bradykinesia) movements, and an inappropriate release and activation of muscles. This can be fast and ballistic (tic), random (chorea), or more sustained (dystonic). There may also be abnormalities of muscle tone (rigidity or hypotonia). There appear to be problems with the automatic execution of movements. Although the overall form of motor programs tends to be intact, there may be problems accessing motor programs, leading to problems in timing and sequencing movements. Moreover, voluntary movements may be disrupted by involuntary movements. Although a general consideration of each syndrome may not reveal this, the initial stages of basal ganglia disorders (or milder forms) may affect a specific side or body part, reflecting the topographic organization of the motor circuit. The presence of contiguous cognitive and limbic circuits in the basal ganglia means that basal ganglia disorders can lead to cognitive and emotional disturbance as well, whether as a result of pathology or as a side effect of pharmacotherapy. Patients may be able to learn (if cognition is intact), but the issue is whether they can appropriately use what they have learned in the face of these disorders.

RECOMMENDED READINGS

Albin, RL, Young, AB, and Penney, JB: The Functional Anatomy of Basal Ganglia Disorders. Trends Neurosci 12:366, 1989.

Cedarbaum, JM and Gancher, ST (eds): Parkinson's Disease. Neurol Clin 10:301, 1992.

Chokroverty, S (ed): Movement Disorders. PMA Publishing, Great Neck, NY, 1990.

Fahn, S: Parkinson's Disease and Other Basal Ganglion Disorders. Chapter 86. In Asbury, AK, McKhann, GM, and McDonald, WI (eds): Diseases of the Nervous System: Clinical Neurobiology, ed 2. WB Saunders, Philadelphia, 1992.

Folstein, SE: Huntington's Disease: A Disorder of Families. The Johns Hopkins University Press, Baltimore, 1989.

Harper, PS (ed): Huntington's Disease. WB Saunders, London, 1991.

Jankovic, J and Tolosa, E (eds): Parkinson's Disease and Movement Disorders, ed 2. Williams & Wilkins, Baltimore, 1993.

Koller, WC (ed): Handbook of Parkinson's Disease. Marcel Dekker, New York, 1987.

Lohr, JB and Wisniewski, AA: Movement Disorders: A Neuropsychiatric Approach. John Wiley, Chichester, 1987.

Marsden, CD: Neurophysiology. In Stern, GM (ed): Parkinson's Disease. Chapman & Hall, London, 1990.

Marsden, CD and Fahn, S (eds): Movement Disorders 2. Butterworth & Co, London, 1987.

Obeso, JA, Rothwell, JC, and Marsden, CD: The Neurophysiology of Tourette Syndrome. Adv Neurol 35:105, 1982.

Shoulson, I: Huntington's Disease. Chapter 87. In Asbury, AK, McKhann, GM, and McDonald, WI (eds): Diseases of the Nervous System: Clinical Neurobiology, ed 2. WB Saunders, Philadelphia, 1992.

Stern, GM (ed): Parkinson's Disease. Chapman & Hall, London, 1990.

Turnbull, GI (ed): Physical Therapy Management of Parkinson's Disease. Churchill Livingstone, New York, 1992.

REFERENCES

1. Lohr, JB and Wisniewski, AA: Movement Disorders: A Neuropsychiatric Approach. John Wiley, Chichester, 1987.
2. Stelmach, GE: Motor Control and Motor Learning: The Closed Loop Perspective. In Kelso, JAS (ed): Human Motor Behavior: An Introduction. Lawrence Erlbaum Associates, Hillsdale, NJ, 1982.
3. Stelmach, GE: Information-Processing Framework for Understanding Human Motor Behavior. In Kelso, JAS (ed): Human Motor Behavior: An Introduction. Lawrence Erlbaum Associates, Hillsdale, NJ, 1982.
4. Marttila, RJ: Epidemiology. In Koller, WC (ed): Handbook of Parkinson's Disease. Marcel Dekker, New York, 1987.
5. Jankovic, J: Pathophysiology and Clinical Assessment of Motor Symptoms in Parkinson's Disease. In Koller, WC (ed): Handbook of Parkinson's Disease. Marcel Dekker, New York, 1987.
6. Jankovic, J and Tolosa, E (eds): Parkinson's Disease and Movement Disorders, ed 2. Williams & Wilkins, Baltimore, 1993.
7. Fahn, S: Parkinson's Disease and Other Basal Ganglion Disorders. Chapter 86. In Asbury, AK, McKhann, GM, and McDonald, WI (eds): Diseases of the Nervous System: Clinical Neurobiology, ed 2. WB Saunders, Philadelphia, 1992.
8. Cedarbaum, JM and Gancher, ST (eds): Parkinson's Disease. Neurol Clin 10:301, 1992.
9. Koller, WC: Classification of Parkinson's Disease. In Koller, WC (ed): Handbook of Parkinson's Disease. Marcel Dekker, New York, 1987.
10. Forno, LS: Pathology of Parkinson's Disease: The Importance of the Substantia Nigra and Lewy Bodies. In Stern, GM (ed): Parkinson's Disease. Chapman & Hall Medical, London, 1990.
11. Calne, DB and Zigmond, MJ: Compensatory Mechanisms in Degenerative Neurologic Diseases: Insights from Parkinsonism. Arch Neurol 48:361, 1991.
12. Kish, SJ, Shannak, K, and Hornykiewicz, O: Uneven Pattern of Dopamine Loss in the Striatum of Patients with Idiopathic Parkinson's Disease: Pathophysiologic and Clinical Implications. N Engl J Med 318:876, 1988.
13. Mitchell, IJ, et al: Neural Mechanisms Underlying Parkinsonian Symptoms Based upon Regional Uptake of 2-deoxyglucose in Monkeys Exposed to 1-methyl-4-phenyl-1,2,3,6-tetrahyropyridine. Neuroscience 32:213, 1989.
14. Stacy, M and Jankovic, J: Current Approaches in the Treatment of Parkinson's Disease. Ann Rev Med 44:431, 1993.
15. King, DB: Diagnosis, Pharmacology, and Medical Management: Drug Management. In Turnbull, GI (ed): Physical Therapy Management of Parkinson's Disease. Churchill Livingstone, New York, 1992.
16. Marsden, CD: Neurophysiology. In Stern, GM (ed): Parkinson's Disease. Chapman & Hall, London, 1990.
17. Stelmach, GE and Phillips, JG: Motor Control in Parkinson's Disease. In Turnbull, GI (ed): Physical Therapy Management of Parkinson's Disease. Churchill Livingstone, New York, 1992.
18. Phillips, JG, et al: Motor Functions of the Basal Ganglia. Psychol Res 55:175, 1993.
19. Stelmach, GE, Worringham, CJ, and Strand, EA: Movement Preparation in Parkinson's Disease: The Use of Advance Information. Brain 109:1179, 1986.
20. Schugens, MM, et al: Proximal and Distal Reaction Times (RTs) Are Not Differentially Affected in Parkinson's Disease. Mov Dis 8:367, 1993.
21. Alexander, GE, DeLong, MR, and Crutcher, MD: Do Cortical and Basal Ganglionic Motor Areas Use "Motor Programs" to Control Movement? Behav Brain Sci 15:656, 1992.
22. Bloxham, CA, Mindel, TA, and Frith, CD: Initiation and Execution of Predictable and Unpredictable Movements in Parkinson's Disease. Brain 10:371, 1984.
23. Bloxham, CA, Dick, DJ, and Moore, M: Reaction Times and Attention in Parkinson's Disease. J Neurol Neurosurg Psychiatry 50: 1178, 1987.
24. Brown, VJ, et al: Dopamine Dependent Reaction Time Deficits in Patients with Parkinson's Disease Are Task Specific. Neuropsychologia 31:459, 1993.
25. Rascol, OJ, et al: Impaired Activity of the Supplementary Motor Area in Akinetic Patients with Parkinson's Disease: Improvement by the Dopamine Agonist Apomorphine. Adv Neurol 60:419, 1993.
26. Narabayashi, H: Three Types of Akinesia in the Progressive Course of Parkinson's Disease. Adv Neurol 60:18, 1993.
27. Hallett, M and Khoshbin, SA: Physiological Mechanism of Bradykinesia. Brain 103:301, 1980.
28. Jordan, N, Sagar, HJ, and Cooper, JA: A Component Analysis of the Generation and Release of Isometric Force in Parkinson's Disease. J Neurol Neurosurg Psychiatry 55:572, 1992.
29. Bennett, KMB, et al: A Kinematic Study of the Reach to Grasp Movement in a Study with Hemiparkinson's Disease. Neuropsychologia 31:709, 1993.
30. Logigian, E, et al: Does Tremor Pace Repetitive Voluntary Motor Behavior in Parkinson's Disease? Ann Neurol 30:172, 1991.
31. Fleminger, S: Control of Simultaneous Movements Distinguishes Depressive Motor Retardation from Parkinson's Disease and Neuroleptic Parkinsonism. Brain 115:1459, 1992.
32. Meara, RJ and Cody, FWJ: Relationship Between Electromyographic Activity and Clinically Assessed Rigidity Studied at the Wrist Joint in Parkinson's Disease. Brain 115:1167, 1992.
33. Deiber, MP, et al: Thalamic Stimulation and Suppression of Parkinsonian Tremor: Evidence of a Cerebellar Activation Using Positron Emission Tomography. Brain 116:267, 1993.
34. Wall, JC and Turnbull, GI: The Kinematics of Gait. In Turnbull, GI (ed): Physical Therapy Management of Parkinson's Disease. Churchill Livingstone, New York, 1992.
35. Kremer, B, Weber, B, and Haydin, MR: New Insights into the Clinical Features, Pathogenesis, and Molecular Genetics of Huntington's Disease. Brain Pathol 2:321, 1992.
36. Penney, JB, Jr and Young, AB: Huntington's Disease. Chapter 12. In Jankovic, J and Tolosa, E (eds): Parkinson's Disease and Movement Disorders, ed 2. Williams & Wilkins, Baltimore, 1993.

37. Shoulson, I: Huntington's Disease. Chapter 87. In Asbury, AK, McKhann, GM, and McDonald, WI (eds): Diseases of the Nervous System: Clinical Neurobiology, ed 2. WB Saunders, Philadelphia, 1992.
38. Harper, PS: Huntington's Disease. WB Saunders, London, 1991.
39. DiFiglia, M: Excitotoxic Injury of the Neostriatum: A Model for Huntington's Disease. Trends Neurosci 13:286, 1990.
40. Folstein, SE: Huntington's Disease: A Disorder of Families. The Johns Hopkins University Press, Baltimore, 1989.
41. Folstein, SE, et al: The Measurement of Abnormal Movement: Methods Developed for Huntington's Disease. Neurobehav Toxicol Teratol 5:605, 1983.
42. Albin, RL, Young, AB, and Penney, JB: The Functional Anatomy of Basal Ganglia Disorders. Trends Neurosci 12:366, 1989.
43. Storey, E and Beal, MF: Neurochemical Substrates of Rigidity and Chorea in Huntington's Disease. Brain 116:1201, 1993.
44. Phillips, JG and Stelmach, GE: The Contribution of Movement Disorders Research to Theories of Motor Control and Learning. In Summers, JJ (ed): Approaches to the Study of Motor Control and Learning. North-Holland, Amsterdam, 1992.
45. Phillips, JG, et al: Motor Functions of the Basal Ganglia. Psychol Res 55:175, 1993.
46. Stelmach, GE and Phillips, JG: Movement Disorders: Limb Movement and the Basal Ganglia. Phys Ther 71:60, 1991.
47. Agostino, R, et al: Sequential Arm Movements in Patients with Parkinson's Disease, Huntington's Disease and Dystonia. Brain 115:1481, 1992.
48. Abbruzzese, G, et al: Impaired Habituation of Long-Latency Stretch Reflexes of the Wrist Muscles in Huntington's Disease. Mov Dis 5:32, 1990.
49. Sandor, P: Gilles de la Tourette Syndrome: A Neuropsychiatric Disorder. J Psychosom Res 37:211, 1993.
50. Robertson, MM: Annotation: Gilles de la Tourette Syndrome: An Update. J Child Psychiatry 35:597, 1994.
51. Shapiro, AK, et al (eds): Gilles de la Tourette Syndrome, ed 2. Raven Press, New York, 1988.
52. Leckman, JF, Walker, DE, and Cohen, DJ: Premonitory Urges in Tourette's Syndrome. Am J Psychiatry 150:98, 1993.
53. Steingard, R and Dillon-Stout, D: Tourette's Syndrome and Obsessive Compulsive Disorder: Clinical Aspects. Psychiatr Clin North Am 15:849, 1992.
54. Bruun, RD and Budman, CL: The Natural History of Tourette Syndrome. Adv Neurol 58:1, 1992.
55. Jankovic, J: The Neurology of Tics. In Marsden, CD and Fahn, S (eds): Movement Disorders 2. Butterworth & Co, London, 1987.
56. Leckman, JF, et al: Pathogenesis of Tourette Syndrome: Clues from the Clinical Phenotype and Natural History. Adv Neurol 58:15, 1992.
57. Stoetter, B, et al: Functional Neuroanatomy of Tourette Syndrome: Limbic–Motor Interactions Studied with FDG PET. Adv Neurol 58:213, 1992.
58. Witelson, SF: Clinical Neurology as Data for Basic Neuroscience: Tourette's Syndrome and the Human Motor System. Neurology 43:859, 1993.
59. Hallett, M: Analysis of Abnormal Voluntary and Involuntary Movements with Surface Electromyography. Adv Neurol 39:907, 1983.
60. Obeso, JA, Rothwell, JC, and Marsden, CD: The Neurophysiology of Tourette Syndrome. Adv Neurol 35:105, 1982.
61. Lang, AE, Consky, E, and Sandor, P: "Signing Tics": Insights into the Pathophysiology of Symptoms in Tourette's Syndrome. Ann Neurol 33:212, 1993.
62. Jankovic, J and Fahn, S: Dystonic Disorders. Chapter 21. In Jankovic, J and Tolosa, E (eds): Parkinson's Disease and Movement Disorders, ed 2. Williams & Wilkins, Baltimore, 1993.
63. Korczyn, AD and Inzelberg, R: Dystonia. Curr Opin Neurol Neurosurg 6:350, 1993.
64. Fahn, S, Marsden, CD, and Calne, DB: Classification and Investigation of Dystonia. In Marsden, CD and Fahn, S (eds): Movement Disorders 2. Butterworth & Co, London, 1987.
65. Obeso, JA and Gimenez-Roldan, S: Clinicopathological Correlation in Symptomatic Dystonia. Adv Neurol 50:113, 1988.
66. Iwata, M: MRI Pathology of Basal Ganglia in Dystonic Disorders. Adv Neurol 60:535, 1993.
67. Ghez, C, Gordon, J, and Hening, W: Trajectory Control in Dystonia. Adv Neurol, 50:141 1988.

CHAPTER 19

■

Disorders of the Cerebellum and Its Connections

Christopher M. Fredericks, PhD

- *Signs and Symptoms of Cerebellar Damage*
- *Extracerebellar Causes of Cerebellar Signs and Symptoms*
- *Localization of Cerebellar Dysfunction*
- *Specific Etiologies*

*T*he cerebellum, which lies just dorsal to the pons and medulla, consists of two highly convoluted lateral cerebellar hemispheres and a narrow medial portion, the vermis. It is connected to the brain by three pairs of dense fiber bundles called the **peduncles.** Although the structure and function of the cerebellum have long been studied, the precise role of the cerebellum in motor control remains to be fully elucidated.

As discussed in Chapter 8, it is clear that the cerebellum receives a tremendous number of inputs from the spinal cord and from many regions of both the cortical and subcortical brain. In this way, the cerebellum receives extensive information from somesthetic, vestibular, visual, and auditory sensory systems, as well as from motor and nonmotor areas of the cerebral cortex. Although afferent connections outnumber efferent projections by about 40 to 1, the cerebellum has extensive outgoing connections to many areas of the brainstem, midbrain, and cerebral cortex.

It is evident that while the cerebellum does not serve to initiate most movement, it does interact with areas of the brain that do.[1-3] In doing so, the cerebellum promotes the synchrony and accuracy of movement required for purposeful motor activity. The cerebellar modulation and coordination of muscular activity are important in skilled voluntary movement, as well as in the movements of posture and equilibrium.

The cerebellum is vulnerable to most of the nonspecific disease processes that affect other areas of the central nervous system, as well as to certain diseases unique to the cerebellum (Table 19–1). When the cerebellum or its direct connections are damaged, a characteristic constellation of symptoms and clinical signs arises. At first glance, the motor deficits produced by such damage are less than one might expect of a structure so centrally located in the neuraxis and so intimately involved in motor control. Extensive damage to the cerebellum, for example, does not abolish movement and rarely even causes muscle weakness. Somesthetic or other sensibilities are not disrupted, nor is cognition. Instead, **the most prominent effects of cerebellar destruction are a type of incoordination or clumsiness**

Table 19–1. *Cerebellar Disorders Organized by Etiology*

- Inherited or idiopathic degenerations
- Nutritional disorders
- Neoplastic and paraneoplastic disorders
- Developmental disorders
- Disorders due to infection
- Vascular disorders
- Intoxications
- Physical or mechanical trauma
- Metabolic disorders
- Demyelinating or dysmyelinating disorders

of movement called *ataxia* **and abnormal muscle tone.** Although cerebellar lesions may delay the initiation of movements and alter their form, they do not prevent their execution. This is very different from the motor deficits that result from damage to the motor cortex or to the systems descending from it, in which the strength and speed of contraction are impaired and the ability to contract individual muscles may be lost altogether. If you recall that the role of the cerebellum is not to initiate motor activity but to modulate and refine motor behaviors initiated elsewhere, then the signs and symptoms of cerebellar damage are not surprising.

Destruction of small portions of the cerebellar cortex rarely causes detectable abnormalities in motor function. **To cause serious and continuing dysfunction, the cerebellar lesion must be extensive and usually involves one or more of the deep cerebellar nuclei in addition to the cerebellar cortex.** It is interesting that the neurologic signs produced even by extensive damage tend to gradually diminish with time, assuming that the underlying disease process does not itself progress. Such improvement is particularly evident following childhood damage. In experimental animals, even after as much as 50% of the cerebellar cortex has been removed, if the deep nuclei are left intact, motor function appears normal as long as the movements are performed slowly.

Signs and Symptoms of Cerebellar Damage

Although the specific neurologic signs associated with cerebellar disease and injury are numerous,[2,4,5] the basic functional deficits producing these signs are relatively few (Table 19–2). Moreover, these basic functional deficits are a logical consequence of the disruption of the motor functions known to be carried out by the cerebellum.

Incoordination of Movement[1,2,4,5]

The cerebellum is responsible for the smoothly integrated coordination of movements. It is needed for movements that require the concerted, synergistic contraction of multiple muscle groups, and it permits such movements to be carried out efficiently and accurately.

The most conspicuous and most common result of cerebellar dysfunction is an incoordination or clumsiness of movement. This incoordination is **referred to by clinicians as** *ataxia,* a term derived from the Greek word meaning "lack of order." Patients with ataxia have difficulty regulating the force, range, direction, velocity, and rhythm of muscle contractions and in maintaining the synergy that normally exists among the various muscles involved in motor activities. Ataxia is a general term and may be manifested in any number of specific clinical signs, depending on the extent and locus of involvement. **Limb movements, gait, speech, and eye movements all may be affected.**

Table 19–2. Basic Characteristics of Cerebellar Signs and Symptoms

- Lesions of the cerebellum produce errors in the planning and execution of movements, rather than paralysis or involuntary movements.
- In general, if symptoms predominate in the trunk and legs, the lesion is near the midline; if symptoms are more obvious in the arms, the lesion is in the lateral hemispheres.
- If only one side of the cerebellum is affected, the symptoms are unilateral and ipsilateral to the lesion.
- The most severe disturbances are produced by lesions in the superior cerebellar peduncle and the deep nuclei.
- Many of the symptoms of cerebellar disease improve gradually with time if the underlying disease process does not itself progress.
- Almost all patients with cerebellar lesions have some type of gait disturbance.
- Speech disturbances occur only with bilateral damage.
- Signs and symptoms similar to those produced by cerebellar lesions can appear with disorders that affect structures adjacent to the cerebellum or affect the afferent or efferent connections of the cerebellum.

If the legs and trunk are affected, difficulty in maintaining posture and coordinating leg movements will result in *ataxia of gait.* Such patients are unsteady during ambulation and attempt to improve their stability by walking with a broad-based gait and lower center of gravity. Their steps are uncertain and irregular, and they may stagger or veer from side to side. Patients with gait ataxia also have a decrease in the normal, free-flowing arm swing that normally accompanies ambulation. Walking heel-to-toe or running the heel of one foot down the shin of the other leg while seated or lying down is difficult and serves as tests for this deficit. Problems with standing or walking are present in almost all patients with cerebellar damage, regardless of the site of the damage, and, when severe, may cause considerable disability.

Ataxia of the arms (limb ataxia) creates its own specific clinical signs. Difficulty in bringing a limb smoothly and accurately to a specific target in space is called **dysmetria.** An involved limb may either overshoot (hypermetria) or undershoot (hypometria) its target. Complex movements, because of errors in the timing and sequencing of their component parts, may deteriorate into a series of successive simple movements, rather than one smooth, coordinated movement. This is termed **decomposition of movement** and is most evident in movements involving multiple joints. At the end of such movements, when the patient is attempting to achieve the greatest precision, a coarse tremor may develop called an **intention tremor.** These tremors do not occur at rest nor during postural fixation, but develop while precise, intentional movements are undertaken. Intention tremors probably reflect impaired coordination of agonists and antagonists, as well as an attempt to correct for overshoot and undershoot.

Dysmetria, decomposition, and tremor all can be demonstrated by simply asking the patient to point from one stationary target to another, such as in bringing the tip of the finger of the extended upper extremity to the nose (Fig. 19–1). As the movement is undertaken, each joint of the shoulder, elbow, wrist, and finger may flex independently in a puppetlike fashion and large errors in the direction and range of movement occur as the target is approached. As the finger nears the nose, the hand and finger exhibit a tremor. Limb ataxia may also be manifested as an impairment of the ability to perform rapidly alternating movements, such as rapid supination and pronation of the forearm. This is termed **dysdiadochokinesia.**

Persistent incoordination of axial muscles may lead to reversible abnormalities of stance and posture, such as head or body tilt, or to more permanent skeletal abnormalities, such as scoliosis. Truncal ataxia may result in swaying of the trunk, staggering gait, and difficulty in sitting unsupported.

Bulbar muscles may also be affected, leading to slurred speech (dysarthria) and numerous disturbances of oculomotor activity, including nystagmus.

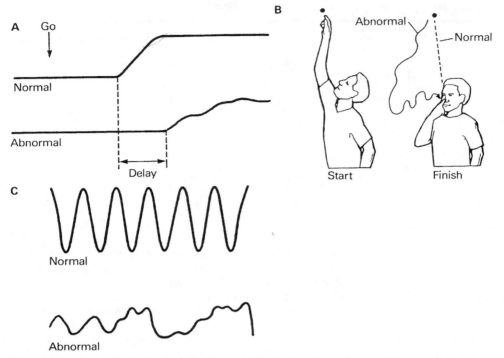

Figure 19–1. *Typical Defects in Cerebellar Diseases.* (*A*) A lesion in the right cerebellar hemisphere causes a delay in the initiation of movement. The patient is told to flex both arms at the same time on a "go" signal. The left arm is flexed later than the right, as evident in the recordings of elbow position. (*B*) A patient moving his arm from a raised position to touch the tip of his nose exhibits dysmetria (inaccuracy in range and direction) and unsmooth movement with increased tremor on approaching the nose. (*C*) Dysdiadochokinesia, an irregular pattern of alternating movements, can be seen in the abnormal position trace. (From Ghez,[1] p 643, with permission.)

Hypotonia[1,2,4–7]

Muscle tone refers to the ease with which a muscle may be lengthened by passive stretch. The normal cerebellum contributes to the maintenance of muscle tone through facilitatory influences on skeletal muscle stretch reflexes.[7] Cerebellar output increases gamma input to muscle spindles, making them more sensitive to stretch and thus increasing overall muscle tone. Without this input, tone diminishes.

Hypotonia refers to a decreased resistance to passive stretch as might occur with passive limb movement. **Although not as common as ataxia, hypotonia may result from cerebellar damage and lead to a number of distinct clinical signs.** Hypotonia is most evident shortly after acute cerebellar injury and tends to decrease with time. In early and severe cases, a distinct **flabbiness of muscle** can be palpated and the muscle accommodates greater stretch without discomfort. Decreased muscle tone may result in a pendular limb, with **pendular deep tendon reflexes.** For example, when the petallar reflex is elicited, the leg will continue to swing back and forth in a pendular fashion. Hypotonia is often associated with an inability to stop a rapidly moving limb (i.e., **lack of check**), resulting in an overshoot, followed by **excessive rebound** in the opposite direction. If such a patient is asked to pull upward strongly with his or her arm while the clinician first holds it back and then releases it, the arm will fly back, unchecked, until it strikes the face instead of being automatically stopped.

Although hypotonia is not as conspicuous as ataxia, it can exacerbate the symptoms produced by ataxia. Decreased tone in postural muscles, for example, contributes to gait disturbances and postural asymmetry. Hypotonia in the muscles of speech promotes abnormalities in pitch and loudness, and in oculomotor muscles results in difficulty in maintaining the gaze.

Dysequilibrium and Vertigo[1,2,4,5]

The most primitive parts of the cerebellum (the floccolonodular lobes) have extensive connections with both the vestibular nuclei and the vestibular apparatus. It is likely that even in the human, the cerebellum plays a significant role in the maintenance of equilibrium and the coordination of head and eye movements.

Lesions in these regions result in **disturbances of equilibrium** that **are particularly evident during rapid changes in body position** or in the direction of movement. **Patients may exhibit unsteadiness of gait or an inability to sit or stand without swaying or falling, as well as abnormalities of head posture and eye movement** (nystagmus). These deficits are specifically related to an inability to carry out motor activities against the force of gravity. The principal defect is in equilibrium, not ataxia or abnormal muscle tone. Moreover, cerebellar infarction and hemorrhage (stroke) have been shown to induce signs and symptoms such as vertigo, nausea, vomiting, and nystagmus, which mimic damage done to the vestibular labyrinth itself.

Delays in the Initiation and Termination of Movement[1,2,4,5]

Lateral portions of the cerebellar hemispheres and the associated dentate nuclei play important roles in the planning and programming of movement. This is particularly so in multijoint movements and in those requiring fine dexterity in the distal extremities. Lesions on either side of the dentate nuclei or the overlying cortex can interfere with this programming, resulting in delays in both the initiation and the termination of movement. **Intentional movements, such as grasping or pointing, may be slowed in both the buildup and the relaxation of force.** Consequently, the movement of an affected limb is delayed and slowed.

Nonmotor Deficits

Although the principal physiologic importance of the cerebellum resides in its contributions to somatic motor control, evidence is accumulating that the cerebellum is also involved in a variety of nonmotor functions (see Chapter 8).

If this involvement is functionally significant, one would expect evidence of this involvement to appear among the sequelae of cerebellar damage. In fact, **nonmotor deficits are now beginning to be discussed in the context of human cerebellar disease.** Studies conducted in both animals and humans provide evidence that the cerebellum plays a role in motor learning.[8,9] Experimental cerebellar lesions in animals and pathologic lesions in humans seem to interfere with these learning processes.[10-12] Evidence is also accumulating through the use of active imaging techniques that the cerebellum is engaged in such mental functions as shape and word recognition.[13,14] Although an association between some developmental disorders of the cerebellum and retarded intellectual development has been reported for some time,[15] cognitive abnormalities are not usually apparent in patients with cerebellar disease. Recently, **subtle defects in verbal and nonverbal intelligence, in memory, and in other "higher functions" in cerebellar patients have been reported.**[16-18] Although anatomic connections exist between the cerebellum and the areas of the brain involved in the expression of emotion and although animal experiments suggest involvement of the cerebellum in various emotion-laden behaviors such as rage, fear, and aggression, little is known of the role the cerebellum may play in mediating or influencing emotions in humans. In this regard, **specific structural abnormalities in the cerebellum of patients with autism**[19-21] **and certain psychological disorders have been revealed** by computed tomography (CT) and magnetic resonance imaging (MRI) scans, as well as by pathologic study.[22-24] As clinical skills and neuroimaging techniques are refined and more attention is focused on nonmotor deficits, these deficits will undoubtedly be found within the constellation of findings associated with cerebellar dysfunction.

Extracerebellar Causes of Cerebellar Signs and Symptoms

Many of the signs and symptoms associated with cerebellar damage can also be caused by lesions outside the cerebellum itself. Ataxia, for example, can be caused or exacerbated by a variety of extracerebellar lesions. Conditions that disrupt the **spinocerebellar tracts** can cause dysmetria and ataxia by depriving the cerebellum of proprioceptive input. These kinds of defects underlie Friedreich's ataxia (discussed later in this chapter) and many of the cerebellar findings of multiple sclerosis (see Chapter 22). By the same token, disruption of **somatosensory nerves** in the peripheral nervous system can impair the proprioceptive sense enough to cause a sensory ataxia, such as might be observed in alcoholic or other types of peripheral neuropathy (see Chapter 15). Disorders of the **vestibular system**, by interfering with balance and equilibrium, can mimic and exacerbate the gait problems associated with cerebellar damage.

Localization of Cerebellar Dysfunction

As discussed in Chapter 8, attempts have been made to functionally compartmentalize the cerebellum into three basic regions, using either phylogenetic or neuroanatomic criteria (Fig. 19–2).[1,2,25] Although not totally congruent, the archicerebellum, paleocerebellum, and neocerebellum of the phylogenetic scheme correspond fairly well to the vestibulocerebellum, spinocerebellum, and cerebrocerebellum, which are defined by their primary afferent and efferent connections. **Attempts have been made over the years to organize the various signs and symptoms that arise from cerebellar disease into distinct syndromes,** which reflect the region of the cerebellum that is damaged.[4,5,25,26] Accordingly, three syndromes have been described, which some consider to be useful models for localizing cerebellar dysfunction.

Vestibulocerebellar, Archicerebellar, or Flocculonodular Lobe Syndrome

The flocculonodular lobe is phylogenetically the oldest division of the cerebellum and receives extensive input from the vestibular system. This is why this portion of the cerebellum is often termed the **archicerebellum** or vestibulocerebellum. The vestibulocer-

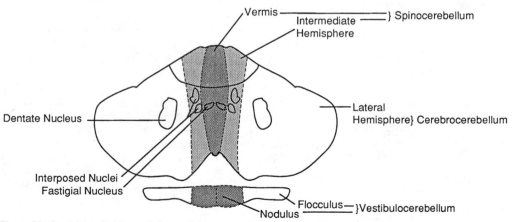

Figure 19–2. Major divisions of the cerebellum.

ebellum receives mossy fiber input chiefly from the vestibular nerve and nuclei and projects back to the vestibular nuclei, which in turn project to the spinal cord (vestibulospinal tracts) and the oculomotor nuclei. This system is important for equilibrium and for control of the axial muscles that are used to maintain balance in the face of gravity. The vestibulocerebellum also controls eye movement and coordinates movements of the head and eyes. Because of the close relationship between the vestibulocerebellum and the vestibular system, **damage to this region of the cerebellum causes clinical findings that mimic vestibular disease itself. Such disorders cause disturbances of locomotion and equilibrium, with prominent truncal and gait ataxia.** Patients with isolated flocculonodular lesions lose their ability to stand or walk without swaying or falling and tend to fall even when sitting with their eyes open. It is interesting that when the effects of gravity are reduced by the patient lying in bed or being physically supported, movements may be completely normal. **Abnormalities of posture and station (e.g., head tilt) and of eye movements also occur.** Tremor is not evident and muscle tone remains normal.

The most common lesion involving the vestibulocerebellum is a special type of tumor, a **medulloblastoma**, which usually occurs in children.

Spinocerebellar or Paleocerebellar Syndrome

Most of the vermal and paravermal (intermediate) regions of the cerebellum receive extensive somatosensory input from the spinal cord and are thus called the *spinocerebellum*. The spinocerebellum also receives input from the auditory, visual, and vestibular systems. The vermal and intermediate portions of the spinocerebellum project to different deep nuclei, controlling different components of the descending motor pathways. The vermis projects to the fastigial nucleus and from there influences cortical and brainstem components of the medial descending systems (axial and girdle muscles). The intermediate part of the cerebellar hemispheres projects to the interposed nucleus to control the lateral descending systems (distal muscles of extremities). **The spinocerebellum receives a continuous flow of somatosensory information regarding the status of the musculoskeletal system, as well as concurrent information from cortical areas about motor commands. It uses this feedback to monitor and refine the execution of movement and to control muscle tone.**

Discrete lesions limited to the spinocerebellum, such as those described in experimental animals, seldom occur in humans. Damage to the human spinocerebellum is most commonly seen in the context of a late degeneration and atrophy of the anterior lobes associated with chronic alcoholism and thiamine deficiency. **The cardinal feature of spinocerebellar disease is involvement of the legs, resulting in abnormal gait and stance.** The gait is wide-based and ataxic, with small hesitant steps. The gait ataxia of spinocerebellar damage is different from that arising from vestibulocerebellar (flocculonodular) damage. Spinocerebellar ataxia reflects a more general deficit in the control of the muscles of ambulation, whereas vestibulocerebellar ataxia reflects a particular inability to control the leg muscles in the presence of the force of gravity. In the case of spinocerebellar damage, the ataxia is not relieved when the patient is freed from the effects of gravity by being physically supported or lying in bed, as it would be with vestibulocerebellar damage.

Cerebrocerebellar, Neocerebellar, or Lateral Cerebellar Syndrome

The cerebrocerebellum, which occupies the lateral zone of the cerebellar hemispheres, is phylogenetically late in developing and is particularly well developed in primates. This region receives most of its input from sensory, motor, and premotor areas of the cerebral cortex that project to the cerebrocerebellum via the pontine nuclei. Most of the output of this area is to the dentate nucleus, which in turn projects back to the cerebral cortex. **Through its extensive connections with the cerebral cortex, the cerebrocerebellum**

is thought to function in the planning and initiation of voluntary movements. It is necessary for achieving precision in rapid limb movements, especially those involving fine dexterity of the distal extremities and movement at multiple joints. **Damage to the lateral hemispheres and dentate nuclei disturbs skilled coordinated movements and speech.** Errors in direction, deviation from proper course, dysmetria, dysdiadochokinesia, and intention tremor all may be present, especially in movements of the upper extremities. The gait may actually be normal, reflecting the relative sparing of the axial muscles and lower limbs. Intentional movements, such as grasping or pointing, may be delayed in their initiation and slowed in both the buildup and the relaxation of intended force. Stretch reflexes and muscle tone are often diminished, resulting in flabbiness, lack of check, and pendular deep tendon reflexes. Muscle weakness and fatigability, although not that common in cerebellar disorders, are most prominent in cerebrocerebellar syndrome. Dysarthric speech may occur with bilateral involvement and can be pronounced. Oculomotor signs may also occur.

When the damage is unilateral, the ipsilateral limb is affected. With limited damage, it is sometimes possible to show impairment only of highly trained movements, such as playing a musical instrument, whereas all other movements appear normal.

Problems with Localization of Dysfunction

Although the divisions of the cerebellum that are based on phylogenetic criteria and comparative anatomic studies (e.g., the archicerebellum, paleocerebellum, and neocerebellum) correspond reasonably well to the divisions of the cerebellum defined by the locus of the termination of the major afferent projections (e.g., the vestibulocerebellum, spinocerebellum, and cerebrocerebellum, respectively). This congruence is not total. Considerable overlap exists between the regions defined by the anatomic sites of afferent terminations. Moreover, the physiologic effects of activating afferent sources project far beyond the boundaries ascribed to these regions. Accordingly, some authors feel that it is misleading to define the clinical scenarios arising from cerebellar damage in terms of these phylogenetic or neuroanatomic regions.

In addition, it should be recognized that **many symptoms of cerebellar dysfunction simply defy limitation to any one division of the cerebellum.** A good example of this is disturbance of gait, which is the most common deficit seen in cerebellar disease. Gait may be disturbed as a consequence of the impairment of equilibrium encountered in disorders involving the flocculonodular lobes. Gait impairment may also result from anterior lobe disorders that adversely affect postural control. Finally, posterior lobe lesions can disturb gait through effects on muscle tone and volitional movement. Accordingly, gait disturbance is to be expected with practically all cerebellar lesions and by itself does little to localize the site of cerebellar damage. In addition, gait can be impaired by disorders of the spinal cord or peripheral nerves that disrupt the flow of proprioceptive information to the cerebellum, as well as by damage to the vestibular system. Lesions in certain cerebral and brainstem areas may likewise interrupt the flow of information to or from the cerebellum, causing gait disturbance similar to that seen in disease of the cerebellum itself.[6]

Specific Etiologies

Although cerebellar disorders as a whole are not very common, **a wide variety of factors, both inherited and acquired, can adversely affect cerebellar function** (see Table 19–1). As with any region of the central nervous system, these conditions may be organized or classified using a number of different criteria, such as prominent clinical features, pathologic criteria, or etiologic factors. For the purposes of this discussion, the major cerebellar disorders are organized along the lines of what is known of their etiology or pathogenesis. It should be noted that because of our incomplete understanding of the causes of many of these disorders, this classification scheme is somewhat arbitrary. Moreover, disorders may logically fall into more than one category.

Inherited or Idiopathic Degenerations[5,27–33]

For unknown reasons, certain regions of the nervous system are particularly vulnerable to degenerative disease. Among these are the cerebellum and its connections. Many of these disorders are genetic or of unknown etiology. These may be distinguished from other degenerative conditions in which underlying toxic, metabolic, infectious, or neoplastic conditions have been identified. These are discussed elsewhere in this chapter.

The genetic and idiopathic degenerations constitute a large group of chronic disorders in which progressive ataxia, disintegration of gait, and dysarthria are the most prominent features.[27–33] This is a complex group of disorders, and numerous attempts have been made to make order of their diversity. Classification schemes have been proposed, based on various clinical, pathologic, biochemical, and genetic criteria. Unfortunately, because of our limited understanding of etiologic factors, the variability of clinical features, and the poor correlation between clinical presentations and pathologic findings, none of these schemes is entirely satisfactory. It is often difficult to discern where one disorder ends and another begins. A more reliable classification of these disorders ultimately depends on a better understanding of the genetics of these disorders and the specific biochemical defects to which they give rise.

Nonetheless, for our descriptive purposes these degenerative diseases may be arbitrarily divided into large clinicopathologic groupings. The entire cerebellar system is vulnerable; **one way to organize these disorders is to divide them into those with a predilection for the cerebellum itself and those with a predilection for the pathways to which it is connected.** With respect to the latter, both peripheral and spinal neurons may be affected. Disorders that primarily involve the peripheral nerves, such as the hereditary sensory motor neuropathies, are discussed in Chapter 15; those with prominent involvement of the spinocerebellar tracts are discussed below. In either case, disruption of the flow of somatosensory (proprioceptive) information to the cerebellum can result in an incoordination of movement. These anatomic distinctions are somewhat arbitrary and although involvement of one particular part of the cerebellar system may be predominant, other regions may also be involved, particularly with disease progression.

Spinal Ataxias

In spinal ataxias the pathology involves primarily the spinocerebellar tracts, whereas the cerebellum itself and the brainstem are relatively spared. Associated degenerative changes in the peripheral nervous system may or may not be evident.

Friedreich's Ataxia[5,27–34]

Friedreich's ataxia is one of the most common hereditary disorders of the nervous system. It is also the most common of the early-onset hereditary spinal ataxias, accounting for at least 50% of these disorders. The symptoms begin to develop in children between 8 and 15 years of age, with clumsiness of gait being the most common presenting symptom. As the condition develops, it is **characterized by relentlessly progressive ataxia, with increasing weakness, loss of tendon reflexes, and impaired proprioceptive sensation in the lower limbs.** The ability to walk is usually lost within 15 years of onset. Ataxia, which begins in the lower limbs, later becomes evident in the arms and then the trunk. **Scoliosis is frequent and may be severe,** particularly if the onset is early (Fig. 19–3). This deformity contributes to

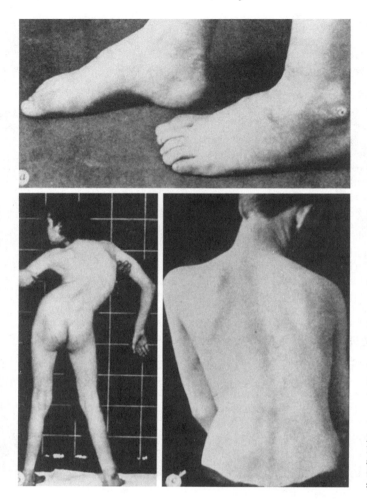

Figure 19–3. *Friedreich's Ataxia.* Note the foot deformity (pes cavus) and kyphoscoliosis in these patients. (From Dow, Kramer, and Robertson,[5] p 56, with permission.)

eventual cardiopulmonary problems. Foot deformities, especially pes cavus, are also common. **Ocular movements are almost always abnormal,** and many patients develop a cerebellar-type dysarthria. Cardiomyopathy with abnormal electrocardiogram (ECG) findings is present in most patients with Friedreich's ataxia, and death from heart failure often occurs late in the disease.

Characteristic pathologic changes are observed in both the peripheral and central nervous systems, particularly in the sensory systems.[33] In the peripheral nervous system, there is degeneration of sensory fibers, sensory ganglion cells, and posterior roots. In the central nervous system, the most conspicuous lesions are in the spinal cord, the posterior columns, and spinocerebellar tracts (Fig. 19–4).[33] Although there may be some patchy loss of cerebellar Purkinje cells and mild degenerative changes in cerebellar nuclei, the ataxia of movement is largely a result of the loss of proprioceptive sense.

The condition most likely to be confused with Friedreich's ataxia is the peroneal atrophy syndrome, in which distal wasting and weakness of the lower limbs (and to a lesser degree the upper limbs) are associated with areflexia.[29–31] This clinical syndrome is associated with type I hereditary sensory and motor neuropathy (see Chapter 15) and distal spinal muscular atrophies (see Chapter 16). In sporadic cases without skeletal deformity, distinguishing between Friedreich's ataxia and multiple sclerosis may also be difficult.

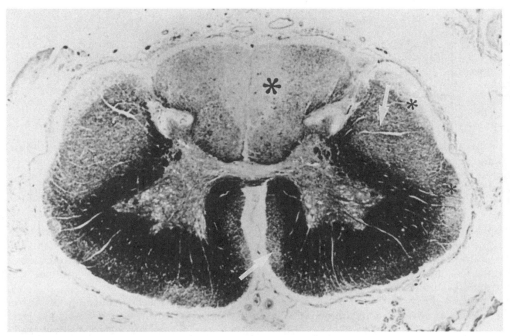

Figure 19–4. *Characteristic Appearance of Lower Cervical Cord in Friedreich's Ataxia.* In this transverse section of the cervical spinal cord in which myelin is darkly stained, a loss of myelin is evident in the posterior columns (*Large* *), spinocerebellar tracts (*Small* *), and the crossed (*Lateral*) and uncrossed (*Anterior*) corticospinal tracts (*Arrows*). (From Oppenheimer, DR: Brain lesions in Friedreich's ataxia. Can J Neurol Sci 6:173, 1979, with permission.)

Cerebellar Ataxias

In the cerebellar ataxias, the predominant pathologic changes occur in the cerebellum and its immediate connections, rather than in the spinal cord tracts.

Olivopontocerebellar Atrophy[5,27–33,35]

In this category are a number of similar disorders characterized by a combined degeneration of the cerebellum, pons, and inferior olives. In general, these disorders are characterized by progressive ataxia with a later onset than Friedreich's ataxia (e.g., between the third and fifth decades of life). The gait is affected first, with progressive ataxia of the trunk and limbs, impairment of equilibrium, slowness of voluntary movement, and abnormal speech. **Although patients often have a pure cerebellar syndrome during the first few years of their illness, pyramidal tract signs, autonomic disturbances, and parkinsonian features with mild dementia may develop later in the illness.** Autonomic disturbances may present as urinary incontinence or orthostatic hypotension. Considerable clinical variability exists among cases of olivopontocerebellar atrophy. Some patients present a picture of relatively pure cerebellar ataxia indistinguishable from that seen in patients with atrophy limited to the cerebellar cortex. Others may have more prominent parkinsonian features and an early dementia.

Pathologic changes are widespread, giving rise to the diverse clinical findings associated with this syndrome. Gross shrinkage of the pons and medulla may be evident, whereas neuronal loss in the inferior olives, cerebellar cortex, and basal ganglia is revealed by microscopic examination. Some degenerative changes may also be evident in the long motor tracts of the spinal cord and the anterior horn cells.[33]

Attempts have been made to define various subtypes of this degeneration, based on the particulars of the mode of inheritance and the predominant clinical features; however, these explorations are beyond the scope of this discussion.

Pure Cerebellar Degeneration[27-33]

In some instances, a relative pure cerebellar syndrome arises, reflecting pathologic changes restricted to just the cerebellum. Unlike Friedreich's ataxia and other spinocerebellar ataxias, there is little evidence of spinal cord involvement. Also, unlike olivopontocerebellar degeneration, there is no prominent involvement of other regions of the brain or brainstem. Although pure cerebellar degeneration can occasionally occur sporadically, in most cases it is evidently inherited as an autosomal-dominant trait. This disorder is less common than Friedreich's ataxia. Its age of onset is later, usually occurring in the fourth decade of life or beyond. The patient first develops gait ataxia (with abnormal stance and instability of gait), progressing to dysarthria and finally to ataxia of the upper extremities and trunk. This disorder is progressive, but may be so gradual that incapacitation does not occur for decades and does not appreciably shorten the life span.

Pathologic changes include a marked loss of neurons (especially Purkinje cells) from the cerebellar cortex, most prominent on the superior surface of the vermis and adjacent parts of the cortex. In advanced cases, atrophy of the cerebellar cortex may be readily apparent with CT scanning. The deep cerebellar nuclei are relatively normal.

Ataxia-Telangectasia[5,27-33,36-38]

Ataxia-telangectasia is the most common cerebellar ataxia of infancy and childhood. This inherited disorder **is unusual to the extent that the cerebellar deficits are accompanied by characteristic vascular lesions (telangectasia) and recurrent pulmonary infections.** The first motor symptom is usually truncal ataxia, which is noted when the child first begins to walk, resulting in an awkward, unsteady gait. When the child reaches 4 or 5 years of age, the limbs become ataxic and dysarthria may be evident. With progression of the disease, extrapyramidal signs such as dystonia and choreoathetosis may develop. Telangectasia is a vascular lesion formed by the dilatation of a small group of blood vessels, which is often observed as a "birthmark." For reasons unknown, these lesions develop in the skin or conjunctiva of the eye in this disorder.

Pathologic changes are noted in many regions of the nervous system, including a severe loss of Purkinje cells in the cerebellum, as well as atrophy of the posterior columns and spinocerebellar tracts of the spinal cord.[33,36-38] Degenerative changes may also be evident in anterior horn cells, sensory and autonomic ganglia, and peripheral nerves.

Nutritional Disorders

Adequate nutrition is necessary for both the normal development and ongoing functioning of the entire nervous system. Nutritional disorders, particularly certain vitamin deficiencies, can adversely affect both the peripheral and central nervous systems, creating a wide range of neurologic manifestations.[39,40] Depending on the deficiency, such findings may include changes in mental status (e.g., coma, mental retardation, psychosis), seizures, cerebellar ataxias, and peripheral motor and sensory disturbances. The few conditions in which cerebellar signs and symptoms are most prominent will be discussed in the following text.[5,29,30,39,40]

Vitamin B$_1$ (Thiamine) Deficiency[5,29,30,39-45]

Of all the vitamin deficiencies, thiamine deficiency is probably the most common in Western society and produces the most severe cerebellar deficits. This deficiency is most often seen in association with chronic alcoholism, but may also be seen in patients with abnormal gastrointestinal activity.

Chronic alcoholics frequently develop a condition termed the Wernicke-Korsakoff syndrome.[41-45] Wernicke's disease is characterized by oculomotor abnormalities, altered mental status, and ataxia of stance and gait. This disease is often associated with Korsakoff's psychosis, a cognitive disorder in which short-term memory is impaired out of proportion to other intellectual functions.

Prominent cerebellar dysfunction occurs in about one third of all alcoholics, and is prominent among those with Wernicke's disease.[41,44] **Stance and gait are primarily affected, the legs being more affected than the trunk or arms.** The ataxia may be so severe in the acute stage of the disease that the patient cannot walk or stand without support. Less severe degrees of the disease are characterized by a wide-based stance and slow, tentative steps. Speech disturbances and abnormal eye movements are relatively infrequent. Pathologic changes in the cerebellum consist of degeneration throughout the cortex, with a striking loss of Purkinje cells.[40] This is most pronounced in the anterior superior aspects of the cerebellum (Fig. 19–5). Signs of peripheral neuropathy are found in most patients with Wernicke-Korsakoff syndrome, but in most cases involvement is mild and does not account for the gait disturbance.

Despite the well-known acute affects of alcohol directly on the cerebellum, it is generally thought that **the chronic cerebellar syndrome observed in alcoholics is caused by thiamine deficiency rather than toxicity of the alcohol itself.**[29,30,41] Alcoholics with this

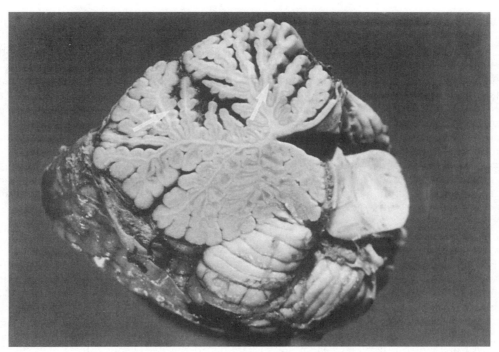

Figure 19–5. *Alcohol-Induced Cerebellar Atrophy.* In this midsaggital section, atrophy is apparent in the anterior and superior aspects of the cerebellum and is most evident in the shrinkage of the vermal folds (*Arrows*). Inferior structures appear grossly normal. (From Victor, M, Adams, RD, and Mancall, EL: A restricted form of cerebellar cortical degeneration occurring in alcoholic patients. AMA Arch Neurol 1:579, 1959, with permission.)

condition are almost always malnourished. That this is not due to alcohol toxicity itself is further suggested by the facts that the ataxia may develop during periods of abstinence, that the symptoms can be relieved by administration of thiamine alone, and that an identical cerebellar degeneration may occur in other (nonalcoholic) states of poor nutrition.

A cerebellar cortical degeneration may also occur in malnourished alcoholics, which is distinct from that associated with Wernicke-Korsakoff syndrome. Truncal instability is the major symptom, often with incoordination of leg movements. The symptoms of this cerebellar degeneration may evolve over weeks or months and may eventually stabilize, even with continued drinking and poor nutrition. In Wernicke's disease, on the other hand, the symptoms are more likely to appear abruptly.

Alcoholics may also develop a sensorimotor polyneuropathy that stabilizes or improves with abstinence and an adequate diet. Although this neuropathy is found in most patients with Wernicke-Korsakoff syndrome, it more often occurs alone. As discussed in Chapter 15, this polyneuropathy is characterized by degeneration of both axons and myelin.

Vitamin B_{12} (Cobalamin) Deficiency[5,39,40]

Vitamin B_{12} deficiency, which is due to an inability to absorb this vitamin from the gut rather than dietary deficiency, **produces a condition called** *pernicious anemia*. The spinal cord, brain, optic nerves, and peripheral nerves all may be involved in pernicious anemia. The spinal cord is affected first and most often and reveals a diffuse degeneration of the white matter. Sensory disturbances, muscle weakness, and spastic ataxia are common. Paresthesias and decreased vibratory and position sense reflect lesions in both spinal and peripheral sensory pathways. Muscle weakness, spasticity, and abnormal tendon reflexes result from lesions in corticospinal tracts. **Ataxia of gait and limbs probably reflects degeneration of spinocerebellar tracts and thus impairments of sensory feedback to the cerebellum.**

Vitamin E Deficiency[5,29,30,39,40,46,47]

Vitamin E, a highly fat-soluble vitamin, is essential for normal neurologic function. **Severe and prolonged vitamin E deficiency produces spinocerebellar degeneration in a number of inherited and acquired disorders.** The most severe vitamin E deficiency state that occurs in humans is due to an inherited failure to synthesis apoprotein B, which is necessary for the intestinal absorption of fat. The result is extremely low levels of circulating lipids and fat-soluble vitamins. Serum vitamin E may be undetectable from birth. Patients with vitamin E deficiency may present in adolescence with progressive ataxia, areflexia, and proprioceptive loss, reflecting the degeneration of posterior column and spinocerebellar tracts in the spinal cord and a loss of large myelinated fibers in the peripheral nervous system. Vitamin E deficiency and similar neurologic symptoms may also occur in patients with diseases affecting bile salt concentrations in the small intestine or disturbing the absorptive surface of the gut.

Neoplastic and Paraneoplastic Disorders

Neoplastic disease, whether located within or near the cerebellum, or at some distant site, can adversely affect cerebellar function.

Paraneoplastic Cerebellar Degeneration[5,29,30,48–51]

All areas of the nervous system are susceptible to the deleterious effects of systemic carcinoma. In addition to effects on the cerebellum, neoplasm may cause encephalopathy, peripheral neuropathy, myopathy, and defects of neuromuscular transmission (e.g., Lambert-Eaton myasthenic syndrome; Chapter 14). **A nonmetastatic paraneoplastic degeneration of** the cerebellar cortex is the most common paraneoplastic syndrome that affects the central nervous system. **Symptoms** may develop before or after discovery of the tumor. They usually **begin with gait ataxia and over a few days or weeks progress to severe truncal and limb ataxia, with dysarthria and often with abnormal ocular movements.** Vertigo is common and patients frequently complain of diplopia. Symptoms may progress in severity for several weeks or months and then stabilize. Unfortunately, by this stage, the patient may already be severely disabled. Often superimposed upon the cerebellar deficits are manifestations of a more diffuse paraneoplastic encephalopathy, including cognitive deterioration, bulbar palsy, and limb weakness.

Pathologic examination usually reveals a severe loss of Purkinje cells throughout the cerebellum, with or without evidence of inflammation.[33,48,49,52,53] Some patients may have more widespread pathologic findings, including degeneration of spinocerebellar tracts, dorsal columns, and corticospinal tracts. Although the pathogenesis of paraneoplastic cerebellar degeneration is poorly understood, theories proposed to explain these remote effects of malignancy focus on nutritional deficiency, viral infections, and autoimmune mechanisms. Evidence such as clinical improvement with plasmapheresis and the presence of anti-Purkinje cell antibodies supports the notion of disturbed immune activity.[52-55] The neurologic status of these patients can improve markedly with treatment of the underlying neoplasm.

Paraneoplastic cerebellar degeneration occurs most often in association with lung, breast, or ovarian cancer or Hodgkin's disease. Up to 50% of all patients over the age of 40 presenting with degenerative cerebellar disease may have an underlying neoplasm.

Primary Tumors[5,28,29,56,57]

The cerebellum and adjacent structures may also constitute the site of primary tumor development. Posterior fossa tumors represent about one third of all intracranial tumors in adults and about two thirds in children. As with other regions of the central nervous system, these tumors may arise from either glial cells (e.g., astrocytomas) or neural cells (e.g., medulloblastomas). No particular type predominates in adults, but in children, most are astrocytomas or medulloblastomas.[56] Lesions limited to just the cerebellum are rare, but are most often due to the presence of a discrete tumor. Cerebellar signs may occur with tumors of the cerebellum itself or with those arising in the fourth ventricle or brainstem.

As with any posterior fossa mass, nonspecific signs and symptoms reflecting increased intracranial pressure or compression of the brainstem may also develop. Headache, nausea, and vomiting may be accompanied to a variable extent by cranial nerve deficits, pyramidal tract signs, sensory disturbances, and decreasing consciousness. An expanding cerebellar mass may compress the medulla and portions of the cervical spine to the extent that infarction occurs and life-threatening abnormalities of cardiovascular and respiratory regulation ensue.

Tumors of the cerebellopontine angle, although they may be considered extracerebellar, are not an uncommon neoplastic cause of cerebellar signs. These tumors damage the inferior cerebellar peduncle, and the usual resulting complaints are impaired balance, ataxia, vertigo, and specific cranial nerve deficits (e.g., hearing loss, oculomotor disturbances, and facial paralysis). The most common tumors in this area are acoustic neuromas, which develop in the vestibulocochlear nerve.

Metastatic Disease[5,28,29,57]

In adults, metastasis is the most common source of neoplasia in the posterior fossa (Fig. 19–6). Common primary tumor sites include the lung (about 50%), followed by the breast, kidney, and melanoma. The effects on the cerebellum reflect the location and extent of involvement. Focal neurologic deficits include limb or truncal ataxia or cranial nerve dysfunction. More generalized symptoms such as headache, nausea, or vomiting may result from obstructive hydrocephalus and elevated intracranial pressure.

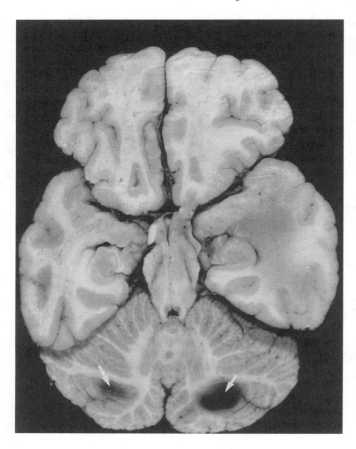

Figure 19–6. *Cerebellar Metastases.* Two hemorrhagic metastases (*Arrows*) from carcinoma of the lung are visible in the cerebellar hemispheres. (From Hirano, A (ed): Color Atlas of Pathology of the Nervous System, ed 2. Igaku-Shoin, Tokyo, p 62, with permission.)

Developmental Disorders[5,29,30,58–62]

Congenital structural anomalies of the cerebellum are not uncommon and probably reflect both genetic (familial) and teratogenic factors. The cerebellum has the longest period of embryologic development of any major structure of the brain and is consequently vulnerable to teratogenic insults longer than most parts of the nervous system. The developing cerebellum is susceptible to the toxic effects of many drugs, chemicals, viral infections, radiation, and ischemic-hypoxic insults.

Malformation of the cerebellum may be focal, confined to the cerebellum, or associated with other brainstem or cerebral abnormalities. Congenital hypoplasia or even the absence of some or most of the cerebellum may occur. Because the vermis forms after the hemispheres, it is more likely to be absent or underdeveloped than other parts of the cerebellum. Although ataxia, hypotonia, tremor, and abnormal eye movements may be present, marked cerebellar hypoplasia has been shown by imaging studies and autopsy to be present in totally asymptomatic individuals (Fig. 19–7). A number of other malformations of the cerebellum have been described. The Dandy-Walker malformation consists of a ballooning of the posterior half of the fourth ventricle and hypoplasia of the cerebellar vermis.[60,61] Swelling of the brain due to excessive cerebrospinal fluid (hydrocephalus) almost always develops and accounts for many of the accompanying clinical manifestations. Hypotonia, cerebellar deficits, pyramidal signs, and seizures are present to varying degrees in about 25% of these cases. The Chiari malformations (the most common developmental abnormality of the posterior fossa) encompass a group of anomalies of the brainstem and cerebellum, in which there is a herniation of part of the cerebellum, medulla, and sometimes

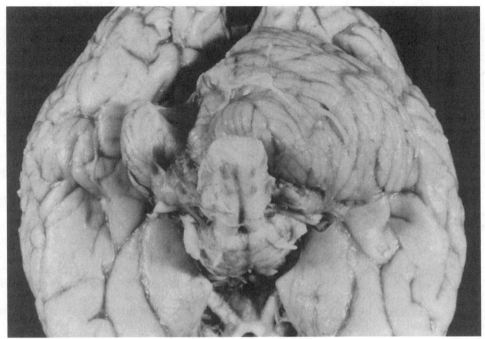

Figure 19–7. *Congenital Aplasia of the Left Cerebellar Hemisphere.* The left hemisphere was almost totally lacking in this brain of an asymptomatic adult. (From Dow, Kramer, and Robertson,[5] p 95, with permission.)

the pons through the foramen magnum into the upper cervical spinal canal.[62] By compressing the cerebellum, lower brainstem, and cervical cord, this herniation may compromise neural function. The Chiari malformations are frequently associated with other malformations of the nervous system, such as spina bifida and hydrocephalus.

Perinatal hypoxia may produce severe cerebellar cortical atrophy, but signs of cerebellar dysfunction are usually overshadowed by evidence of damage to the cerebral cortex and other areas of the brain.

Disorders Due to Infection[5,29,30,63]

A variety of organisms can infect the central nervous system, and in certain infectious disorders cerebellar signs and symptoms may be preeminent. Both slow and conventional viruses may produce a cerebellar syndrome.[63] Creutzfeldt-Jakob disease, for example, is an encephalopathy resulting from infection with a so-called slow virus. It is now thought that almost 50% of affected patients may have a cerebellar or ataxic form of this disease, in which cerebellar deficits dominate the clinical picture for the first several months. Encephalitis produced by a wide range of conventional viruses can also give rise to cerebellar findings. Viral cerebellitis has been associated with polio, mumps, rubella, chickenpox, and herpesviruses. The most common cerebellar syndrome attributed to viral infection is an acute cerebellar ataxia that occurs in young children. Children may develop over hours or a few days severe truncal ataxia, with less prominent limb involvement. Recovery is usually complete, although it can take up to 6 months. **Bacteria, fungi, and other parasites may also infect the cerebellum.** Cerebellitis may accompany bacterial meningitis or be secondary to a variety of systemic bacterial infections. Ataxic syndromes, in association with meningitis or systemic bacterial infection, are usually transient and resolve within weeks. Cerebellar syndromes as a sole result of fungal infection are rare. Amebas, tapeworms, and other parasites may create cerebellar cysts or masses.

Vascular Disorders[5,29,30,64–68]

Ischemic disease and hemorrhage in the posterior fossa seldom give rise to cerebellar signs alone. Cerebellar deficits are usually accompanied by brainstem and cranial nerve findings, including nausea, vomiting, vertigo, and visual disturbances, which may dominate the clinical picture.

Cerebellar hemorrhage is estimated to account for about 10% of all intracranial hemorrhages and a few percent of all strokes (Fig. 19–8). **Cerebellar hemorrhage typically manifests as an acute onset of headache, repeated vomiting, vertigo and dizziness, and an inability to walk or stand.**[64,65] Coma develops over hours or days in about 50% of these patients. In many cases, cerebellar hemorrhage is not suspected until neuroimaging or autopsy. The typical patient is hypertensive and older than 60 years of age, and frequently has a prior history of transient neurologic symptoms.

Although cerebellar infarction is more common than cerebellar hemorrhage, it represents only about 1% of all strokes (see Chapter 21).[66–68] **Infarction in this region, however, has one of the highest mortality rates**, estimated to be 20% to 50%. Diagnosis is often missed because of the wide range of clinical presentations. Actually, many patients have few cerebellar signs, despite radiologic evidence of cerebellar infarction. New imaging techniques have greatly increased the accuracy of diagnosis and suggest that its incidence is greater than heretofore suspected. The cerebellum is supplied by distal branches of the posterior inferior cerebellar artery, the anterior inferior cerebellar artery, and the superior cerebellar artery, all of which are supplied by the basilar artery. Although cerebellar infarction usually involves multiple vessels, occlusion of any one of the three principal arteries supplying the

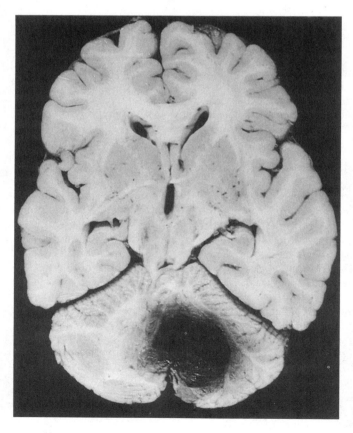

Figure 19–8. Large hemorrhage (hematoma) of the cerebellum. From Hirano, A (ed): Color Atlas of Pathology of the Nervous System, ed 2. Igaku-Shoin, Tokyo, 1988, p 69, with permission.)

cerebellum may give rise to specific signs and symptoms. **Many different clinical patterns may develop, but unsteadiness of gait, dizziness, nausea, and vomiting are common early symptoms.** Cerebellar infarction with edema formation can lead to sudden respiratory arrest due to increased intracranial pressure in the posterior fossa.

Intoxications[29,30,69,70]

Cerebellar dysfunction may occur in association with exposure to a wide variety of toxins, including drugs, solvents, and heavy metals. These toxins may adversely affect the cerebellum directly or as part of a more generalized encephalopathy.

Practically all drugs given at high enough doses can cause neurologic signs and symptoms, including those indicating cerebellar dysfunction.[69,70] The *drug-induced cerebellar syndrome* **is characterized by transient gait ataxia, dysarthria, and nystagmus.** Symptoms usually subside with discontinuation of the offending agent. The most common form of this syndrome is that associated with anticonvulsant medications.[71] Certain cardiac agents, antineoplastic agents, and lithium may produce similar findings.

Recreational or accidental exposure to a wide variety of volatile solvents may cause ataxia along with other neurologic problems, including psychoses, cognitive impairment, and pyramidal signs.[69,70,72,73] As with drug toxicity, these deficits are usually reversible unless exposure has been heavy and prolonged. These volatile chemicals are ubiquitous in our society and are found in many products, such as adhesives, solvents, aerosols, and fire extinguishers. Unfortunately, they are increasingly a choice for recreational abuse, with devastating neurologic consequences.

Poisoning with heavy metals such as mercury, manganese, bismuth, thallium, and lead **can also result in neurologic syndromes, including prominent ataxia.**[29,30,69,70]

Injury Due to Physical or Mechanical Trauma[5]

Direct mechanical trauma to the head, particularly in the area of the occiput, can produce cerebellar hemorrhage and tissue disruption (see Chapter 20).[5] In most physical trauma resulting in closed-head injury, however, cerebellar dysfunction is not particularly apparent clinically and is overshadowed by the sequelae of the rest of the central nervous system damage. As some patients emerge from the acute phase of closed-head injury, cerebellar deficits may become more prominent.

The cerebellum has one of the highest rates of oxygen consumption in the nervous system and **is particularly sensitive to oxygen deprivation.**[5] Following severe brain hypoxia, however, signs of cerebellar dysfunction may be overshadowed by diffuse cerebral dysfunction. **The cerebellum is also particularly sensitive to thermal injury.**[5] Cerebellar dysfunction is known to occur following hyperthermia, whether it is due to heat stroke or prolonged fever. Radiation-induced injury to the cerebellum can result from both therapeutic and accidental exposure to ionizing radiation, manifested as diffuse atrophy and various functional deficits.

Metabolic Disorders[29–31]

A number of inherited and acquired metabolic disorders are associated with cerebellar dysfunction. Disorders of lipids, the urea cycle, pyruvate and lactate metabolism, and some aminoacidurias are associated with cerebellar symptoms. Some of these disorders manifest in infancy or early childhood; others are not evident until later in life. They vary markedly in their severity and the extent to which they are progressive. Genetically determined metabolic disorders may give rise to either intermittent bouts of ataxia, due to the accumulation of circulating neurotoxic substances such as ammonia, or to persistent progressive ataxia.[29–31] These metabolic disorders often cause disordered function at multiple sites in the nervous system. Accordingly, affected patients may present, in addition to cerebellar signs and symptoms, additional symptoms such as vomiting, headache, involuntary movements, seizures, confusion, and varying degrees of mental retardation.

Acquired disturbances of liver function, electrolyte balance (e.g., hyponatremia), and endocrine activity may also produce cerebellar findings. For example, hypothyroidism may be associated with an ataxic syndrome in both children and adults, as well as an accompanying peripheral neuropathy described in Chapter 15.

Demyelinating and Dysmyelinating Disorders[74–76]

Many of the nerve fibers of both the peripheral and central nervous systems are myelinated and depend on this myelin for normal impulse propagation. **Myelin is disturbed in a variety of disorders, both acquired and inherited,** with resultant abnormalities in both the speed and the quality of impulse conduction (see Chapter 22). In some of these disorders, normal myelin may be damaged or destroyed (demyelinating diseases). In others, myelin is never properly formed (dysmyelinating diseases). Both the spinocerebellar pathways and the cerebellum contain abundant myelin and may be damaged by these types of disorders.

The most common of the demyelinating diseases of the CNS is multiple sclerosis (see Chapter 22), which is characterized by multisystem demyelination and clinical features encompassing spasticity, visual and oculomotor disturbances, urinary dysfunction, and cerebellar deficits.[74–76] **The classic signs of cerebellar dysfunction are common in multiple sclerosis** in a variety of combinations, which may include dysarthria, instability of head and trunk, intention tremor, and incoordination of voluntary movements and gait. Cerebellar signs such as nystagmus and ataxia may appear early in the disease. Although most patients with multiple sclerosis have clinical manifestations referable to damage to many areas of the nervous system, in a few patients, cerebellar deficits predominate throughout much of the course of the disease. The cerebellar deficits may be severe and may make a significant contribution to patient disability.

Cerebellar dysfunction may result from the direct involvement of the cerebellum or may be due to involvement of spinocerebellar tracts. Demyelinating lesions (plaques) may be found randomly distributed throughout the cerebellar hemispheres, the peduncles, in the vicinity of the dentate nuclei, and in the spinocerebellar tracts.

Certain dysmyelinating diseases are also associated with progressive cerebellar dysfunction. Although cerebellar deficits are not a predominant component of the leukodystrophies, pathologic examination often reveals areas of demyelination throughout the cerebellar system, as well as in the cerebrum.

RECOMMENDED READINGS

Adams, RD and Victor, M: Principles of Neurology, ed 5. Chapter 36. Multiple Sclerosis and Allied Demyelinating Diseases. McGraw-Hill, New York, 1993.

Brooks, VB: The Neural Basis of Motor Control. Chapter 13. The Cerebellum. Oxford University Press, New York, 1986.

Conner, KE and Rosenberg, RN: The Hereditary Ataxias. Chapter 45. In Rosenberg, RN, et al (eds): The Molecular and Genetic Basis of Neurological Disease. Butterworth-Heinemann, Boston, 1993.

Dow, RS, Kramer, RE, and Robertson, LT: Disorders of the Cerebellum. Chapter 37. In Joynt, RJ (ed): Clinical Neurology, vol 3. JB Lippincott, Philadelphia, 1991.

Ghez, C: The Cerebellum. Chapter 41. In Kandel, ER, Schwartz, JH, and Jessell, TM (eds): Principles of Neural Science, ed 3. Appleton & Lange, Norwalk, CT, 1991.

Gilman, S: Cerebellum and Motor Dysfunction. Chapter 23. In Asbury, AK, McKhann, GM, and McDonald, WI (eds): Diseases of the Nervous System. Clinical Neurobiology, ed 2. WB Saunders, Philadelphia, 1992.

Gilman, S, Bloedel, JR, and Lechtenberg, R: Disorders of the Cerebellum. FA Davis, Philadelphia, 1981.

Harding, AE: The Hereditary Ataxias and Related Disorders. Churchill Livingstone, Edinburgh, 1984.

Harding, AE: Cerebellar and Spinocerebellar Disorders. Chapter 77. In Bradley, WG, et al (eds): Neurology in Clinical Practice, vol II. Butterworth-Heinemann, Boston, 1990.

Harding, AE and Deufel, T (eds): Inherited Ataxias. Adv Neurol 61:1, 1993.

Ito, M: The Cerebellum and Neural Control. Raven Press, New York, 1984.

King, JS (ed): New Concepts in Cerebellar Neurobiology. Alan R. Liss, New York, 1988.

Lechtenberg, R (ed): Handbook of Cerebellar Diseases. Marcel Dekker, New York, 1993.

Matthews, WB, et al (eds): McAlpine's Multiple Sclerosis, ed 2. Churchill Livingstone, Edinburgh, 1991.

Stumpf, DA: Cerebellar Disorders. In Rosenberg, RN (ed): Comprehensive Neurology. Raven Press, New York, 1991.

REFERENCES

1. Ghez, C: The Cerebellum. Chapter 41. In Kandel, ER, Schwartz, JH, and Jessell, TM (eds): Principles of Neural Science, ed 3. Appleton & Lange, Norwalk, CT, 1991.

2. Gilman, S: Cerebellum and Motor Dysfunction. Chapter 23. In Asbury, AK, McKhann, GM, and McDonald, WI (eds): Diseases of the Nervous System: Clinical Neurobiology, ed 2. WB Saunders, Philadelphia, 1992.

3. Ito, M: The Cerebellum and Neural Control. Raven Press, New York, 1984.

4. Lechtenberg, R: Signs and Symptoms of Cerebellar Disease. Chapter 4. In Lechtenberg, R (ed): Handbook of Cerebellar Diseases, Marcel Dekker, New York, 1993.

5. Dow, RS, Kramer, RE, and Robertson, LT: Disorders of the Cerebellum. Chapter 37. In Joynt, RJ (ed): Clinical Neurology, vol 3. JB Lippincott, Philadelphia, 1991.

6. Thompson, PD, and Day, BL: The Anatomy and Physiology of Cerebellar Disease. Adv Neurol 61:15, 1993.

7. Rothwell, JC: Control of Human Voluntary Movement. Chapter 9. The Cerebellum. Aspen Publishers, Rockville, MD, 1987.

8. LaLonde, R and Botez, MI: The Cerebellum and Learning Processes in Animals. Brain Res Rev 15:325, 1990.

9. Glickstein, M and Yeo, C: The Cerebellum and Motor Learning. J Cogn Neurosci 2:69, 1990.

10. Lye, RH, et al: Effects of a Unilateral Cerebellar Lesion on the Acquisition of Eye-Blink Conditioning in Man. J Physiol (Lond) 403:58P, 1988.

11. Topka, H: Deficit in Classical Conditioning in Patients with Cerebellar Degeneration. Brain 116(Pt 4):961, 1993.

12. Sanes, JN, Dimitrov, B, and Hallett, M: Motor Learning in Patients with Cerebellar Dysfunction. Brain 113(Pt 1):103, 1990.

13. Decety, J, et al: The Cerebellum Participates in Mental Activity: Tomographic Measurement of Regional Blood Flow. 535:313, 1990.

14. Petersen, SE, et al: Position Emission Tomographic Studies of the Cortical Anatomy of Single-Word Processing. Nature 331:585, 1988.

15. Sarnet, HB and Alcala, H: Human Cerebellar Hypoplasia. Arch Neurol 37:300, 1980.

16. Fiez, JA, et al: Impaired Non-Motor Learning and Error Detection Associated with Cerebellar Damage: A Single Case Study. Brain 115 (Pt. 1):155, 1992.

17. Akshoomoff, NA, et al: Contribution of the Cerebellum to Neuropsychological Functioning: Evidence from a Case of Cerebellar Degenerative Disorder. Neuropsychologia 30:315, 1992.

18. Ackermann, H, et al: Speech Deficits in Ischaemic Cerebellar Lesions. J Neurol 239:273, 1992.

19. Murakami, JW, et al: Reduced Cerebellar Hemisphere Size and Its Relationship to Vermal Hypoplasia in Autism. Arch Neurol 46:689, 1989.

20. Kemper, TL and Banman, ML: The contribution of neuropathologic studies to the understanding of autism. Neurol Clin 11:175, 1993.

21. Holroyd, S, Reiss, AL, and Bryan, RN: Autistic Features in Jouberts Syndrome: A Genetic Disorder with Agenesis of the Cerebellar Vermis. Biol Psychiatry 29:287, 1992.

22. Snider, SR: Cerebellar Pathology in Schizophrenia: Cause or Consequence? Neurosci Biobehav Rev 6:47, 1982.

23. Volkow, ND, et al: Low Cerebellar Metabolism in Medicated Patients with Schizophrenia. Am J Psychiatry 149:686, 1992.

24. Sandyk, R, Kay, SR, and Merriam, AE: Atrophy of the Cerebellar Vermis: Relevance to the Symptoms of Schizophrenia. Int J Neurosci 57:205, 1981.

25. Martin, JH: Neuroanatomy: Text and Atlas. Appleton & Lange, Norwalk, CT, 1989.

26. Dichgans, J, and Diener, HC: Clinical Evidence for Functional Compartmentalization of the Cerebellum. In Bloedel, JR, Dichgans, J, and Precht, W (eds): Cerebellar Functions. Springer-Verlag, Berlin, 1985.

27. Chadwick, D, Cartlidge, N, and Bates, D: Medical Neurology. Chapter 15. Inherited and Degenerative Disorders of the Central Nervous System. Churchill Livingstone, Edinburgh, 1989.

28. Conner, KE and Rosenberg, RN: The Hereditary Ataxias. Chapter 45. In Rosenberg, RN, et al (eds): The Molecular and Genetic Basis of Neurological Disease. Butterworth-Heinemann, Boston, 1993.

29. Harding, AE: Cerebellar and Spinocerebellar Disorders. Chapter 77. In Bradley, WG, et al (eds): Neurology in Clinical Practice, vol II. Butterworth-Heinemann, Boston, 1990.

30. Harding, AE: Hereditary Ataxias and Related Disorders. Chapter 88. In Asbury, AK, McKhann, GM, and McDonald, WI (eds): Diseases of the Nervous System: Clinical Neurobiology, ed 2. WB Saunders, Philadelphia, 1992.

31. Harding, AE: Clinical Features and Classification of Inherited Ataxias. Adv Neurol 61:1, 1993.

32. Rosenberg, RN and Grossman, A: Hereditary Ataxia. Neurol Clin 7:25, 1989.

33. Oppenheimer, DR and Esiri, MM: Diseases of the Basal Ganglia, Cerebellum, and Motor Neurons. Chapter 15. In Adams, JH and Duchen, LW (eds): Greenfield's Neuropathology, ed 5. Oxford University Press, New York, 1992.

34. Manyam, BV: Friedreich's Disease. Chapter 33. In Lechtenberg, R (ed): Handbook of Cerebellar Diseases. Marcel Dekker, New York, 1993.

35. Duvosin, RC and Plaitakis, A (eds): The Olivopontocerebellar Atrophies. Adv Neurol 41:1, 1984.

36. Gatti, RA: Candidates for the Molecular Defect in Ataxia Telangiectasia. Adv Neurol 61:127, 1993.

37. Jeret, JS and Lechtenberg, R: Ataxia-Telangiectasia. Chapter 40. In Lechtenberg, R (ed): Handbook of Cerebellar Diseases. Marcel Dekker, New York, 1993.

38. Taylor, AMR, et al: Variant Forms of Ataxia Telangiectasia. J Med Genet, 24:669, 1987.

39. So, YT and Simon, RP: Deficiency Diseases of the Nervous System. Chapter 62. In Bradley, WG, et al (eds): Neurology in Clinical Practice, vol 2. Butterworth-Heinemann, Boston, 1990.

40. Adams, RD and Victor, M: Principles of Neurology, ed 4. Chapter 39. Diseases of the Nervous System Due to Nutritional Deficiency. McGraw-Hill Information Services, New York, 1989.

41. Worner, TM: Effects of Alcohol. Chapter 46. In Lechtenberg, R (ed): Handbook of Cerebellar Diseases. Marcel Dekker, New York, 1993.

42. Butterworth, RF: Pathophysiology of Cerebellar Dysfunction in the Wernicke-Korsakoff Syndrome. Can J Neurol Sci 20(suppl 3):S123, 1993.

43. Neiman, J, et al: Movement Disorders in Alcoholism: A Review. Neurology 40:741, 1991.

44. Lindboe, CF and Loberg, EM: The Frequency of Brain Lesions in Alcoholics: Comparison Between the 5-year Periods 1975–1979 and 1983–1987. J Neurol Sci 88:107, 1988.

45. Pratt, OE, et al: Genesis of Alcoholic Brain Tissue Injury. Alcoholism 25:217, 1990.

46. Muller, DPR, Lloyd, JK, and Wolff, OH: Vitamin E and Neurological Function. Lancet 1:225, 1983.

47. Harding, AE: Vitamin E and the Nervous System. CRC Crit Rev Neurobiol 3:89, 1987.

48. Dropcho, EJ: Paraneoplastic Cerebellar Disorders. Chapter 15. In Lechtenberg, R (ed): Handbook of Cerebellar Diseases. Marcel Dekker, New York, 1993.

49. Posner, JB: Paraneoplastic Syndromes. Chapter 83. In Asbury, AK, McKhann, GM, and McDonald, WI (eds): Diseases of the Nervous System: Clinical Neurobiology, ed 2. WB Saunders, Philadelphia, 1992.

50. Waterhouse, DM, Natale, RB, and Cody, RL: Breast Cancer and Paraneoplastic Cerebellar Degeneration. Cancer 78:1835, 1991.

51. Posner, JB: Paraneoplastic Cerebellar Degeneration. Can J Neurol Sci 20(suppl 3):S117, 1993.

52. Posner, JB: Pathogenesis of Central Nervous System Paraneoplastic Syndromes. Rev Neurol 148:502, 1992.

53. Graus, F and Rene, R: Clinical and Pathological Advances on Central Nervous System Paraneoplastic Syndromes. Rev Neurol 148:496, 1992.

54. Anderson, NE, Rosenblum, MK, and Posner, JB: Paraneoplastic Cerebellar Degeneration: Clinical-Immunological Correlations. Ann Neurol 24:559, 1988.

55. Dropcho, EJ: Autoimmune Aspects of Paraneoplastic Cerebellar Degeneration. Prog Neuro Endocrin Immunol 3:90, 1990.

56. Roberts, RO, et al: Medulloblastoma: A Population-Based Study of 532 Cases. J Neuropathol Exp Neurol 50:134, 1990.

57. Lechtenberg, R (ed): Handbook of Cerebellar Diseases. Part IV. Neoplastic Disease. Marcel Dekker, New York, 1993.

58. Lechtenberg, R (ed): Handbook of Cerebellar Diseases. Part III. Structural Disease. Marcel Dekker, New York, 1993.

59. Harding, BN: Malformations of the Nervous System. Chapter 10. In Adams, JH, and Duchen, LW (eds): Greenfield's Neuropathology, ed 5. Oxford University Press, New York, 1992.

60. Bordarier, C and Aicardi, J: Dandy-Walker Syndrome and Agenesis of the Cerebellar Vermis: Diagnostic Problems and Genetic Counselling. Dev Med Child Neurol 32:285, 1990.

61. Johanson, CE: The Dandy-Walker Syndrome. In Myrianthopoulos, N-C (ed): Handbook of Clinical Neurology, vol 6. Malformations. Elsevier, New York, 1987, pp 323–336.

62. Banberger, BC: The Chiari II Malformation. In Myrianthopoulos, N-C (ed): Handbook of Clinical Neurology, vol 6. Malformations. Elsevier, New York, 1987, pp 403–42.

63. Tateishi, J, Kita Moto, T, and Doh-ura, K: Slow Transmissible Diseases Affecting the Cerebellum. In Lechtenberg, R (ed): Handbook of Cerebellar Diseases. Marcel Dekker, New York, 1993.

64. Shafer, SQ and Brust, JCM: Cerebellar Hemorrhage. Chapter 17. In Lechtenberg, R (ed): Handbook of Cerebellar Diseases. Marcel Dekker, New York, 1993.

65. Dunne, JW, Chakera, T and Kermode, S: Cerebellar Hemorrhage—Diagnosis and Treatment: A Study of 75 Consecutive Cases. QJ Med 64:739, 1987.

66. Amarenco, P, Hauw, JJ, and Caplan, LR: Cerebellar Infarctions. Chapter 16. In Lechtenberg, R (ed): Handbook of Cerebellar Diseases. Marcel Dekker, New York, 1993.

67. Amarenco, P, Hauw, JJ, and Gautier, JC: Arterial Pathology in Cerebellar Infarction. Stroke 21:1299, 1990.

68. Kase, CS, et al: Cerebellar Infarction. Clinico-Anatomic Correlations. J Neurol 237:160, 1990.

69. Johnson, LM, Hubble, JP, and Koller, WC: Effect of Medications and Toxins on Cerebellar Function. Chapter 45. In Lechtenberg, R (ed): Handbook of Cerebellar Diseases. Marcel Dekker, New York, 1993.

70. Goetz, CG and Cohen, MM: Neurotoxic Agents. Chapter 20. In Joynt, RJ (ed): Clinical Neurology, vol 2. JB Lippincott, Philadelphia, 1992.

71. McLain, LW, Martin, JT, and Allen, JH: Cerebellar Degeneration Due to Chronic Phenytoin Therapy. Ann Neurol 7:18, 1980.

72. Lolin, Y: Chronic Neurological Toxicity Associated with Exposure to Volatile Substances. Hum Toxicol 8:293, 1989.

73. Fornazzari, L, et al: Cerebellar, Cortical, and Functional Impairment in Toluene Abusers. Acta Neurol Scand 67:319, 1983.

74. Troiano, R: Multiple Sclerosis and Other Demyelinating Diseases. Chapter 43. In Lechtenberg, R (ed): Handbook of Cerebellar Diseases. Marcel Dekker, New York, 1993.

75. Matthews, WB, et al (eds): McAlpine's Multiple Sclerosis, ed 2. Churchill Livingstone, Edinburgh, 1991.

76. Adams, RD and Victor, M: Principles of Neurology, ed 5. Chapter 36. Multiple Sclerosis and Allied Demyelinating Diseases. McGraw-Hill, New York, 1993.

CHAPTER 20

■

Traumatic Brain Injury

Lisa K. Saladin, BMR(PT), MSc

*I*n the United States, about 2 million traumatic brain injuries occur annually, with 500,000 severe enough to require hospital admission.[1] In the past 20 years, the mortality rate from traumatic head injuries has been declining as emergency care has improved. As a result, the number of disabled survivors has increased. Many will be mildly injured and discharged in a few days with minimal residual deficits. However, a significant percentage of those who survive will experience some degree of permanent disability. An estimated 13% to 16% or about 65,000 of these injuries will result in severe physical and mental disability, whereas another 30% to 50% will suffer moderate disability.[2]

To understand the nature of traumatic brain injury and its staggering socioeconomic impact, knowledge of general patient characteristics is required. The average age of traumatically brain-injured individuals is 30, with the highest incidence in those 15 to 24 years old.[3] **Brain injury is the leading cause of disability in children and adolescents, and the psychological and financial effects on the family may be devastating.** Traumatic brain injuries occur two to four times more frequently in males than females, with athletic or aggressive individuals having a greater risk. Finally, the high incidence of students, the unemployed, and those from lower socioeconomic backgrounds has significant repercussions on the financial burden associated with this type of injury. **It is estimated that the economic costs related to traumatic brain injury will approach $25 billion per year.**[1]

Rehabilitation professionals are challenged with the task of understanding, evaluating, and treating the often radical alterations in multiple functions that confront a traumatically brain-injured person and their families. The human nervous system directs all aspects of movement, cognition, emotion, and behavior. A traumatic brain injury may produce deficits in all these areas and has the potential to significantly alter a person's ability to function. The effects of such an injury on motor control are complex and vary greatly from one patient to the next.

Factors such as the mechanism of injury, the extent and location of central nervous system damage, the presence of secondary complications, and the presence of accompanying

467

Table 20–1. *Mechanisms of Traumatic Brain Injury*

Injury	Cause
Head in motion strikes a relatively immobile solid object	Traffic accident, fall
Head struck by objects in motion	Bullet wound, blow to head, falling object
Compression of the head	Crush injury

musculoskeletal trauma all influence the clinical presentation following a traumatic brain injury. Knowledge of the mechanisms of injury and the pathophysiology associated with traumatic brain injury is critical to an understanding of the clinical manifestations and subsequent management of this disorder. Therefore, this chapter first reviews mechanisms of injury and the pathophysiologic effects of traumatic brain injury. This is followed by a description of the clinical manifestations, with a focus on those that influence motor control.

Mechanisms of Traumatic Brain Injury

The nature, direction, and magnitude of the forces applied to the head determine the extent of ensuing brain dysfunction. Various mechanisms that typically produce traumatic brain injuries are listed in Table 20–1. Most (48%) adult injuries are caused by traffic accidents, with accidental falls being the next major cause of injury.[4] In contrast, most (64%) infant head injuries are the result of child abuse.[5]

Craniocerebral injuries may be classified as penetrating (open) or nonpenetrating (closed), depending on whether the integrity of the dura is maintained or violated. Bullet wounds, for example, produce a penetrating injury in which the dura is disrupted, exposing the brain or spinal cord to the external environment. The presence of dural tearing is associated with an increased risk of brain infection. These penetrating injuries often produce focal deficits localized to the area of invasion. In contrast, the dural integrity is maintained in nonpenetrating or closed injuries such as blunt trauma. Although the dura and often the skull remain intact, brain damage may be more severe and diffuse. Injuries related to both traffic accidents and falls, which typically involve a sudden acceleration or deceleration of the head, are in this category.

To understand the nature of the damage inflicted by these forces, it is necessary to review the structural anatomy of the brain and its outer coverings. The **cranial vault** is divided into cavities or fossae that accommodate different cerebral lobes (Fig. 20–1). The **dura mater** is a dense inelastic membrane, which covers the brain and extends deep into the major sulci to provide structural support (Fig. 20–2). It is possible for the brain to move within the skull and dural envelope to a limited extent. At impact or with sudden arrest of an acceleration or deceleration force, the momentum of the brain can propel it against the inner surface of the skull. The movement of the gelatinous brain against the sharp edges of the dura mater and the rough interior of the skull can cause **lacerations or bruising.** In addition to these focal areas of damage, movement of the brain about the relatively fixed brainstem can create shearing forces that produce diffuse damage.

Pathophysiology of Traumatic Brain Injury

Impact Damage to Scalp and Skull

Structures that surround the brain are often damaged at the time of injury. Scalp lacerations and contusions are common and serve to increase suspicion that underlying brain trauma is present. However, the absence of scalp trauma does not rule out brain injury.

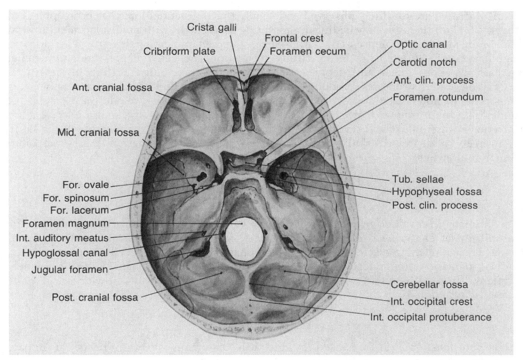

Figure 20–1. The three cranial fossae of the skull. (From Leeson, RC and Leeson, TS: Human Structure. BC Decker, Inc., Toronto, 1989; p 92, with permission.)

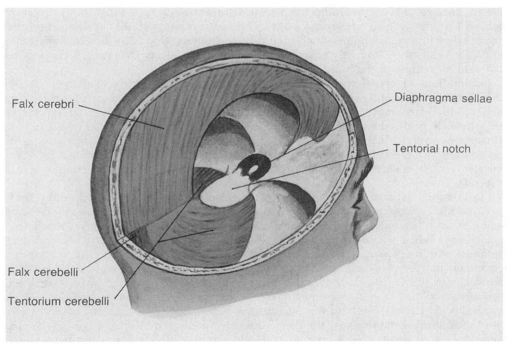

Figure 20–2. Schematic view of the cranial dura mater and its folds from the posterolateral aspect. (From Leeson, RC and Leeson, TS. Human Structure. BC Decker, Inc., Toronto, 1989, p 103, with permission.)

Skull fractures are routinely observed and signify that substantial force has been applied to the skull. Skull fractures may be **linear**, presenting as a "crack" with no displacement toward the brain surface, or **depressed**, with bone fragments projecting inward. The primary significance of skull injuries is the strong correlation between fractures and intracranial hematomas. Both linear and depressed skull fractures may cause tearing of superficial arterial or venous structures, producing intracranial bleeding and hematoma formation. It is important to note that the absence of a skull fracture does not exclude the existence of underlying brain trauma. For example, a sudden high-magnitude acceleration/deceleration force may cause diffuse and severe brain injury without disturbing the integrity of the skull. Conversely, a depressed skull fracture may produce focal damage and preserve brain function elsewhere.

Primary Brain Damage

Primary brain damage reflects the degree of immediate brain pathology due to the initial impact of the head injury and may be classified as either focal or diffuse. Focal brain damage refers to discrete areas of brain damage, generally localized to sites of impact. Diffuse damage, often referred to as **diffuse axonal injury,** is characterized by widely scattered shearing of axons within their myelin sheaths, which results in widespread white matter degeneration.

Focal Brain Damage

Contusions or *bruises* **caused by physical distortion of brain tissue at impact constitute the most frequently observed type of focal brain lesion.** A cerebral contusion is an area in which hemorrhage into the brain parenchyma has occurred and is dispersed throughout the brain tissue. These lesions are characterized by diffuse nerve cell and axonal damage, multiple punctate capillary hemorrhages, and edema. Although cerebral **contusions typically occur at sites where the brain impacts against the bony cranial cavity or the unyielding dural reflections**, they may appear anywhere within the brain parenchyma. The inferior surfaces of the frontal and temporal lobes that rest against rough bony structures such as the cristae galli, the roof of the orbit, or the wing of the sphenoid bone are particularly vulnerable and routinely contused bilaterally (Fig. 20–3). Small petechiae (contusions) are also frequently observed in the dorsal brainstem structures because of the rotational movement of the brain within the skull.

Lacerations or actual tears in the cortical surface represent a second type of focal brain damage. Penetrating injuries that disrupt both the skull (skull fracture) and the dura often produce lacerations of the underlying tissue. Clinically significant lacerations are generally well localized and are often found in the dorsal and lateral aspects of the cerebral hemispheres. Interior irregularities of the skull may also cause surface lacerations as the brain moves within the dural envelope during acceleration/deceleration injuries. Lacerations typically result in tearing of cerebral blood vessels, as well as localized destruction of cortical neurons.

Intracranial hemorrhages are associated with lacerations and contusions and reflect a third and final type of primary focal brain damage. Arteries and veins that supply the skull, meninges, and cerebral tissue may be torn or penetrated at the time of injury, resulting in hemorrhage. When a hemorrhage results in a localized mass of blood that is relatively contained within a space, it is referred to as a **hematoma**. Intracranial hemorrhages and hematomas may be classified as epidural (extradural), subdural, or intracerebral, based on their location (Table 20–2). **Epidural hemorrhages** are almost invariably associated with skull fractures that lacerate superficial vessels and are most frequently observed in the temporal region. These account for the smallest percentage of hematomas observed after injury. **Subdural hemorrhages** are often due to bleeding from the edges of cerebral lacerations or to the tearing of bridging vessels between the dura and the brain during acceleration/deceleration injuries. The resulting acute hematoma is associated with severe

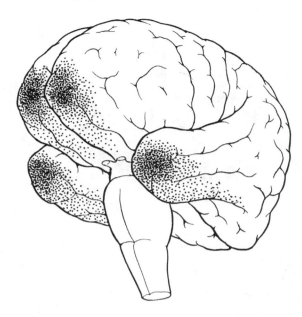

Figure 20–3. Diagrammatic illustration of the cortical areas vulnerable to contusion. (From Fletcher et al (eds): Rehabilitation Medicine: Contemporary Clinical Perspectives. Lea & Febiger, Philadelphia, 1992, p 65, with permission.)

cerebral edema and a very high mortality rate. **Intracerebral hemorrhages** are often associated with contusions or tearing of vessels deep within the brain parenchyma and reflect a more diffuse type of injury.

Disruption of the arterial blood supply may induce ischemia in the areas normally supplied by the affected vessels, causing neuronal dysfunction and possible cell death. Furthermore, hematomas occupy space within the cranial vault and may raise intracranial pressure and compress brain tissue. If bleeding continues, additional brain damage may occur as the brain shifts to accommodate the growing mass (Fig. 20–4).

The primary predictor of the neurologic signs and physical dysfunction associated with focal brain damage is the location of the lesion. To some extent, impairments may be predicted based on an understanding of functional anatomy. For example, a focal lesion involving the parietal sensory cortex typically manifests as a contralateral impairment of sensation, whereas a lesion in the frontal motor cortex is associated with contralateral paresis. However, it is important to note that a focal lesion may also produce deficits at anatomic sites distant from the initial lesion. **Transneuronal degeneration** is a process whereby degenerative changes may occur in cells that synapse on or receive synaptic input from a damaged neuron. In this way, even a focal lesion has the potential to adversely affect distant cells and to create nonfocal clinical deficits.

Table 20–2. *Classification of Intracranial Hemorrhages*

Type of Hemorrhage	Source of Bleeding	Location
Epidural	Middle meningeal artery Dural sinus Temporal veins	Between skull and dura over temporal lobe
Subdural	Surface or bridging veins Cerebral lacerations	In subdural space between dura and arachnoid
Intracerebral	Intracerebral arteries and veins	Within brain parenchyma

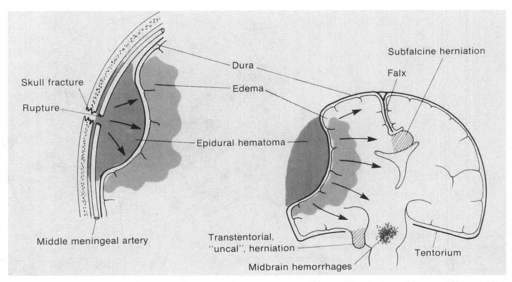

Figure 20–4. *A Fracture of the Parietal Bone Resulting in Rupture of the Middle Meningeal Artery and an Epidural Hematoma.* This intracranial mass may compress brain tissue and result in herniation. (Artist: Dimitri Karetnikov; from PATHOLOGY, ed 1, edited by Emanuel Rubin, MD and John L. Farber, MD. Copyright © 1988, by JB Lippincott Co, Philadelphia, PA [USA].)

Diffuse Axonal Injury

Movement of a part of the brain at a different speed or angle than surrounding tissues imparts a shearing or torsional force to the adjacent white matter tracts connecting various cell bodies. This causes diffuse stretching and tearing of axons and interrupts the normal flow of information necessary for function. Microscopic examination reveals axon retraction balls scattered throughout white matter tracts, often accompanied by demyelination and degeneration of the pathways. This type of primary brain injury has been demonstrated in the subcortical white matter, corpus callosum, and cerebellar peduncles, as well as throughout the brainstem (Fig. 20–5).

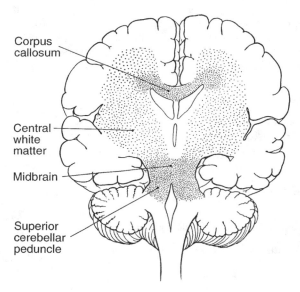

Figure 20–5. Diagrammatic illustration of the areas predisposed to diffuse axonal injury. (From Fletcher et al (eds): Rehabilitation Medicine: Contemporary Clinical Perspectives. Lea & Febiger, Philadelphia, 1992, p 66, with permission.)

Diffuse axonal injury often occurs in the absence of skull fractures or any focal lesion and yet may have a significant clinical impact. It represents the most common structural abnormality underlying the severe neurologic disability observed subsequent to a brain injury.[6] Patients with severe diffuse axonal injury are usually rendered immediately comatose due to impairment in the reticular activating system and may remain in that state for a prolonged period of time.

Secondary Brain Damage

The primary lesions are often so widespread or so severe that they are inconsistent with any return of neurologic function. In many brain-injured patients, however, the initial impact damage is not severe enough to preclude a satisfactory functional recovery. Yet, some of these patients may become severely disabled because of secondary processes that create additional brain injury. *Secondary brain damage* **refers to any process that evolves as a consequence of the initial injury and that generates additional brain dysfunction.** The cumulative effects of these secondary processes often cause more serious deficits than the primary injury itself, so that acute management of the traumatic brain injury patient is aimed at preventing these secondary insults. **Secondary brain injury may be systemic or intracranial.**

Secondary Systemic Insults

The brain has a very large metabolic requirement and is highly vulnerable to conditions that reduce its supply of nutrients. Despite accounting for only 2% of the total body weight, the brain consumes 20% of the oxygen and 25% of the body glucose. Since the brain lacks the capacity to store the energy required to function, it depends on a continuous supply of oxygen and glucose from the arterial system. Interruption or reduction of this supply may produce permanent neurologic dysfunction. **Secondary insults of systemic origin often reduce the critical supply of oxygen and glucose to the injured brain and produce widespread ischemic damage.**

Cerebral blood flow consumes 15% to 20% of the cardiac output and complex autoregulatory mechanisms serve to maintain cerebral blood flow within adequate limits. These autoregulatory mechanisms are often disrupted following traumatic brain injury. **Arterial hypoxemia is the most common form of systemic secondary brain insult.** Hypoxemia occurs when the arterial partial pressure of oxygen (Po_2) falls below 55 mm Hg. At this point, oxygen desaturation occurs, and there is a decrease in the volume of oxygen carried per unit volume of blood. The response of a normal brain to this threat is compensatory cerebral vasodilation, which serves to increase the cerebral blood flow and hence the oxygen supply. This compensatory cerebrovascular autoregulation is often impaired following traumatic brain injury, resulting in an inability to compensate for oxygen deprivation. Neuronal death accompanies any persistent and significant reduction in oxygen and is referred to as **ischemic damage.** Hypoxemia is most often caused by obstruction of the airway (i.e., by blood or foreign objects) or by the impairment in respiration frequently induced by the primary brain trauma. Oxygen saturation is routinely monitored in the acute phase after injury, and any activity that significantly reduces the Pao_2 is avoided or terminated.

Other systemic insults that have the potential to cause secondary brain pathology and their mechanisms of action are listed in Table 20–3. The combined presence of arterial hypotension and hypoxemia after injury has been shown to be associated with a 150% increase in mortality rate.[7]

Secondary Intracranial Insults

The intracranial insults that have the potential to cause secondary brain pathology are listed in Table 20–4. **Brain edema and increased intracranial pressure occur frequently** and may have significant deleterious effects on the injured brain. Therefore, these factors are discussed in detail.

Table 20–3. *Systemic Insults Causing Secondary Brain Damage*

Insult	Mechanisms of Action
Arterial hypotension	Cerebral ischemia
Hypercapnia	Increased cerebral blood flow, resulting in increased intracranial pressure
Anemia	Cerebral ischemia
Hyponatremia	Cerebral edema

The brain edema associated with traumatic brain injury may be classified as either *vasogenic* or *cytotoxic*. Vasogenic edema presents as a localized increase in extracellular water content due to an increased fluid permeability in damaged blood vessels and is often a sequela of cerebral contusions and lacerations. This type of edema is often observed surrounding a primary lesion and typically produces focal neurologic signs and symptoms. Cytotoxic edema appears as intracellular swelling in response to cell injury and tissue necrosis. This diffuse form of edema is often associated with systemic hypoxemia. The clinical manifestations of cytotoxic edema are less localized, with drowsiness as a prominent feature. Cerebral edema of either type typically results in increased intracranial pressure.

The cranial vault is a rigidly enclosed space with a fixed capacity. The contents within this space include brain tissue, cerebrospinal fluid within the ventricular system, and blood located in the intravascular compartment. The capacity of this system to accommodate an increase in volume is limited. Any expanding mass or volume at first is accommodated by displacement of the cerebrospinal fluid within the ventricular system and compression of neural tissue. Once a critical volume is reached, however, the intracranial pressure begins to rise, creating its own deleterious effects on the brain.

Normal intracranial pressure ranges from 5 to 10 mm Hg. Intracranial pressure higher than this level results in a reduction in cerebral blood flow and contributes to ischemic brain damage. Pressures that exceed 40 mm Hg are associated with impairment of electrical activity and corresponding neurologic dysfunction. Severe elevations are associated with an increase in mortality due to brain herniation. Even moderate elevations (20 to 40 mm Hg) may contribute significantly to disability after injury. **The clinical manifestations associated with increased intracranial pressure include headache, nausea, drowsiness, weakness, and papilledema.**

The mechanisms by which increased intracranial pressure produces neural dysfunction are not clear. It is likely that increased intracranial pressure may cause brain injury by directly decreasing cerebral blood flow. Increased intracranial pressure may also cause additional dysfunction as a result of displacement of the brain. Physical displacement of the brain occurs with any intracranial mass lesion and results in flattening of the gyri, compression of surface blood vessels, and possibly herniation of the brain beneath the falx cerebri through the tentorial notch or through the foramen magnum.

Table 20–4. *Secondary Intracranial Insults*

- Increased intracranial pressure
- Cerebral edema
- Intracranial infection
- Hydrocephalus
- Cerebral arterial vasospasm
- Post-traumatic epilepsy

Brain Shift and Herniation

The most significant consequence of mass cerebral lesions and concomitantly increased intracranial pressure is brain displacement and herniation. Some increase in the volume within the cranial cavity due to factors such as cerebral edema or hemorrhage can be accommodated by displacement of the cerebrospinal fluid and obliteration of the ventricular and subarachnoid spaces. Further expansion may cause cerebral and brainstem structures to shift or herniate from one intracranial compartment to another. Certain structures are more likely to herniate than others. The principal types of herniation (see Fig. 20–4) are the shift of the cingulate gyrus beneath the falx cerebri (subfalcial herniation) (Fig. 20–6), the medial temporal lobe through the tentorial hiatus (tentorial herniation), and the cerebellar tonsils into the foramen magnum (tonsillar herniation). Each such shift has the potential to cause additional specific neurological dysfunction.

Subfalcial herniation is usually not associated with specific clinical features. However, the potential exists for damage to the anterior cerebral arteries that supply the medial aspect of the hemispheres. This can cause ischemic injury, resulting in contralateral lower extremity weakness and sensory loss.

Tentorial herniation is characterized by herniation of the medial temporal lobe, which displaces the midbrain to the opposite side. The oculomotor nerve is compressed against the midbrain, generating a dilated fixed pupil, a drooping eyelid (ptosis), and lateral deviation of the eye on the same side as the lesion. As the temporal lobe herniation progresses, the brainstem is displaced downward. This often results in a shearing of the arteries supplying the brainstem and is associated with damage to the reticular nuclei, manifesting in irreversible coma.

Tonsillar herniation is associated with compression of critical medullary structures involved in cardiovascular regulation and typically results in death.

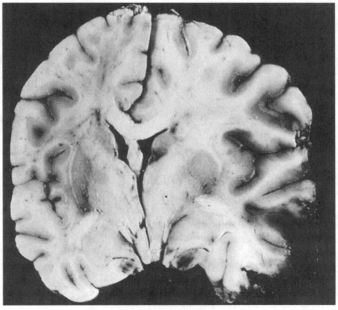

Figure 20–6. *Acute Subdural Hematoma Overlying Extensive Cortical Contusions and Lacerations.* As a result of the hematoma and swelling of the right cerebral hemisphere, there was herniation of the right cingulate gyrus beneath the falx, compression and distortion of the right third ventricle, and bilateral uncal herniation. This 31-year-old woman died 1½ days after falling from a moving truck. (From Schochet, SS, Jr and Nelson, J: Atlas of Clinical Neuropathology. Appleton & Lange, Norwalk, CT, 1989, p 195, with permission.)

Motor Impairments Associated with Traumatic Brain Injury

A vast number of signs and symptoms reflecting disturbance of multiple central nervous system functions are observed subsequent to a traumatic brain injury. A description of all the potential deficits is beyond the scope of this chapter; only those that contribute to disorders of posture and movement will be emphasized.

The neurologic impairments associated with traumatic brain injury that result in abnormal motor control vary according to the location and extent of the injury. The clinical presentation following a diffuse brain injury is a reflection of damage to multiple systems and typically includes a decreased level of consciousness and extensive neurologic deficits. In contrast, the deficits observed following focal damage reflect dysfunction of particular regions in the central nervous system. Table 20–5 lists some of the frequently observed impairments associated with craniocerebral injury localized to specific functional areas of the brain. The general cause and presentation of the disorders of central motor control have been discussed in detail in Chapter 12. Therefore, the purpose in this section is to provide a brief review of the motor impairments specifically associated with traumatic brain injuries.

Table 20–5. *Clinical Manifestations Associated with Localized Craniocerebral Injury*

Site of Damage	Signs and Symptoms
Basal ganglia	Akinesia, bradykinesia Dystonia Choreiform movements Ballistic movements Tremor
Primary motor cortex	Contralateral paresis, distal more than proximal Contralateral hypertonia Positive Babinski's reflex Problems with force modulation and trajectory, during active movements
Supplementary motor cortex	Motor apraxia Difficulty with bimanual tasks
Premotor cortex	Motor apraxia Difficulty with tasks that require sensory guidance
Cerebellum	Hypotonia Ataxia Dysmetria Disdiadochokinesia Disequilibrium

Parietal lobe	Contralateral sensory disorders
	Ideational and ideomotor apraxia
	Perceptual disorders
	  Depth perception
	  Spatial relations
	  Figure/ground

Reticular activating formation	Decreased consciousness
Broca's area	Expressive aphasia
Wernicke's area	Receptive aphasia
Primary visual cortex	Contralateral hemianopsia

The clinical manifestations associated with damage to the cerebellum and basal ganglia are described in Chapters 19 and 18, respectively, and will not be covered in detail here.

Abnormal Muscle Tone

Rigidity

Decorticate rigidity and decerebrate rigidity are extreme forms of hypertonus frequently observed immediately following traumatic brain injury and are indicative of extensive central nervous system damage (see Figure 12–9). Decerebrate rigidity is manifested as rigid extension of the upper and lower extremities, which in its most severe form may also include arching of the back and extension of the neck (opisthotonos). Decorticate rigidity presents as rigid flexion of the upper extremities and extension of the lower extremities. **Both are characterized by marked resistance to passive movement,** with involvement of the trunk and neck, as well as the extremities.

These forms of rigidity are often present immediately following a traumatic brain injury and indicate that extensive damage has occurred within the central nervous system. The abnormal postures may occur spontaneously, or they may be evoked by various forms of stimulation. Caution must be taken to avoid unnecessarily eliciting a decerebrate or decorticate posture in a patient with unstable intracranial pressure, since this may further elevate the intracranial pressure and possibly contribute to further secondary brain damage.[8]

Rigidity that persists is correlated with a poor prognosis for functional recovery. In patients whose neurologic recovery is evident, these manifestations gradually diminish over a period of days, weeks, or months. **The most significant functional consequence of this severe hypertonus is muscle contracture,** which in turn may result in altered biomechanics, musculoskeletal deformity, and functional disability. The incidence of contractures following craniocerebral trauma has been noted to be as high as 84% in a sample of patients admitted to rehabilitation facilities.[9] Rigidity and contractures have been associated with and may contribute to the high incidence of heterotopic ossification in this patient population[10] (see Chapter 23).

Spasticity

The rigidity may be replaced over time by spasticity. *Spasticity* **is another form of hypertonia** and is one of the most common motor deficits associated with traumatic brain injuries.[11,12] Clinically, **spasticity is manifested as a velocity-dependent increase in resistance to passive stretch.** This form of hypertonia presents in a classic pattern typically involving flexor muscles of the upper extremity and extensors of the lower extremity (see Table 12–5 and Fig. 12–7). It may be unilateral or bilateral, depending on the extent of cerebral damage.

Like rigidity, the most significant functional consequence of spasticity is muscle contractures. The most common site for contracture development is the ankle plantarflexors, associated with severe spasticity in the gastrocnemius muscle. Treatment is often focused on the prevention of secondary reductions in joint range of motion associated with spastic muscle groups.[13] However, alleviating the spasticity may not significantly enhance volitional movements (see Chapter 12).

Hypotonia

Hypotonia, **or a reduction in muscle tone, is not a common sequela of traumatic brain injury.** Immediately after injury, it may be present for a few days or weeks associated with cerebral shock. However, this is usually replaced as time progresses by spastic hypertonia. Hypotonia is characterized by decreased resistance to passive movement, such that the limb feels heavy and falls when dropped. **The presence of significant hypotonia is associated with joint instability,** particularly when dynamic muscle activity contributes to joint integrity.

Abnormal Reflexes

The hypertonia that is evident after traumatic brain injury is also associated with alterations in the deep tendon reflexes. Decreased threshold and increased amplitude of deep tendon reflexes and clonus may be present in the involved limbs. Ankle clonus is common and manifests as rapid involuntary muscle contractions in the plantarflexors of the ankle in response to a quick stretch. In addition to hyperactive deep tendon reflexes, cutaneous reflexes such as the palmar grasp and plantar grasp (Babinski's reflex) may be present. The palmar grasp reflex, in which tactile stimulation on the palmar surface of the hand and fingers produces a mass activation of the finger flexors, may significantly impair hand function.

Primitive motor reflexes are spontaneous stereotypical movement patterns that are generally evoked by a certain stimulus. These reflexes are normally present in the developmental years and may be observed in infants and young children. However, they are generally integrated early and are not normally present in adults or adolescents. In a traumatically brain-injured person, these primitive reflexes may reappear and influence both movement and muscle tone. Table 20–6 briefly describes the clinical picture associated with some of these primitive reflexes.

Weakness and Decreased Endurance

A frequently observed motor deficit associated with traumatic brain injuries is weakness or the inability to generate tension, force, or torque.[14,15] Weakness may range in severity from an inability to achieve any visible muscle contraction to minimal impairment, which is evident only upon thorough objective testing. The degree of weakness is dependent on the extent of the central nervous system damage. **The most common distribution of weakness is hemiparesis,** with involvement of the upper and lower extremity on one side of the body. **Quadriparesis** is characteristic of severe injuries that are more diffuse in nature. Distal muscles are typically affected to a greater extent than proximal muscles due to the strong bilateral innervation of most proximal muscles.

If the injury has affected the cranial nerve nuclei in the brainstem or the descending corticobulbar pathways, weakness in the muscles of the face, jaw, tongue, eyes, pharynx, and larynx may be present. For example, interruption of bilateral corticobulbar pathways or the cranial nerve nuclei in the medulla oblongata often causes weakness in the muscles of the tongue, pharynx, and larynx. **This weakness may cause *dysphagia,* an impairment in the ability to swallow, or *dysarthria,* a motor speech impairment.** The damage to the oculomotor nuclei or nerve in the midbrain often associated with increased intracranial pressure may produce weakness in the muscles that control the opening of the eyelid and

Table 20–6. *Primitive Motor Reflexes*

Reflex	Stimulus	Response
Asymmetric tonic neck	Rotation of head	Extension of arm and leg on side toward which head is turned Flexion of arm and leg on side away from which head is turned
Symmetric tonic neck	Neck flexion Neck extension	Arms flex and legs extend Arms extend and legs flex
Labyrinthine	Supine position Prone position	Increased extensor tone Increased flexor tone

movement of the eye in tracking an object. **The resultant drooping of the eyelid is referred to as** *ptosis,* **and the double vision that occurs with abnormal tracking is called** *diplopia.*

Note that the muscle weakness observed during isolated muscle testing does not always correlate with the ability to generate tension during a functional activity. For example, although the quadriceps muscle may test as a 1 on a manual muscle testing scale of 1 to 5 in sitting, the influence of factors such as reflexes and automatic motor programs may allow the patient to easily support their body weight in standing with fair quadriceps control. The most important question to ask is how the observed muscle weakness actually contributes to functional disability.

One element of motor control that is often associated with strength is muscle endurance or the ability to sustain a force over time. Sufficient endurance is particularly critical in the musculature involved in postural control or proximal stabilization. **Increased fatigability has been observed in both hypertonic and hypotonic muscles following traumatic brain injuries.**

Altered Timing and Sequencing of Muscle Activation

Although strength and endurance are important factors in motor control, other parameters of movement such as **the sequence of muscle activation and the timing of a movement may also be disturbed by traumatic brain injury.**

To produce an efficient and effective movement, the recruitment or activation of muscles must occur in the proper progression and pattern. For example, to achieve a concentric contraction resulting in elbow extension, the elbow flexors must be inhibited as the extensors are activated. Often as a result of a traumatic brain injury, this timing of activation and inhibition is disrupted, producing co-contraction in which there is no inhibition of the antagonist. This failure in reciprocal inhibition is one factor that may impair voluntary movement.[16]

Another of the motor deficits observed in traumatic brain-injured patients is the presence of abnormal muscle synergies.[17] A **muscle synergy** is a pattern of movement produced by the cooperation of various muscle groups. Subsequent to brain injury, isolated joint movement or the ability to produce fractionated movement is often difficult due to the simultaneous activation of muscles at multiple joints. Dominant muscle synergies emerge in which voluntary activation of one joint movement is invariably accompanied by predictable movements at other joints, forming a specific pattern or synergy (see Figure 12–10). The mechanisms accounting for the presence of these abnormal motor patterns remain to be determined. However, they illustrate another abnormality of muscle activation that has the potential to adversely affect volitional functional movements.

The **timing of a movement** has three basic components: the reaction time, the speed of the actual movement, and the time necessary to stop the movement. **An increased reaction time has been documented** in many brain-injured patients and results in delays in the initiation of movement.[18] **The speed of voluntary movements is also affected,** with patients unable to achieve high velocities of movement or with impaired accuracy at high velocities.[19] Finally, **the time necessary to halt a movement in progress is increased.** This contributes to difficulties in checking rapid movements. These abnormalities in movement timing have the potential to significantly affect functions such as balance, gait, and skilled movement, but are often not directly addressed in the rehabilitation process.

Ataxia

The **trajectory of a movement** is the path that a limb or body segment follows in performing that motor activity. The smoothness of the trajectory may be influenced by all of the variables noted thus far. However, **the most significant motor deficit contributing to** altered trajectories is *ataxia*. Motor ataxia is characteristic of damage to the cerebellum or its afferent or efferent pathways and is manifested as uncoordinated, halting movements. Diffuse axonal injury without a focal lesion in the cerebellum may also produce this disorder.[20] Movements of individual limbs or of the entire trunk are jerky and lack fluidity. The presence of ataxia can have a significant impact on the patient's functional level. Ataxia of the lower extremities or trunk is associated with an unsteady gait and impaired sitting and standing balance. Ataxia of the upper extremities results in impaired coordination and difficulty with activities such as eating and writing. Other movement impairments associated with ataxia and cerebellar dysfunction are described in Chapters 12 and 19.

Apraxia

The disorders of voluntary movement discussed in the preceding sections relate almost exclusively to problems associated with the **execution** of a voluntary motion. In contrast, *apraxia* **is best described as a disorder of motor planning**, which results in the inability to perform a purposeful motor activity. An extremity with normal tone, strength, and coordination may be functionally ineffective in the presence of apraxia, because of an inability to organize the movement components and translate them into appropriate actions. Although automatic motor tasks that are performed habitually may remain intact, **complicated or sequential tasks that require motor planning and an understanding of abstract concepts may be severely impaired.** Apraxia is a common manifestation of traumatic brain injury and may seriously interfere with self-care, mobility, and vocational activities.

Balance Disorders

Disorders of both static and dynamic sitting and standing balance are routinely observed following traumatic brain injury.[21] **Static balance** refers to the ability to maintain a static position without the use of external support. The maintenance of stability during activities such as reaching or ambulating is referred to as **dynamic balance.**

Multiple factors may contribute to the impairment in balance noted following traumatic brain injury, including dysfunction in any component of the vestibular system that may alter the integration of sensory input and motor commands, weakness, sensory loss, and visual impairment. Furthermore, indirect effects of the injury, such as muscle contractures, may adversely affect a person's ability to execute an appropriate balance response. Treatment of a balance dysfunction will vary according to the factors that are contributing to the dysfunction.

Other Clinical Manifestations of Traumatic Brain Injury

Decreased Consciousness and Alertness

One of the most consistent effects observed following a moderate-to-severe traumatic brain injury is impairment of consciousness. This impairment is usually due to damage to the reticular activating formation in the brainstem or its connections and may range from drowsiness to persistent coma. *Coma* **is defined as a state of unresponsiveness characterized by persistent eye closure (even in response to pain), inability to follow commands, and no comprehensible verbalization.**[22] Although coma is usually characterized by the

Table 20-7. Glasgow Coma Scale

Category	Response	Assigned Score
Eye opening	Opens eyes spontaneously	E4
	Opens eyes to loud voice	3
	Opens eyes to pain	2
	Does not open eyes	1
Motor response	Follows simple commands	M6
	Localizes to pain	5
	Withdraws to pain	4
	Abnormal flexion to pain	3
	Abnormal extension to pain	2
	No response to pain	1
Verbal response	Oriented, carries conversation	V5
	Confused conversation	4
	Inappropriate words	3
	Incomprehensible sounds	2
	Makes no noise	1

absence of voluntary and purposeful movements, spontaneous involuntary movements and reflexive responses to stimuli may be present. The duration and degree of altered consciousness are the best indicators of the severity of brain damage. The most popular universal objective measure of consciousness is the **Glasgow Coma Scale** (Table 20-7). A score consisting of eye opening = 1, motor response ≤ 5, and verbal response ≤ 2 indicates that the patient is in a comatose state.

Although the motor deficits associated with coma are well defined and obvious, the impact of less severe degrees of altered consciousness on motor behavior is more difficult to define. A certain amount of concentration is required to process the information necessary to complete a voluntary motor task. The various degrees of drowsiness and reduced alertness observed after injury have been correlated with poor motor performance on specific tasks, even in the absence of specific motor deficits. For example, a patient with altered consciousness may present with apparent weakness, decreased balance, and inaccurate movements. These may be transient motor deficits, which reflect a reduced level of consciousness rather than pathology within the motor systems. The degree to which a reduced level of consciousness may be influencing motor behavior must be accounted for when evaluating motor dysfunction.

Dysfunction in Other Systems

Dysfunction in cognition, communication, behavior, and sensation may also be manifested after injury.[23] These deficits significantly affect potential outcome and the patient's ability to participate in rehabilitation. In fact, it is often the cognitive and behavioral difficulties that preclude return to vocational and social activities.[24] Table 20-8 outlines some of the major deficits in these areas and their clinical implications. The clinical presentation of patients' traumatic brain injury is often further complicated by the presence of trauma to other organ systems incurred at the time of the injury and iatrogenic complications that develop at a later date.[25] Therefore, a thorough evaluation of the musculoskeletal, integumentary, and cardiopulmonary systems is necessary to obtain a complete clinical picture.

Table 20–8. *Communication, Cognitive, Behavioral, and Sensory Deficits Associated with Traumatic Brain Injury*

Deficit	Presentation	Clinical Implications
Communication		
Broca's aphasia (expressive aphasia)	Unable to communicate either verbally or in writing Comprehension usually good Telegraphic speech Patient usually aware of deficit	Often frustrated with speech Requires alternative communication
Wernicke's aphasia (receptive aphasia)	Disturbance in comprehension of verbal or written language Patient may be unaware of deficit Verbal speech may not make sense	Difficulty following instructions Impedes learning new skills
Dysarthria	Motor speech disorder resulting in poor articulation Comprehension intact	Difficulty communicating
Cognition		
Impaired memory	Short-term memory affected more significantly than long-term	Problems remembering instructions Forgets commitments Difficulty remembering names and conversation
Disorientation confusion	Inability to discriminate between and recognize people Confusion regarding date and time Confusion regarding location	Does not remember appointments Gets lost easily Confusion often heightens agitation
Concentration and attention deficits	Easily distracted Unable to sustain attention	Learning impeded Influences academic and vocational potential
Problem-solving deficits	Difficulty with abstract concepts Difficulty reasoning	Discussions must remain concrete
Judgment deficits	May be impulsive Difficulty discriminating right from wrong Limited insight into disability May be socially inappropriate	Often unsafe Requires supervision May interfere with social interactions

Outcome Following Traumatic Brain Injury

The outlook for recovery following traumatic brain injury is often difficult to predict. Factors such as the extent of injury,[26,27] the age of the patient,[26,27] the length of time in coma,[26,27] the presence of other medical complications, and patient motivation[28] all influence the functional outcome. Evidence suggests that comprehensive postacute rehabilitation programs may significantly improve function[29] and increase the number of individuals who are able to return to independent living.[30] The functional recovery following "permanent brain lesions" may be due to modification of intact brain structures and various mechanisms that may account for this neural plasticity have been described.[31] However, the rehabilitation process may be slow, with functional changes continuing as long as 2 years after injury.[32] Although most patients achieve a good recovery, as identified by the Glasgow Outcome Scale developed by Jennett and Bond,[33] lifestyles, vocations, and relationships are often permanently altered.

Table 20–8. *Continued*

Deficit	*Presentation*	*Clinical Implications*
Behavioral/Emotional		
Agitation/irritability	Exhibits verbal and physical aggression Hyperactivity Associated with reduced attention	Easily frustrated with difficult tasks
Sexual disinhibition	Verbally or physically inappropriate Engages in public self-stimulation	Socially unacceptable behavior may be reduced through behavior modification
Decreased motivation	Decreased initiative Often flat affect Extreme passivity Easily fatigued	Interferes with rehab and vocational potential
Emotional lability	Inappropriate outbursts of laughter, tears, or anger	
Sensory		
Decreased somesthetic sensation	Decreased ability to detect and localize touch, movement, pain, and temperature	At risk for injury May interfere with coordination
Spatial relations deficits	Difficulty perceiving the position of objects in relation to each other or to self	May be unsafe guiding wheelchair or ambulating in crowded environment
Unilateral neglect	Decreased awareness of one side of the body and the environment Does not attend to one side May deny the existence of one arm and leg	Bumps into objects Potential trauma of neglected side Contributes to motor problems on neglected side
Hemianopsia	Unable to see objects in half of the visual field without turning head	Contributes to neglect Bumps into objects Compromises safety
Diplopia	Double vision	Interferes with balance Difficulty reading

Summary

The clinical presentation of traumatically brain-injured patients is affected by factors such as the extent and location of the lesion, the mechanism of injury, and the presence of secondary complications that cause additional brain dysfunction. The signs and symptoms will vary greatly from patient to patient and may encompass cognitive, behavioral, emotional, sensory, and motor functions. Motor dysfunction ranges from a complete inability to voluntarily produce movement to a minor loss of fine motor control. However, a comprehensive understanding of both the pathophysiology of the injury and the functional neuroanatomy will enable the rehabilitation professional to predict motor impairments and prevent the complications that often arise secondary to movement dysfunction.

RECOMMENDED READINGS

Bach-y-Rita, P (ed): Traumatic Brain Injury. Demos, New York, 1989.

Becher, DP and Gudeman, SK (eds): Textbook of Head Injury. WB Saunders, Philadelphia, 1989.

Cooper, PR (ed): Head Injury. Williams & Wilkins, Baltimore, 1993.

Crompton, R: Closed Head Injury: Its Pathology and Legal Medicine. Edward Arnold, London, 1985.

Esiri, MM and Oppenheimer, DR: Diagnostic Neuropathology: A Practical Manual. Blackwell Scientific, Chicago, 1989.

Finger, S et al (eds): Brain Injury and Recovery: Theoretical and Controversial Issues. Plenum Press, New York, 1988.

Grossman, RG and Gildenberg, PL (eds): Head Injury: Basic and Clinical Aspects. Raven Press, New York, 1982.

James, HE, Nicholas, GA, and Perkin, RM (eds): Brain Insults of Infants and Children: Pathophysiology and Management. Grune & Stratton, Orlando, 1985.

Kovich, KM and Berman, DE: Head Injury: A Guide to Functional Outcomes in Occupational Therapy. Aspen Publishers, Rockville, MD, 1988.

Long, CJ, and Ross, LK (eds): Handbook of Head Trauma: Acute Care to Recovery. Plenum Press, New York, 1992.

Montgomery, J (ed): Physical Therapy for Traumatic Brain Injury. Churchill Livingstone, New York, 1994.

Okazaki, H: Fundamentals of Neuropathology: Morphologic Basis of Neurologic Disorders, ed 2. Igaku-Shoin, New York, 1989.

Okazaki, H and Scheithauer, BW: Atlas of Neuropathology. Gower Medical Publishers, Philadelphia, 1988.

Parker, RS: Traumatic Brain Injury and Neuropsychological Impairment: Sensorimotor, Cognitive, Emotional and Adaptive Problems of Children and Adults. Springer-Verlag, New York, 1990.

Rosenthal, M et al (eds): Rehabilitation of the Adult and Child with Traumatic Brain Injury. FA Davis, Philadelphia, 1989.

Ylvisaker, M (ed): Head Injury Rehabilitation: Children and Adolescents. College-Hill Press, San Diego, CA, 1985.

REFERENCES

1. Miller, J: Handbook of Head Trauma. Chapter 1. In Long, CH and Leslie, K (eds): Handbook of Head Trauma: Acute Care to Recovery. Plenum Press, New York, 1992.
2. Taylor, D: TBI: Outcomes and Predictors of Outcome. Chapter 17. In Long, CH and Leslie, K (eds): Handbook of Head Trauma: Acute Care to Recovery. Plenum Press, New York, 1992.
3. Hardman, JM: Cerebrospinal Trauma. Chapter 17. In Davis, RL and Robertson, DM (eds): Textbook of Neuropathology. Williams & Wilkins. Baltimore, 1991.
4. Parker, RS: Traumatic Brain Injury and Neuropsychological Impairment. Chapter 5. Springer-Verlag, New York, 1990.
5. Kreutzer, FS: Neuromedical and Psychosocial Aspects of Rehabilitation After Traumatic Brain Injury. Chapter 3. In Fletcher, GF et al (eds): Rehabilitation Medicine: Contemporary Clinical Perspectives. Lea & Febiger, Philadelphia, 1992.
6. Blumbergs, PC, Jones, NR, and North, JB: Diffuse Axonal Injury in Head Trauma. J Neurol Neurosurg Psychiatry 52:838, 1989.
7. Chestnut, RM, et al: The Role of Secondary Brain Injury in Determining Outcome from Severe Head Injury. J Trauma 34:216, 1993.
8. Smith, SL: Continuous Intracranial Pressure Monitoring: Implications and Applications for Critical Care. Crit Care Nurse 4:42, 1981.
9. Yarkony, G and Sahgal, V: Contractures: A Major Complication of Craniocerebral Trauma. Clin Orthop 219:93, 1987.
10. Marinissen, JC: Management of Heterotopic Ossification Following Traumatic Brain or Spinal Cord Injury. Orthop Phys Ther Clin North Am 2:71, 1993.
11. Rifici, C, et al: Intrathecal Baclofen Application in Patients with Supraspinal Spasticity Secondary to Severe Traumatic Brain Injury: Functional Neurology. 9:29, 1994.
12. Glenn, MB: Case Example: The Management of Spasticity After Traumatic Brain Injury. Chapter 14. In Glenn, MB and Whyte, J (eds): The Practical Management of Spasticity. Lea & Febiger, Philadelphia, 1990.
13. Glenn, MB and Whyte, J (eds): The Practical Management of Spasticity. Lea & Febiger, Philadelphia, 1990.
14. Craik, R: Abnormalities of Motor Behavior. Chapter 16. In Lister, M (ed): Contemporary Management of Motor Control Problems: Proceedings of the II Step Conference. Bookcrafters, Fredericksburg, VA, 1991.
15. Jennett, B, et al: Disability After Severe Head Injury: Observations on the Use of the Glasgow Coma Scale. J Neurol Neurosurg Psychiatry 44:285, 1981.
16. el-Abd, MA, Ibrahim, IK, and Dietz, V: Impaired Activation Pattern in Antagonistic Elbow Muscles of Patients with Spastic Hemiparesis: Contribution to Movement Disorder. Electromyogr Clin Neurophysiol 33:247 1993.
17. Davies, PM; Steps to Follow: A Guide to the Treatment of Adult Hemiplegia. Springer-Verlag, New York, 1985.
18. Stuss, DT, et al: Reaction Time After Head Injury: Fatigue, Divided and Focused Attention, and Consistency of Performance. J Neurol Neurosurg Psychiatry 52:742, 1989.
19. Chaplin, D, Deitz, J, and Jaffe, KM: Motor Performance in Children After Traumatic Brain Injury. Arch Phys Med Rehabil 74:161, 1993.

20. Mysiw, WJ, Corrigan, JD, and Gribble, MW: The Ataxic Subgroup: A Discrete Outcome After Traumatic Brain Injury. Brain Inj 4:247, 1990.

21. Newton, RA: Recovery of Balance Abilities in Individuals with Traumatic Brain Injuries. In Duncan, P (ed): Balance: Proceedings of the APTA forum. American Physical Therapy Association, Alexandria, VA, 1989.

22. Snyder-Smith, S and Winkler, PA: Traumatic Brain Injuries. Chapter 13. In Umphred, DA (ed): Neurological Rehabilitation. CV Mosby, St. Louis, 1990.

23. Charness, A: Stroke/Head Injury Outcome: A Guide to Functional Outcomes in Physical Therapy Management. Unit 2. Aspen Publishers, Gaithersburg, MD, 1986.

24. Levin, HS: Behavioral Outcome 1 Year After Severe Head Injury. Experience of the Traumatic Coma Data Bank. J Neurosurg 73:688, 1990.

25. Kaufman, HH, et al: Medical Complications of Head Injury. Contemp Clin Neurol 77:43, 1993.

26. Jones, CL: Recovery From Head Trauma: A Curvilinear Process? Chapter 20. In Long, CH and Leslie, K (eds): Handbook of Head Trauma: Acute Care to Recovery. Plenum Press, New York, 1992.

27. Vollner, D: Prognosis and Outcome of Severe Injury. Chapter 23. In Cooper, PR (ed): Head Injury. Williams & Wilkins, Baltimore, 1993.

28. Prigatano, GP: Emotion and Motivation in Recovery and Adaptation After Brain Damage. Chapter 21. In Finger, S, et al (eds): Brain Injury and Recovery: Theoretical and Controversial Issues. Plenum Press, New York, 1988.

29. Mills, VM, et al: Outcomes for Traumatically Brain-Injured Patients Following Post-Acute Rehabilitation Programmes. Brain Inj 6:219, 1992.

30. Malec, JF, et al: Outcome Evaluation and Prediction in a Comprehensive-Integrated Post-Acute Outpatient Brain Injury Rehabilitation Programme. Brain Inj 7:15, 1993.

31. Boyeson, MG, Jones, JL, and Harmon, RL: Sparing of Motor Function after Cortical Injury: A New Perspective on Underlying Mechanisms. Arch Neurol 51:405, 1994.

32. Panikoff, LB: Recovery Trends of Functional Skills in the Head Injured Adult. Am J Occup Ther 37:735, 1983.

33. Jennett, B and Bond, M: Assessment of Outcome After Severe Brain Damage: A Practical Scale. Lancet 1:480, 1975.

CHAPTER 21

∎

Cerebrovascular Disease: Stroke

Lisa K. Saladin, BMR(PT), MSc

- *Classification of Cerebrovascular Disease*
- *Pathophysiology of Cerebrovascular Disease*
- *Clinical Course of Cerebrovascular Disease*
- *Medical Management of Cerebrovascular Disease*
- *Motor Impairments Associated with Strokes*
- *Distribution of Motor Deficits*
- *Laterality of Motor Control*
- *Neurovascular Clinical Syndromes*
- *Risk Factors Associated with Cerebrovascular Disease*
- *Stroke Outcomes*
- *Summary*

*T*he National Institute of Neurological Disorders and Stroke has defined *cerebrovascular disease* as any disorder in which an area of the brain is transiently or permanently affected by ischemia or bleeding or in which one or more blood vessels of the brain are primarily impaired by a pathologic process.[1] The clinical terms often used to represent the expression of cerebrovascular disease are stroke and cerebrovascular accident (CVA). *Stroke (or CVA) is defined as the sudden and convulsive onset of a focal neurologic deficit and refers to the syndrome that results from the vascular disease of the brain.*[2] The characteristic signs and symptoms of stroke vary according to the area of central nervous system damaged and may include changes in the level of consciousness, motor control, sensory perception, and visual and speech function.

To be classified as a stroke, the focal neurologic deficits must be present for at least 24 hours and take longer than 3 weeks to resolve. When the duration of signs and symptoms is less than 24 hours, the event is classified as a **transient ischemic attack (TIA)** and is considered a warning that a stroke may occur in the future. **Reversible ischemic neurologic deficit** refers to neurologic signs and symptoms that last longer than 24 hours but resolve within 3 weeks. This chapter focuses on the pathophysiology and clinical implications of the stroke syndrome.

The incidence of mortality and morbidity from stroke has been declining over the last 20 years.[3,4] This may be due to multiple factors, the most notable of which is the improved treatment of hypertension, a well-known risk factor associated with stroke.[4] Despite this decline, stroke remains the third leading cause of death in the United States and is a major source of disability.[5] The economic impact of this disorder is staggering, with financial costs associated with stroke estimated at 7 billion dollars per year.[6]

An estimated 500,000 new cases of stroke occur annually, with the incidence increasing steadily with age.[3] Although the incidence is highest in persons 65 years of age and older, a considerable proportion of strokes occurs in active young adults under the age of 45.[7] This is particularly significant when one considers the potential financial and social impact of chronic disability that begins at such a young age.

After the initial period of high mortality is over, the chance for survival after stroke is good, with mean survival time exceeding 7 years.[8] However, the quality of life is often reduced by the presence of residual physical and mental disabilities. There are about 1.5 million stroke survivors in the United States, 50% of whom have residual neurologic impairments and disabilities. In addition, stroke survivors constitute the largest group admitted to inpatient rehabilitation hospitals, where rehabilitation efforts focus on restoring disabled persons to their maximum possible level of physical, mental, and social function.

To maximize the potential for recovery after stroke, rehabilitation professionals need to understand the mechanisms underlying cerebrovascular disease and the potential effects that a stroke may impose on movement and function. Therefore, the purpose of this chapter is to review the pathophysiology of cerebrovascular disease, the prominent motor signs and symptoms associated with strokes, the clinical syndromes associated with strokes (in specific cerebral vessels), risks factors that influence the development of cerebrovascular disease, and outcomes following stroke.

Classification of Cerebrovascular Disease

The pathogenesis, treatment and recovery from a stroke vary according to the mechanism or mechanisms that precipitated the event. There are two main classifications of cerebrovascular disease. *Ischemic strokes* **are caused by a lack of blood flow, which deprives brain tissue of necessary oxygen and metabolites.** This classification can be further divided into the subtypes of thrombosis, embolism, and decreased systemic perfusion in accordance with the mechanism that causes the ischemia. *Hemorrhagic strokes* **represent the second major category and result from the release of blood into the extravascular space of the brain, which causes localized or generalized pressure injuries to the brain tissue.** Subtypes of this classification are subarachnoid and intracerebral hemorrhages. The prevalence of stroke subtypes has been difficult to ascertain. However, it is generally agreed that most strokes are ischemic, that is, caused by thrombosis and embolism, whereas hemorrhagic strokes account for only 16% to 21% of the total number of cases.[9]

Pathophysiology of Cerebrovascular Disease

Ischemic Strokes

Ischemia **is the complete loss of blood flow to a tissue.** The definitive physiologic lesion in ischemic cerebrovascular disease is a failure to deliver adequate oxygen and glucose to the brain tissue, resulting in neuronal dysfunction and possible cell death. Although the brain has high energy requirements, it possesses almost no metabolic reserves and depends on a continuous supply of oxygen and glucose in order to function. During an ischemic episode in the brain, the glucose and oxygen reserves are depleted within minutes, and neuronal dysfunction rapidly becomes evident, with the onset of neurologic impairments.

Evidence from a variety of animal studies suggests that **ischemic damage may be reversible, if the ischemia lasts less than 1 to 3 hours.**[10]

Brain ischemia can be categorized as either focal or global. *Focal ischemia* **reflects the loss of blood flow to a particular vascular territory** and is due to an interruption or severe reduction of blood flow in one or several individual cerebral arteries. The cause of focal ischemia is invariably embolic or thrombotic vascular occlusion and the neurologic impairments may be predicted from the anatomic distribution of the affected artery. In contrast, *global ischemia* **occurs when there is a severe reduction or interruption of blood supply to all or a major portion of the brain.** This type of ischemia is usually caused by generalized hypoperfusion. Neurologic deficits associated with this type of ischemic injury are typically unpredictable, widespread, and more severe.

The structural damage that results from irreversible ischemia varies according to the duration and distribution of the reduced blood flow. The most common forms of damage are infarction and selective neuronal necrosis. *Cerebral infarction* **describes an area of damage that involves all cell types including neurons, glia, and endothelial cells.** Thrombotic and embolic focal ischemia typically produce this type of cerebral destruction. *Selective neuronal necrosis* **refers to neuronal necrosis in specific central nervous system regions that are more susceptible to ischemia.** This type of structural damage is frequently observed following episodes of global ischemia; the hippocampus and cerebellum appear to be the most vulnerable central nervous system regions.[11]

Another sequela associated with ischemic stroke is brain edema. Tissue osmolality increases during severe ischemia and, upon recirculation, water moves from the blood into the brain to restore the osmotic pressure. **Ischemic brain edema develops within minutes of arterial occlusion and reaches a maximum level in the following 3 to 4 days.** Brain swelling or edema may cause an increase in intracranial pressure and often leads to progressive neurologic deterioration and secondary structural damage.

Thrombotic Strokes

Thrombosis **is the development or existence of a blood clot or thrombus within the vascular system.** In most patients who present with this type of stroke, the cerebral thrombus has developed in association with atherosclerotic vascular disease. *Atherosclerosis* **is the most common form of vascular disease and is associated with the accumulation of lipids, complex carbohydrates, fibrous tissue, and calcium deposits on the arterial walls.** These substances form plaques that begin to obstruct the lumen of arteries causing stenosis (narrowing) (Fig. 21–1). The plaques develop preferentially at bifurcations and curvatures in the arterial system and are most common in the internal carotid and vertebral arteries, followed by the basilar and middle cerebral arteries (Fig. 21–2). Platelets aggregate around the plaques and produce clots, especially following degeneration or hemorrhage in a sclerotic vessel. The acute formation of a thrombus may occlude the lumen of the artery and produce focal ischemia and infarction.

Embolic Strokes

Embolism **is a term used to refer to a substance formed elsewhere in the vascular system, which travels in the bloodstream to lodge in a vessel and obstruct blood flow.** Table 21–1 lists the common causes of cerebral embolism. Occasionally, the embolic material is air, fat, or tumor cells that enter the vascular system and embolize to cerebral vessels. **The most common types of cerebral emboli are cardiogenic in nature.** Fragments from a thrombus within the heart, such as on a diseased heart valve or on damaged myocardium overlying a myocardial infarction, often become dislodged and enter the cerebral circulation. Seventy-five percent of cardiac emboli lodge in the brain and there is a twofold to fivefold increased incidence of stroke in patients with ischemic heart disease. Another source of cerebral emboli is intra-arterial thrombi, which consist of atheromatous material that breaks away from the arterial walls of proximal arteries and lodges in distal locations.

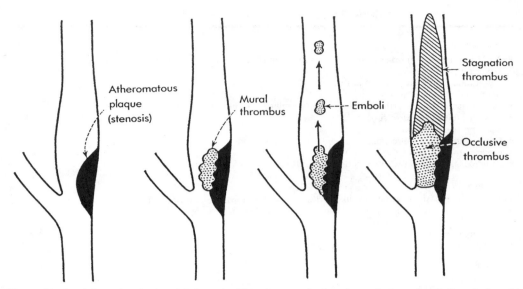

Figure 21–1. *Atherosclerotic Arterial Stenosis.* This diagram depicts the evolution of emboli and thrombi associated with an atherosclerotic narrowing of a large artery. (From Escourolle, R, Poirier, J, and Rubin Stein, LJ: Manual of Basic Neuropathology. WB Saunders, Philadelphia, 1973, p 108, with permission.)

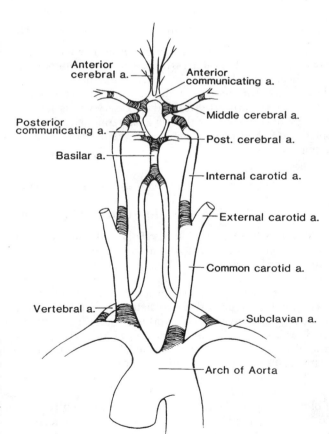

Figure 21–2. *Cerebrovascular Atherosclerosis.* The *shaded areas* indicate the sites where atherosclerosis and obstruction is most likely to occur in cerebral blood vessels. (From Branch, EF: The Neuropathology of Strokes. In Duncan, PW and Badke, MB: Stroke Rehabilitation: The Recovery of Motor Control. Year Book Medical Publishers, Chicago, 1987, p 51, with permission.)

Table 21-1. *Causes of Cerebral Embolism*

Cardiac Origin

- Atrial fibrillation and other arrhythmias (with rheumatic, atherosclerotic, hypertensive, congenital or syphilitic heart disease)
- Myocardial infarction with mural thrombus
- Acute and subacute bacterial endocarditis
- Heart disease without arrhythmia or mural thrombus (mitral stenosis, myocarditis, and others)
- Complications of cardiac surgery
- Valve protheses
- Nonbacterial thrombotic (marantic) endocardial vegetations
- Prolapsed mitral valve
- Paradoxical embolism with congenital heart disease

Noncardiac Origin

- Atherosclerosis of aorta and carotid arteries (mural thrombus, atheromatous material)
- From sites of cerebral artery thrombosis (basilar, vertebral, middle cerebral)
- Thrombus in pulmonary veins
- Fat, tumor, or air
- Complications of neck and thoracic surgery

Undetermined Origin

The progression of the embolus is often arrested at sites of bifurcation or where the lumen is already narrowed and ischemic infarction follows. **Although any vessel may be affected by emboli, the middle cerebral artery is most frequently involved.**

Strokes Related to Decreased Systemic Perfusion

Ischemic stroke related to systemic perfusion is caused by conditions that produce low systemic perfusion pressures. The most common causes are cardiac pump failure (due to myocardial infarction or arrhythmia) and systemic hypotension (due to significant blood loss). Any dramatic reduction in systemic blood pressure may reduce cerebral blood flow below the critical threshold necessary for tissue survival. The ischemia associated with this type of stroke is global, with a bilateral distribution. The effects are most notable in areas called **watershed regions,** which denote the border zones between the distribution of major cerebral vessels.

Hemorrhagic Strokes

Intracerebral Hemorrhage

Primary intracerebral hemorrhage is defined as a nontraumatic hemorrhage within the parenchyma of the brain, which most commonly manifests as a sequela of hypertensive cerebrovascular disease. Although the exact nature of the vascular lesion that leads to rupture of a cerebral vessel remains uncertain, the predominant view is that hemorrhage is caused by the rupture of small arterial or arteriolar aneurysms associated with hypertension. These Charcot-Bouchard microaneurysms are found in the small cerebral vessels of about 50% of hypertensive patients and may burst under the influence of chronic hypertension.[12] **The vessel involved in an intracerebral hemorrhage is typically a small penetrating artery located in the basal ganglia and thalamus (70%), the brainstem (13%), the cerebral white matter (10%), or the cerebellum (9%).**[12]

The neurologic damage associated with hemorrhage is highly variable and depends on the location, speed, and volume of the bleeding. In mild cases in which only a small amount of blood is released, local damage is produced with a resultant cavity or lacuna developing as blood is reabsorbed. The prognosis for neurologic recovery may be better than that following an ischemic infarct, since these lesions are characterized by tissue compression rather than

Table 21–2. *Common Causes of Subarachnoid Hemorrhage*

- Traumatic
- Aneurysm rupture (saccular, atherosclerotic, mycotic)
- Vascular malformation (arteriovenous, cavernous, angioma)
- Bleeding disorders (leukemia, anticoagulation treatment)
- Vasculitis (polyarteritis nodosa, systemic lupus erythematosus, granulomatous arteritis)
- Drug abuse (cocaine, amphetamines)
- Infections (sepsis, bacterial meningitis)
- Thrombosis of cerebral sinus
- Secondary to intraparenchymatous bleeding
- Undetermined (20%)

tissue destruction. In contrast to a mild hemorrhage, sudden and severe arterial bleeding into the brain parenchyma results in a rapid accumulation of blood that compresses and displaces adjacent brain tissue. The resultant hematoma may rupture into the ventricles or through the surface of the brain into the subarachnoid space. These rapidly expanding lesions are associated with significant elevations in intracranial pressure and are often fatal as vital centers are displaced and compressed leading to coma and death. If the patient survives, the mass of blood gradually decreases, and the site of the former hemorrhage is marked by a cleft or slit deep in the cerebral hemisphere. The prognosis may be good if tissue destruction is minimal.

Subarachnoid Hemorrhage

Nontraumatic subarachnoid hemorrhage occurs when blood hemorrhages into the subarachnoid space and constitutes approximately 6% to 8% of all strokes.[13] These hemorrhages are most frequently due to rupture of an aneurysm on one of the major cerebral vessels or to rupture of a vessel involved in an arteriovenous malformation (Table 21–2).

The aneurysms associated with subarachnoid hemorrhage are different from those that contribute to intracerebral hemorrhage. These saccular or berry aneurysms are located on large blood vessels, with the most common sites illustrated in Figure 21–3. Although multiple factors contribute to the formation of an aneurysm, they are thought to result primarily from developmental defects in the media and elastica of cerebral vessels. The

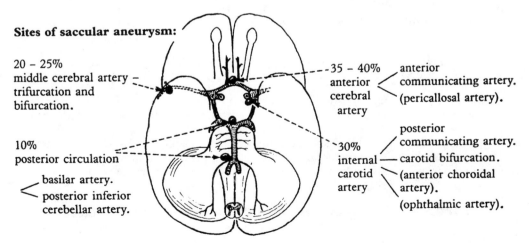

Figure 21–3. *Cerebrovascular Aneurysm.* Diagram indicates the sites where saccular aneurysms are likely to form in cerebral blood vessels. (From Lindsay, KW, Bone, I, and Callander, R: Neurology and Neurosurgery Illustrated. Section IV. Localized Neurological Disease and Its Management, ed 2. Churchill Livingstone, Edinburgh, 1991, p 274, with permission.)

Table 21–3. *Grading for Subarachnoid Hemorrhage*

Grade   I—Asymptomatic or slight headache and stiff neck
Grade II—Moderate-to-severe headache and nuchal rigidity but no focal or lateralizing neurologic signs
Grade III—Drowsiness, confusion, and mild focal deficit
Grade IV—Persistent stupor or semicoma, early decerebrate rigidity, and vegetative disturbances
Grade V—Deep coma and decerebrate rigidity

intima of the vessels bulges outward, enlarges, and may eventually rupture. The ensuing subarachnoid hemorrhage may be limited to the immediate vicinity of the aneurysm. However, more frequently extensive bleeding occurs throughout the subarachnoid space. The presence of the blood in the subarachnoid space elicits an inflammatory and fibrotic response in the meninges and vascular system and the secondary complications often prove fatal in these patients. The sudden hemorrhage often induces extreme elevations in intracranial pressure due to obstruction of cerebrospinal fluid circulation and brain edema. **Lethal brain herniation may occur as a result of the increased pressure and mass within the cranial cavity.** Ischemic cerebral infarctions are also common complications because of the reduction in cerebral blood flow associated with increased intracranial pressure and cerebral vasospasm. The severity of subarachnoid hemorrhage is traditionally rated on a scale of 1 to 5, with increasing mortality associated with increased severity (Table 21–3). The overall mortality rate for subarachnoid hemorrhage due to ruptured aneurysms is 50% within the first 30 days after onset.

Arteriovenous malformations **consist of a tangle of arteries and veins that represent the persistence of an embryonic pattern of blood vessels.** The thin-walled vessels of these malformations do not have the structure of either arteries or veins, and their abnormal connections cause the shunting of blood from the arterial to the venous circulation. Arteriovenous malformations vary tremendously in size and location and may occur on the surface or within the brain parenchyma in all regions of the brain, brainstem, and spinal cord. Hemorrhage of these thin-walled vessels occurs most often in persons between the ages of 20 and 30, and bleeding may occur within the subarachnoid space or the brain tissue. Since a large number of hemorrhages are due to the rupture of veins and the bleeding is less intense, **the long-term prognosis for ruptured arteriovenous malformations is generally better than that for subarachnoid hemorrhage resulting from a ruptured aneurysm.** Although the first hemorrhage may be fatal, about 90% of patients survive and bleeding stops. Since the hemorrhage is often slow and restricted to brain tissue in the immediate vicinity, **focal neurologic deficits are common.**

Clinical Course of Cerebrovascular Disease

Knowledge regarding the initial signs and symptoms and the general progression of each condition that causes a stroke is imperative for the safe implementation of appropriate treatment strategies. For example, the fact that a high percentage of patients with subarachnoid hemorrhage rebleed should influence decisions regarding the rigor of activities initiated during the rehabilitation phase. Table 21–4 presents a summary of the salient clinical findings associated with each subtype of stroke discussed in the previous section.

Medical Management of Cerebrovascular Disease

The primary goals of acute treatment for a patient immediately after stroke are to minimize the extent of irreversible brain damage and to prevent secondary complications. There is a paucity of controlled clinical trials regarding the effectiveness of selective

Table 21-4. *Clinical Picture of Various Subtypes of Cerebrovascular Disease and Strokes*

Disease Subtype	Clinical Picture
Ischemic Strokes	
Thrombosis	Variable onset
	Often preceded by one or more transient ischemic attacks
	Most often manifests as a single attack of focal neurologic deficits within a few hours
	May manifest with **intermittent** deficits that evolve over several hours or days
	Often (60%) during sleep
	Not usually accompanied by headaches
	Associated with hypertension, diabetes mellitus, and atherosclerosis in other areas
	Many deteriorate over the first few days because of associated edema
Embolism	Rapid onset (hallmark) within seconds or minutes
	There is rarely is a warning signal
	Typically focal neurologic deficits
	Corresponding to the anatomic area supplied by the affected vessel
	May produce severe deficits followed by resolution if embolus breaks up
	Most associated with heart disease
Decreased perfusion	Sudden onset
	Often bilateral global neurologic deficits
	Associated with blood loss and cardiac arrest
Hemorrhagic Strokes	
Intracerebral hemorrhage	Abrupt onset of symptoms that evolve gradually and **steadily** over minutes, hours, or days
	Typically occurs during physical activity in daytime
	Associated with hypertension
	Generally minimal occurrence of rebleeding
	Massive hemorrhage possibly fatal because of increased intracranial pressure
Subarachnoid hemorrhage Ruptured aneurysm	
	Mild
	Sudden onset with minimal warning
	Consciousness regained quickly if lost
	Stiff neck, headache, drowsiness, and confusion possibly persisting for weeks
	Minimal focal neurologic signs
	Moderate
	Sudden onset with or without loss of consciousness
	Survivors of initial coma often have focal neurologic signs associated with ischemia
	May have delayed onset of focal signs owing to onset of vasospasm 4-12 days after rupture
	Significant chance of rebleeding
	Severe
	Sudden onset of severe headache and loss of consciousness
	Persistent coma and death often
	Associated with infarcts and increased intracranial pressure
Arteriovenous malformation	Onset of symptoms between 10 and 30 years of age
	May be preceded by recurrent headaches or seizures
	Symptom progression and outcome less severe than with ruptured aneurysm

treatments, but advances have been made in recent years. The following is a brief description of some specific therapies and the rationale for their use.

Ischemic Strokes

Although neuronal dysfunction develops within minutes of an ischemic episode, cell death or infarction appears to take from 1 to 3 hours to occur. Therefore, the rapid institution of any therapy that can successfully restore cerebral circulation or prevent cell injury during this time has the potential to minimize permanent damage.

A massive influx of calcium into neurons has been documented during ischemic conditions, and this intracellular calcium is thought to mediate enzymatic processes that lead to cell death.[14] One strategy for the prevention of tissue destruction has been the administration of nimodipine, a calcium channel antagonist. Although far from conclusive, a meta-analysis of five double-blind studies reported that nimodipine reduced both mortality and impairments after stroke.[15] These effects were most evident in patients older than 65 with moderate-to-severe deficits who were treated within 12 hours of onset.

Anticoagulant therapy is routinely used in the treatment of acute cerebral infarction.[16] However, the efficacy of this treatment remains to be determined and controversy surrounds its use. **Early anticoagulation has been shown to reduce recurrence of cardioembolic strokes,[17] but the studies examining its effectiveness in preventing stroke evolution have failed to demonstrate a significant effect.**[18] Intravenous heparin is the agent most frequently used immediately after stroke, followed by oral warfarin. Potential complications of this therapy are hemorrhage and thrombocytopenia.

One of the newest therapeutic strategies for stroke is to administer, within 6 hours after stroke, thrombolytic agents (such as streptokinase) in an effort to break up the thrombus and restore circulation. This form of therapy appears to be effective in reducing the ischemic damage following myocardial infarction, but its effectiveness in stroke patients remains to be determined.

Antiplatelet agents such as aspirin are routinely administered to prevent the occurrence or recurrence of a stroke, but they play no significant role in the reduction of ischemic damage immediately following a stroke.

Hemorrhagic Strokes

Specific therapies for hemorrhagic stroke, such as surgical evacuation of the clot and decreasing systemic blood pressure, have failed to produce any significant effects. In fact, pharmacologically reducing the blood pressure may actually contribute to the ischemia. Treatment has focused primarily on the reduction of potentially fatal secondary complications, such as increased intracranial pressure and brain edema, through the use of drugs such as dexamethasone and mannitol. **The best strategy for the treatment of intracerebral hemorrhage is prevention.** Improvements in the treatment of essential hypertension have been a significant factor leading to the decreased incidence of this subtype of stroke.[4]

Motor Impairments Associated with Strokes

A vast number of signs and symptoms reflecting the disturbance of multiple central nervous system functions are observed subsequent to a stroke. The clinical presentation varies, depending on the anatomic distribution of the affected vessel, the extent of the lesion, and the presence of secondary complications such as edema. Common clinical syndromes that describe the potential communication, behavioral, sensory, and motor deficits associated with the disturbance of blood flow in individual cerebral vessels are outlined in a subsequent section. The focus of this segment is to provide a more detailed discussion of the motor manifestations. The general etiology and presentation of these disorders of central motor control have been discussed in detail in Chapter 12. The purpose here is to provide a brief review and to refer to the literature that specifically addresses the presentation of these impairments in stroke patients. The motor incoordination and involuntary movements associated with strokes affecting the cerebellum or basal ganglia are addressed in Chapters 19 and 18, respectively.

Although this chapter describes the impairments, or clinical signs and symptoms, associated with stroke, it is important for clinicians to determine the resultant functional limitations or disabilities. Rehabilitation should focus on remediating or compensating for those impairments that adversely affect functional activities such as transfers or ambulation and quality of life.

Prerequisites for Normal Movement

To better understand the influence of various impairments on the production of a movement, one must first recognize the basic requirements necessary for normal volitional movement. According to DeLong,[19] **three conditions must be met to achieve a normal coordinated movement: (1) the proper muscles must be selected; (2) the selected muscles must be activated and inactivated in the proper sequence and at the correct time; and (3) the muscles must be activated with the correct amount of tension.** All these parameters of movement may be impaired after a stroke. In addition to these essentials, many volitional tasks require interlimb coordination, motivation, attention, sensory guidance, conceptual understanding of the task, and intact problem-solving abilities. Deficits in any of these areas may seriously impair movement and the ability to learn a motor skill (see Chapter 11).

Abnormal Muscle Tone

Hypotonia, **which manifests as a decreased resistance to passive muscle stretch, may be present immediately after a CVA associated with cerebral shock.** However, this is a temporary state that is often replaced by progressively increased muscle tone in the form of spasticity. Although persistent hypotonia is not common, it may occur if the lesion associated with the stroke is restricted to the primary motor cortex, the corticospinal pathways, or the cerebellum or its connections. The presence of hypotonia is often associated with joint instability, decreased endurance, and weakness.

Spasticity, **a form of hypertonia that typically is manifested as a velocity-dependent increased resistance to passive movement, is one of the most common motor abnormalities observed subsequent to a stroke.** Patients with lesions that affect multiple motor cortical areas or upper motor neuron inhibitory pathways, such as the medullary reticulospinal tracts, often exhibit spasticity. **The classic distribution of spasticity is a unilateral presentation on the side of the body contralateral to the lesion, which predominantly affects the antigravity muscles (Table 12–5; see Fig. 12–7).** Moderate-to-severe spasticity is associated with the development of soft tissue contractures, which may seriously impede rehabilitation efforts and limit functional abilities and which must be addressed in treatment. However, **controversy exists regarding the effects of spasticity on volitional movement** (see Chapter 12). Therefore, it is important to reexamine traditional methods of stroke rehabilitation that emphasize reducing spasticity to achieve improvements in active movement.

Abnormal Reflexes

Hyporeflexia of the deep tendon reflexes is uncommon and typically associated with the lesions that produce hypotonia discussed in the previous section. **Hyperactive tendon reflexes or hyperreflexia is a more common manifestation subsequent to a stroke. Clonus,** a series of rapid involuntary muscle contractions in response to abrupt muscle stretch, may also be present and has the potential to interfere with function, especially when present in the ankle plantarflexors. A positive Babinski's sign is likely to be elicited if there has been damage to upper motor neuron pathways such as the pyramidal tracts.

Muscle Weakness and Decreased Endurance

A frequently observed motor deficit associated with stroke is weakness, or the inability to generate tension, force, or torque.[20-22] Weakness or paresis may range in severity from an inability to achieve any visible muscle contraction to minimal impairment that is evident only through sensitive objective testing and generally is the result of damage in the primary motor cortex or its descending pathways. The degree of weakness is usually dependent on the extent of the central nervous system damage. **The most common distribution of weakness is contralateral hemiparesis, which is involvement of the upper and lower extremity on one side of the body (Fig. 21–4). Quadriparesis, which is**

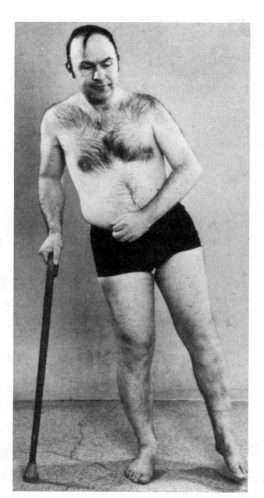

Figure 21–4. *Hemiparesis.* This patient has a left hemiparesis subsequent to a right cerebral infarct. Note the postural and movement abnormalities evident as he attempts to step with his left foot. (From DeJong, RN and Haerer, AF: Case taking and the neurologic examination. In Joynt, RJ: Clinical Neurology, vol. 1. JB Lippincott, Philadelphia, 1993, p 48, with permission.)

involvement of all four limbs, is uncommon and characteristic of lesions that affect the brainstem or are more diffuse in nature. **Distal muscles are typically affected to a greater extent than proximal muscles.** This may be due to numerous factors including the greater degree of bilateral innervation of the proximal muscles.

It is important to understand some of the mechanisms that appear to be contributing to this weakness in order to effectively treat the impairment. In normal persons, an increase in muscle force is achieved by increasing the number of motor units activated (recruitment) and by increasing the firing rate of already activated motor units (rate coding). Recent evidence suggests that both of these force control mechanisms are altered following a CVA.

Several researchers have reported a loss of motor units in patients within the first few months after stroke.[23,24] The proposed mechanism producing this reduction is one of transynaptic degeneration of motor neurons secondary to degeneration of descending corticospinal fibers.[23,24] This reduction in motor units, which has been reported to be as high as 50% for certain muscles[24] reduces the available potential recruitment pool. Furthermore, **there is evidence that there is selective loss of high force motor units associated with type II muscle fibers.**[23-25] The selective loss of type II muscle fibers would specifically create difficulty in the initiation and achievement of rapid, high-force movements.

Although the data remain inconclusive, **there is also evidence suggesting that persons exhibiting spasticity after stroke demonstrate a decrease in mean firing rates of motor units.**[26,27] This alteration in rate coding, suggested by an increase in the mean duration of the interspike intervals, may also contribute to the clinical presentation of weakness.

Another clinical problem, related to the lack of ability to generate adequate force, is the inability to respond quickly to changes in force requirements. This impairment in force modulation may be related to abnormal motor unit discharge patterns. Normal subjects have a negative serial correlation of motor unit interspike intervals in which a long interval between successive firings is followed by a short one. Recently, positive interspike serial correlations have been identified in hemiplegic patients; these correlations represent a decrease in the variability in motor unit firing.[26,28] **Clinically, this may be manifested as difficulty in maintaining a steady force or in adapting to rapid changes in force requirements.**

In contrast to the lack of a significant correlation between spasticity and function, numerous researchers have demonstrated strong correlations between decreased muscle strength and impaired ability to perform activities such as gait,[29] **standing,**[30] **balance,**[31] **and upper extremity functional tasks.**[32,33] Although the presence of weakness has been acknowledged, it has not been the focus of treatment for the last 20 years. This is especially true in the treatment of patients presenting with spasticity. An exhaustive review of the literature revealed very few studies investigating the effectiveness of "strengthening" activities in stroke- or brain-injured patients. The prevalence of weakness in this patient population and the increasing evidence demonstrating the negative impact of weakness on active movement and function highlight the need to reevaluate treatment strategies that focus on the primary goal of reducing spasticity to improve motor control.

A decrease in muscular endurance reflected in an inability to sustain force over time or through repetitions is also frequently observed in association with weakness and abnormal tone.

Altered Muscle Activation Patterns

Another characteristic motor impairment is a reduction in the ability to produce fractionated movements in the hemiparetic limbs. *Fractionation* **means the ability to move a single joint without simultaneously producing movements in other joints.** This inability to isolate joint movement or muscle contraction contributes to the stereotypical dominant active motor synergies often observed after stroke (Table 12–6; see Fig. 12–10). This loss of fractionation illustrates that the accurate selection or sequencing of muscle activation/inactivation necessary to perform a task is impaired. In other words, muscles are not activated in appropriate functional groups. The presence of associated reactions may reflect a similar dysfunction in the selection of appropriate motor programs. **An associated reaction involves the unintentional movement of one limb during the intentional movement of another limb** (see Fig. 12–12). In this situation, the patient has difficulty isolating movement in one limb from the others. The loss of fractionation typically results in a loss of fine motor control and may seriously affect function, especially in the hand.

The timing of muscle activation and contraction, which includes the reaction time, the speed of the actual movement or movement time, and the time necessary to stop the movement, may also be impaired subsequent to a stroke. **An increased reaction time has been documented in patients diagnosed with stroke.**[34–37] This impairment has been demonstrated in the nonparetic ipsilateral limb, as well as in the contralateral paretic limb,[34,45] and appears to be more prevalent and severe in patients with right hemispheric lesions.[35] **Movement time, or the time taken to complete a task after it has been initiated, may also be increased in this patient population.**[38,39] Finally, **the time necessary to halt a movement in progress may be increased.** This contributes to difficulties in checking rapid movements and in performing rapidly alternating movements, which require fast termination of agonist activity prior to activation of the antagonist. All these timing abnormalities may significantly disturb function, and it is essential to evaluate and address these impairments during treatment.

Deficits in Motor Planning

Lesions in the premotor, supplementary motor, or parietal cortices in the dominant hemisphere may produce deficits in motor planning or apraxias. Although the patients may have the strength and other physical components necessary to produce movement, they are unable to conceptualize and organize or plan complex movement sequences to achieve specific goals. The deficits are especially evident when imitating others or when performing sequential movements. The ability to perform automatic functional movements may remain intact.

Abnormal Balance Reactions

The ability to statically sit or stand unsupported, to maintain balance when displaced by an external force, and to safely react to self-imposed movement may be impaired after a stroke.[40–42] **A few of the specific balance abnormalities demonstrated in stroke patients include a reduction in voluntary sway during standing,**[43] **the inappropriate selection of muscles to produce an appropriate response,**[43] **a reduced amplitude of reactive force in the paretic limb,**[40] **and increased latencies of balance reactions in the paretic limb.**[44] In addition, somatosensory dysfunction, visual impairments, muscle weakness, and contracture and postural abnormalities all may contribute to balance impairments and increase the risk of falling. Each of these components must be evaluated and its contribution to balance dysfunction assessed.

Distribution of Motor Deficits

A unilateral cerebral lesion typically results in contralateral motor deficits that may include most of the impairments discussed. The extremities ipsilateral to the lesion have generally been considered "unaffected" and have been labeled as such. **Recently, impairments in ipsilateral sensory motor function following unilateral cerebral lesion have been reported.** Jones and associates[45] investigated the performance of the ipsilateral limb on 12 computerized tests. Although there was no impairment noted on clinical evaluation, **there were significant reductions in arm strength, reaction time, speed, steadiness, and tracking in the ipsilateral limb of stroke subjects compared with a group of controls.** Ipsilateral impairments in reaction and movement time,[34] finger tracking,[35] fast tapping, and peg-board performance have also been demonstrated.[46,47] Generally, these impairments are not severe enough to be identified on a clinical evaluation. However, this may reflect the lack of sensitivity of the clinical tests, rather than the potential clinical significance of these deficits. The functional implications of these ipsilateral impairments in the "unaffected" extremities have not yet been examined.

Laterality of Motor Control

Laterality refers to the tendency for the cerebral hemispheres to specialize in function. For example, the dominance of the left hemisphere for speech and language in the majority of individuals and the dominance of the right hemisphere for visuospatial orientation are well documented.[48] **Recent evidence suggests that certain aspects of motor control may also demonstrate hemispheric dominance.** For example, right-sided brain lesions have been associated with "motor impersistence" or the inability to maintain a steady grip or posture.[49,50] Conversely, motor deficits associated with left-sided brain damage include difficulty in performing fast-paced repetitive movements[51,52] and difficulty in sequencing movements.[36,53] The laterality of cerebral functions implies that each hemisphere exerts a degree of bilateral control over its specialized functions and most of these lateralized motor functions have been documented in the bilateral extremities. If this laterality for motor control is confirmed, implications for rehabilitation may exist. Treatment for right-sided lesions may focus greater attention on the ability to sustain contractions and increase endurance, whereas that for left-sided lesions may emphasize fast-paced, repetitive activities to remediate these dysfunctions.

Neurovascular Clinical Syndromes

Although there are some minor variations among patients, there are characteristic signs and symptoms associated with occlusion of specific cerebral vessels. The clinical manifestations may include sensory, motor, autonomic, and communication dysfunctions. Clinical syndromes have been established based on knowledge of the vascular anatomy, the functional localization in the central nervous system, and the typical clinical presentations. The syndromes reflect the deficits associated with ischemic infarcts due to embolism or thrombosis, in which occlusion is usually limited to a single vessel. Although hemorrhagic strokes may produce many of the same deficits, the extent of bleeding and the secondary effects often complicate the clinical picture. These descriptions may be far from exact and variability may exist, but they can help a therapist to predict impairments and identify possible mechanisms accounting for dysfunction. The following is a description of some of

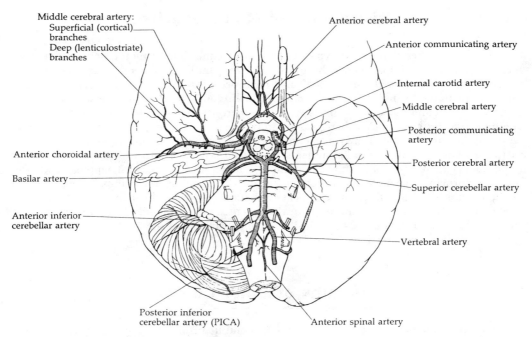

Figure 21–5. *Cerebral Vasculature.* Diagram of the ventral surface of the brainstem and cerebral hemispheres illustrating the key components of the anterior (carotid) and posterior (vertebral-basilar) circulation. (From Martin, JH: Neuroanatomy: Text and Atlas. Appleton & Lange, Norwalk, CT, 1989, p 83, with permission.)

the more common vascular syndromes associated with disruption of blood supply to the cortex and brainstem. The clinical syndromes associated with strokes in the cerebellum and basal ganglia have been presented in Chapters 19 and 18, respectively.

Internal Carotid Artery Syndrome

The common carotid artery branches to form the internal and external carotid artery. The internal carotid ascends through the neck, enters the skull, gives off an ophthalmic branch, and continues on to pierce the dura and bifurcate into the terminal anterior and middle cerebral arteries (Fig. 21–5). This vessel is highly susceptible to atherosclerosis, but the manifestations associated with its occlusion are the most variable of all vascular syndromes (Fig. 21–6).

A large percentage of patients present with a history of transient ischemic attacks. **One frequent early symptom is the temporary fading of vision or blindness in the ipsilateral eye. This is referred to as** *amaurosis fugax.* The retinal arterioles are fairly vulnerable to decreased flow in the ophthalmic artery and this visual deficit often precedes other focal neurologic signs. However, this symptom is temporary, and the eye is seldom permanently damaged during ischemic episodes.

The most common presentation of internal carotid occlusion is the middle cerebral artery syndrome, which is discussed in the following text. If the distribution of the anterior cerebral artery is also affected, there will be additional signs and symptoms and the patient will probably experience a reduced level of consciousness resulting from the massive extent of the lesion and associated edema.

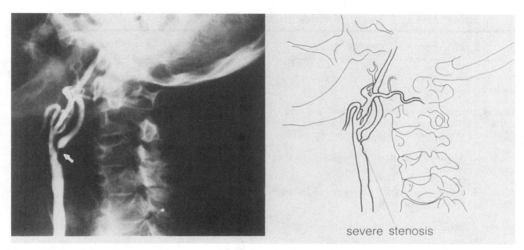

Figure 21–6. *Severe Stenosis at the Origin of the Left Internal Carotid Artery.* This 69-year-old patient had had numerous vertebrobasilar ischemic attacks, with deafness, vertigo, and ill-defined visual blurring. An X-ray study (arteriogram) made with radiopaque dye present in the blood reveals a marked narrowing of the left internal carotid (*Arrow*). (From Atlas of Clinical Neurology by GD Perkins, et al. Mosby-Wolfe, an imprint of Times Mirror International Publishers, Ltd, London, UK, 1986.)

Middle Cerebral Artery Syndrome

The middle cerebral artery is the artery most often occluded as a result of cerebrovascular disease. It is the largest terminal branch of the internal carotid artery and supplies almost the entire lateral surface of the brain (cortical branches; Figs. 21–5 and 21–7), as well as the basal ganglia and large portions of the internal capsule (deep penetrating branches). Occlusion of the main stem of the artery is generally associated with extensive neurologic dysfunction and decreased consciousness. Table 21–5 lists the classic signs and symptoms associated with a disruption of blood flow in the middle cerebral artery.

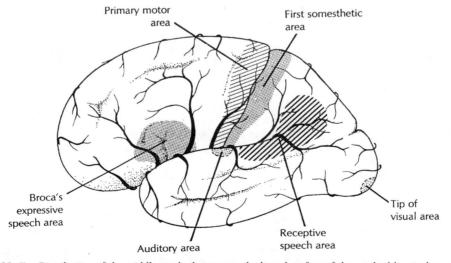

Figure 21–7. Distribution of the middle cerebral artery on the lateral surface of the cerebral hemisphere. (From Barr, ML and Kiernan, JA: The Human Nervous System: An Anatomical Viewpoint, ed 5. JB Lippincott, Philadelphia, 1988, p 367, with permission.)

Table 21–5. *Clinical Manifestations—Middle Cerebral Artery Syndrome*

Signs and Symptoms	Structures Involved
Paresis of contralateral face, arm, and leg (leg is least affected)	Primary motor cortex and internal capsule
Sensory impairment over the contralateral face, arm, and leg (pain, temperature, touch, vibration, position, two-point discrimination, stereognosis)	Primary sensory cortex and internal capsule
Motor speech disorder (expressive-aphasia-telegraphic halting speech)	Broca's cortical area in the dominant hemisphere
Wernicke's or receptive aphasia (fluent but often jargon speech, poor comprehension)	Wernicke's cortical area in the dominant hemisphere
Perceptual problems such as unilateral neglect, apraxias, depth perception problems, spatial relation difficulties	Parietal sensory association cortex
Homonymous hemianopia	Optic radiation in internal capsule
Loss of conjugate gaze to the opposite side	Frontal eye fields or their descending tracts
Ataxia of contralateral limb(s) (sensory ataxia)	Parietal lobe

Adapted from Adams and Victor,[2] p 677.

The most frequently observed manifestations of the middle cerebral artery syndrome are contralateral spastic paresis that predominantly affects the distal musculature of the upper extremity, contralateral sensory impairments, expressive or receptive aphasia, and homonymous hemianopia, a visual field deficit (Fig. 21–8). The clinical presentation varies, depending on factors such as the location and extent of infarction and the adequacy of collateral circulation.

Anterior Cerebral Artery Syndrome

This smaller terminal branch of the internal carotid artery supplies the anterior two thirds of the medial cerebral cortex (Fig. 21–9), as well as portions of the basal ganglia, corpus callosum, and the anterior limb of the internal capsule. This artery is less frequently affected by cerebrovascular disease, and the impact of an occlusion in the main stem is often reduced by the presence of the collateral circulation provided by the anterior communicating artery (see Fig. 21–5). Characteristic signs and symptoms associated with anterior cerebral artery strokes are described in Table 21–6. The contralateral lower extremity is predominantly affected, since the functional area of the primary and sensory motor cortex for the lower extremity is on the medial aspect of the cortex (Fig. 21–10).

Vertebral Artery Syndrome

The two vertebral arteries arise as branches from the subclavian arteries and ascend through the neck in the foramina of the transverse processes of the upper six cervical vertebrae (see Fig. 21–5). These arteries enter the skull at the foramen magnum and lie on the ventral surface of the medulla where they join to form the single basilar artery just caudal to the junction of the pons and medulla (see Fig. 21–5). The vertebral arteries and their branches form the main source of blood flow to the medulla and also supply the posterior inferior aspect of the cerebellum.

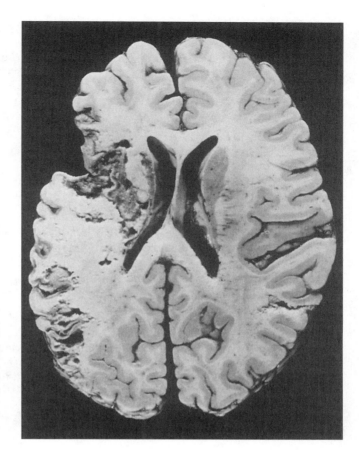

Figure 21–8. Middle Cerebral Infarct. This 59-year-old man developed right hemiplegia, aphasia, and homonymous visual field defects. These deficits persisted until his death 2 months later. A massive infarct within the distribution of the left middle cerebral artery was found at autopsy. (From Schochet, SS and Nelson, J: Atlas of Clinical Neuropathology. Appleton & Lange, Norwalk, CT, 1989, p 127, with permission.)

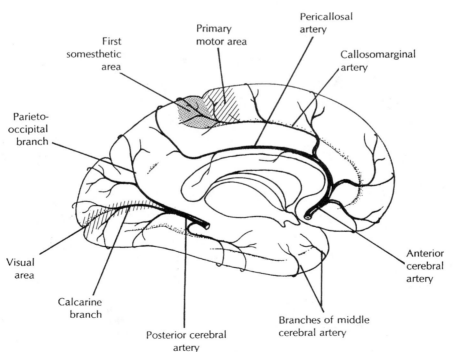

Figure 21–9. Distribution of the anterior and posterior cerebral arteries on the medial surface of the cerebral hemisphere. (From Barr, ML and Kiernan, JA: The Human Nervous System. An Anatomical Viewpoint, ed 5. JB Lippincott, Philadelphia, 1988, p 368, with permission.)

Table 21–6. *Clinical Manifestations—Anterior Cerebral Artery Syndrome*

Signs and Symptoms	Structures Involved
Paresis of opposite foot and leg and to a lesser extent the arm	Primary motor area, medial aspect of cortex, internal capsule
Mental impairment (perseveration, confusion, and amnesia)	Localization unknown
Sensory impairments primarily in lower extremity	Primary sensory area, medial aspect of cortex
Urinary incontinence	Posteromedial aspect of superior frontal gyrus
Problems with imitation and bimanual tasks, apraxia	Corpus callosum
Abulia (akinetic mutism), slowness, delay, lack of spontaneity, motor inaction	Uncertain localization

Adapted from Adams and Victor,[2] p 680.

Although atherosclerosis is the most common type of pathology that disrupts blood flow in this system, **the extracranial portion of these arteries that course through the neck are susceptible to trauma, such as forced neck rotation and hyperextension.** The most common cause of traumatic infarction in these vessels is automobile accidents. However, aggressive neck manipulations such as those administered by a chiropractor, have also produced vertebrobasilar insufficiency and strokes.[54,55]

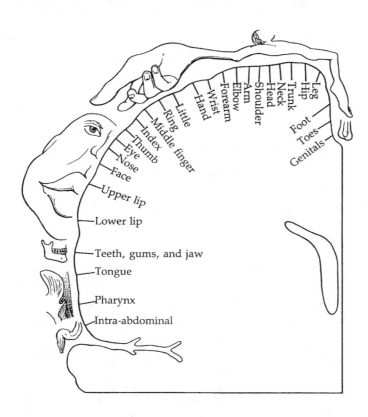

Figure 21–10. *Somatotopic Organization of the Primary Sensory Cortex.* This figure illustrates a schematic coronal section through the postcentral gyrus. (From Martin, JH: Neuroanatomy: Text and Atlas. Appleton & Lange Norwalk, CT, 1989, p. 129, with permission.)

Table 21–7. *Clinical Manifestations—Vertebrobasilar Artery Syndrome*

Signs and Symptoms	Structures Involved
Medial medullary syndrome (occlusion of vertebral artery or branch of vertebral or lower basilar artery)	
Ipsilateral to lesion	
Paralysis with atrophy of half the tongue	CNXII, hypoglossal nucleus or nerve
Contralateral to lesion	
Paralysis of arm and leg	Corticospinal tract
Impaired tactile and proprioceptive sense over 50% of the body	Medial lemniscus
Lateral medullary syndrome (occlusion of vertebral, posterior inferior cerebellar, basilar)	
Ipsilateral to lesion	
Decreased pain and temperature sensation in face	Descending tract and nucleus of fifth nerve
Ataxia of limbs, falling to side of lesion	Vestibular nuclei and connections
Vertigo, nausea, vomiting	Vestibular nuclei and connections
Nystagmus	Vestibular nuclei and connections
Horner's syndrome (miosis, ptosis, decreased sweating)	Descending sympathetic tract
Dysphagia, hoarseness, paralysis of vocal cord, diminished gag reflex	CNIX and CNX nuclei or nerve fibers
Sensory impairment of ipsilateral arm, trunk, or leg	Cuneate and gracile nuclei
Contralateral to lesion	
Impaired pain and thermal sense over 50% of body, sometimes face	Spinothalamic tract
Basilar artery syndrome—a combination of the various brainstem syndromes plus those arising in the posterior cerebral artery distribution	
Paralysis or weakness of all extremities, plus all bulbar musculature	Corticobulbar and corticospinal tracts bilaterally
Diplopia, paralysis of conjugate lateral or vertical gaze, internuclear ophthalmoplegia, horizontal or vertical nystagmus	Ocular motor nerves, apparatus for conjugate gaze, medial longitudinal fasciculus
Blindness, impaired vision, various visual field defects	Primary visual cortex
Bilateral cerebellar ataxia	Cerebellar peduncles and the cerebellar hemispheres
Coma	Reticular activating system
Sensation may be strikingly intact in the presence of almost total paralysis (locked in)	Sparing of tegmentum of pons
Thalamic pain syndrome	Thalamic nuclei
Medial inferior pontine syndrome (occlusion of paramedian branch of basilar artery)	
Ipsilateral to lesion	
Paralysis of conjugate gaze to side of lesion (preservation of convergence)	Pontine "center" for lateral gaze paramedian pentine reticular formation (PPRF)
Nystagmus	Vestibular nuclei and connections
Ataxia of limbs and gait	Middle cerebellar peduncle
Diplopia on lateral gaze	Abducens nerve or nucleus

(continued)

Adapted from Adams and Victor[2] p 691.

Various syndromes may occur with occlusion of the vertebral arteries or their branches and some of the more common presentations are presented in Table 21–7 and illustrated in Figure 21–11. **The most common and well-documented syndrome is the lateral medullary or Wallenberg's syndrome.** This represents the typical clinical manifestation associated with disruption of the posterior inferior cerebellar branch or the main vertebral artery.

Table 21–7. *Clinical Manifestations—Vertebrobasilar Artery Syndrome—Continued*

Signs and Symptoms	Structures Involved
Contralateral to lesion	
Paresis of face, arm, and leg	Corticobulbar and corticospinal tract in lower pons
Impaired tactile and proprioceptive sense over 50% of the body	Medial lemniscus
Lateral inferior pontine syndrome (occlusion of anterior inferior cerebellar artery)	
Ipsilateral to lesion	
Horizontal and vertical nystagmus, vertigo, nausea, vomiting	Vestibular nerve or nucleus
Facial paralysis	Seventh nerve or nucleus
Paralysis of conjugate gaze to side of lesion	Pontine "center" for lateral gaze (PPRF)
Deafness, tinnitus	Auditory nerve or cochlear nucleus
Ataxia	Middle cerebellar peduncle and cerebellar hemisphere
Impaired sensation over face	Main sensory nucleus and descending tract of fifth nerve
Contralateral to lesion	
Impaired pain and thermal sense over half the body (may include face)	Spinothalamic tract
Medial midpontine syndrome (paramedian branch of midbasilar artery)	
Ipsilateral to lesion	
Ataxia of limbs and gait (more prominent in bilateral involvement)	Middle cerebellar peduncle
Contralateral to lesion	
Paralysis of face, arm, and leg	Corticobulbar and corticospinal tract
Deviation of eyes	PPRF
Lateral midpontine syndrome (short circumferential artery)	
Ipsilateral to lesion	
Ataxia of limbs	Middle cerebellar peduncle
Paralysis of muscles of mastication	Motor fibers or nucleus of cranial nerve V
Impaired sensation over side of face	Sensory fibers or nucleus of cranial nerve V
Medial superior pontine syndrome (paramedian branches of upper basilar artery)	
Ipsilateral to lesion	
Cerebellar ataxia	Superior or middle cerebellar peduncle
Internuclear ophthalmoplegia	Medial longitudinal fasciculus
Contralateral to lesion	
Paralysis of face, arm, and leg	Corticobulbar and corticospinal tract
Lateral superior pontine syndrome (syndrome of superior cerebellar artery)	
Ipsilateral to lesion	
Ataxia of limbs and gait, falling to side of lesion	Middle and superior cerebellar peduncles, superior surface of cerebellum, dentate nucleus
Dizziness, nausea, vomiting	Vestibular nuclei
Horizontal nystagmus	Vestibular nuclei
Paresis of conjugate gaze (ipsilateral)	Uncertain
Loss of optokinetic nystagmus	Uncertain
Miosis, ptosis, decreased sweating over face (Horner syndrome)	Descending sympathetic fibers
Contralateral to lesion	
Impaired pain and thermal sense of face, limbs, and trunk	Spinothalamic tract
Impaired touch, vibration, and position sense, more in leg than arm (tendency to incongruity of pain and touch deficits)	Medial lemniscus (lateral portion)

Adapted from Adams and Victor,[2] p 693.

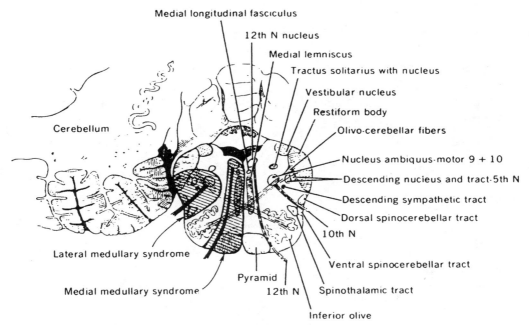

Medial longitudinal fasciculus
12th N nucleus
Medial lemniscus
Tractus solitarius with nucleus
Vestibular nucleus
Restiform body
Olivo-cerebellar fibers
Cerebellum
Nucleus ambiguus-motor 9 + 10
Descending nucleus and tract-5th N
Descending sympathetic tract
Dorsal spinocerebellar tract
10th N
Lateral medullary syndrome
Ventral spinocerebellar tract
Medial medullary syndrome
Pyramid
12th N
Spinothalamic tract
Inferior olive

Figure 21–11. *Syndromes Associated with Obstruction of the Vertebral Artery or Its Branches.* The lateral medullary syndrome is probably the most frequent consequence of occlusion of one vertebral artery; the medial medullary syndrome is rare. Cross-hatching indicates the areas of infarction. (From Adams, RD and Victor, M: Principles of Neurology, ed 5. McGraw-Hill, New York, 1993, p 690, with permission.)

Basilar Artery Syndrome

The basilar artery continues up the ventral aspect of the pons and bifurcates to form the two terminal posterior cerebral branches (see Fig. 21–5). The basilar artery and its branches (excluding the posterior cerebral) supply the lateral two thirds of the pons, the middle and superior cerebellar peduncles, and portions of the cerebellum, midbrain, and diencephalon.

Occlusion of the basilar artery often is a catastrophic event, resulting in bilateral damage to the basal and tegmental regions of the pons. The patient is often comatose and quadriplegic with a poor prognosis. A particularly tragic result may be the "locked-in" syndrome, characterized by intact consciousness and sensation with the almost total absence of voluntary movements in the face or limbs. Eye movements may provide the only means of communication, and while many patients succumb to secondary complications, those who survive remain severely disabled. Characteristic presentations associated with strokes in the basilar artery or its branches are described in Table 21–7 and illustrated in Figure 21–12.

Posterior Cerebral Artery Syndrome

The posterior cerebral arteries constitute the terminal branches of the basilar artery and are connected to the internal carotid system by the posterior communicating arteries (see Fig. 21–5). These arteries and their various tributaries supply large portions of the midbrain, temporal lobe, and diencephalon, as well the posterior third of the medial cortex (Fig. 21–9). Similar to the anterior cerebral artery, occlusion proximal to the posterior communicating artery usually results in minimal deficits due to the presence of adequate collateral circulation.

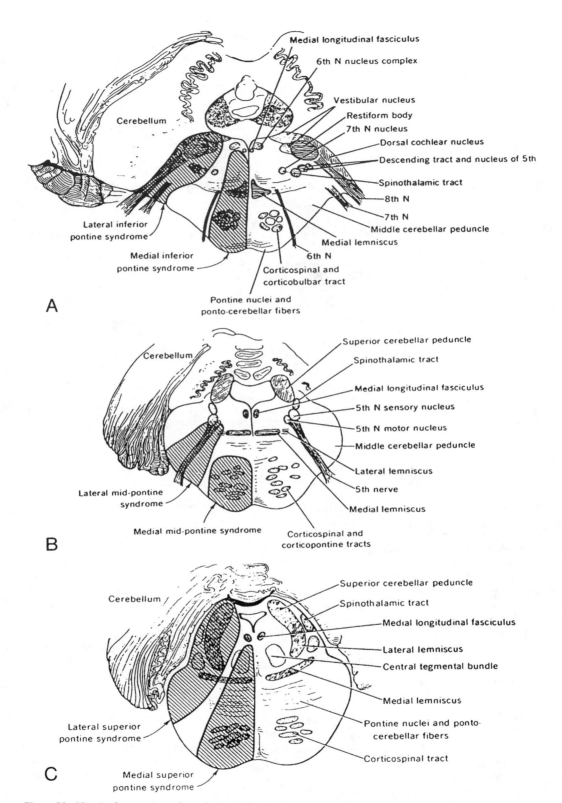

Figure 21-12. In these sections through the (A) lower, (B) mid, and (C) upper pons, the cross-hatching indicates the area of infarction associated with occlusion of the basilar artery or its branches. (Adapted from Adams, RD and Victor, M: Principles of Neurology, ed 5. McGraw-Hill, New York, 1993, p 693–695, with permission.)

Table 21–8. *Clinical Manifestations of Posterior Cerebral Artery Syndrome*

Signs and Symptoms	Structures Involved
Peripheral Territory	
Contralateral homonymous hemianopia	Primary visual cortex or optic radiation
Prosopagnosia (difficulty naming people on sight)	Visual association cortex
Dyslexia (difficulty reading) without agraphia (difficulty writing), color naming (anomia), and color discrimination problems	Dominant calcarine lesion and posterior part of corpus callosum
Memory defect	Lesion of inferomedial portions of temporal lobe bilaterally or on the dominant side only
Topographic disorientation	Nondominant primary visual area, usually bilaterally
Central Territory	
Thalamic syndrome: sensory impairments (all modalities), spontaneous pain, and dysesthesias	Ventral posterolateral nucleus of thalamus
Involuntary movements; choreoathetosis, intention tremor, hemiballismus	Subthalamic nucleus or its pallidal connections
Contralateral hemiplegia	Cerebral peduncle - midbrain
Weber's syndrome—Oculomotor nerve palsy and contralateral hemiplegia	Third nerve and cerebral peduncle of midbrain
Paresis of vertical eye movements, slight miosis and ptosis, and sluggish pupillary light response	Supranuclear fibers to third nerve

Adapted from Adams and Victor,[2] p 685.

One of the most common signs associated with occlusion in the cortical branch is contralateral homonymous hemianopia. The affected patient presents with a visual field deficit, wherein a patient looking straight ahead is unable to see objects in 50% of his or her visual field. These patients ignore objects placed in that field, and safety becomes an issue since they are unable to see obstacles when ambulating. The typical clinical manifestations associated with posterior cerebral circulation deficits are delineated in Table 21–8.

Risk Factors Associated with Cerebrovascular Disease

It has been clear for some time that the recent reduction in mortality and disability following stroke is attributed to improved prevention, not treatment. Multiple risk factors have been described that correlate with an increased incidence of cerebrovascular disease. Although the etiology of stroke is often multifactorial, reductions in risk factors that predispose an individual to stroke will help to reduce the incidence of both new and recurrent strokes.

Hypertension is a significant risk factor that contributes to the pathogenesis of both ischemic and hemorrhagic strokes.[56] Both diastolic (>90 mm Hg) and systolic (>160 mm Hg) hypertension are associated with cerebrovascular disease, and the improved detection and treatment of this variable has resulted in a decreased incidence of both initial and recurrent strokes.[57,58] **Several investigators have identified diabetes as a significant risk factor for stroke.** This may be a direct correlation or it may be secondary to a strong correlation between diabetes and hypertension. However, the controlled treatment of diabetes does not appear to influence the incidence of stroke.[59] **Other factors that have been implicated in the pathogenesis of cerebrovascular disease are smoking,[60] oral contraceptives,[61] obesity,[62] hypercholesterolemia,[63] alcohol abuse,[64] and elevated hemoglobin concentrations.[65]**

Stroke Outcomes

Immediate post-stroke survival is influenced by multiple factors such as age, stroke type, stroke location, and the presence of secondary complications. Increased age, hemorrhagic lesions, large infarcts or hemorrhages affecting the brainstem, and significant edema and elevated intracranial pressure, all are correlated with increased mortality in the acute stage. Fatality rates for the initial 30-day period following stroke range from 15% for thrombotic infarcts to 82% for intracerebral hemorrhages. The presence of concurrent cardiac disease and hypertension is significantly correlated with death in both acute and chronic stages.

Functional recovery subsequent to a stroke is highly variable from one patient to another. The percentage of patients regaining functional independence is reported to range between 43% and 68%[66] and to increase to 75% in patients younger than 45 years old.[7] To provide cost-effective rehabilitation services and to assist with program planning, numerous investigators have attempted to delineate those factors that assist in the prediction of recovery. **Factors such as advanced patient age, profound motor or sensory loss, visuospatial perceptual deficits, and incontinence are perceived as negative prognostic variables.**[67] In addition, the single most significant predictor of eventual outcome is probably the magnitude of the initial lesion.[68] Mathematical equations are currently being developed to provide an objective measure of predictive variables that can then be used for rehabilitation program planning, resource management, and family education.

Summary

Although the incidence of stroke resulting from cerebrovascular disease is declining, it remains a leading cause of mortality and morbidity, with staggering economic, physical, social, and emotional impacts. This chapter has attempted to identify the various mechanisms and risk factors that contribute to the etiology of strokes, as well as to describe certain classic clinical syndromes that result from disruption of the cerebral circulation. A thorough understanding of these principles should allow the therapist to be aware of factors that might contribute to further secondary brain injury, to predict and plan rehabilitation for resultant neurologic impairments, and to comprehend the typical clinical course and management of these patients.

RECOMMENDED READINGS

Adams, JH, Graham, DI, and Harriman, DGF: An Introduction to Neuropathology. Churchill Livingstone, Edinburgh, 1988.

Adams, RD and Victor, M: Principles of Neurology, ed 5. McGraw-Hill Information Services, New York, 1993.

Barnett, HJM, et al (ed): Stroke: Pathophysiology, Diagnosis and Management, ed 2. Churchill Livingstone, New York, 1992.

Brandstater, ME and Basmajian, JV (eds): Stroke Rehabilitation. Williams & Wilkins, Baltimore, 1987.

Caplan, LR: Stroke: A Clinical Approach, ed 2. Butterworth & Company, Boston, 1993.

Duncan, PW and Badke MB: Stroke Rehabilitation: The Recovery of Motor Control. Year Book Medical Publishers, Chicago, 1987.

Ebrahim, S: Clinical Epidemiology of Stroke. Oxford University Press, Oxford, 1990.

Greenberg, DA, Aminoff, MJ, and Simon, RP: Clinical Neurology, ed 2. Appleton & Lange, Norwalk, CT, 1993.

Gunderson, CH: Essentials of Clinical Neurology. Raven Press, New York, 1990.

Kaplan, PE and Cerullo, LJ (eds): Stroke Rehabilitation. Butterworth & Company, Boston, 1986.

Kottke, FJ and Lehmann, JF (eds): Krusen's Handbook of Physical Medicine and Rehabilitation, ed 4. WB Saunders, Philadelphia, 1990.

Mori, K (ed): MRI of the Central Nervous System: A Pathology Atlas. Springer-Verlag, Tokyo, 1991.

REFERENCES

1. Licata-Gehr, EE: Etiology of Stroke Subtypes. Nurs Clin Am 26:943, 1991.
2. Adams, RD and Victor, M: Principles of Neurology, ed 5. McGraw-Hill Information Services, New York, 1993.
3. Wolf, PA: An Overview of the Epidemiology of Stroke. Stroke 21(suppl II):II4, 1990.
4. Klag, MJ, Whelton, PK, and Seidler, AJ: Decline in US Stroke Mortality, Demographic Trends and Antihypertensive Treatment. Stroke 20:14, 1989.
5. Wolf, PA, Cobb, JL, and D'Agostino, RB: Epidemiology of Stroke. Chapter 1. In Barnett, HJM, et al (eds): Stroke: Pathophysiology, Diagnosis and Management, ed 2. Churchill Livingstone, New York, 1992.
6. Adelman, SM: Economic Impact. Stroke 12(suppl 1):69,1981.
7. Bogousslavsky, J and Pierre, P: Ischemic Stroke in Patients Under Age 45. Neurol Clin 10:113, 1992.
8. Garraway, WM, Whisnant, JP, and Drury, I: The Changing Pattern of Survival Following Stroke. Stroke 14:699, 1983.
9. Wolf, PA, et al: Probability of Stroke: A Risk Profile from the Framingham Study. Stroke 22:312, 1991.
10. Kaplan, B, Brint, S, and Tanabe, J: Temporal Thresholds for Neocortical Infarcts in Rats Subjected to Reversible Focal Cerebral Ischemia. Stroke 22:1032, 1991.
11. Pulsinelli, WA: Selective Neuronal Vulnerability: Morphological and Molecular Characteristics. Prog Brain Res 63:29, 1985.
12. Garcia, JH, Ho, KL, and Caccamo, DV: Pathology of Stroke. Chapter 7. In Barnett, HJM, et al (eds): Stroke: Pathophysiology, Diagnosis and Management, ed 2. Churchill Livingstone, New York, 1992.
13. Kurtzke, JF: Epidemiology of Cerebrovascular Disease. In McDowell, F and Caplan, L (eds): Cerebrovascular Survey Report 1985 for the National Institute of Neurological and Communicative Disorders and Stroke. Bethesda, MD, 1985.
14. Picone, CM, et al: Immunohistochemical Determination of Calcium-Calmodulin Binding Predicts Neuronal Damage After Global Ischemia. J Cereb Blood Flow Metab 9:805, 1989.
15. Gelmers, HJ and Hennerici, M: Effect of Nimodipine on Acute Ischemic Stroke: Pooled Results from Five Randomized Clinical Trials. Stroke 21(suppl IV):81, 1990.
16. Foulkes, MA, et al: The Stroke Data Bank: Design, Methods and Baseline Characteristics. Stroke 19:547, 1988.
17. Cerebral Embolism Study Group: Immediate Anticoagulation of Embolism Stroke: A Randomized Trial. Stroke 14:668, 1983.
18. Duke, RJ, et al: Intravenous Heparin for the Prevention of Stroke Progression in Acute Partial Stable Stroke: A Randomized Clinical Trial. Ann Intern Med 105:825, 1986.
19. DeLong, M: Central Patterning of Movement. Neurosci Res Bull 9:10, 1972.
20. Colebatch, JG, Gandevia, SC, and Spira, PJ: Voluntary Muscle Strength in Hemiparesis: Distribution of Weakness at the Elbow. J Neurol Neurosurg Psychiatry 49:1019, 1986.
21. Watkins, MP, Harris, BA, and Kozlowski, BA: Isokinetic Testing in Patients with Hemiparesis: A Pilot Study. Phys Ther 64:184, 1984.
22. Bohannon, RW and Smith, MB: Assessment of Strength Deficits in Eight Paretic Upper Extremity Muscle Groups of Stroke Patients with Hemiplegia. Phys Ther 67:522, 1987.
23. Dattola, R, et al: Muscle Rearrangement in Patients with Hemiparesis After Stroke: An Electrophysiological and Morphological Study. Eur Neurol 33:109, 1993.
24. McComas, AJ, et al: Functional Changes in Motorneurones of Hemiparetic Subjects. J Neurol Neurosurg Psychiatry 36:183, 1976.
25. Dietz, V, et al: Motor Unit Involvement in Spastic Hemiparesis: Relationship Between Leg Muscle Activation and Histochemistry. J Neurol Sci 75:89, 1986.
26. Andreassen, S and Rosenfalck, A: Regulation of Firing Pattern of Single Motor Units. J Neurol Neurosurg Psychiatry 43:897, 1980.
27. Tang, A and Rymer, WZ: Abnormal Force-EMG Relations in Paretic Limbs of Hemiparetic Human Subjects. J Neurol Neurosurg Psychiatry 44:690, 1980.
28. Shahani, BT, Wierzbicka, MM, and Parker, SW: Abnormal Single Motor Unit Behavior in Upper Motor Neuron Syndrome. Muscle Nerve 14:64, 1991.
29. Bohannon, RW: Selected Determinants of Ambulatory Capacity in Patients with Hemiplegia. Clin Rehab 3:47, 1989.
30. Bohannon, RW: Correlation of Lower Limb Strengths and Other Variables in Standing Performance in Stroke Patients. Physiother Can 41:198, 1989.
31. Hamrin, E, et al: Muscle Strength and Balance in Post Stroke Patients. Ups J Med Sci 87:11, 1982.
32. Wilson, DJ, Baker, LL, and Craddock, JA: Functional Test for the Hemiparetic Upper Extremity. Am J Occup Ther 38:159, 1984.
33. Bohannon, RW, Warren, ME, and Cogman, KA: Motor Variables Correlated with Hand-to-Mouth Maneuver in Stroke Patients. Arch Phys Med Rehabil 72:682, 1991.
34. Dickstein, R, et al: Reaction and Movement Times in Patients with Hemiparesis for Unilateral and Bilateral Elbow Flexion. Phys Ther 73:37, 1993.
35. Buonocore, M, Casale, R, and Arrigo, A: Psychomotor Skills in Hemiplegic Patients: Reaction Time Differences Related to Hemispheric Lesion Side. Neurophysiol Clin 20:203, 1990.
36. Harrington, DL and Haaland, KY: Hemispheric Specialization for Motor Sequencing: Abnormalities in Levels of Programming. Neuropsychologia 29:147, 1991.
37. Kaizer, F, et al: Response Time of Stroke Patients to a Visual Stimulus. Stroke 19:335, 1988.
38. Segal, RL and Youssef, EL: Wrist Movements in Able Bodied and Brain Injured Individuals. Arch Phys Med Rehabil 72:454, 1991.
39. Rosecrance, JC and Guiliani, CA: Kinematic Analysis of Lower-Limb Movement During Ergometer Pedaling in Hemiplegic and Non-Hemiplegic Subjects. Phys Ther 71:334, 1991.

40. Di Fabio, RP, Badke, M, and Duncan, PW: Adapting Human Postural Reflexes Following Localized Cerebrovascular Lesion: An Analysis of Bilateral Long Latency Responses. Brain Res 363:259, 1986.
41. Lee, WA, Deming, L, and Sahgal, V: Quantitative and Clinical Measures of Static Standing Balance in Hemiparetic and Normal Subjects. Phys Ther 68:970, 1988.
42. Horak, FB, et al: The Effects of Movement Velocity, Mass Displaced, and Task Certainty on Associated Postural Adjustments Made by Normal and Hemiplegic Individuals. J Neurol Neurosurg Psychiatry 47:1020, 1984.
43. Dettmann, MA, Linder, MT, and Sepic, SB: Relationships Among Walking Performance, Postural Stability, and Functional Assessments of the Hemiplegic Patient. Am J Phys Med Rehabil 66:77, 1987.
44. Diener, HC, et al: Medium and Long Latency Responses to Displacement of the Ankle Joint in Patients with Spinal and Central Lesions. Electroencephalogr Clin Neurophysiol 60:407, 1985.
45. Jones, RD, Donaldson, IM, and Parkin, PJ: Impairment and Recovery of Ipsilateral Sensory-Motor Function Following Unilateral Cerebral Infarction. Brain 112:113, 1989.
46. Halaney, ME and Carey, JR: Tracking Ability of Hemiparetic and Healthy Subjects. Phys Ther 69:342, 1989.
47. Smutok, MA, et al: The Effects of Unilateral Brain Damage on Contralateral and Ipsilateral Upper Extremity Function in Hemiplegia. Phys Ther 69:195, 1989.
48. Springer, SP and Deutsch, G: Left Brain, Right Brain, rev ed. WH Freeman, New York, 1985.
49. Joynt, RJ, Benton, AL, and Fogel, ML: Behavioral and Pathological Correlates of Motor Impersistence. Neurology 12:876, 1962.
50. Kertesz, A, et al: Motor Impersistence: A Right Hemisphere Syndrome. Neurology 35:663, 1985.
51. Kimura, D and Archibald, Y: Motor Functions of the Left Hemisphere. Brain 97:22, 1974.
52. Robinson, LM: Laterality of Performance in Finger Tapping and Grip Strength by Hemisphere of Stroke and Gender. Arch Phys Med Rehabil 71:695, 1990.
53. Haaland, KY and Harrington, DL: Limb Sequencing Deficits After Left But Not Right Hemisphere Damage. Brain Cogn 24:104, 1994.
54. Kreuger, B and Okazaki, H: Vertebral-Basilar Distribution Infarction Following Chiropractic Cervical Manipulation. Mayo Clin Proc 55:322, 1980.
55. Robertson, J: Neck Manipulation as a Cause of Stroke. Stroke 12:1, 1981.
56. Kannel, WB, et al: Systolic Blood Pressure, Arterial Rigidity, and Risk of Stroke: The Framingham Study. JAMA 245:1225, 1981.
57. MacMahon, S: Blood Pressure, Stroke, and Coronary Heart Disease. Part 1. Lancet 335:765, 1990.
58. Wikstrand, J, Warnold, I, and Olsson, G: Primary Prevention with Metoprolol in Patients with Hypertension: Mortality Results from a MAPHY Study. JAMA 259:1976, 1988.
59. Goldner, MG, Knatterud, GL, and Prout, TE: Effects of Hypoglycemic Agents on Vascular Complications in Patients with Adult Onset Diabetes. JAMA 218:1400, 1971.
60. Higa, M, and Davanipour, Z: Smoking and Stroke. Neuroepidemiology 10:211, 1991.
61. Collaborative Group for the Study of Stroke in Young Women: Oral Contraceptives and Stroke in Young Women: Associated Risk Factors. JAMA 231:718, 1975.
62. Ostfeld, AM, et al: Epidemiology of Stroke in an Elderly Welfare Population. Am J Public Health 64:450, 1974.
63. Kannel, WB, Gordon, T, and Dawber, TR: Role of Lipids in the Development of Brain Infarction: The Framingham Study. Stroke 5:679, 1974.
64. Hillborn, M and Kaste, M: Alcohol Intoxication: A Risk Factor for Primary Subarachnoid Hemorrhage. Neurology 32:706, 1982.
65. Harrison, MJG, et al: Effect of Hematocrit on Carotid Stenosis and Cerebral Infarction. Lancet 2:114, 1981.
66. Duncan, PW, et al: Measurement of Motor Recovery After Stroke: Outcome Assessment and Sample Size Requirements. Stroke 23:1084, 1992.
67. Jongbloed, L: Prediction of Function After Stroke: A Critical Review. Stroke 17:765, 1986.
68. Lincoln, NB, et al: An Investigation of Factors Affecting the Progress of Patients on a Stroke Unit. J Neurol Neurosurg Psychiatry 52:493, 1989.

CHAPTER 22

■

Multiple Sclerosis and Other Disorders of Central Nervous System Myelin

Christopher M. Fredericks, PhD

- ■ *Normal Myelination*
- ■ *Classification of Diseases of Demyelination*
- ■ *Multiple Sclerosis*
- ■ *Closely Related Variants of Multiple Sclerosis*
- ■ *Acute Disseminated Encephalomyelitis*
- ■ *Demyelination Associated with Systemic Disease*
- ■ *Dysmyelinating Diseases*

Many of the nerve fibers of both the peripheral and central nervous system are covered by a protective sheath of fatty material, called **myelin.** This insulating covering makes possible the process of saltatory conduction and is necessary for normal impulse propagation in these nerve cells (see Chapter 1). **A variety of disorders exists in which this myelin sheath is abnormal, resulting in adverse changes in both the speed and quality of impulse conduction.** Abnormalities of myelin may occur with or without concurrent involvement of the axon or other cellular elements of the nervous system. **This chapter is specifically concerned with the demyelinating diseases of the central nervous system in which the primary pathologic defect is in the myelin itself.** The demyelinating peripheral neuropathies are discussed in Chapter 15.

Normal Myelination

Myelin is largely composed of phospholipids, long-chain fatty acids, cholesterol, and other lipids, as well as several proteins. Although the composition of myelin itself is essentially the same in the peripheral and central nervous systems, its origins and the manner in which it is produced differ.[1-4] As discussed in Chapters 1 and 15, in the peripheral nervous system the myelin sheath is deposited around each axon by Schwann cells. In the central nervous system, it is produced by oligodendrocytes (Fig. 22-1). In

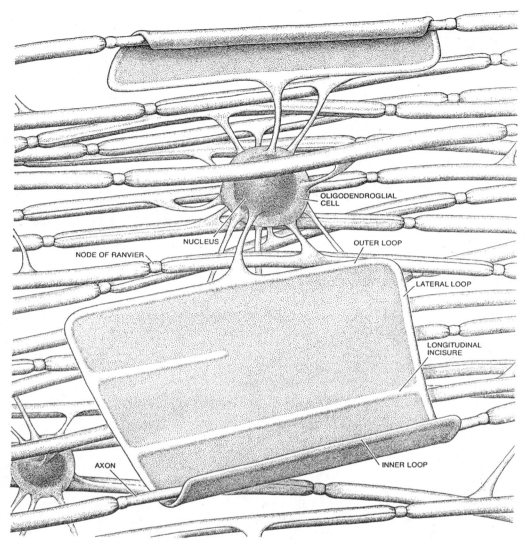

Figure 22–1. *Myelin Formation in the Central Nervous System.* Myelin sheaths in the brain or spinal cord are formed by oligodendrocytes that extend their surface membranes to provide segments of sheath for numerous axons. (From Morrell and Norton,[2] p 90, with permission.)

either case, the myelin sheath forms as a multilayered extrusion of the cell membrane of its cell of origin (i.e., Schwann cell or oligodendrocyte), which wraps around the axon in concentric, spiraling layers. The more layers, the thicker the myelin sheath. Although each Schwann cell in the peripheral nervous system provides the myelin sheath for only a single axon, within the central nervous system each oligodendrocyte provides the myelin for up to 20 or 30 axons. The thickness of the myelin coating in the periphery seems to be primarily determined by axon diameter, whereas that of the central nervous system is more variable and may be more related to the number of axons subserved by a single oligodendrocyte.

The most active synthesis of myelin begins in utero and continues for the first 2 years of life. Slower synthesis continues until the adult nervous system is fully formed. Both developing and mature myelin are susceptible to injury by disease.

Table 22-1. *Classification of Diseases Associated with Loss of Myelin*

Demyelinating Disorders (Damage or Destruction of Normal Myelin)
- Primary demyelinating diseases (idiopathic, presumably autoimmune)
    Multiple sclerosis and closely related disorders
    Acute disseminated encephalomyelitis (including postviral and postvaccinal)
- Demyelinating disorders associated with systemic disease (nutritional or immunologic deficiency)
- Demyelination associated with infection, toxic exposure, anoxia, or ischemia

Dysmyelinating Disorders (Failure to Form or Maintain Myelin)
- Leukodystrophies

Classification of Diseases of Demyelination

Many conditions are associated with central nervous system demyelination (Table 22–1).[5-12] The term *demyelinating disease,* however, is used to designate a relatively small, narrowly defined group of disorders. **All these disorders are characterized by extensive destruction of myelin sheaths in the central nervous system, along with evidence of an inflammatory response.** The demyelination characteristic of these disorders is accompanied by a relative sparing of the axons, nerve cells, and supporting cellular elements. With a few exceptions, no specific cause of these disorders has been determined, although autoimmunity or viral infection is suspected. **The demyelinating diseases make up a group of neurologic disorders that are important both because of the frequency of their occurrence and because of the severity of the disability that they may cause.**

Without a clear-cut understanding of the pathogenesis of the demyelinating diseases, a rigorous, defensible classification scheme is not possible. To some extent, the disorders termed the primary demyelinating diseases are defined by the exclusion of other disorders involving demyelination.[9-12] The **primary demyelinating diseases** are considered distinct from the genetic disorders of myelin formation (the dysmyelinating diseases) and from diseases in which myelin breakdown occurs as a consequence of dysfunction of neurons, blood vessels, or other components of the nervous system. Other conditions in which demyelination occurs as a consequence of certain known factors, such as malnutrition and exposure to toxins or opportunistic viral infections, are also excluded. In these conditions, the characteristic inflammatory response is lacking and demyelination is not the sole or predominant histologic abnormality. What remains are essentially two groups of demyelinating diseases: (1) multiple sclerosis and its closely related disorders and (2) acute disseminated encephalomyelitis. Although the pattern of myelin loss is considerably different in these two groups of disorders (irregular and patchy in the former and widely disseminated in the latter), central nervous system demyelination is the predominant, if not sole pathologic process in both. These two groups are also the most important clinically among the demyelinating diseases. **Of all the primary demyelinating diseases, multiple sclerosis is by far the most common** and is the primary focus of this chapter.

Multiple Sclerosis[5-19]

Although rare in the tropics, multiple sclerosis is the most common demyelinating disease in moderate climates and one of the more common diseases of the central nervous system in general. **In its most common form, multiple sclerosis is characterized by a course of recurring relapses and remissions, upon which is superimposed gradual neurologic deterioration.** In most patients, this disease follows a protracted course spread over several decades. Other forms of multiple sclerosis also occur with a more relentless course and

Table 22–2. *Common Initial Symptoms of Multiple Sclerosis*

Symptoms	Approximate Incidence (%)
Sensory symptoms	25–35
Paresthesias, numbness	
Visual loss	25–30
Central vision	
Muscle weakness	35–40
One or more limbs	
Brainstem and cerebellar symptoms	15–20
Ataxia	
Diplopia	
Vertigo, vomiting, nystagmus	

varying rates of progression. Onset of this disease is rare in childhood or old age, with most patients developing their first symptoms between 20 and 40 years of age. Multiple sclerosis is twice as common in women as in men.

In many of the disorders described in previous chapters in this book, pathologic changes were limited to a relatively circumscribed area of the nervous system, the result being that the associated clinical signs and symptoms arising from this pathology were relatively few and relatively uniform. Multiple sclerosis is not like this. **In this disease, almost any elements of the central nervous system, brain or spinal cord, can be involved, and multiple sclerosis is characterized by a constellation of signs and symptoms of almost unlimited variety.**

Onset and Initial Clinical Features[8,10,12,16–24]

It is perhaps simplest to describe the clinical features of multiple sclerosis by beginning with the onset and earliest stages of the disease, at which time the lesions (and hence the clinical manifestations) are fewest. In about 40% of patients, the initial occurrence of multiple sclerosis is monosymptomatic, even though many other signs and symptoms arise with its progression.

Patients with the classic form of multiple sclerosis usually present with focal neurologic signs and symptoms developing over a period of several days. Although the white matter in any area of the central nervous system may be affected, there are a number of favored sites and hence certain symptoms are more common initially than others (Table 22–2). **Common initial problems are unilateral visual disturbances (optic neuritis), sensory abnormalities, weakness of one or more extremities, and incoordination.** Visual loss can vary in degree from a slight loss in acuity to total blindness and is often associated with pain in or behind the eye. Sensory disturbances range from vague "pins and needles" or numbness in the trunk or limbs to the pain of classic trigeminal neuralgia (tic douloureux). Weakness most often affects the lower extremities and may produce a range of dysfunction from slight fatigue to paralysis. Incoordination as a result of cerebellar lesions or a loss of positional sense may occur independent of weakness and often leads to ataxia of the extremities and gait impairment.

Common Signs and Symptoms in Established Disease

The demyelinating lesions of multiple sclerosis can occur almost anywhere in the brain and spinal cord (Fig. 22–2). **Accordingly, the potential clinical manifestations of this disorder are innumerable** (Table 22–3).[8,10,12,16–24] These lesions, however, tend to be most numerous in the white matter of the cerebrum, brainstem, cerebellum, and spinal cord,

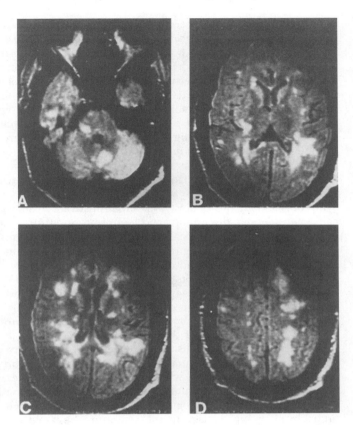

Figure 22–2. *MRI Scan of the Brain in Multiple Sclerosis.* Numerous periventricular, cerebellar, and brainstem lesions are evident as white areas on the MRI. (From Herndon, and Rudick,[10] p 14, with permission.)

Table 22–3. *Multiple Sclerosis: Common Sites of Pathology and Associated Neurologic Disturbances*

Optic Nerve

  Central loss of vision, often accompanied by pain associated with the eye (optic neuritis)
  Painless progressive loss of visual acuity

Brainstem

  Diplopia (III, IV, VI)
  Facial hypesthesia or trigeminal neuralgia (V)
  Bell's palsy or hemifacial spasm (VII)
  Vertigo, vomiting, nystagmus (VIII)

Cerebellum and Spinocerebellar Pathways

  Ataxia of speech, head, trunk, or limbs; abnormal stance and gait

Spinal Cord

  Upper motor neuron syndrome of weakness, spasticity, hyperreflexia, clonus, Babinski's sign
    (i.e., corticospinal tracts)
  Paresthesias or sensory loss (i.e., posterior columns)
  Abnormal or diminished pain and temperature sensation (i.e., lateral spinothalamic tracts)
  Urinary bladder and bowel dysfunction (i.e., autonomic tracts)

Cerebral Cortex

  Intellectual impairment and memory loss
  Emotional changes, especially depression

with a predilection for certain specific areas. This narrows somewhat the signs and symptoms most likely to occur over the course of the disease. The clinical features of any specific patient depend on both the location and the severity of these lesions.

In multiple sclerosis, **a clear predilection exists for the optic nerves and chiasms, creating an assortment of visual disturbances,** including blurred vision and abnormal visual fields. An acute optic neuritis in which patients suffer monocular loss of central vision, and eye-associated pain is common. A painless, more slowly progressing loss of visual acuity may also occur, particularly in older patients. **The corticospinal (pyramidal) tracts are frequently involved, producing a typical upper motor neuron syndrome of spastic muscle weakness, hyperreflexia, and Babinski's response.** Any or all of the extremities may be affected, with varying degrees of severity. **Lesions are also common in the spinal sensory tracts, especially the posterior columns, giving rise to paresthesias, numbness, and loss of proprioception.** Sensory symptoms in one or more extremities are common as early symptoms and are nearly always apparent in advanced stages of the disease. Paresthesias can cause considerable discomfort, and loss of proprioceptive feedback contributes to incoordination of movement. Pain is also common in multiple sclerosis, particularly in the back, hip, and legs. Although the origins of this pain are not well understood, it is in part related to muscle spasms, cramps, and gait disturbances.

The cerebellum and its connections with the brainstem are ultimately involved in most cases, causing nystagmus, dysarthria, ataxia, and considerable disability. Axial instability may cause severe gait disturbance. Appendicular ataxia may result in intention tremor, dysmetria, or dysrhythmias. **Disturbances of autonomic function frequently develop in the later stages of the disease.** Urinary bladder dysfunction is a primary cause of patient distress and social disability. As descending pathways are disrupted, a spastic bladder with incontinence and frequency or urgency of urination may develop. A spastic bowel may cause severe constipation, which is a source of considerable discomfort and morbidity. Sexual dysfunction is common in men in the form of impotence and loss of libido and has both physical and psychological origins. Finally, **neurobehavioral problems are common,** probably reflecting damage to the cerebrum. Impaired cognition and memory, as well as emotional changes (especially depression), are common.

Fatigue may be the most common single complaint in multiple sclerosis patients and is often disabling. However, because fatigability is difficult to describe and to objectively assess, it is often underemphasized in discussions of the signs and symptoms of multiple sclerosis. Nonetheless, fatigability is an early and frequent symptom of this disorder and in some cases may create significant disability.[21-23] In a study reported by Reingold[22] in 1990, for example, fatigue was listed as the most common symptom in 80% of cases and as the most serious symptom in 40% of cases. Simple tasks such as dressing may be exhausting to some patients, even in the presence of normal or near-normal muscle strength. The impaired performance produced by fatigue creates an additional burden for patients, because it is often misconstrued as laziness or malingering. The fatigability of multiple sclerosis takes various forms, including persistent fatigue, transient fatigue following modest physical exertion, and increased fatigue with elevated environmental temperature.

Fatigue may also be manifested as disturbed psychological or cognitive function. The etiology of this fatigue is poorly understood and, unlike many of the other signs and symptoms of multiple sclerosis, it is difficult to ascribe to pathologic lesions in specific regions of the central nervous system. Since most patients report an increase in fatigue before and during a flare-up, some component may relate to immune system abnormalities. In multiple sclerosis, as the pattern and severity of lesions change with the progression of the disease, old signs and symptoms tend to recur, new ones appear, and residual disability increases.

Course of the Disease

One of the characteristic features of multiple sclerosis is the extent to which the course of the disease varies among individuals and thus the degree to which it is unpredictable in any particular individual. **The course of multiple sclerosis varies markedly in the frequency**

Table 22-4. Temporal Patterns of Multiple Sclerosis

Benign (20%–30%)	A few, mild early exacerbations followed by complete or nearly complete recovery; little residual disability
Relapsing/remitting (50%–60%)	More frequent exacerbations followed by less complete recovery than in the benign form
Stable	Long periods of quiescence between exacerbations with some disability
Progressive	Fewer remissions as the disease progresses, with more cumulative disability
Chronic/progressive (15%–20%)	Insidious relatively late onset and steady progression of symptoms and disability; few significant remissions
Acute/progressive (<5%)	Acute onset with rapid deterioration leading to severe impairment and often early death

and severity of attacks, the extent to which recovery is made from these attacks, and the progression of disability (Table 22–4).[10,17,18,20–24] Whether or not a particular person will improve or deteriorate, and to what extent, is as unpredictable as where and when more lesions will appear.

Most patients with multiple sclerosis experience a disease pattern characterized by a long series of relapses and remissions. This pattern is particularly common among those manifesting the disease prior to age 40. The initial neurologic signs and symptoms develop over a period of a few days. Typically, these symptoms improve spontaneously in a matter of days and are followed months or years later by an attack of new signs and symptoms. Improvement following the initial attack ranges from slight to a total disappearance of any evidence of neurologic dysfunction. Although there may be long periods of clinical stability, the disease advances as a series of attacks, each resolving but tending to leave some residual deficit. The cumulative effect of these deficits is growing disability. After a number of years of exacerbations and remissions, there is an increasing tendency for the patient to enter a phase of slow, progressive deterioration of neurologic function, attributable to the cumulative effect of increasing numbers of lesions.

About 20% of all patients with multiple sclerosis experience a chronically progressive course of accumulating disability in which significant remissions do not occur. This type of pattern most often begins insidiously with slowly progressing symptoms and occurs most often in patients with an onset later in life (40 to 60 years old) than is typical for relapsing-remitting multiple sclerosis (20 or 40 years old).

Occasionally, multiple sclerosis occurs in a highly malignant form, in which a combination of cerebral, brainstem, and spinal manifestations evolve quickly. Rapid deterioration occurs and severe impairment or death may ensue within a few weeks to months. This form of the disease is most common in relatively young patients and is often preceded by a febrile illness. Occasionally, an acute fulminating attack like this may occur as the terminal event late in a more classic case of multiple sclerosis. The pathologic lesions found in these patients are similar to the acute plaques of multiple sclerosis, differing only in the fact that they have all occurred at about the same time.

About 20% to 30% of patients experience multiple sclerosis as a relatively benign disorder. These individuals may have one or two minor episodes of abnormal vision, paresthesia, or weakness, only to recover completely with no subsequent clinical evidence of the disease. Postmortem studies have revealed the presence of scattered demyelinated lesions in patients showing no clinical evidence of multiple sclerosis in life, suggesting that even a greater percentage of those with the disease may experience a benign or subclinical course.

As multiple sclerosis progresses temporally, the distribution of the symptoms may coalesce into one of several neuroanatomic patterns.[8,10,11] About 50% of patients present a classic picture of widespread, generalized involvement of the optic nerves, oculomotor systems, pyramidal tracts, cerebellum, and posterior columns, producing a variety of clinical manifestations including ocular disturbances, spastic weakness, ataxia, and sensory symptoms. Other patients may exhibit primarily signs and symptoms of spinal cord involvement (myelopathy) with varying degrees of spastic weakness, ataxia, abnormal tendon reflexes in the extremities, and bladder dysfunction. Less common patterns are a predominantly cerebellar or brainstem-cerebellar form, characterized by axial, appendicular, and oculomotor cerebellar symptoms, and an optic neuritis (amaurotic form), characterized by progressive visual loss without other manifestations. In some patients, progressive cognitive impairment is an early and predominant characteristic.

Overall, the clinical course of multiple sclerosis is remarkably variable and unpredictable, and any individual may experience considerable overlap of the clinical patterns just described. In most individuals, the severity of the disease is intermediate, with the disease characterized by fluctuating and varied symptoms, a wide range of disability, and a course spanning decades. The average interval from clinical onset to death is 30 to 35 years. In about 50% of patients in whom the cause of death is known, death is directly attributable to the complications of multiple sclerosis. In the final stages of this disease, most patients are wheelchair-bound or bedridden, with infections and the many complications of immobility (see Chapters 23 and 24).[25,26] Death is usually due to respiratory failure or pneumonia, pulmonary embolism, or bacterial sepsis arising from infection of the urinary tract or decubiti. Other causes of death are suicide, cancer, acute myocardial infarction, and stroke. It is a source of great concern that the proportion of suicides among multiple sclerosis deaths is many times more than that for the age-matched general population.

Risk Factors and Prognosis[10,16,20,24,28–31]

One of the most troubling aspects of multiple sclerosis is the inability to predict who will acquire this disease and what the course and severity of this disease will be. Although hundreds of studies have been undertaken in an effort to define factors that might precipitate the onset or influence the course of this disorder, few consistent indicators of real prognostic value have been identified.[29–31] This failure is partly due to our lack of understanding of the pathogenesis of the disorder and our almost total reliance on retrospective epidemiologic studies, many of which have significant methodologic flaws.[27]

A few factors have been identified that are associated with an increased probability of acquiring multiple sclerosis.[10,16,20,24,28–31] Gender is a factor, since females are more than twice as likely as males to be afflicted. Age is also an influence, with multiple sclerosis developing most often at about 30 years of age, while seldom appearing prior to puberty or after 60 years of age. Geographic and ethnic factors also influence its occurrence, with its prevalence varying significantly among locations and ethnic groups. Kinship may also create an element of risk, which is greatest between monozygotic twins.

Numerous attempts have been made to define specific factors that might precipitate the onset of the disease, with particular attention focused on prior viral infection, dietary factors (e.g., high fat), socioeconomic conditions, and trauma to the brain or spinal cord. The results of these studies are contradictory, and it has not been possible to unequivocally link any prior event or condition with the onset of multiple sclerosis.[20,24,28–31]

Considering the enormous variability of the clinical course of multiple sclerosis, **innumerable attempts have been made to identify early predictors of the course of this disease.**[10,16,20,24,28–31] Recognition of these factors has implications for both the treatment of this disorder and for our understanding of its causes. Moreover, the uncertainty surrounding its prognosis creates a tremendous psychological burden for many patients. When the outcome of the disease is defined in terms of the resultant disability, **certain demographic and disease-related features appear to be associated with a more favorable prognosis.** An acute onset of the disease, female gender, young age at onset, a high degree of remission after the first attack, an initial presentation limited to optic neuritis or other sensory symptoms, and an initial involvement of only one region of the nervous system all are associated with a favorable long-term outlook. The poorest prognosis is suggested by a high age at onset (i.e., >35 years of age), early cerebellar or lower brainstem symptoms, and a chronically progressive course (unremitting). No specific prior illness, surgery, trauma, or known environmental or socioeconomic factor has been shown conclusively to affect the course of multiple sclerosis. Pregnancy, which was once thought to strongly influence this disease, does not influence the prognosis, regardless of whether it occurs before or after the onset of multiple sclerosis.

With respect to survival itself, multiple sclerosis is a relatively benign disorder. Many patients have near-normal life spans, with the average interval from clinical onset to death being 25 to 35 years in many studies. Data suggest that survival is negatively influenced by male gender, an advanced level of disability in the initial stage, and an older age at onset.[20,25]

It is important to remember that all the predictors of multiple sclerosis are derived from statistical correlations developed from the study of large groups of patients. **It is still impossible to provide any individual patient with an accurate prognosis.**

Pathologic Findings

Although the pathogenesis of multiple sclerosis is poorly understood, the typical pathologic features accompanying this disorder have been well described.[9–12,17,32] **Multiple sclerosis, as the name might suggest, is characterized by numerous demyelinated lesions, called *plaques*, which are scattered throughout the central nervous system.** Although these plaques may be found anywhere in the white matter of the brain, they are most often found in the periventricular regions of both cerebral hemispheres (Fig. 22–3). The optic nerves, brainstem, and spinal cord (especially cervical) may also be severely affected, and in some

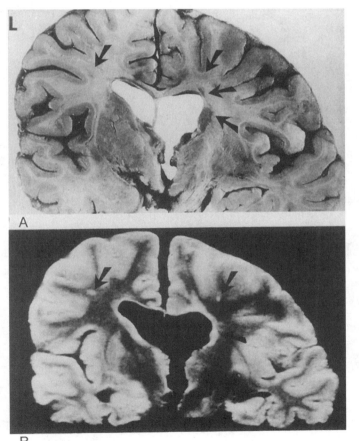

Figure 22–3. Demyelinating Lesions in Multiple Sclerosis. (*A*) Distinct, discolored lesions (*Arrows*) are evident in an unstained, fixed brain slice. In (*B*), an MRI scan of (*A*) visualizes these same subcortical and periventricular lesions as small pale areas. (From Allen and Kirk,[9] p. 490, with permission.)

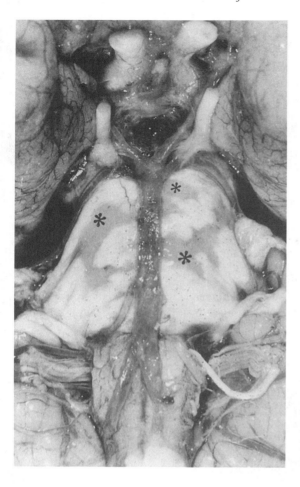

Figure 22–4. *Demyelinating Lesions in Multiple Sclerosis.* Large discolored lesions (*) are evident on the surface of the pons of a 40-year-old man with an 11-year history of multiple sclerosis. The leptomeninges have been removed. (Allen and Kirk,[9] p 464, with permission.)

patients these sites may be far more involved than the hemispheres (Fig. 22–4). The plaques seem to follow the venous drainage of the brain and spinal cord. The peripheral nervous system is not affected. No particular part of the central nervous system is exempt, and the distribution of plaques varies considerably from case to case.

The gross appearance of the external surface of most of the brain in multiple sclerosis is usually normal, although irregular, distinct plaques may be observed on the surface of the optic nerves, brainstem, and spinal cord (see Fig. 22–4).[9–12,32] Unstained sections of the brain and spinal cord, reveal numerous small, irregular areas of pinkish-gray discoloration, which are scattered throughout the white matter (see Fig. 22–3). Sections of the central nervous system that have been stained, making myelin darker in color, show a depletion of myelin in the areas that were discolored in the unstained specimens. The plaques are readily visualized by computed tomography (CT scans) and magnetic resonance imaging (MRI) techniques (see Figs. 22–2 and 22–3). Although the increased signal density that makes these lesions so evident with MRI is probably related more to the presence of inflammation, edema, and an increased local water content than to demyelination, these imaging techniques are powerful clinical tools. In fact, these techniques (especially MRI) have created a remarkable capability for both diagnosing this disorder and following its progression. This ability has profound implications for our understanding of the clinical significance of these lesions, as well as for monitoring treatment outcomes.

The lesions in the cerebral hemispheres vary in size from a few millimeters to many centimeters across (see Figs. 22–2 and 22–3). Large plaques form by the growth and

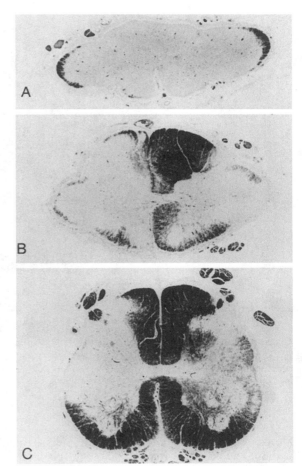

Figure 22–5. *Spinal Cord Involvement in Multiple Sclerosis.* In most cases of multiple sclerosis, evidence of spinal cord involvement can be found, particularly in the cervical cord. These sections from different levels of the cord (*A,* cervical/thoracic; *B,* midthoracic; *C,* lumbar) in which myelin is darkly stained demonstrate regions of varying degrees of demyelination as large pale areas. Note the almost total loss of myelin in *A,* the large lesions in *B,* and the disseminated involvement in *C.* (From Raine,[11] p 550, Copyright © Williams & Wilkins, with permission.)

coalescence of smaller ones. Although the lesions typically occur in the midst of the heavily myelinated white matter, a significant proportion occurs at the junction of white and gray matter and may extend into the gray matter. In the spinal cord, lesions vary from small defects to an almost complete loss of myelin in the entire cross section of the cord (Fig. 22–5).

Microscopic examination of the lesions shows areas of circumscribed demyelination with relatively well-preserved axons, gliosis (scarring), and varying degrees of inflammation. The specific histologic appearance of a lesion depends on its age.[8,9,11,32] In this regard, plaques range from relatively recent lesions rich in inflammatory infiltrates and macrophages loaded with lipid and other myelin degeneration products to long-standing, inactive lesions associated with thick acellular fibroglial tissue (scars) with few lymphocytes and macrophages. Although the associated axons tend to be preserved, the extent of axonal loss in the demyelinated areas is variable, with some loss occurring in almost all lesions. In the chronic stages of the disease, significant axonal loss occurs and evidence of wallerian degeneration is seen, for example, in long tracts of the spinal cord.[9,11] In the center of a plaque, oligodendrocytes may be diminished or lost, which may explain the limited regeneration of myelin in multiple sclerosis.

The correlation of anatomically established lesions with clinical symptomatology is not always possible.[9,33–36] Serial MRI scans have shown that specific lesions may rapidly appear and disappear, often without apparent clinical consequences (Fig. 22–6). Although MRI shows that new symptoms lasting more than 24 to 48 hours are usually associated with one or more new lesions or enlargement of old lesions, this is not always the case.[17]

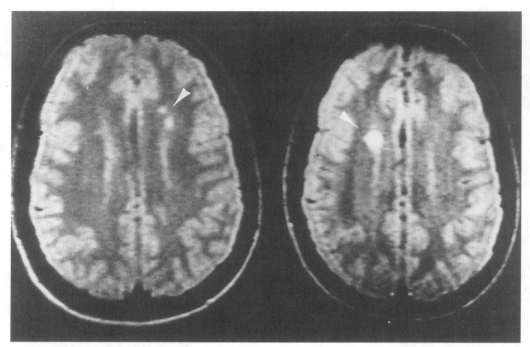

Figure 22–6. ***Evolution of Multiple Sclerosis Lesions.*** Individual lesions visualized by MRI can often be seen to come and go over a matter of a few weeks or months. In these two MRI scans, a new white matter lesion (*Arrow*) has appeared 8 months after an acute attack of optic neuritis without any clinical change; two lesions (*Arrow*) in the left hemisphere on the earlier scan have disappeared. (From Kesselring, J, et al: Magnetic Resonance Imaging in Multiple Sclerosis. Copyright © Thieme Medical Publishers, Inc., New York, 1989, p 21, with permission.)

Moreover, in patients with stable multiple sclerosis, new lesions may often appear on MRI without any change in symptomatology. It is interesting that the number of plaques found at autopsy is invariably greater than that expected on the basis of history and physical signs. Therefore, numerous plaques are probably clinically silent or possibly bear some relationship to aspects of the disease that are poorly understood, such as emotional or cognitive disturbances. Occasionally, typical plaques are found in a totally asymptomatic person (Fig. 22–7). Lesions on MRI similar to those of multiple sclerosis may also be seen in a variety of other encephalopathies, as well as in aging patients with no other apparent disease.

Exactly how the demyelinated lesions (plaques) disrupt neuronal activity and create functional deficits is not completely understood. Ultimately, functional loss is due to distortion or blockade of impulse traffic. However, it is not entirely clear which specific features of these lesions actually interfere with impulse transmission. Demyelination can slow or distort conduction, preventing nerve fibers from faithfully transmitting long trains of impulses, or it can prevent transmission altogether—either of which may account for many of the clinical deficits.[16] However, some symptoms in multiple sclerosis may reverse so quickly that remyelination of the involved pathways cannot have taken place. This suggests the involvement of other factors in the acute lesions of this disorder. In this regard, some evidence suggests that the inflammatory process itself may contribute to transient conduction block.[16] The functional effects of chronic lesions and the persistent deficits that they produce are also complex. In chronic lesions, remyelination is progressively less complete, demyelination is more widespread and persistent, and entire axons are lost. Compensation becomes less effective as more of the nerve fibers subserving a particular function disappear. In addition, like the infarcts caused by stroke or trauma, persistent multiple sclerosis lesions may produce deleterious changes in remote parts of the brain.[16] Reduced cerebral blood flow and oxygen utilization have also been reported in chronic multiple sclerosis and may contribute to neuronal dysfunction.

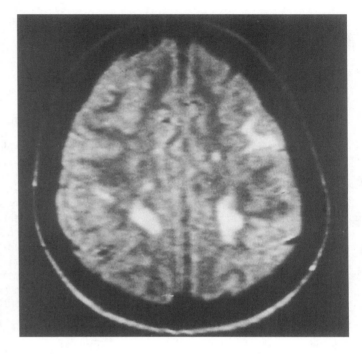

Figure 22–7. MRI Scan of the Brain in Multiple Sclerosis. Multiple lesions are evident as white areas in the cerebral hemispheres of a 34-year-old woman with definite multiple sclerosis who was asymptomatic at the time of the scan. (Reprinted with permission from Kesselring, J et al: Magnetic Resonance Imaging in Multiple Sclerosis, p 21, 1989. Copyright © Thieme Medical Publishers Inc.)

Etiology and Pathogenesis[8,9,12,16,17,37–44]

Although multiple sclerosis may be one of the most extensively studied of all neurologic disorders, its pathogenesis remains poorly understood. Until relatively recently, hypotheses formulated to explain the etiology of multiple sclerosis tended to focus on a single causative agent (e.g., a virus). This perspective has given way to the realization that **multiple factors are probably involved in the pathogenesis of multiple sclerosis.**[37–39,44] It is now widely believed that, although multiple sclerosis is fundamentally an abnormal immune-related process, this process is strongly influenced by both genetic and environmental factors.

Considerable evidence suggests that abnormal immunologic activity is a fundamental component of multiple sclerosis.[7,10,12,16,40,41] Pathologic studies show that the demyelination occurring in this disease occurs in the presence of an active immune response and is associated with infiltration by immunocompetent cells, including T and B lymphocytes and macrophages.[9,11,16,32] There is also a striking similarity between the lesions of multiple sclerosis and those of certain autoimmune disorders in humans (e.g., postvaccinal encephalomyelitis) and autoimmune models established in various animals (e.g., experimental allergic encephalomyelitis). Patients with multiple sclerosis demonstrate a wide array of immunologic abnormalities of both cell-mediated and humoral systems. The most common abnormalities are the presence of excessive numbers of inflammatory cells and elevated levels of IgG in the cerebrospinal fluid. The latter are produced by lymphocytes within the central nervous system. Impaired immunoregulatory mechanisms are further indicated by an abnormal distribution of lymphocyte phenotypes (e.g., fewer suppressor lymphocytes) and abnormal lymphocyte function.[16,40,41] Clearly, the immune system is abnormal in patients with multiple sclerosis. Relatively little is known, however, about what causes this dysfunction, the antigen(s) to which it is directed, or precisely how this derangement causes central nervous system lesions to form.

The specific factors that "trigger" the abnormal immunologic activity are not known. It is widely believed, however, that among these triggers are certain environmental factors.[37] In this regard, considerable evidence suggests that **multiple sclerosis may have infective origins, with several common viruses being the most likely causative agents.**[9,10,12,41]

Epidemiologic studies, which have established the geographic distribution of multiple sclerosis, strongly implicate environmental factors.[27,28,37,38] This is particularly true of migration studies. Migration to a low-risk area before the age of 15 decreases the risk of developing multiple sclerosis. Migration after that age, however, does not produce any change in risk. This suggests that some exogenous factor operates during adolescence, which permanently alters the susceptibility to this disease. Disease clusters and "epidemics" also provide evidence of environmental influences.

Considerable evidence suggests that microbial agents may be the environmental factors specifically involved, with several common viruses being the most likely culprits.[16,40,41] The serum and cerebrospinal fluid from patients with multiple sclerosis, for example, have high titers of antibodies to common viruses (e.g., measles, rubella, and herpes simplex), and there is evidence of viral antibody synthesis within the central nervous system. Abnormalities also exist in the way patients respond to various viruses, and evidence is accumulating that these abnormalities may be related to prior viral infection and possibly to viral persistence. In fact, recent studies suggest the persistence of viral genetic material in some patients. Experimental animal models indicate that viruses can induce demyelination, either by direct effects on the oligodendrocytes or by a variety of immune-mediated mechanisms. Although most studies have failed to isolate actual viruses from the tissues of established cases of multiple sclerosis, there are many mechanisms by which viruses may have long-lasting effects on the immune system without their actual persistence within the tissues. These and many other observations suggest that the specific cause of the immune abnormalities observed in multiple sclerosis may be prior viral infection.

Several lines of evidence have established that genetic factors are also important in the etiology of multiple sclerosis.[10,12,38,39,42-46] First, epidemiologic studies of the incidence and prevalence of this disease have revealed significant differences in susceptibility among racial and ethnic groups.[27,28,38,39] For example, multiple sclerosis is more common among Caucasians than any other ethnic group living within the same geographic area. It is least common among people of African and Asian origins. Second, studies of its incidence in families confirm an increased incidence of multiple sclerosis among the immediate relatives of patients with this disease.[42-46] The strongest evidence for this link comes from studies of disease concordance between twins. Twin studies have shown that the risk of developing multiple sclerosis for a patient's monozygotic (identical) twin is more than 500 times that of the normal population, and for a dizygotic twin, it is almost 300 times normal.[41] Third, certain findings suggest that multiple sclerosis is associated with certain specific genetic markers. In particular, an association has been found with certain classes of histocompatibility (HLA) genes.[42] One or more genetic factors are clearly involved in the pathogenesis of multiple sclerosis, most likely predisposing individuals to the effects of factors triggering this disease.

It is likely that many factors, both genetic and environmental, interact to produce multiple sclerosis. An interesting hypothesis that reconciles much of what is known about multiple sclerosis has been proposed by Poser.[47] He suggests that multiple sclerosis is acquired as a systemic trait characterized by hyperactive immunoresponsiveness. This trait is acquired by individuals who are genetically susceptible and develops as a result of an antigenic challenge posed by a viral protein, either in the context of a viral infection or a vaccination. This immune hyperactivity does not initially involve the central nervous system but does so when the integrity of the blood-brain barrier is somehow disrupted (e.g., by another viral infection or trauma). As a result, the multiple sclerosis lesion, which consists of edema and inflammation, occurs. This focus of inflammatory activity may or may not lead to demyelination and the neurologic consequences that follow.

Treatment

The treatment of multiple sclerosis, like the disorder, is complex and full of controversy.[12,16,48-55] For the sake of discussion, **a distinction is often made between measures designed to affect the course of the underlying disease and those concerned** primarily with symptomatic relief or rehabilitation. This is an arbitrary distinction, however, with considerable overlap between the two. The status of the disease is judged primarily by its symptoms, and many forms of symptomatic treatment may influence the underlying disease process.

To date, **no treatment has been developed that significantly modifies the progression of multiple sclerosis.**[48–55] This is due in part to our lack of understanding of its cause or causes. Moreover, the therapeutic trials required in the search for such an agent are made extremely difficult because of the unpredictability and variability of the course of multiple sclerosis.

Based on the premise that multiple sclerosis is mediated by an abnormal immune response, many forms of immunotherapy have been tried. Common approaches have included suppression of autoimmunity (e.g., immunosuppressive drugs, total lymphoid irradiation, and thymectomy), removal of circulating antibodies or immune complexes (e.g., plasma exchange), desensitization to myelin-related antigens, and stimulation of immuno-responsivity (e.g., interferon).[51–55] Unfortunately, none of these treatments has been shown to predictably slow the course of the disease or to be of sufficient clinical benefit to justify their routine usage. Except for the use of adrenocorticotropic hormone and corticosteroids in acute exacerbations, current use of immunosuppressive agents is largely limited to clinical trials.[51–55]

Symptomatic treatment and rehabilitative measures for patients with multiple sclerosis have proved to be the most effective.[52,56,57] Symptomatic relief is of great importance in the management of multiple sclerosis and is focused on ameliorating spasticity, intention tremor, urinary, bowel and sexual dysfunction, pain, fatigue, cognitive disturbances, and psychological disorders, all of which may contribute to the development of disability and discomfort. Although rehabilitative therapy cannot alter the course of the disease, it is continually necessary to maintain mobility and to counteract the many detrimental effects of inactivity (see Figs. 12–7 and 24–10). Optimal care for these patients requires a multidisciplinary approach that uses physical, occupational, speech, and recreational therapy.[56,57] Physical and occupational therapy become particularly important after a severe relapse or when important functional activities such as walking or standing are threatened.[16,50]

Long-term comprehensive management must also include adequate psychosocial services in support of patient vocational, financial, and familial responsibilities. These aspects of patient life are often neglected with the emphasis on medical management.

Closely Related Variants of Multiple Sclerosis

In addition to the more typical forms of multiple sclerosis previously described, several rarer variants have been recognized and merit some discussion. Most of these conditions involve an acute onset in children or young adults, a rapidly progressive course, and a poor prognosis.

Devic's Disease (Neuromyelitis Optica)[8–11,18,32,58]

Devic's disease is characterized by a sudden onset of bilateral optic neuritis, followed or preceded within days or weeks by manifestations of a transverse myelitis. Both eyes are affected with central loss of vision or, in severe cases, total blindness. The spinal cord lesions lead to the usual symptoms of transverse myelitis, with paraplegia, loss of all or some forms of sensation, and loss of bowel and bladder control. Neuromyelitis optica frequently occurs in children or young adults as a single episode. In about 50% of cases, death ensues within months, although in some cases there is partial or total recovery. Although the combination of visual loss with paraplegia is not unusual in chronic multiple sclerosis, these symptoms would most likely be accompanied by more generalized involvement of the central nervous system. Although the histologic appearance of the lesions in Devic's disease is similar to that of the lesions of multiple sclerosis, this disorder is characterized by more extensive involvement of the optic nerves, chiasm, and spinal cord. Although Devic's disease is usually a form of multiple sclerosis, it may also be caused by other diseases of myelin (e.g., encephalomyelitis) and by systemic disorders such as lupus erythematosus.

Schilder's Disease (Schilder's Diffuse Cerebral Sclerosis)[8-10,17,18,32]

If the hereditary leukodystrophies and various other childhood disorders of the cerebral white matter are excluded, a fairly distinct group of cases remains that probably represents a single variant of multiple sclerosis.[58] These are identified by the designation, Schilder's disease. All these conditions are nonfamilial and are most common in children or young adults in whom they produce severe neurologic deficits, including progressive motor, visual, and mental deterioration. Death occurs in most patients within a few months or years. Necropsy typically reveals a large demyelinating lesion involving much of one or both cerebral hemispheres as well as smaller, discrete lesions (reminiscent of multiple sclerosis) in the optic nerves, brainstem, and spinal cord (Fig. 22–8). Histologically, the large single lesion, as well as the smaller widely disseminated lesions, resemble those of multiple sclerosis.

Baló's Concentric Sclerosis[8,9,11,58,59]

Baló's sclerosis is an extremely rare form of multiple sclerosis, with an acute onset, usually occurring in young adults, and a rapid course of progressive neurologic deterioration. Motor symptoms are prominent. This disease is unremitting, with few patients surviving more than 5 years. The distinctive pathologic feature of Baló's sclerosis is the presence of concentric, alternating zones of myelinated and demyelinated tissue visible in the white matter of the cerebral hemispheres. Baló's sclerosis may be a variety of Schilder's disease, which it resembles clinically and in the cerebral distribution of its lesions.

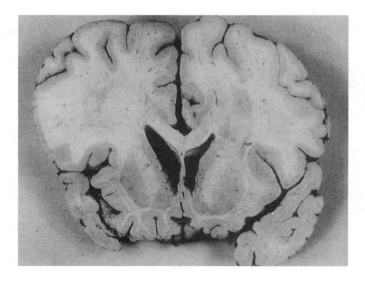

Figure 22–8. Multiple Sclerosis: Schilder Type. In this brain slice in which myelin is darkly stained, widespread, confluent, pale areas of demyelination are evident involving both cerebral hemispheres asymmetrically. (From Allen and Kirk,[9] p 487, with permission.)

Acute Disseminated Encephalomyelitis

The term *acute disseminated encephalomyelitis* (ADEM) **and a number of interrelated synonyms** (postinfectious encephalomyelitis, postvaccinal encephalomyelitis, acute demyelinating encephalomyelitis, perivenous encephalitis) **are used to designate a group of conditions that are characterized by central nervous system demyelination and share many of the pathologic and clinical features of multiple sclerosis.**[8-12,60] Although definition of the ADEM disorders is somewhat confused by the large assortment of names used to describe them, they share certain basic clinical and pathologic features, and probably are fundamentally the same pathologic entity. **ADEM, like multiple sclerosis, is distinguished pathologically by numerous regions of** perivenous inflammation and demyelination scattered throughout both the brain and spinal cord (Fig. 22–9).[9,11] The lesions of ADEM are histologically very similar to the newly formed lesions of multiple sclerosis. The lesions of ADEM are also indistinguishable from those of multiple sclerosis in their appearance on MRI, but they may be somewhat more symmetric and diffuse in their pattern of distribution.[60]

Patients with **ADEM present with signs and symptoms indicative of widespread central nervous system disturbance.**[8-12] These include headache, fever, stiffness, and other signs of meningeal irritation; paralysis, areflexia, and other manifestations of spinal cord involvement; confusion, stupor, and coma indicative of cerebral dysfunction; and nystagmus, ocular palsies, and pupillary changes indicative of brainstem involvement. Some patients experience only mild symptoms lasting a few weeks, whereas others have an explosive course proceeding to coma and death within 2 or 3 days. Typically, ADEM progresses for days to weeks after onset; the patient then stabilizes and gradually recovers. Mortality rate may be as high as 20%, with significant residual neurologic and intellectual impairment in survivors.

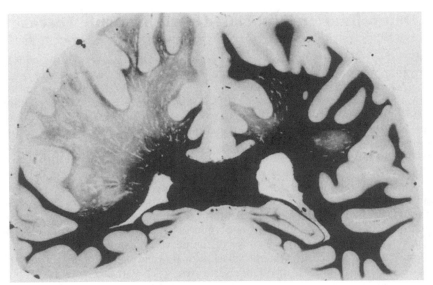

Figure 22–9. *Acute Disseminated Encephalomyelitis (ADEM).* In this section through the parietal lobes in which myelin is darkly stained, the widespread (pale) areas of demyelination characteristic of ADEM are apparent. This fatal disease developed in a middle-aged woman following a flulike illness. (From Okazaki, H: Fundamentals of Neuropathology: Morphological Basis of Neurological Disorders, ed 2. Igaku-Shoin, New York, p 150, with permission.)

The ADEM syndromes are distinguished from multiple sclerosis largely on clinical grounds. ADEM is usually a monophasic illness and typically involves presentations such as fever, headache, stiff neck, and altered consciousness, which are only rarely seen in multiple sclerosis. Moreover, ADEM occurs predominantly in children and is characteristically preceded or accompanied by a viral illness or inoculation.

Within the ADEM group, several more specific syndromes may be identified, with their own particular features.[8-12] Postinfectious encephalomyelitis is a syndrome that appears shortly after certain viral infections. This disorder is seen most frequently following measles infection, but is also occasionally observed after chickenpox, rubella, and smallpox. Symptoms typically develop 2 to 4 days after the appearance of the rash associated with these infections. Postinfectious encephalomyelitis is increasingly uncommon, probably because of the increased use of the measles vaccine. Postvaccinal encephalomyelitis is a similar condition, which may follow within 1 or 2 weeks of inoculation with certain types of vaccines, especially the rabies vaccine. With improved vaccines, postvaccinal encephalomyelitis is now rare. The mortality rate for postvaccinal encephalomyelitis is high (30% to 50%). Most patients who survive show residual neurologic and intellectual impairment. Acute hemorrhagic encephalitis is a particularly fulminant form of ADEM, which tends to occur within 1 to 2 weeks of an upper respiratory tract infection (possibly viral). Autopsy reveals extensive hemorrhage and necrosis of the white matter in the cerebrum, cerebellum, and spinal cord. This condition is typified by an abrupt onset of headache, fever, motor and sensory disturbances, and decreasing consciousness rapidly progressing to stupor and coma. Most patients die within a few days of onset of symptoms. Unlike postviral and postvaccinal encephalomyelitis, acute hemorrhagic encephalitis occurs primarily in young adults and is rarely seen in children.

The pathogenesis of ADEM is poorly understood, although an autoimmune etiology is suggested. In spite of the fact that a direct viral infection of the central nervous system has not been demonstrated, a virus may play a role by altering host antigenicity or by provoking a host antibody response against central nervous system antigens.

Demyelination Associated with Systemic Disease

There are a number of disorders unrelated to multiple sclerosis in which central nervous system demyelination is a prominent feature and which are usually not included among the primary demyelinating disorders.[9,11,12] Although these conditions are characterized by prominent demyelinating lesions with appreciable axonal sparing, pathologically they generally lack the perivenous distribution of lesions and the associated inflammation typical of multiple sclerosis. Clinically, these demyelination disorders are distinct from multiple sclerosis in the age at onset, the course of the disease, and the presence of various peripheral features associated with the other disease processes. Unlike multiple sclerosis and closely related disorders in which causes remain obscure, these disorders arise in the presence of obvious systemic disease. Demyelination disorders are found in association with various infectious, nutritional, and metabolic conditions (Table 22–5).

Without going into much detail, it might be useful to consider several examples of demyelination disorders associated with systemic disease. **Progressive multifocal leukoencephalopathy** is a rare progressive disorder of the nervous system, which usually occurs in adults immunocompromised by systemic disease or its treatment and which may be due to an opportunistic viral infection of oligodendrocytes.[9,11,12] Pathologically, this condition is characterized by diffuse, asymmetric involvement of the cerebral hemispheres. Varied neurologic signs and symptoms rapidly develop and progress, terminating in death within 3 to 6 months of onset. **Central pontine myelosis**, which may be the most common of these disorders, is associated with alcoholism and the accompanying malnutrition, as well as a number of other chronic systemic disorders and neoplasia.[9,61,62] As the name suggests, the demyelinating lesions of this disorder are found primarily within the pons, although the

**Table 22–5. Demyelinating Disorders
Associated with Systemic Disease**

Viral
    Progressive multifocal leukoencephalopathy
Nutritional/metabolic
    Central pontine myelosis
    Marchiafava-Bignami disease
    Pernicious anemia (vitamin B_{12} deficiency)
Anoxic/ischemic
    Delayed anoxic encephalopathy
    Progressive subcortical ischemic encephalopathy
    Carbon monoxide intoxication (anemic anoxia)

white matter of other parts of the brain may be affected (i.e., cerebrum and tegmentum). Central pontine myelosis is typified by rapidly progressing corticospinal and corticobulbar dysfunction expressed as flaccid tetraplegia and bulbar paralysis. Death ensues within days or weeks of onset. **Marchiafava-Bignami disease** is an exceedingly rare disorder character-ized by well-defined lesions of the corpus callosum.[9,61,63] This condition is also associated with alcoholism, although this association is not invariable. Nonspecific mental changes are the most common presentation. In **pernicious anemia** caused by vitamin B_{12} deficiency, demyelination of the peripheral nervous system may be accompanied by demyelination of spinal cord large fiber tracts, optic nerves, and deep cerebral white matter. These lesions give rise to various neurologic presentations, which often fail to improve with treatment of the underlying vitamin deficiency. Finally, certain conditions causing **generalized or focal brain anoxia** (or ischemia) may lead to selective destruction of myelin.

Dysmyelinating Diseases

In contrast to the demyelinating diseases previously described, in which myelin is formed normally and then damaged or destroyed by some acquired mechanism, **the dysmyelinating diseases are genetic disorders in which the formation of myelin is abnormal.**[5,6,64–68] Dysmyelinating diseases also differ to the extent that to a varying degree the axons themselves are involved in the disease process, and there is a significant loss in the number of oligodendrocytes. Dysmyelination is a somewhat nonspecific designation and encompasses improperly constituted myelin, slowed or arrested myelin formation, or failure of myelin maintenance.[5,6]

Although dysmyelination has been shown to be associated with a variety of disturbances in lipid and amino acid metabolism, in most cases the underlying metabolic deficiency is unknown.[64–68] With few exceptions, these diseases are familial and are frequently associated with other genetically determined conditions. The dysmyelinating diseases are characterized by widespread symmetric involvement of myelin of the white matter in both the cerebrum and cerebellum and occasionally of the peripheral nerves. The extent to which myelin is affected varies, and preferential involvement of certain specific tracts has been noted. The dysmyelinating diseases have been largely classified according to neuropathologic criteria. Recent advances in the understanding of the metabolic abnormali-ties underlying these disorders have prompted the proposal of biochemical classifications.

The leukodystrophies are the most common of the dysmyelinating diseases, but they are still relatively rare.[49,64–69] These are a heterogeneous group of incurable disorders, usually affecting individuals in infancy or early childhood. These disorders are characterized clinically by extensive neurologic impairment, including rapidly progressive visual failure, mental deterioration, and spastic paralysis; pathologically they are characterized by massive

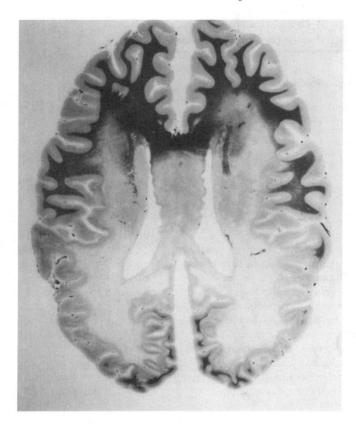

Figure   22–10. Adrenoleukodys- trophy. In this section of the cerebral hemispheres in which myelin is darkly stained a striking occipital-to-frontal progression of myelin loss (i.e., pallor) is evident. (From Okazaki, H: Funda- mentals of Neuropathology: Morpho- logical Basis of Neurological Disor- ders, ed 2. Igaku-Shoin, New York, 1989, p 159, with permission.)

degeneration of the white matter of the cerebral hemispheres (Fig. 22–10). The leukodys- trophies have historically been subdivided according to various clinical and histopathologic criteria. As the underlying biochemical abnormalities of specific leukodystrophies have been elucidated, they have been reclassified more accurately as specific metabolic disorders. Three leukodystrophies (Krabbe's leukodystrophy, adrenoleukodystrophy, and metachromatic leu- kodystrophy) are now known to be associated with specific enzyme deficiencies.[66–69] As further discoveries are made regarding the biochemical and genetic bases of the leukodys- trophies, additional specific disorders will undoubtedly be reclassified as well.

RECOMMENDED READINGS

Adams, RD and Victor, M: Principles of Neurology, ed 5. Chapter 36. Multiple Sclerosis and Allied Demyelina- tive Diseases. McGraw-Hill, New York, 1993.

Allen, IV and Kirk, J: Demyelinating Diseases. Chapter 9. In Adams, JH and Duchen, LW (eds): Greenfield's Neuropathology, ed 5. Oxford University Press, New York, 1992.

Bannister, Sir R: Brain and Bannister's Clinical Neurol- ogy, ed 7. Chapter 26. Multiple Sclerosis and Demy- elinating Diseases. Oxford University Press, Oxford, 1992.

Bauer, HJ and Hanefeld, FA: Multiple Sclerosis: Its Impact from Childhood to Old Age. WB Saunders, London, 1993.

Cook, SD (ed): Handbook of Multiple Sclerosis. Marcel Dekker, New York, 1991.

Francis, GS, Antel, JP, and Duquette, P: Inflammatory Demyelinating Diseases of the Central Nervous Sys- tem. Chapter 61. In Bradley, WG, et al (eds): Neurol- ogy in Clinical Practice. Butterworth-Heinemann, Boston, 1990.

Herndon, RM and Rudick, RA: Multiple Sclerosis and Related Conditions. Chapter 33. In Joynt, RJ (ed): Clinical Neurology, vol 3. JB Lippincott, Philadelphia, 1987.

Kesselring, J, et al: Magnetic Resonance Imaging in Multiple Sclerosis. Thieme Medical Publishers, New York, 1989.

Matthews, WB, et al (ed): McAlpine's Multiple Sclerosis, ed 2. Churchill Livingstone, Edinburgh, 1991.

Poser, C: The Dysmyelinating Diseases. Chapter 34. In Joynt, RJ (ed): Clinical Neurology, vol 3. JB Lippincott, Philadelphia, 1983.

Quarles, RH, Morell, P, and McFarlin, DE: Diseases Involving Myelin. Chapter 37. In Siegel, GJ, et al (eds): Basic Neurochemistry: Molecular, Cellular and Medical Aspects, ed 5. Raven Press, New York, 1994.

Raine, CS: Demyelinating Diseases. Chapter 12. In

Davis, RL and Robertson, DM: Textbook of Neuropathology, ed 2. Williams & Wilkins, Baltimore, 1990.

Rudick, RA and Goodkin, DE (eds): Treatment of Multiple Sclerosis: Trial Design, Results, and Future Perspectives. Springer-Verlag, London, 1992.

Thompson, AJ and McDonald, WI: Multiple Sclerosis and Its Pathophysiology. Chapter 90. In Asbury, AK, McKhann, GM, and McDonald, WI (eds): Diseases of the Nervous System: Clinical Neurobiology, ed 2. WB Saunders, Philadelphia, 1992.

REFERENCES

1. Peters, A, Palay, SL, and Webster, H deF: The Fine Structure of the Nervous System: Neurons and Their Supporting Cells, ed 3. Chapter 6. The Cellular Sheaths of Neurons. Oxford University Press, New York, 1991.

2. Morell, P and Norton, WT: Myelin. Sci Am 242(5):88, 1980.

3. Morell, P, Quarles, RH, and Norton, WT: Myelin Formation, Structure, and Biochemistry. Chapter 6. In Siegel, GT, et al (eds): Basic Neurochemistry: Molecular, Cellular and Medical Aspects, ed 5. Raven Press, New York, 1994.

4. Raine, CS: Oligodendrocytes and Central Nervous System Myelin. Chapter 3. In Davis, RL and Robertson, DM: Textbook of Neuropathology, ed 2. Williams & Wilkins, Baltimore, 1990.

5. Quarles, RH, Morell, P, and McFarlin, DE: Diseases Involving Myelin. Chapter 37. In Siegel, GJ, et. al. (eds): Basic Neurochemistry: Molecular, Cellular, and Medical Aspects, ed 5. Raven Press, New York, 1994.

6. Hauw, JJ, et al: Morphology of Demyelination in the Human Central Nervous System. J Neuroimmunol 40(2–3):139, 1992.

7. Martin, R, McFarland, HF, and McFarlin, DE: Immunological Aspects of Demyelinating Diseases. Ann Rev Immunol 10:153, 1992.

8. Adams, RD and Victor, M: Principles of Neurology, ed 5. Chapter 36. Multiple Sclerosis and Allied Demyelinative Diseases. McGraw-Hill, New York, 1993.

9. Allen, IV and Kirk, J: Demyelinating Diseases. Chapter 9. In Adams, JH and Duchen, LW (eds): Greenfield's Neuropathology, ed 5. Oxford University Press, New York, 1992.

10. Herndon, RM and Rudick, RA: Multiple Sclerosis and Related Conditions. Chapter 33. In Joynt, RJ (ed): Clinical Neurology, vol 3. JB Lippincott, Philadelphia, 1987.

11. Raine, CS: Demyelinating Diseases. Chapter 12. In Davis, RL and Robertson, DM: Textbook of Neuropathology, ed 2. Williams & Wilkins, Baltimore, 1990.

12. Francis, GS, Antel, JP, and Duquette, P: Inflammatory Demyelinating Diseases of the Central Nervous System. Chapter 61. In Bradley, WG, et al (eds): Neurology in Clinical Practice: The Neurological Disorders. Butterworth-Heinemann, Boston, 1990.

13. Bauer, HJ and Hanefeld, FA: Multiple Sclerosis: Its Impact from Childhood to Old Age. WB Saunders, London, 1993.

14. Matthews, WB, et al (ed): McAlpine's Sclerosis, ed 2. Churchill Livingstone, Edinburgh, 1991.

15. Cook, SD (ed): Handbook of Multiple Sclerosis. Marcel Dekker, New York, 1991.

16. Thompson, AJ and McDonald, WI: Multiple Sclerosis and Its Pathophysiology. Chapter 90. In Asbury, AK, McKhann, GM, and McDonald, WI (eds): Diseases of the Nervous System: Clinical Neurobiology, ed 2. WB Saunders, Philadelphia, 1992.

17. Sibley, WA, Poser, CM, and Alter, M: Multiple Sclerosis. Chapter 137. In Rowland, LP (ed): Merritt's Textbook of Neurology, ed 8. Lea & Febiger, Philadelphia, 1989.

18. Chadwick, D, Cartridge, N, and Bates, D: Medical Neurology. Chapter 16. The Demyelinating Diseases. Churchill Livingstone, Edinburgh, 1989.

19. Matthews, WB, et al: McAlpine's Multiple Sclerosis. Section 2. Clinical Aspects, ed 2. Churchill Livingstone, Edinburgh, 1991.

20. Goodkin, DE: The Natural History of Multiple Sclerosis. Chapter 2. In Rudick, RA and Goodkin, DE (eds): Treatment of Multiple Sclerosis: Trial Design, Results, and Future Perspectives. Springer-Verlag, London, 1992.

21. Bauer, HJ and Hanefeld, FA: Multiple Sclerosis: Its Impact from Childhood to Old Age. Chapter 3. Multiple Sclerosis in the Adult. WB Saunders, London, 1993.

22. Reingold, St C: Fatigue and Multiple Sclerosis. M.S. News. Br MS Soc 142:30, 1990.

23. Kemp, BA and Gora, ML: Amantadine and Fatigue of Multiple Sclerosis. Ann Pharmacother 27:893, 1993.

24. Matthews, WB, et al: McAlpine's Multiple Sclerosis, ed 2. Chapter 5. Course and Prognosis. Churchill Livingstone, Edinburgh, 1991.

25. Bauer, HJ and Hanefeld, FA: Multiple Sclerosis: Its Impact from Childhood to Old Age. Chapter 4. Old Age, Mortality, and Cause of Death in Multiple Sclerosis. WB Saunders, London, 1993.

26. Sadovnick, AD, et al: Cause of Death in Patients Attending Multiple Sclerosis Clinics. Neurology 41:1193, 1991.

27. Sadovnick, AD and Ebers, GC: Epidemiology of Multiple Sclerosis: A Critical Overview. Can J Neurol Sci 20:17, 1993.

28. Matthews, WB, et al: McAlpine's Multiple Sclerosis, ed 2. Chapter 1. Epidemiology. Churchill Livingstone, Edinburgh, 1991.

29. Runmarker, B and Anderson, O: Prognostic Factors in a Multiple Sclerosis Incidence Cohort with

Twenty Five Years of Follow-Up. Brain 116(Pt 1): 117, 1993.

30. Riise, T, et al: Early Prognostic Factors for Disability in Multiple Sclerosis: A European Multicenter Study. Acta Neurol Scand 85(3):212, 1992.

31. Lauer, K and Firnhaber, W: Prognostic in an Epidemiological Group of Patients with Multiple Sclerosis: An Exploratory Study. J Neurol 239:93, 1992.

32. Matthews, WB, et al: McAlpines Multiple Sclerosis, ed 2. Chapter 12. Pathology of Multiple Sclerosis. Churchill Livingstone, Edinburgh, 1991.

33. Engell, T: A Clinical Patho-Anatomical Study of Clinically Silent Multiple Sclerosis. Acta Neurol Scand 79:428, 1989.

34. Harris, JO, et al: Serial Gadolinium-Enhanced Magnetic Resonance Imaging Scans in Patients with Early, Relapsing-Remitting Multiple Sclerosis: Implications for Clinical Trials and Natural History. Ann Neurol 29:548, 1991.

35. Gilbert, JJ and Sadler, M: Unsuspected Multiple Sclerosis. Arch Neurol 40:535, 1983.

36. Matthews, WB, et al: McAlpine's Multiple Sclerosis, ed 2. Chapter 8. Pathophysiology. Churchill Livingstone, Edinburgh, 1991.

37. Murrell, TG, Harbige, LS, and Robinson, IC: A Review of the Aetiology of Multiple Sclerosis: An Ecological Approach. Ann Hum Biol 18:95, 1991.

38. Granieri, E, et al: Multiple Sclerosis: Does Epidemiology Contribute to Providing Etiological Clues. J Neurol Sci 115(Suppl):S16, 1993.

39. Compston, A and Sadovnick, AD: Epidemiology and Genetics of Multiple Sclerosis. Curr Opin Neurol Neurosurg 5(2):175, 1992.

40. Matthews, WB, et al: McAlpine's Multiple Sclerosis, ed 2. Chapter 11. Immunological Aspects of Multiple Sclerosis. Churchill Livingstone, Edinburgh, 1991.

41. Allen, I and Brankin, B: Pathogenesis of Multiple Sclerosis: The Immune Diathesis and the Role of Viruses. J Neuropathol Exp Neurol 52:95, 1993.

42. Matthews, WB, et al: McAlpine's Multiple Sclerosis, ed 2. Chapter 10. Genetic Susceptibility to Multiple Sclerosis. Churchill Livingstone, Edinburgh, 1991.

43. Sadovnick, AD, et al: A Population-Based Study of Multiple Sclerosis in Twins: Update. Ann Neurol 33(3):281, 1993.

44. Poser, CM (ed): Multiple Sclerosis: Epidemiology and Genetics. Ann Neurol 36 (suppl 2):S163, 1994.

45. Sadovnick, AD: Familial Recurency Risks and Inheritance of Multiple Sclerosis. Curr Opin Neurol Neurosurg 6(2):189, 1993.

46. Sadovnick, AD, Baird, PA, and Ward, RH: Multiple Sclerosis: Updated Risks for Relatives. Am J Med Genet 29:533, 1988.

47. Poser, CM: The Pathogenesis of Multiple Sclerosis: Additional Considerations. J Neurol Sci 115(suppl): 53, 1993.

48. Rudick, RA and Goodkin, DE (eds): Treatment of Multiple Sclerosis: Trial Design, Results, and Future Perspectives. Springer-Verlag, London, 1992.

49. Matthews, WB, et al: McAlpine's Multiple Sclerosis. Chapter 9. Treatment, ed 2. Churchill Livingstone, Edinburgh, 1991.

50. Bauer, HJ and Henefeld, FA: Multiple Sclerosis: Its Impact from Childhood to Old Age. Chapter 5. Long-term Management of Multiple Sclerosis. WB Saunders, London, 1993.

51. Whitaker, JN: Rationale for Immunotherapy in Multiple Sclerosis. Ann Neurol 36 (Suppl 1):S103, 1994.

52. Mitchell, G: Update on Multiple Sclerosis Therapy. Med Clin North Am 77:231, 1993.

53. Francis, DA: The Current Therapy of Multiple Sclerosis. J Clin Pharmacol Ther 18:77, 1993.

54. Noseworthy, JH: Clinical Trials in Multiple Sclerosis. Curr Opin Neurol Neurosurg 6:209, 1993.

55. Compston, A: Future Prospects for the Management of Multiple Sclerosis. Ann Neurol 36 (suppl): S146, 1994.

56. Maloney, FP, Burks, JS, and Ringel, SP: Interdisciplinary Rehabilitation of Multiple Sclerosis and Neuromuscular Disorders. JB Lippincott, Philadelphia, 1985.

57. Bohannon, RW: Physical Rehabilitation in Neurologic Diseases. Curr Opin Neurol 6:765, 1993.

58. Sibley, WA: Devic Syndrome and Balo Disease. Chapter 138. In Rowland, LP (ed): Merritt's Textbook of Neurology, ed 8. Lea & Febiger, Philadelphia, 1989.

59. Moore, GRW, et al: Balo's Concentric Sclerosis: New Observations on Lesion Development. Ann Neurol 17:604, 1985.

60. Kesselring, J, et al: Acute Disseminated Encephalomyelitis: MRI Findings and the Distinction from Multiple Sclerosis. Brain 113(Pt 2):291, 1990.

61. Poser, CM: Demyelination in the Central Nervous System in Chronic Alcoholism, Central Pontine Myelinolysis and Marchiafava-Bignami's Disease. Ann NY Acad Sci 215:373, 1973.

62. Mancall, EL: Central Pontine Myelinolysis. Chapter 140. In Rowland, LP (ed): Merritt's Textbook of Neurology, ed 8. Lea & Febiger, Philadelphia, 1989.

63. Mayer, J, et al: Computerized Tomography and Nuclear Magnetic Resonance Imaging in Marchiafava-Bignami Disease. J Neuroradiol 14:152, 1987.

64. Poser, C: The Dysmyelinating Diseases. Chapter 34. In Joynt, RJ (ed): Clinical Neurology, vol 3. JB Lippincott, Philadelphia, 1983.

65. Kolodny, EH: Dysmyelinating and Demyelinating Conditions in Infancy. Curr Opin Neurol Neurosurg 6:379, 1993.

66. Lake, BD: Lysosomal and Peroxisomal Disorders. Chapter 12. In Adams, JH and Duchen, LW (eds): Greenfield's Neuropathology, ed 5. Oxford University Press, New York, 1992.

67. Becker, LE and Yates, AJ: Inherited Metabolic Disease. Chapter 9. In Davis, RL and Robertson, DM (eds): Textbook of Neuropathology, ed 2. Williams & Wilkins, Baltimore, 1990.

68. Suzuki, K: Genetic Disorders of Lipid, Glycoprotein, and Mucopolysaccharide Metabolism. In Siegel, B, et al (eds): Basic Neurochemistry, ed 4. Raven Press, New York, 1989.

69. Moser, HW, et al: Adrenoleukodystrophy: Survey of 303 Cases: Biochemistry, Diagnosis, and Therapy. Ann Neurol 16:628, 1989.

CONSEQUENCES OF IMMOBILIZATION

Overview

Many of the locomotor disorders considered in this text cause patients to endure long periods of decreased physical activity or immobilization. Although most of these disorders are of neurogenic or myogenic origins, many other conditions may directly or indirectly curtail movement. Orthopedic problems, burns, and inflammatory conditions can directly restrict musculoskeletal mobility. By the same token, chronic illness, post-traumatic or postsurgical states, old age, severe pain, and even psychiatric disturbances can necessitate prolonged bed rest or confinement to a bed or wheelchair. Whatever the primary condition, the outcome is a significant period of inactivity and often recumbency.

It has become increasingly clear in recent years that inactivity and immobilization create many deleterious changes in the human body and constitute a significant impediment to rehabilitation. Much of the morbidity and mortality of patients with locomotor disorders arises primarily from the adverse effects of immobilization on musculoskeletal and visceral systems. The purpose of the chapters in this section is to describe these complications and the deleterious effects that they may inflict on a patient's health.

The human body is designed to be mobile (after all, it is 40% skeletal muscle) and is dependent on physical activity for its well-being. The mechanical stresses of daily living are necessary for the maintenance of muscle strength and stamina, the growth and remodeling of bone, and the integrity and mobility of joints. As we shall see in this section, immobilization rapidly leads to muscle atrophy, contractures, joint deterioration, and osteoporosis. In addition, many visceral systems are also adversely affected. Cardiopulmonary insufficiency, thromboembolic conditions, and gastrointestinal and urinary tract stasis all may rapidly develop. The adverse effects of immobilization are all the worse when specific neural pathways or regulatory centers are damaged, in geriatric or chronically ill patients, and when recumbency is prolonged.

The pathophysiologic changes accompanying immobilization begin rapidly, and the most severe decrements in function usually occur during the initial phases of inactivity. Although many of these deleterious changes are reversible, the longer the inactivity persists, the more likely it is that permanent alterations will have occurred in tissues and organ systems. Even when these changes are reversible, the period of recovery from these effects is usually appreciably longer than the period of immobilization.

It is ironic that the complications arising from immobilization may ultimately create greater disability than the initial underlying disorder. These complications impede rehabilitation and may make patients dependent who would otherwise be self-sufficient. At the extreme, respiratory insufficiency, thrombosis, infections, and gastrointestinal or urinary tract obstruction may become life-threatening. The tragedy is that most of these complications are largely preventable with careful medical management and proper physical therapy.

CHAPTER 23

■

Adverse Effects of Immobilization on the Musculoskeletal System

Christopher M. Fredericks, PhD

- *Muscle Atrophy and Deconditioning*
- *Contractures*
- *Disuse Osteoporosis (Osteopenia)*
- *Joint Deterioration*
- *Heterotopic Bone Formation (Ossification)*
- *Osteomyelitis*
- *Skeletal Deformity*

All components of the musculoskeletal system are dependent on physical activity for their well-being. The mechanical stresses produced by weight-bearing and muscle tension are necessary for the maintenance of both muscle and the bony skeleton to which it is attached. The mechanical stresses of daily activity sustain the strength, endurance, and coordination of muscle, modulate the deposition and remodeling of bone, and maintain the integrity and mobility of joints. Immobility, particularly when accompanied by prolonged recumbency, has a wide range of adverse effects on the musculoskeletal system, among which muscle weakness, contracture, degenerative joint disease, and osteoporosis are the most prominent. Impairment of musculoskeletal function in turn threatens a cascade of deleterious changes in cardiopulmonary and other visceral functions (see Chapter 24).

Muscle Atrophy and Deconditioning

Lack of use (as in bed rest, inactivity, or limb or body casts) **and loss of innervation** (as in disease or injury) **both promote a marked decline in muscle mass, strength, and endurance** (Fig. 23–1).[1-7] Disuse atrophy is particularly severe with prolonged recumbency. In the recumbent position, not only is muscle activity minimal but also the force exerted by gravity on the musculoskeletal system is reduced. With complete bed rest, muscle bulk may

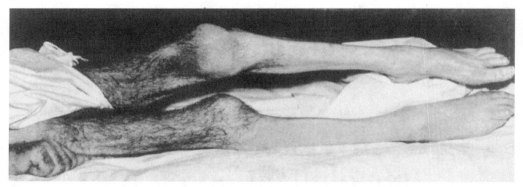

Figure 23–1.   Atrophy of thigh and leg muscles in an ALS patient. (From Rowland, LP (ed): Merritt's Textbook of Neurology, ed 7. Copyright © Lea & Febiger, Philadelphia, 1984, p 550, with permission.)

shrink to half its original size in less than 2 months.[4–6] If neural connections to a muscle are destroyed, the muscle atrophies even more rapidly (denervation atrophy), and eventually its volume may be only 5% to 10% of normal. **Rapid declines in muscle strength accompany muscle atrophy**, reflecting both the decrease in muscle fiber size and a decrease in the tension-producing capacity per unit of fiber cross-sectional area. With complete bed rest, a muscle may lose 10% to 15% or more of its strength per week and 50% within 3 to 5 weeks.[2,4,5] Muscle atrophy begins within hours of immobilization, and the greatest declines in size and strength are observed during the first week or so, the rate of decline diminishing beyond that point. **Muscle stamina and fatigability are also adversely affected**, reflecting deleterious changes in muscle metabolism.[1–5] Oxidative (aerobic) enzyme systems in particular are adversely affected, resulting in decreased muscle endurance. Glycolytic enzymes are relatively unaffected. Intracellular fuel sources are also depleted. Endogenous carbohydrate and high-energy stores (glycogen and creatine) are lower at the start of work and depleted to even lower levels during work. The adverse effects of inactivity on muscle stamina are compounded by cardiac deconditioning and possible changes in the muscle vasculature itself.

Certain muscles atrophy more quickly than others.[1–3,6] With inactivity and recumbency, the muscles most susceptible to atrophy are those composed of predominantly oxidative or slow-twitch fibers. Because of this, the antigravity muscles of the lower extremities and trunk, with their high proportion of oxidative fibers, are most vulnerable and atrophy first. The quadriceps and back extensor muscles are particularly affected, which may significantly impair functional activities such as stair climbing and ambulation.

The exact mechanisms by which disuse or denervation promote muscle wasting are not known. Muscle, like other tissues, is maintained by balancing the rate of protein synthesis with that of protein degradation.[3] How the functional demands of muscle load and activity regulate this balance is not yet clear. It appears that **immobilization decreases contractile protein synthesis while increasing protein degradation**, thus causing a net catabolism of muscle to occur.[1–3] Inactive or denervated muscle may also become less responsive to endogenous growth-promoting factors, through changes in receptor numbers or affinities. In addition, catabolism of contractile proteins may be caused by the release of calcium-activated proteolytic enzymes from muscle itself. Although somatic motor neurons clearly mediate a beneficial, trophic influence on muscle, the mechanisms of this effect are poorly understood. By the same token, which denervation clearly produces markedly deleterious effects on muscle, the mechanisms accounting for this effect are not clear either.

Muscle disuse atrophy can be reversed with exercise after short periods of immobilization, but the longer the atrophy exists, the longer the time needed to reverse the problem. After too long a period, muscle disintegration from disuse is no longer reversible.[3,6] Reactivation after 2 years rarely results in the return of any function at all. Muscle fibers will have degenerated and are replaced by collagen and fatty tissue. With preexisting neurologic or musculoskeletal disease, atrophy is more difficult to prevent and reverse and may have devastating functional consequences.

Difficulty in performing activities of daily living, poor work tolerance, and compromised cardiovascular and pulmonary function all may result from muscle weakness and atrophy (see Chapter 24). Rehabilitation efforts must focus on their prevention.

Contractures[4,8–11]

As the word implies, *contracture* **refers to a tightness or restricted range of motion across a joint** (Fig. 23–2). Contractures usually limit motion in a particular direction, most often imposing an abnormal degree of flexion on the extremities. Contractures may occur rapidly, particularly after trauma to a joint, or insidiously over a long period of time. Although all joints can be adversely affected by immobilization, **the hip, knee, and ankle are most susceptible** because of the effect of gravity, the strength of flexor muscles, and the difficulty of full extension or range of motion while in a sitting or recumbent position.[12] When the body is supine or is in a lateral recumbent or sitting position, partial flexion of the hip and knee is almost always present.

Three basic types of pathologic changes promote the development of contracture: those that occur in the structures of the joint itself (arthrogenic contracture), those that are in the

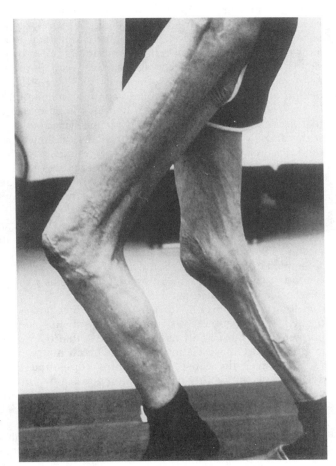

Figure 23–2. Patient with hip and knee flexion contractures having difficulty in ambulation. (From Kottke, FJ and Lehmann, JF (eds): Krusen's Handbook of Physical Medicine and Rehabilitation, ed 4. WB Saunders, Philadelphia, p 118, with permission.)

Table 23-1. *Major Factors in the Development of Contractures*

Muscle conditions	Joint conditions	Soft tissue conditions
Intrinsic factors	Cartilage damage	Skin, subcutaneous fibrosis (burns)
Trauma	Trauma	Tendon, aponeurosis
Inflammation	Inflammation	Trauma
Degeneration	Infection	Inflammation
Extrinsic factors	Immobilization	Calcifications (heterotopic)
Spasticity	Capsular fibrosis	
Flaccid paralysis	Joint soft tissue, ligaments	
Positional, mechanical		

Adapted from Halar and Bell.[4]

associated skeletal muscles (myogenic contracture), and those that are in the adjacent soft tissues (Table 23–1).[4,8] Although other conditions may promote the development of contracture, the most common cause is immobilization.

Myogenic contractures may arise from both intrinsic and extrinsic factors.[4,8] Intrinsic structural changes in muscle itself may occur as a result of inflammatory, degenerative, ischemic, or traumatic processes and directly contribute to muscle shortening or fibrosis. Myositis and other inflammatory disorders lead rapidly to the development of fibrotic changes in muscle. Muscular dystrophies result in degenerative changes in muscle tissue and muscle shortening. Extrinsic factors such as muscle imbalance or abnormal mechanical forces can also promote contracture development.[11] Spastic muscles, by producing heightened tonic activity on one side of a joint, and paralyzed muscles, by not providing adequate balance to opposing muscles, may create abnormal joint positions. If these positions are allowed to persist and full range of motion is not provided, contracture will result. By the same token, external mechanical factors may promote ill-adapted joint positions and restricted range of motion in individuals who are restricted to a bed or wheelchair. Abnormal flexion of extremities is particularly common among immobilized patients. For patients on bed rest, the tendency to develop tightness is promoted by the typical position of comfort, that is, flexed hips and knees and plantar-flexed ankles (Fig. 23–3).[10] Similarly, patients with painfully inflamed joints spontaneously assume a position of minimum joint pressure (and discomfort), namely, 30 to 45 degrees of flexion for hip and knee and 15 degrees of plantar flexion at the ankle.[10] Likewise, amputees tend to develop flexor contractures as a result of prolonged sitting with flexion at the hip and knees.

In addition to muscle contractures, **arthrogenic contractures** result from tightness of the connective tissues of the joint itself, as may occur with inflammation, infection, trauma, and immobilization.[4,8] Pain and effusion, for example, can result in reduced joint mobilization. Contracture of the capsule and ligaments results, further compromising the range of motion. The shoulder is a common site of capsular tightening, which can ultimately lead to a completely immobilized shoulder and to loss of arm function. The posterior knee capsule is another common area for capsular shortening as a consequence of prolonged flexion (e.g., in wheelchair-restricted patients).[4,8]

Joint motion may be further restricted by changes in the distensibility of **adjacent soft tissue**.[4,8] For example, overlying skin and subcutaneous tissues may be severely scarred and fibrosed from burns. Soft tissues may be stiffened by regions of heterotopic ossification, as might develop in association with spinal cord injury.

Whatever the cause, contractures compound the disability accompanying motor dysfunction. Immobility not only promotes contracture formation but is exacerbated by its development. The development of contractures reduces mobility and the ability to perform activities of daily living, especially in persons already disabled by motor deficits. Contractures of the lower extremities (hip, knee, and ankle) are common, and the required postural adjustments distort gait, making it slower, more difficult, and less efficient. Overall energy consumption during ambulation is increased, and endurance is decreased.[10] Persons who

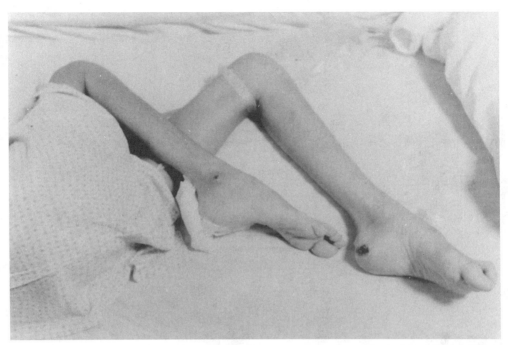

Figure 23–3. Contractures and pressure sores in head trauma patients. (From Goodgold, J (ed): Rehabilitation Medicine. CV Mosby, St. Louis, 1988, p 125, with permission.)

have the added disability of muscle weakness from disuse atrophy or paralysis may lose the ability to walk altogether. Wheelchair use and car transfers may be difficult (Fig. 23–4).[8] Contractures of the upper extremities may impair functions such as reaching, dressing, grooming, eating, maintaining proper hygiene, and the performance of fine motor tasks.[4,8] Contractures may also make proper positioning in a bed or chair difficult or impossible and may promote the development of pressure sores (see Chapter 24).

Because contractures may significantly increase disability and adversely impact a patient's independence and quality of life, one focus of rehabilitation should be aggressive treatment designed to prevent their occurrence. Prevention of contractures by joint mobilization is a particularly important goal in the management of patients with spasticity. Once established, contractures can usually be treated by conservative measures (e.g., stretching, splints, and so on). However, some well-established contractures may require surgical correction and occasionally ligamentous, bony, and skin reconstruction.

Disuse Osteoporosis (Osteopenia)[13–19]

The growth, maintenance, and remodeling of bone depend on the stresses applied to the bone by both muscle contraction and the force of gravity. When weight bearing and physical activity (movement) are reduced, whether due to prolonged recumbency or paralysis, significant bone atrophy (osteopenia) results. Patients with diffuse osteoporosis due to complete bed rest can lose about 1% of their total bone mass per week and ultimately up to 30% to 40% of their total bone mass.[7,17] As with skeletal muscle atrophy, bone atrophy is greatest during the early phase of immobilization. Bone loss increases rapidly from the third day to the third week of immobilization and peaks during the fifth or sixth week.[17] This is almost equivalent to the loss of bone in patients with primary osteoporosis (i.e.,

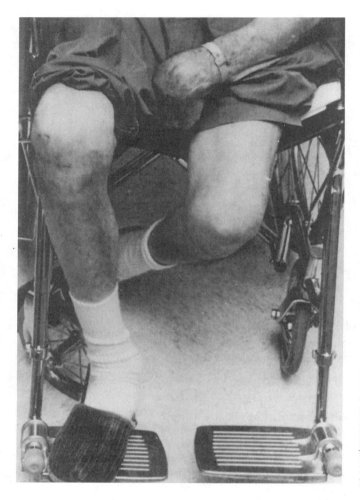

Figure 23–4. Hemiplegic Patient with Multiple Contractures. This advanced knee flexion contracture limits this patient's wheelchair mobility, since it prevents him from keeping his leg on the leg rest. (From Delisa, JA and Gans, BM (ed): Rehabilitation Medicine: Principles and Practice, ed 2. JB Lippincott, Philadelphia, 1993, p 688, with permission.)

hormonal), which occurs over a lifetime. Although the bone loss is intense initially, after a certain amount of bone has been lost, a new equilibrium will be established at a reduced bone mass. Disuse osteopenia does not lead to total bone loss but rather to a new steady state at a reduced bone mass. [13,14]

Not all bones are equally affected by immobilization. **The greatest loss of bone is in rapidly remodeling, weight-bearing trabecular bone.**[12,15] Loss of compact bone from the weight-bearing skeleton occurs at a slower rate. In non–weight-bearing structures, there is little loss of compact bone. **The long bones of the lower extremities, the heel, and the spinal vertebrae are the most vulnerable.**

Bone loss can be generalized in individuals whose motor activity is significantly impaired by neurologic or orthopedic disorders or by prolonged bed rest.[12] On the other hand, a more localized osteopenia may accompany the injury and immobilization of a single extremity (Fig. 23–5). For example, both of the involved extremities of a hemiplegic stroke victim may be osteoporotic.[13,19] Similarly, if a bone is fractured, atrophy may involve just that one extremity, being most pronounced in the bones distal to the fracture site. Immobilization osteopenia is particularly evident in the presence of neurogenic paralysis, such as accompanies spinal cord injury.[18] Radiographically apparent disuse osteoporosis develops in about 50% of all spinal cord–injured patients.[18] Individuals with preexisting abnormalities of bone metabolism, such as occur in postmenopausal osteoporosis or Paget's

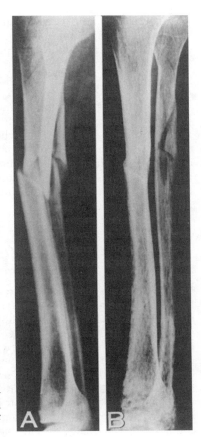

Figure 23–5. Osteoporosis Following Limb Immobilization. (*A*) Spiral fracture of the tibia and fibula in a young adult. (*B*) Three months later, the fractures are uniting but note the marked osteoporosis, particularly in the distal fragments. (From Salter, RB: Textbook of Disorders and Injuries of the Musculoskeletal System, ed 2. Copyright © Williams & Wilkins, Baltimore, 1983, p 412, with permission.)

disease, are also at increased risk for bone loss during immobilization. The bone loss resulting from inactivity is compounded by the loss resulting from age-related osteoporosis.[7,17] In older women, osteoporosis is heightened by the effects of estrogen loss.

The skeletal atrophy that accompanies immobilization is not simply a decalcification of bony tissue, but is a true osteoporosis, reflecting a loss of both organic and inorganic constituents of bone.[13–15] Loss of the organic component is reflected in elevated excretion of hydroxyproline during immobilization. The inorganic loss is reflected in the elevated urinary loss of calcium. The fact that the rise in hydroxyproline excretion precedes the hypercalciuria suggests that bone collagen resorption actually precedes demineralization.

Calcium released from the immobilized skeleton is excreted in the urine, resulting in hypercalciuria. In most patients, plasma calcium is within normal limits or only slightly elevated, depending on the extent of immobilization. Patients in whom one extremity is paralyzed do not usually develop hypercalciuria or hypercalcemia, but quadriplegic patients may develop both. Hypercalcemia is most pronounced in young patients (especially adolescent males) in whom bone growth and remodeling are occurring at a high rate.

Immobilization, regardless of whether it arises from paralysis or prolonged bed rest, results in a negative calcium balance and loss of skeletal mass. Although it is generally agreed that this bone loss reflects an imbalance in bone formation and resorption, the exact causes of this imbalance are not known.[7,11–15] Osteoclastic activity is increased, but it is not clear why. Parathyroid hormone is known to stimulate osteoclastic resorption of bone. In immobilized patients, however, there is minimal hypercalcemia or hyperphosphatemia, which actually implies a decrease in parathyroid hormone activity.[13–15] Local factors related to immobilization may sensitize the affected bone to circulating low levels of parathyroid hormone. Bone loss may be independent of parathormone altogether and reflect the direct effects of unknown local factors. For example, a number of animal studies have shown that limb immobilization produces regional stagnation of bone blood flow, which may in turn promote bone resorption.[13,14] In the case of more general paralysis and bed rest, some evidence suggests that altered intestinal absorption and renal excretion of calcium may contribute to the overall negative calcium balance.

Bone that is osteoporotic from immobilization is more likely to fracture than normal bone. A fracture can further immobilize the patient and impede rehabilitation. Minor trauma, during transfer and wheelchair activities, for example, can cause fracture of osteoporotic bone (frequently a femur) in chronic spinal cord–injured patients. Otherwise, an osteoporotic limb does not cause tenderness, pain, or any other symptoms. It is important to make every attempt to minimize the osteoporosis that often accompanies immobility. Early weight-bearing activities such as standing are encouraged, even in patients who are comatose.

Joint Deterioration

Like bone, synovial joints are dependent on the regular stimulation of physical activity for their well-being. **Immobility,** even for relatively short periods of time, **will have deleterious effects on the morphologic, biochemical, and biomechanical characteristics of synovial joints.**[4,7,12,19–21] Changes in joint structure may occur after as few as 5 days of immobilization, with measurable changes in the range of motion within 1 week.[17]

As immobility or inactivity persists, contracture of the joint capsule and the periarticular muscles develops, physically restricting movement of the joint. **Within the joint cavity, fibrofatty connective tissue proliferates,** adhering to cartilaginous surfaces, further limiting movement and ultimately obliterating the joint cavity (Table 23–2, Fig. 23–6).[20,21] **Cartilage deteriorates,** appearing pitted and ulcerated in areas where the joint surfaces are in contact.[20,21] Eventually, the cartilage is replaced by fibrofatty tissue, which penetrates to the subchondral bone. The cellular and fibrillar elements of the associated ligaments may change, resulting in increased distensibility and decreased strength. Ligament insertions may be weakened by increased osteoclastic activity.

Immobilization is particularly destructive if the joint surfaces are under pressure. The pressures of weight-bearing may be exacerbated by the undue pressures exerted by muscle and connective tissue contractures or by muscle spasticity.[20,21] Not only do spastic muscles restrict joint movement, but they also add to the damage of articular structures by exerting continual pressure on opposing joint surfaces.

Table 23–2. *Gross and Microscopic Changes in Synovial Joints Observed After Prolonged Immobilization*

Type of Structure	Changes
Synovium	Proliferation of fibrofatty connective tissue into joint space
	Adhesions between synovial folds
	Tearing of cartilage surface by adhesions with forced manipulation
Cartilage	Adherence of fibrofatty connective tissue to cartilage surfaces
	Atrophy of cartilage
	Pressure necrosis at points of cartilage-cartilage contact
Ligament	Disorganization of the parallel arrays of fibrils and cells
Ligament insertion site	Destruction of ligament fibers attaching to bone as the result of osteoclastic activity
Bone	Generalized osteoporosis of cancellous and cortical bone

Adapted from Akeson, et al.[20]

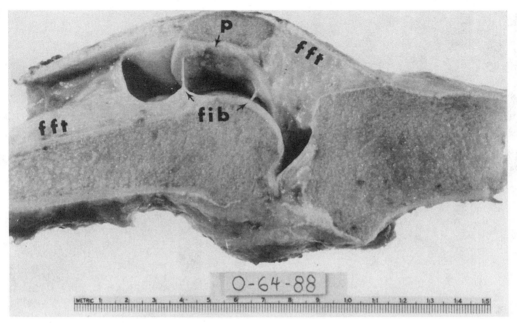

Figure 23–6. *Effects of Immobilization on the Human Knee.* This 59-year-old man sustained a fracture of the neck of the femur ultimately resulting in a hip disarticulation due to infection. This sagittal section reveals fibrofatty connective tissue filling the anterior joint cavity (FFT), fibrous adhesions (Fib), and degeneration of the articular cartilage of the patella (p). (From Enneking and Horowitz,[21] p 973, with permission.)

Although all the mechanisms responsible for the deleterious changes occurring in joints when they are immobilized are not known, ischemia is probably an important factor. Although the deep layers of cartilage are nourished by the blood vessels of the subchondrial bone, the superficial layers are dependent on the synovial fluid for their nutrition. Joint motion causes alternating compression and distention of cartilage, promoting the flow of synovial fluid and the diffusion of fluid in and out of the cartilage. Absence of these pressure fluctuations causes stagnation of the intercellular fluid of the cartilage and decreases its nutrition.

In addition to neuromuscular disorders, restricted range of motion is promoted by fracture treatment by casts, joint pain, prolonged bed rest, and a variety of disturbances that result in mechanical incongruity of joint surfaces. Whatever the cause, this restraint leads to joint contracture and the whole process of immobility-induced joint deterioration.

Heterotopic Bone Formation (Ossification)[4,18,22–25]

Heterotopic ossification **is a term used to describe the formation of bone in abnormal anatomic locations,** usually in the muscles and other soft tissues surrounding major joints. This condition is not common with all types of immobilization but occurs **frequently following severe neurologic injury.** It is often seen after paraplegia and head injury and occasionally following stroke. Heterotopic ossification is estimated to occur in 15% to 50% of spinal cord–injured patients, in whom the hip is most often involved (Fig. 23–7); next in frequency of involvement is the knee.[18,22,23] Heterotopic ossification also occurs in 10% to 20% of traumatic brain-injured patients, with the hip, shoulder, and elbow being the most common sites (Fig. 23–8).[24]

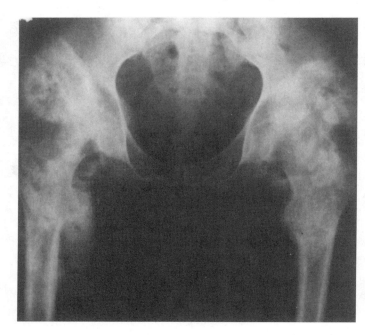

Figure 23–7. Severe Heterotopic Ossification of the Hips in a Quadriplegic Patient. Diffuse heterotopic bone formation is apparent as the radiopaque areas enveloping both hip joints. (From Goodgold, J (ed): Rehabilitation Medicine. CV Mosby, St. Louis, 1988, p 161, with permission.)

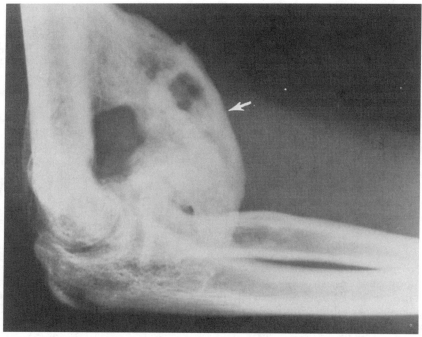

Figure 23–8. Heterotopic Ossification of the Elbow. This traumatic brain-injured patient had marked elbow flexor spasticity. A bridge of periarticular heterotopic bone had formed anterior to the elbow joint, which further restricted elbow movement. (From Nickel, VL and Botte, MJ (eds): Orthopaedic Rehabilitation, ed 2. Churchill Livingstone, New York, 1992, p 367, with permission.)

Unlike soft tissue calcification, which simply involves a deposition of amorphous calcium phosphate into the tissue, **heterotopic ossification involves true osteoblastic activity and bone formation.**[23-25] This bone has the lamellar structure of normal bone, with occasional haversian systems. The new bone is formed in planes between connective tissue layers. Although the cause of this process is poorly understood, tissue hypoxia due to circulatory stasis (or some unknown factor) is believed to induce a transformation of multipotential connective tissue cells into osteoblasts. Theories regarding the cause of heterotopic ossification suggest that local factors such as venous thrombosis, chronic venous insufficiency, decubitus ulcers, infection, and trauma all may cause localized edema, circulatory stasis, and finally tissue hypoxia.[23-25] Patients with limb spasticity, trauma to a joint or surgical repair of a fracture, or decubitus ulcers adjacent to a proximal joint all are at increased risk of developing heterotopic ossification.[22,25]

Anatomically, the heterotopic lesion is extra-articular and extracapsular, but may be firmly attached to the joint capsule or aponeurosis and, even at times, to the adjacent bone.[23,24] The lesion may develop in tendons, in connective tissue between muscles, in aponeurotic tissue, or in the peripheral aspects of muscle. Heterotopic ossification develops in most instances in association with proximal joints.

Heterotopic ossification is often asymptomatic and only incidentally noted on x-ray. When symptomatic, it is associated with the classic inflammatory signs of swelling, redness, and local warmth, pain upon movement, and loss of range of passive motion. As heterotopic ossification progresses, it can result in the immobilization of an affected joint and can be disabling. Restriction of joint range of motion to even a modest degree can then result in deterioration of joint structure and function. In addition, pressure sores may occur as a secondary complication. This may result from difficulty in positioning and weight bearing (e.g., increased pressure on the ischial tuberosity contralateral to an involved hip) or the presence of an ossification directly overlying a bony prominence (e.g., trochanter or ischial tuberosity). When heterotopic ossification is extensive and has caused joint deterioration, surgery may be required. Physical therapy is important in maintaining range of motion and preventing deformity. However, range-of-motion exercises should not include aggressive, forceful movement of the involved joint, since this may traumatize the soft tissue and increase the deposition of heterotopic bone.[24]

Heterotopic ossification is distinct from myositis ossificans (post-traumatic ossification), which results from injury to a muscle and is characterized by bony deposits within the muscle tissue.[26] Heterotopic ossification develops between rather than within the injured muscles. Myositis ossificans may occur after a fracture, a dislocation, or even an isolated muscle injury, particularly in the region of the elbow or thigh of children and young adults.

Osteomyelitis[18,27]

Osteomyelitis is an inflammation of bone due to infection. Although many types of microorganisms, including fungi and viruses, may cause osteomyelitis, it is usually bacterial in origin. One of the routes by which infecting organisms may reach bone is by extension from some adjacent site of infection, such as a burn or pressure sore in the overlying tissue. As will be discussed in Chapter 24, pressure sores are a common complication in immobilized and debilitated persons, especially those with spinal cord injury or other neurologic deficits. Pressure sores are often infected and thus threaten underlying bone with infection. In one study of 154 spinal cord–injured patients, 29 developed osteomyelitis, which in most cases was associated with a pressure sore.[27] **Osteomyelitis is a potential complication of any immobilizing condition that fosters the development of pressure sores.**

Osteomyelitis is a serious medical condition, which is most treatable with early diagnosis. Therapists should be aware of its existence and its manifestations. Pain may be its most common symptom, but in spinal cord–injured patients this sensation may be lost. The presence of osteomyelitis is suggested by persistent drainage from a wound, swelling of an

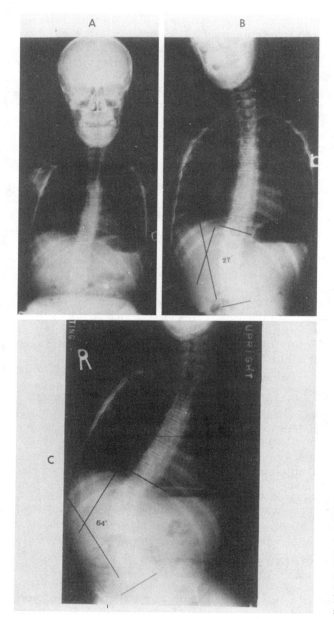

Figure 23–9. *Progressive Scoliosis in a Wheelchair Patient.* (*A*) Spine in patient with muscular dystrophy on first assuming wheelchair existence. (*B*) Spine after 18 months in wheelchair. (*C*) Spine 2 years later after refusing spine-stabilizing operation. (From Crenshaw, AH (ed): Campbell's Operative Orthopaedics, ed 8. Mosby Year Book, St. Louis, 1991, p 2472, with permission.)

extremity, unexplained fever, or increased white blood cell count.[27] Diagnosis of this type of infection is difficult and is best confirmed by bone biopsy. Because osteomyelitis is often difficult to cure with antibiotics, surgery (including amputation) may be necessary.

Skeletal Deformity

The relative positions and even the actual shapes of the bones of our skeleton are largely determined by the mechanical forces exerted on the skeleton by muscle and gravity. If the muscular balance that normally controls the position of joints and influences the remodeling

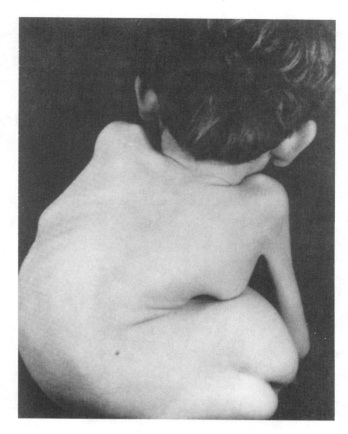

Figure 23–10. *Extensive Musculoskeletal Deformity.* This 7-year-old boy with a chronic inherited motor neuronopathy has generalized muscle wasting and weakness and a severe scoliosis. (From Dyck, PJ and Thomas, PK (eds): Peripheral Neuropathy, ed 3. WB Saunders, Philadelphia, 1993, p 1056, with permission.)

of bone is upset, skeletal deformity results. In fact, skeletal deformity ultimately develops in association with any locomotor disorder characterized by significant muscle weakness or spasticity. **Weak muscles yielding to antagonists, spastic muscles overriding normal opposing forces, and contractures limiting joint mobility all distort body shape and position.** Skeletal deformity is particularly evident in the hands and feet (e.g., talipes calcaneus, planus, valgus, and varus). It is also common in the shoulders (e.g., winging) and spine (e.g., kyphosis, lordosis, scoliosis, and torsion) (Fig. 23–9). As deformity evolves, ambulation becomes more difficult, increasingly abnormal sitting and sleeping postures develop, and pulmonary function is made less efficient and more difficult, all of which further immobilize the patient and threaten new complications (Fig. 23–10). The anticipation of potential deformities and the use of treatment strategies (such as providing external support with orthotics, splints, braces, and adaptive equipment) to minimize their occurrence constitute important elements of any rehabilitation plan.

RECOMMENDED READINGS

Browse, NL: The Physiology and Pathology of Bed Rest. Charles C Thomas, Springfield, IL, 1965.

Coletta, EM and Murphy, JB: The Complications of Immobility in the Elderly Stroke Patient. J Am Board Fam Pract 5:389, 1992.

Goodgold, J (ed): Rehabilitation Medicine. CV Mosby, St. Louis, 1988.

Halar, EM and Bell, KR: Contracture and Other Deleterious Effects of Immobility. Chapter 33. In Delisa, JA and Gans, BM (eds): Rehabilitation Medicine: Principles and Practice, ed 2. JB Lippincott, Philadelphia, 1993.

Halar, EM and Bell, KR: Rehabilitation's Relationship to Inactivity. Chapter 52. In Kottke, FJ and Lehmann, JF (eds): Krusen's Handbook of Physical Medicine and Rehabilitation, ed 4. WB Saunders, Philadelphia, 1990.

Harper, C and Lyles, Y: Physiology and Complications of Bed Rest. J Am Geriatr Soc 36:1047, 1988.

Milde, FK: Physiological Immobilization. Chapter 5. In Hart, LK, Reese, JL, and Fearing, MD (eds): Concepts Common to Acute Illness: Identification and Management. CV Mosby, St. Louis, 1981.

Mobily, PR and Kelly, LS: Iatrogenesis in the Elderly: Factors of Immobility. J Gerontol Nurs, 17(9):25, 1991.

Nickel, VL and Botte, MJ (eds): Orthopaedic Rehabilitation, ed 2. Churchill Livingstone, New York, 1992.

Olson, EV: The Hazards of Immobility. Am J Nurs 67:780, 1967.

Salter, RB: Textbook of Disorders and Injuries of the Musculoskeletal System, ed 2. Williams & Wilkins, Baltimore, 1983.

Sandler, H and Vernikos, J (eds): Inactivity: Physiological Effects. Academic Press, Orlando, 1986.

Steinberg, FV (ed): Immobilized Patient: Functional Pathology and Management. Plenum Medical Book Company, New York, 1980.

Sugarman, B: Medical Complications of Spinal Cord Injury. Quart J Med Series 54(213):3, 1985.

REFERENCES

1. Lieber, RL: Skeletal Muscle Adaption to Decreased Use. Chapter 5. Skeletal Muscle Structure and Function. In Williams & Wilkins, Baltimore, 1992.

2. Appell, H-J: Muscular Atrophy Following Immobilization: A Review. Sports Med 10(1):42, 1990.

3. Sandler, H: Effects of Inactivity on Muscle. Chapter 4. In Sandler, H and Vernikos, J (eds): Inactivity: Physiologic Effects. Academic Press, Orlando, 1986.

4. Halar, EM and Bell, KR: Rehabilitation's Relationship to Inactivity. Chapter 52. In Kottke, FJ and Lehmann, JF (eds): Krusen's Handbook of Physical Medicine and Rehabilitation, ed 4. WB Saunders, Philadelphia, 1990.

5. Booth, FW: Physiological and Biochemical Effects of Immobilization on Muscle. Clin Orthop 219:15, 1987.

6. Steinberg, FU (ed): Immobilized Patient: Functional Pathology and Management. Plenum Medical Book Company, New York, 1980. Chapter 4.

7. Harper, C and Lyles, Y: Physiology and Complications of Bed Rest. J Am Geriatr Soc 36:1047, 1988.

8. Halar, EM and Bell, KR: Contracture and Other Deleterious Effects of Immobility. Chapter 33. In Delisa, JA and Gans, BM (eds): Rehabilitation Medicine: Principles and Practice, ed 2. JB Lippincott, Philadelphia, 1993.

9. Duthie, RB and Young, A (eds): Pathophysiology of Joint Contractures and Their Correction: A Symposium. Clin Orthop 219:1, 1987.

10. Perry, J: Contractures: A Historical Perspective. Clin Orthop 219:8, 1987.

11. Olson, EV: The Hazards of Immobility. Am J Nurs 67:780, 1967.

12. Milde, FK: Physiological Immobilization. Chapter 5. In Hart, LK, Reese, JL, and Fearing, MO (eds): Concepts Common to Acute Illness: Identification and Management. CV Mosby, St. Louis, 1981.

13. Steinberg, FU (ed): Immobilized Patient: Functional Pathology and Management. Plenum Medical Book Company, New York, 1980. Chapter 3.

14. Arnaud, SB, Schneider, VS, and Morey-Hilton, E: Effect of Inactivity on Bone and Calcium Metabolism. Chapter 3. In Sandler, H and Vernikos, J (eds): Inactivity: Physiologic Effects. Academic Press, Orlando, 1986.

15. Mazess, RB and Whedon, GD: Immobilization and Bone. Calcif Tissue Int 35:265, 1982.

16. LeBlanc, AD, et al: Bone Loss and Recovery After 17 Weeks of Bed Rest. J Bone Min Res 5(8):843, 1990.

17. Mobily, PR and Kelly LS: Iatrogenesis in the Elderly: Factors of Immobility. J Gerontol Nurs 17(9):25, 1991.

18. Sugarman, B: Medical Complications of Spinal Cord Injury. Q J Med 54(213):3, 1985.

19. Coletta, EM and Murphy, JB: The Complications of Immobility in the Elderly Stroke Patient. J Am Board Fam Pract 5:389, 1992.

20. Akeson, WH, et al: Effects of Immobilization on Joints. Clin Orthop 219:28, 1987.

21. Enneking, WF and Horowitz, M: The Intra-Articular Effects of Immobilization on the Human Knee. J Bone Joint Surg 54A:973, 1972.

22. Lal, S, et al: Risk Factors for Heterotopic Ossification in Spinal Cord Injury. Arch Phys Med Rehabil 70:387, 1989.

23. Stover, SL: Heterotopic Ossification After Spinal Cord Injury. Chapter 11. In Bloch, RF and Basbaum, M (eds): Management of Spinal Cord Injuries. Williams & Wilkins, Baltimore, 1986.

24. Davies, PM: Starting Again: Early Rehabilitation After Traumatic Brain Injury or Other Severe Brain Lesion. Chapter 6. Overcoming Limitation of Movement, Contracture, and Deformity. Springer-Verlag, Berlin, 1994.

25. Garland, DE: Heterotopic Ossification. Chapter 35. In Nickel, VL and Botte, MJ (eds): Orthopaedic Rehabilitation, ed 2. Churchill Livingstone, New York, 1992.

26. Schmitz, TJ: Traumatic Spinal Cord Injury. Chapter 26. In O'Sullivan, SB and Schmitz, TJ: Physical Rehabilitation: Assessment and Treatment, ed 2. FA Davis, Philadelphia, 1988.

27. Sugarman, B: Osteomyelitis in Spinal Cord Injury. Arch Phys Med Rehabil 65:132, 1984.

CHAPTER 24

■

Adverse Effects of Immobilization on Visceral Function

Christopher M. Fredericks, PhD

- ■ *Effects on the Respiratory System*
- ■ *Effects on the Cardiovascular System*
- ■ *Effects on the Urinary Tract*
- ■ *Effects on the Skin*
- ■ *Effects on the Gastrointestinal Tract*

The morbidity and mortality associated with locomotor dysfunction do not arise from impaired neuromuscular activity per se, but from the impact that disordered motor activity has on other physiologic systems. Neuromuscular dysfunction, whether it is due to disease or injury, can exert a variety of adverse effects on visceral activity (Fig. 24–1). **First, the primary motor disorder may have direct effects on specific visceral systems.** For example, both central and peripheral neurologic disorders by disrupting autonomic nervous system pathways may impair specific visceral activities. Prominent among the complications of such diseases are abnormalities of vasomotor, urogenital, and gastrointestinal function. **Second, chronic impairment of motor function, by causing immobilization, may give rise to a whole cascade of medical complications due to inactivity and recumbency.** The clinical manifestations of immobilization are multiple and reflect the fact that prolonged inactivity causes marked physiologic and biochemical changes in practically all organs and systems of the body.[1-8] With prolonged immobilization, even a healthy person will develop a range of complications, including cardiovascular inefficiency, impaired respiration, urinary tract infections, and skin breakdown (Table 24–1). These complications are most severe with prolonged recumbency and are worse in the chronically ill or elderly patient.

Although this discussion is focused on patients whose physical activity is restricted by neuromuscular dysfunction, it should be remembered that **many different types of patients are also subjected to prolonged bed rest or inactivity and are thus susceptible to developing these same medical consequences.** Physical therapists are involved in the management of these complications in orthopedic, transplant, burn, surgical, geriatric, psychiatric, and chronically ill patients. Regardless of the cause of the immobilization, the medical complications may often lead to a greater degree of disability than that caused by the

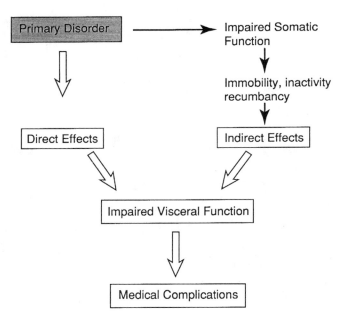

Figure 24–1. Direct and indirect effects of motor disorders upon visceral function.

initial illness or injury. It is tragic that although modern medicine can, in many cases, do little to correct the underlying motor deficit, most of the immobility-related complications are readily preventable.

Effects on the Respiratory System

Respiratory complications of immobility and motor dysfunction are common and often severe.[1,3,5,6,8–10] After prolonged immobilization, many patients suffer from chronic respiratory insufficiency. Ultimately, additional acute respiratory problems, such as infection or aspiration, may be superimposed and become life-threatening.

Impaired Respiratory Movements (Ventilatory Mechanics)

The pressure/volume changes that are necessary for ventilation of the lungs are dependent on adequate respiratory muscle strength and coordination, and adequate mobility in the thoracic cage, all of which **can be significantly impaired in the immobilized patient.** The mechanical restriction of ventilation caused by recumbency itself reduces tidal volume, minute volume, and maximum breathing capacity.[1,4,5,9,10] In the supine position, the vital capacity of the lungs may be decreased by 4%.[1] Protracted sitting and lying postures directly restrict diaphragmatic and thoracic movement and increase the work of breathing. Moreover, the shifting of abdominal contents toward the head elevates the diaphragm and restricts its descent, whereas the external pressure exerted by the bed or chair impedes chest expansion. In the immobilized patient, other factors may also contribute to impeded respiratory movement.[6] For example, decreased thoracic mobility can result from skeletal deformity (e.g., scoliosis), progressive stiffness or ankylosis of rib cage joints, or abnormalities in intercostal muscle tone. Decreased respiratory muscle strength and coordination can result from both disuse and denervation. Decreased central respiratory drive may result from concomitant neurologic damage (e.g., stroke), attenuated responsiveness due to chronic hypoxemia, or centrally active drugs such as sedatives and narcotics. As a result, breathing

Table 24–1. *Adverse Effects of Prolonged Immobilization on Visceral Function*

Respiratory System

    Impaired ventilatory movements
    Decreased vital capacity and maximal minute ventilation
    Changes in ventilation/perfusion ratio
    Impaired coughing
    Stasis and pooling of secretions
    Atelectasis
    Infections
    Pneumonia
    Aspiration

Cardiovascular System

    Alterations in the volume and distribution of body fluids
    Cardiac deconditioning and exercise intolerance
    Orthostatic hypotension
    Deep venous thrombosis and pulmonary embolism

Urinary System

    Stasis of urine
    Renal stones (calculi)
    Infections
    Neurogenic bladder; detrusor/external sphincter dyssynergia
    Urinary retention or incontinence
    Autonomic hyperreflexia

Integumentary System

    Pressure sores
    Infections
    Malignancy

Gastrointestinal System

    Loss of appetite
    Decreased food intake and absorption
    Fecal incontinence
    Gas trapping
    Constipation, impaction, obstruction
    Poor nutrition and loss of weight

in the immobilized patient tends to be more shallow, to occur with increased rate, and to expend more energy than that of the normal person.

Ventilatory problems may be particularly severe in spinal cord–injured patients.[9–12] All patients with quadriplegia and those with high paraplegia have significant impairment of ventilation (see Chapter 17). The higher the level of the spinal cord lesion, the greater the loss of respiratory function. Ventilation is particularly ineffective in quadriplegics, in whom difficulties in both inspiration and expiration exist. As the level of the lesion rises, the primary muscles responsible for inspiration (diaphragm and external intercostals) are progressively lost, resulting in ventilation becoming increasingly difficult and uncoordinated, and increasingly dependent on the accessory muscles. By the same token, the muscles that assist in expiration (abdominals and internal intercostals) may also be lost. Although normal expiration is largely a passive process caused by the elastic recoil of the lungs and thorax, with spinal cord lesions at the T-12 level and above expiration becomes an increasingly active and labored process. Musculoskeletal trauma to the thoracic cage and shoulder girdle can further compromise ventilation on an acute basis, as well as create long-term impairment of thoracic mobility. Lung contusions and other soft tissue injury can leave residual lung and intrathoracic scarring that can further impede ventilation. As a consequence of all these factors, ventilation in the high spinal cord–injured patient is insufficient and requires a much greater expenditure of energy than normal.

Stasis and Pooling of Secretions

The respiratory tract is lined by ciliated mucous membrane, which produces protective, sticky secretions. In a healthy individual, these secretions are continually cleared from the respiratory system. **In immobilized patients, these secretions tend to accumulate because cleansing mechanisms are impaired.**[1] Recumbency in particular makes the clearance of pulmonary secretions difficult. Just being in the supine position interferes with the efficiency of the pulmonary cilia, which under normal conditions sweep mucus from the bronchi to the trachea and larynx. In a person in the upright position, the bronchioles run vertically and their epithelium is covered by a thin, even layer of mucus. In a person in the supine position, the same bronchioles are horizontal. Gravity now makes the mucus collect on the lower side of the bronchiole, whereas the upper wall loses its covering of mucus and may become dry.[8,10] Both the excessive pooling of mucus on the bottom and the desiccation of the mucous membrane on the top interfere with the cleansing action of the cilia. In addition, because the diaphragm is elevated by the pressure of the abdominal viscera and the large thoracic vessels are engorged while recumbent, intrathoracic pressure is less negative and bronchiolar diameter is reduced. As a consequence, the mucous layer lining the bronchioles becomes proportionately thicker, increasing the chance of obstruction (Fig. 24–2). Moreover, the restriction of diaphragmatic and intercostal motion that is inherent in the supine position and the muscle weakness caused by immobilization impair coughing, which is the primary mechanism for clearing secretions.[1,4]

Clearing of pulmonary secretions is all the more difficult in immobilized patients in whom muscle and nerve dysfunction create additional muscle weakness. Chest expansion is further reduced, coughing more impaired, and postural changes, which facilitate the clearance of secretions, may be impossible. In quadriplegics, for example, coughing is markedly impaired and the clearance of secretions is an ongoing objective of medical management.[9,11,12]

The eventual result of the accumulation of secretions is the formation of thick mucus plugs at the ends of the bronchial tubes, which impede gaseous exchange, are very difficult to expectorate, and provide an ideal medium for bacterial growth. Airways may eventually be occluded, leading to regional lung collapse (atelectasis) and pneumonia. The dependent pulmonary segments of immobilized patients are especially poorly ventilated. Since blood perfusion of these regions continues at a normal rate, the ventilation/perfusion ratio is distorted, leading to increasing arteriovenous shunting.[8]

The combination of impaired ventilatory mechanics and the accumulation of pulmonary secretions can significantly impair the alveolar exchange of oxygen and carbon dioxide. Chronic hypoxemia, hypercapnia, and respiratory acidosis can result. Although these disturbances may initially serve to stimulate ventilation, they ultimately lead to further depression of respiratory drive and impair the function of all body organs.[6] Moreover, inefficient ventilation and bronchiolar obstruction can so increase the work of breathing that little capacity for increased respiratory effort is available to meet any increased metabolic demands exerted by the patient. Respiratory exhaustion can lead to catastrophic respiratory failure.

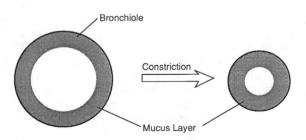

Bronchiole

Constriction

Mucus Layer

Figure 24–2. Cross Section of a Mucus-Lined Bronchiole. As the bronchiolar diameter decreases an increasing percentage of the cross section is occupied by the unchanging layer of mucus.

Pharyngeal, epiglottal, and esophageal weakness creates an additional hazard to the extent that aspiration of fluid, food, and oronasopharyngeal secretions predispose infection and may cause choking.

Many of these serious respiratory complications can be prevented or their effects minimized if they are anticipated and treated aggressively. Strategies that include mobilization of the trunk, postural support, respiratory muscle training, assistive coughing techniques, and teaching the patient more efficient breathing patterns should be initiated in those at risk.

Effects on the Cardiovascular System

Immobilization and inactivity have significant effects on the cardiovascular system. These effects are all the more pronounced when prolonged periods of recumbency accompany inactivity.[1-8,13]

Increased Cardiac Workload

When a patient is placed in the supine position, about 11% of the total blood volume shifts from the lower extremities into the thoracic circulation. As a result, **cardiac workload is increased about 20% when the body is recumbent,** even in normally healthy individuals.[1-3]

Redistribution of Body Fluids

Recumbency, even in healthy individuals, leads to significant alterations in the volume and distribution of various body fluids. During standing, the force of gravity on the blood in the vessels of the trunk and lower extremities results in a shift of about 700 mL of blood into the legs. In the supine position, this hydrostatic pressure is eliminated, causing 500 to 700 mL of blood to return to the lungs and the right side of the heart.[1,4,7] This increases the central blood volume and pressure stimulating baroreceptors, which results in suppression of antidiuretic hormone release. As a result, **recumbency leads to a diuresis, which during the first few days of bed rest can cause an 8% to 10% loss of plasma volume.** Plasma volume ultimately tends to stabilize with a 15% to 20% decrease after 2 to 4 weeks. Red blood cell volume shrinks proportionately less than the plasma volume, so that the hematocrit increases.

The initial response to this redistribution of blood volume differs from the long-term response. Initially, the augmentation of central blood volume that occurs with lying down causes an increase in heart rate, stroke volume, and cardiac output. However, the continual activation of baroreceptors and more chronic changes in myocardial performance cause reversal of these initial cardiogenic responses and result in a progressive reduction of stroke volume and cardiac output.

Deconditioning and Exercise Intolerance

Prolonged bed rest and inactivity result in a progressive decline in basal cardiac activity. During periods of bed rest, heart size, left ventricular end-diastolic volume, stroke volume, and cardiac output all decrease, while the resting pulse rate increases (about 1 beat per minute every 2 days).[4,7,8,14] These deleterious changes in cardiac function are a reflection of reduced blood volume, reduced venous return, and the reduced metabolic demands associated with inactivity and loss of muscle mass.

Tolerance to both supine and upright exercise also progressively declines. A reduced capacity for work is reflected in significantly reduced maximum oxygen uptake, lower stroke volume during submaximal exercise, and a higher than normal heart rate at any given level of oxygen uptake.[14] Although diminished myocardial performance itself contributes to the reduced capacity for exercise, other factors are probably also involved. Reduced venomotor tone, reduced muscular pumping in the lower extremities, reduced venous return, skeletal muscle deconditioning, alterations in oxygen utilization by tissues, and poor ventilatory dynamics all may play a role in deconditioning.[14]

Orthostatic (Postural) Hypotension

When a person moves from a recumbent to an upright position, 10% to 15% of the blood volume shifts into the lower extremities due to gravity. The immediate effects of this fluid shift are reductions in venous return, heart stroke volume, and cardiac output. In a normal individual, compensatory mechanisms such as vasoconstriction and increased heart rate allow such changes in position to be made with little change in blood pressure or oxygen delivery to the brain. **Following prolonged bed rest or inactivity, assumption of an upright position may be accompanied by sudden reductions in systolic and diastolic blood pressure and marked elevation of heart rate. This is termed** *orthostatic intolerance or postural hypotension.*[1,4,7,8,10,15] Excessive pooling of blood in the lower extremities and a resultant hypotension may cause dizziness, light-headedness, and even sudden loss of consciousness (syncope) on rising. In patients with coronary artery disease, angina may also be triggered.

Orthostatic hypotension is one of the most common hazards of prolonged bed rest and inactivity, even in otherwise normal individuals. In healthy individuals, the ability to adjust to the upright position is lost after only 1 or 2 weeks of bed rest. It may be particularly severe in higher-level (generally above T-6) spinal cord–injured patients, especially quadriplegics, in whom numerous autonomic pathways are disrupted. In either case, such episodes may be largely prevented by shifting a patient to the upright position gradually, while monitoring the effect on their blood pressure.

Although all the mechanisms by which immobilization promotes orthostatic intolerance are not fully understood, a major contributor is the excessive pooling of venous blood in the lower extremities that is caused by changes in both skeletal muscle and autonomic nervous system activity. Skeletal muscles in the lower extremities normally apply pressure to the venous system and serve to "pump" venous blood back to the heart. With decreased skeletal muscle tone and strength, either due to the deconditioning of inactivity or denervation, venous return is impaired and pooling promoted. In many immobilized patients, autonomic reflexes are impaired, and the normal compensatory changes in vasoconstriction and heart rate that normally compensate for shifting to an upright posture cannot be made. In patients with high spinal cord lesions, for example, the areas of the brainstem that promote peripheral vasoconstriction in compensation for reduced blood pressure are disconnected from much of the peripheral vasculature. In addition, beta-sympathetic activity is increased during bed rest and may contribute to the orthostatic loss by promoting peripheral vasodilation.

As mentioned earlier, salt and water diuresis and a resultant reduction in total blood volume often accompany prolonged recumbency. Although not proven, it has been suggested that a reduced effective circulating blood volume may also contribute to orthostatic hypotension.[8]

Deep Venous Thrombosis and Pulmonary Embolus

A thrombus is an abnormal blood clot that has formed at some site within a blood vessel. Each thrombus has the potential to break free from this site and to float freely within the bloodstream. These mobile clots, which are known as **emboli,** are particularly prone to lodging in and obstructing pulmonary blood vessels (pulmonary embolism).

Deep venous thrombosis and pulmonary embolism are among the most common and most serious complications occurring in immobilized patients.[1,3–5,8,13,16] In patients who are immobilized or are recovering from surgery, most thrombi arise in the veins of lower extremities, especially the calf, and often remain localized and asymptomatic. However, if untreated, extension into the popliteal, femoral, or iliac veins may occur, creating the risk of significant obstruction of venous return or the occurrence of pulmonary embolism. For reasons not entirely understood, deep venous thrombosis is particularly common following spinal cord injury.[10,16–19] It has been reported to occur in 15% to 60% of spinal cord–injured patients and is a major cause of early morbidity and mortality. The period of greatest risk seems to be during the several months after injury, but thrombosis can appear within days of injury. Deep venous thrombosis develops more frequently in complete than incomplete lesions and with greater frequency in thoracic and cervical injury. The reported incidence of fatal pulmonary emboli in spinal cord–injured patients ranges from 2% to 16%, within the first 2 to 3 years following the injury.[16]

Three basic factors create a predisposition for thrombus formation: changes in blood flow, changes in the coagulability of the blood, and changes in the vessel wall. All these factors may be present to varying degrees in the immobilized patient. As we have seen, venous stasis often occurs in the lower extremities of these patients because of the lack of skeletal muscle pumping. In addition, mechanical compression of leg veins during bed rest exacerbates this stasis. With decreased blood flow, thrombi are more likely to be initiated and propagated. Prolonged inactivity and recumbency, by reducing the volume and increasing the viscosity of the blood, may make it hypercoagulable. Moreover, blood factors directly involved in clotting may be abnormal. For example, it is known that changes in plasma procoagulants and fibrinogen, increases in the number and reactivity of platelets,[8,16] and alterations in fibrinolysis all are common in patients after injury or surgery. The vessel endothelium ordinarily does not support the formation of thrombi. However, in certain patients this endothelium seems to be damaged, predisposing platelet adherence and the initiation of thrombogenesis.[16]

A number of additional factors are thought to increase the risk of deep venous thrombosis in bedridden patients, such as trauma, increasing age, obesity, malignancy, heart disease, the use of oral contraceptives, or a history of prior venous thromboembolism.[16] Several of these risk factors may coexist and multiply the usual risk to the patient.

Although deep venous thromboses are often clinically silent, they may manifest as deep pain in the calf, unilateral limb edema, locally increased temperature, and a positive Homans' sign (pain in the leg when the foot is passively dorsiflexed). Clinical manifestations of pulmonary emboli vary widely and reflect the size of the embolism and the preexisting condition of the heart and lungs. Pulmonary emboli may be indicated by pleuritic chest pain, rapid (tachypnea) or labored (dyspnea) breathing, bloody expectorate, or tachycardia. All therapists should be familiar with the clinical signs of these serious conditions. Because they may foster thrombus progression or embolization, weight-bearing and range-of-motion activities should be performed with care in patients with thromboembolic disease or at particular risk for thrombus formation (e.g., following orthopedic surgery, myocardial infarction, stroke, or spinal cord injury).

Effects on the Urinary Tract

Inactivity, particularly when accompanied by prolonged periods of recumbency, can lead to deleterious changes in urinary tract function. The end result of these alterations is an increased incidence of bladder or renal stones (calculi) and urinary tract infections.[1,2,4]

Calculi

With immobilization and recumbency, several factors combine to promote stone formation (lithiasis).[4,6,10] First, both calcium and phosphates are present in the urine in increased amounts owing to osteopenia (see Chapter 23), creating an overabundance of the minerals involved in stone formation. Second, stagnation of urine may exist in both the upper and lower urinary tract. Not only is urine flow from the renal pelvis and ureters slowed without the normal assistance of gravity, but it is more difficult to empty the bladder in the supine position. The restricted diaphragmatic movements of recumbency and weakened abdominal muscles make it more difficult to generate the increased intra-abdominal pressure necessary for complete bladder emptying. Third, with prolonged immobilization, the urine becomes more alkaline because of the lack of the acidic metabolites of muscle metabolism. **Stasis of alkaline urine combined with hypercalciuria provides an ideal environment for stone formation** (Fig. 24–3).

Infection

Incomplete bladder emptying promotes infection, which further promotes stone development.[4,10] Once formed, these stones provide a locus for further bacterial growth, creating a self-propelling cycle of stone and bacterial proliferation. Irritation and trauma to the mucosa by stones can further increase the likelihood of bacterial infection. Calculi may become large enough to damage the kidney or to obstruct the flow of urine from the kidney through the ureter or from the urinary bladder. As obstruction develops, further urinary

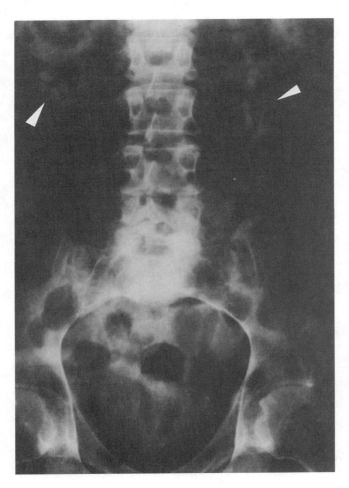

Figure 24–3. Kidney Stones. In this radiograph of the abdomen of a quadriplegic person 8 months after a cervical spinal cord injury, kidney stones are evident as small radiopaque shapes in both the right and left kidney areas. There is also extensive osteoporosis of the spine and pelvis. (From Kottke, FJ, Stillwell, GK, and Lehmann, JF (eds): *Krusen's Handbook of Physical Medicine and Rehabilitation*, ed 3. WB Saunders, Philadelphia, 1982, p 972, with permission.)

stasis and distention may develop facilitating additional bacterial growth and threatening renal infection.

Long-term catheterization of immobilized patients further increases the likelihood of urinary tract infections. Fecal incontinence and inadequate perianal hygiene are also predisposing factors, particularly in women, in whom the short urethra provides easy access for pathogenic organisms (especially *Escherichia coli*).

Neurogenic Bladder

All the complications of the urinary tract are aggravated by the presence of neurologic diseases affecting the bladder innervation, such as spinal cord injury, multiple sclerosis, or diabetes mellitus.[19-22] Spinal cord–injured patients are at particular risk for developing of urinary tract complications, which represent a major cause of morbidity and death (see Chapter 17). An estimated two thirds of all paraplegics develop urinary tract infections. **In patients with neurologic disorders, the urinary complications of immobilization are made all the worse by the disruption of nervous pathways necessary for the contraction of the detrusor muscle in coordination with relaxation of the urinary sphincters.**

Neural dysfunction can affect urinary function in many different ways, depending on the location and extent of the injury.[19-22] In the case of spinal cord injury, the first few weeks following injury are generally characterized by a period of markedly reduced neural activity, **spinal shock**, during which the bladder is paralyzed and flaccid, resulting in urinary retention and often overflow incontinence. Once spinal shock begins to resolve, the extent of the residual neurologic deficit becomes evident. Injury to the spinal cord that occurs above the level of the sacral cord, thereby leaving the major bladder reflex arcs intact, is termed an **upper motor neuron lesion.** An automatic, reflex, or spastic bladder results. With this disruption of the neural connections to higher centers, conscious awareness of fullness and voluntary motor control is lost. Reflex pathways below the level of the lesion become disinhibited and hyperirritable, resulting in hyperactivity and hypertrophy of the detrusor, spasms of the striated urethral sphincters, and dyssynergy between contraction of the detrusor and relaxation of the outlet (urethral) sphincters (Fig. 24–4). As a result, bladder capacity is reduced and high intravesical pressure may develop. Such a bladder can often be retrained to respond to stimuli such as tapping the suprapubic area or pulling pubic hairs. Injury that actually disrupts the sacral reflex pathways is termed a **lower motor neuron lesion** and results in a paralytic or areflexic bladder. With disruption of the sacral reflexes themselves, the detrusor remains flaccid and striated muscle tone is diminished. As a result, the bladder capacity is increased with low intravesical pressure and high residual volumes. Although the detrusor cannot contract, in some cases fairly efficient bladder emptying can be accomplished by using unparalyzed abdominal muscles to raise intra-abdominal pressure or by manual suprapubic pressure.

In the case of either an upper or lower motor neuron lesion, if adequate bladder emptying is not possible, long-term catheterization will be necessary.

A neurogenic bladder makes the common complications of infections and stones all the more likely. Catheterization facilitates the entry of bacteria into the bladder. Reflux of urine up the ureters to the kidneys may result from outflow obstruction (e.g., due to sphincter spasms), elevated intravesical pressure, or faulty ureterovesical valves. This may lead ultimately to renal damage and impaired renal function. Renal failure is a common late cause of death in male spinal cord–injured patients.[19]

Autonomic Dysreflexia (Hyperreflexia)

Although autonomic dysreflexia is not a consequence of immobilization per se, it often accompanies spinal cord injury and may be triggered by the sequelae of immobilization.

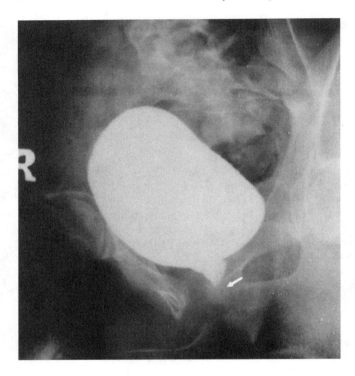

Figure   24–4. Detrusor/External Sphincter Dyssynergia. In this radiograph in which the bladder is filled with radiopaque dye, it is apparent that the hyperreflexic bladder is contracting but not emptying because there is a concurrent spasm in the area of the external sphincter (*Arrow*). The patient is an 18-year-old man with complete paraplegia 12 months after a spinal lesion at T-8. (From Goodgold, J (ed): Rehabilitation Medicine. CV Mosby, St. Louis, 1988, p 185, with permission.)

Autonomic dysreflexia is a paroxysmal syndrome of excessive autonomic activity, which is manifested by hypertension, bradycardia, excessive sweating (hyperhidrosis), facial flushing, and headache (Table 24–2).[15,19,33] Increases in blood pressure are marked and may reach 100 to 200 mm Hg systolic and 50 to 100 mm Hg diastolic, or higher. Many other symptoms of abnormal autonomic activity may occur including piloerection, nasal conges-

Table 24–2. Autonomic Dysreflexia

Stimuli	Clinical Manifestations
Bladder distention	Paroxysmal hypertension
Bladder infection	Bradycardia or tachycardia
Urethral/bladder irritation	Cardiac arrhythmia
Defecation and rectal distention	Pounding headache
Bowel impaction	Vasoconstriction (below the level of the lesion)
Rectal stimulation	Vasodilatation: flushing, blotching of skin, cold sweating
Noxious cutaneous stimulation	(above the level of the lesion)
Gastric irritation	Piloerection
Menstrual cramps	Pupillary dilatation and other eye signs
Labor and delivery	Blurring of vision
Genital stimulation	Anxiety, apprehension
Range-of-motion exercises	Unresponsiveness
Muscle spasm	Nasal congestion
Changes in environmental temperature	Nausea, vomiting
Infected pressure sores	Syncope
Surgery	Paresthesias
	Penile erection
	Dyspnea
	Convulsions
	Intracranial hemorrhage

Adapted from Schneider.[11]

tion, and pupillary dilation. Severe complications, although rare, include retinal hemorrhage and visual loss, convulsions, aphasia, and death as a result of massive intracranial bleeding.

Autonomic dysreflexia is elicited by noxious stimuli to the body, especially to the skin and viscera below the level of the spinal cord injury (see Table 24–2). It frequently occurs in response to distention of the urinary bladder (e.g., cystoscopy) or rectum (e.g., defecation).

Autonomic hyperreflexia is bladder-related in more than 85% of cases, resulting from overdistention, catheter blockage, urinary tract infection, stones, decubitus ulcers, ingrown toenails, cutaneous stimulation, spontaneous and induced muscle spasms, range-of-motion exercises, electrical stimulation for the collection of semen for artificial insemination, labor and delivery, menstrual cramps, and genital stimulation during sexual activity.

Most instances of autonomic dysreflexia occur within the first year after injury with an incidence as high as 85% in adult quadriplegics.[15,19] Frequently, it subsides within several years of injury, but it can recur even after many years of quiescence. The incidence is lower in children.

The pathophysiology of autonomic dysreflexia is not fully understood. It occurs primarily in spinal cord–injured patients with complete and incomplete lesions at the T-6 spinal level or higher and reflects dissociation of the sympathetic spinal reflexes still active below the lesion from supraspinal inhibitory control above the lesion (Fig. 24–5). Afferent impulses from organs such as the rectum or bladder reach the spinal cord where they may initiate segmental reflexes or ascend to synapse with neurons in the thoracic cord, initiating autonomic vasoconstrictor reflexes. The resulting rise in blood pressure stimulates the aortic and carotid sinus reflexes; however, a coordinated readjustment of the peripheral resistance cannot be achieved through the autonomic nervous system because of the spinal cord lesion. A marked bradycardia and irregularities of heart rhythm may occur. Other mechanisms that might contribute to this response are denervation hypersensitivity of sympathetic spinal, ganglionic, or peripheral receptor sites and the formation of abnormal synaptic connections due to axonal sprouting.

The physical therapist should be aware of the types of noxious stimuli common to a physical therapy setting, which might precipitate autonomic dysreflexia, and of the established protocols for medical management of this problem. The therapist should be

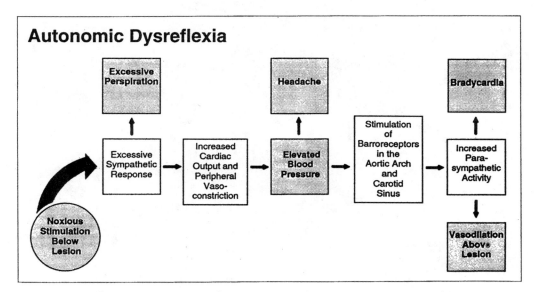

Figure 24–5. Schematic Representation of Autonomic Dysreflexia. Clinical signs and symptoms are in the darkened boxes. (From Somers, MF: Spinal Cord Injury. Functional Rehabilitation. Appleton & Lange, Norwalk, CT, 1991, p 31, with permission.)

aware that simple factors such as blockage or twisting of a urinary catheter, traction on a catheter or pressure on the penis, scrotum, or urethra, painful cutaneous stimuli below the level of the lesion, and even muscle stretch can trigger autonomic dysreflexia.

Treatment of autonomic dysreflexia includes identification and removal of the trigger stimulus, elevating the patient's torso to induce venous pooling in the legs and thereby decreasing cardiac output, and antihypertensive medication.

Effects on the Skin

Deleterious changes in the skin create much of the morbidity associated with immobilization and promote infections that can become life-threatening.

Decubitus Ulcers

Decubitus ulcers, also known as bed sores, pressure sores, pressure ulcers, and pressure necroses, constitute the major hazards confronting any patient with restricted mobility (Fig. 24–6).[8,24–30] The largest group at risk for developing pressure sores are patients with spinal cord injury. However, many other patients with impaired sensation or mobility are susceptible. The prevalence of pressure sores is estimated to range from 4% to 14% among hospitalized persons, 9% to 19% among those cared for in their homes, and 12% to 23% among persons cared for in long-term care facilities.[27] In patients with spinal cord injury, an incidence of 24% to 85% has been reported.[19,29] Elderly and hemiplegic patients (i.e., stroke) and those with multiple sclerosis or hip replacement also frequently develop pressure sores.

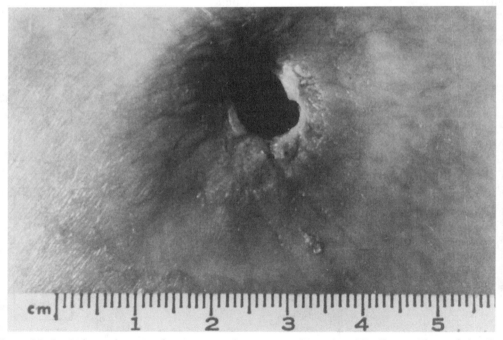

Figure 24–6. Right trochanteric ulcer in a paraplegic patient. (From Lee, BY: Chronic Ulcers of the Skin. McGraw-Hill, New York, 1985, p 159, with permission.)

Decubitus ulcers are open wounds created by the local necrosis of skin and underlying tissues. These sores vary markedly both in their size and in the extent to which underlying structures are involved (Fig. 24–7). Pressure sores range in severity from erythema to massive lesions involving joint structures, which can lead to profound osteomyelitis with subsequent amputation (Fig. 24–8). They can be remarkably deceiving in that the visible skin wound may be small, whereas the subcutaneous tissue destruction may be extensive. They may form sinus tracts that connect with a large abscess cavity or an adjacent joint.

Any areas of skin that are exposed to prolonged or excessive pressure are likely sites for ulcer development, especially where bony prominences are close to the surface. The most frequently involved areas are the sacrum, the trochanters of the hip, the ischial rami, the malleoli, and the heels. All these are sites at which the greatest pressures are exerted in the supine position and sites with relatively little tissue interposed between the skin and bone (Fig. 24–9).[26]

Although the exact mechanisms of soft tissue breakdown and ulcer formation are not completely understood, as the name implies, **pressure sores are thought to be due primarily to pressure-induced ischemia depriving tissues of the oxygen and nutrients they require for survival.** The dermis has a richer blood supply than the underlying subcutaneous fat, which may explain why larger areas of the fatty tissue may be involved (necrosed) than of the overlying skin.

Under normal circumstances, the skin is protected by frequent movements that shift the body weight from one area to another. The immobilized patient, however, is incapable of performing these weight shifts, so the same skin areas remain under pressure for long periods of time. If these forces are great enough to disrupt capillary flow, cellular metabolism will be impaired, leading to tissue necrosis. The extent of ischemic injury and the likelihood of ulcer formation reflect of both the magnitude of the pressure and the time for which the tissue is exposed to that pressure. Decubitus ulcers can develop very quickly. One episode of intense pressure applied over a bony prominence can result in tissue necrosis. By the same token, repeated ischemia from pressures insufficient to cause acute tissue necrosis may result in gradual replacement by fibrotic tissue. This is noted first in the subcutaneous fat layer, and

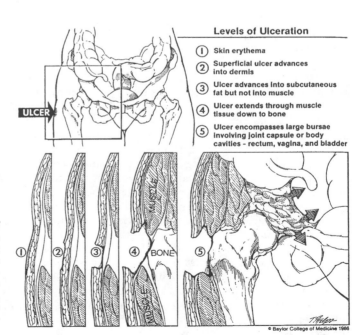

Levels of Ulceration

1. Skin erythema
2. Superficial ulcer advances into dermis
3. Ulcer advances into subcutaneous fat but not into muscle
4. Ulcer extends through muscle tissue down to bone
5. Ulcer encompasses large bursae involving joint capsule or body cavities – rectum, vagina, and bladder

Figure 24–7. Classification of Pressure Ulcers. This figure depicts the depth of tissue involvement for each grade of pressure ulcer. (From Delisa, JA and Gans, BM (eds): Rehabilitation Medicine: Principles and Practice, ed 2. JB Lippincott, Philadelphia, 1993, p 722, with permission. Copyright © Baylor College of Medicine 1986.)

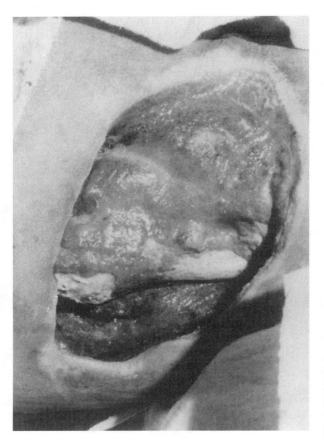

Figure 24–8. Large Decubitus Ulcer in the Hip Region with Exposed Greater Trochanter. Osteomyelitis commonly develops when bone is exposed. (From Nickel, VL and Botte, MJ: Orthopaedic Rehabilitation, ed 2. Churchill Livingstone, New York, 1992, p 450, with permission.)

later in the dermis. Eventually, a stage will be reached at which thin fragile skin overlies dense fibrous tissue and constitutes a site vulnerable for future injury and ulcer formation.

Direct compressive forces may be brought to bear upon the skin. During normal activities such as lying, sitting, or leaning against another surface, relatively small volumes of tissue are compressed between bony prominences and the external surface. Since nearly all the weight is supported at these sites, extremely high pressures can be generated in the tissues compressed between the weight-bearing bone and the external surface. A poorly fitting wheelchair, cast, bandage, clothing, or shoes may also cause direct pressure on an area of skin. In addition, **shearing forces** may be imposed on the skin as one surface slides over another. These forces place blood vessels under stretch and may cause multiple small-vessel thromboses, compounding the ischemia produced by external pressure. Sliding down in bed against the sacral skin, poor turning and transfer techniques, and sliding rather than lifting, all increase shearing forces. **Friction**, which develops when patients are pulled across bed linens, may damage the protective epidermis of the skin. **Spasticity**, which is common in spinal cord–injured, stroke, and other neurologically impaired patients, may aggravate these pressures by interfering with turning and body positioning, and promoting the development of contractures. Limbs may be caused to slide repeatedly across a surface or press directly against another part of the body for a prolonged period of time. Multiple joint contractures also tend to create areas of accentuated pressure on the skin, leading to pressure sores. In some instances, decubitus ulcers may be impossible to treat without first reducing the spasticity and contractures that hastened their formation (Fig. 24–10).

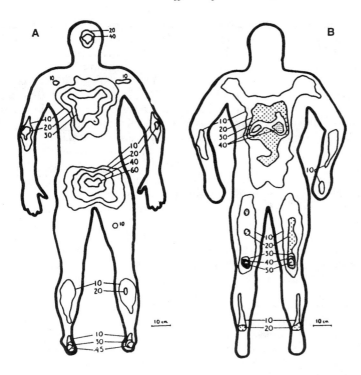

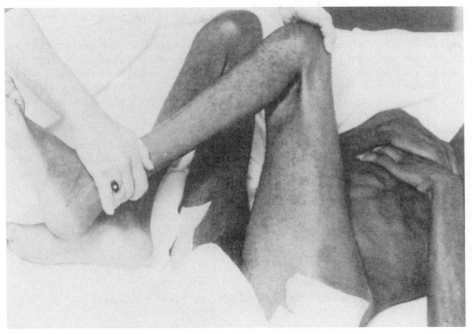

Figure 24–9. *Pressure on the Body Surface.* This figure compares the surface pressure distribution in a healthy adult man lying (A) supine and (B) prone with his feet hanging over the edge of the bed. Isobar values are in millimeters of mercury. (From Lindan, O, Greenway, RM, and Piazza, JM: Pressure distribution on the surface of the human body. Arch Phys Med Rehabil 46:378, 1965, with permission.)

Figure 24–10. *Pressure Sores with Spasticity and Contractures.* In this patient with multiple sclerosis, severe spasticity and contractures made treatment of the pressure sores over the trochanters difficult. Surgical repair was deferred until the contractures could be reduced. Nerve blockade was considered to reduce the spasticity. (From Delisa, JA and Gans, BM (eds): Rehabilitation Medicine: Principles and Practice, ed 2. JB Lippincott, Philadelphia, 1993, p 687, with permission. Copyright © Baylor College of Medicines, 1986.)

The development of decubitus ulcers is aggravated by many of the conditions that often accompany immobilization. For example, individuals with disruption of sensory pathways will not feel the discomfort resulting from excessive or protracted pressure and therefore will be even less likely to regularly change body position. Disruption of autonomic pathways can disturb vasomotor tone, further compromise regional blood flow, and heighten sensitivity to pressure. Decreased venous return may lead to the development of tissue edema, further impairing the delivery of oxygen and nutrients to the tissues. Increased skin temperature may exacerbate tissue breakdown by increasing the metabolic demands of tissues that are already vascularly compromised. Excessive moisture, whether due to prolonged contact with sweat, urine, or feces, will make the skin more susceptible to maceration. Wet skin is also more likely to adhere to clothing and bed linens, thus enhancing the generation of shearing forces. A warm, moist environment provides an optimal environment for bacterial growth, especially as might arise from urinary or fecal incontinence. Seat cushions and mattress surfaces are especially troublesome because they tend to retain both heat and moisture.

Poor nutrition among immobilized patients is well documented and may result in weight loss and emaciation, thereby reducing the padding over bony prominences and making the overlying tissue more susceptible to pressure. Poor nutrition may also cause deleterious changes in connective tissue synthesis, resulting in reduced tensile strength and atrophy of the skin.[8,27-29] Inadequate nutrition is accompanied by impaired healing in general. Ironically, if pressure sores are allowed to develop, the loss of body protein through the ulcer and the metabolic demands posed by healing and combating infection will place further nutritional demands on the patient. Obesity may interfere with the ability to perform pressure relief techniques, and equipment such as a wheelchair or braces may no longer fit, resulting in skin breakdown in high-pressure areas. Anemia, which is also common in immobilized patients, reduces the oxygen carrying capacity of the blood, and impairs the ability of the body to heal and react to the ischemic effects of pressure. Chronic anemia may accompany malnutrition. Diabetic patients, because of various metabolic and vascular abnormalities associated with diabetes, are at particular risk for developing decubiti (even without immobilization) and require careful monitoring.

Infection of decubitus ulcers is common, especially in the presence of urinary tract infection or fecal incontinence.[27] If infection is not controlled, further tissue destruction may result, with abscess formation and osteomyelitis of the underlying bone. Infected pressure sores are a major cause of fever and sepsis in patients with impaired mobility. Chronic long-standing ulcers may occasionally undergo malignant transformation, but in general 10 to 15 years is required for this to occur. In such cases, the prognosis is poor.

Although **pressure sores are totally avoidable**, they remain a common complication, which prolongs hospital stays, markedly increases the cost of care, and threatens the lives of patients with impaired mobility. All personnel working with patients must be taught to recognize the skin changes that indicate an impending breakdown of the skin and to carry out the management techniques that minimize their occurrence. Once a sore has developed, treatment ranges from local wound care with débridement of necrotic tissue to operative measures involving wound closure through the use of skin grafts, skin flaps, and muscle flaps (Fig. 24–11).

Frictional Sores and Other Minor Trauma

In addition to pressure sores, the presence of muscle weakness, sensory loss, and decreased vasomotor tone all make the skin more susceptible to frictional sores and other minor trauma. Poorly fitting shoes or appliances, rough or tight clothes, buckles, and buttons all can erode soft tissue (Fig. 24–12). Cuts and burns, easily avoided by others, are common. All injuries to the skin are made all the more hazardous by impaired healing.

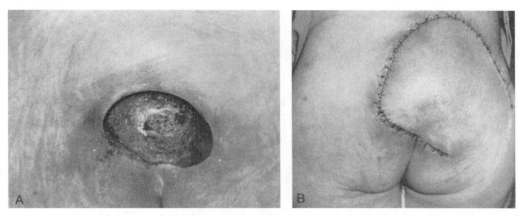

Figure 24–11. *Surgical Repair of a Pressure Sore.* (*A*) Preoperative view of a sacral pressure sore. (*B*) View after the defect has been reconstructed using a gluteal maximus myocutaneous flap. (From McCarthy, JG, May, JW, Jr, and Littler, JW (eds): Plastic Surgery. WB Saunders, Philadelphia, 1990, p 3820, with permission.)

Effects on the Gastrointestinal Tract

Deterioration of gastrointestinal tract function often accompanies immobilization and can result in impairment of overall health, considerable discomfort, and ultimately necessitate surgical intervention and threaten life itself.[1,5,6,31–33] As the mortality rate among immobilized patients has decreased with improved overall care and better pulmonary and genitourinary management, gastrointestinal complications have become increasingly prominent. Gastrointestinal complications now account for up to 10% of fatalities among spinal cord–injured patients.[19,33]

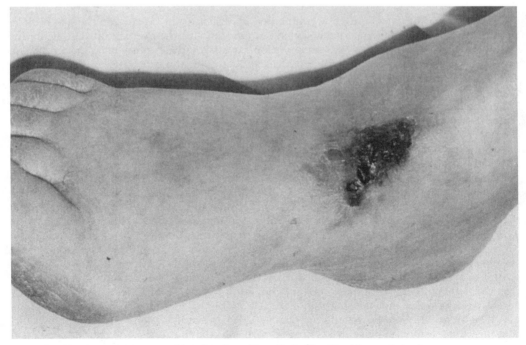

Figure 24–12. Pressure sore caused by a bandage. (From Bader,[24] p 67, with permission.)

In many locomotor disorders, deleterious changes in alimentary tract function that arise from inactivity and recumbency alone are exacerbated by the disruption of specific somatic and autonomic pathways.

Decreased Intake and Absorption of Food

Immobilization is often accompanied by a loss of appetite (anorexia), especially for protein-rich foods. Hunger is regulated by a complex interplay between psychological and physiologic factors, and the loss of appetite is equally complex. In most instances, the immobilized patient just doesn't "feel" like eating. Such individuals are stressed, often beyond their coping abilities, resulting in fear and depression and often the unpleasant consequences of excessive parasympathetic stimulation, including dyspepsia, hyperacidity, gastric stasis, and distention. The decreased physical and metabolic activity and the prolonged negative nitrogen balance observed in these patients further contribute to their lack of hunger. Damage to the brain may injure areas mediating hunger and thirst, as well as overall arousal.

In addition to loss of desire to eat, the actual mechanics of feeding may be impaired. Loss of skeletal muscle strength and coordination may make feeding difficult and exhausting. Bulbar weakness (labioglossopharyngeal) may impede feeding, drinking, chewing, and swallowing. Prolonged recumbency itself, by distorting the effects of gravity, may impede feeding secondary to the sagging of the tongue into the throat, the aspiration of food, difficulty swallowing and moving food down the esophagus, gas trapped in the stomach, and esophageal reflux.

Whatever the cause, decreased food intake may lead to malnutrition (especially hypoproteinemia). In spite of reduced energy requirements, the immobilized individual requires appropriate and sufficient nutrients to meet his or her basal metabolic needs and to compensate for loss due to immobility-induced catabolism.

Constipation, Impaction, and Obstruction

Immobilization is also often accompanied by difficulty in evacuating the gastrointestinal tract.[1,6] Defecation depends on skeletal muscle activity, the primary muscles being the abdominals, diaphragm, and levator ani. Contraction of these muscles is necessary for raising intra-abdominal pressure prior to defecation and for the expulsion of the fecal mass. The muscle weakness, hypotonia, and atrophy that occurs as a consequence of both inactivity and denervation can therefore markedly impair the effectiveness of defecation. Loss of sensory pathways can deny the patient the sensation of fullness (of the colon and rectum) that normally signals the need to defecate and triggers the onset of this process. Moreover, the increased sympathetic nervous system response to bed rest and the disruption of specific autonomic pathways can distort the normal balance between parasympathetic and sympathetic influences regulating the gastrointestinal tract. This often results in decreased peristalsis and disruption of the reflexes that promote the propulsion of material along the tract and the expulsion of feces from the rectum. The reduced intake of fluid and appropriate foods, which accompanies immobilization, and the loss of plasma volume and dehydration that occurs with bed rest, both serve to reduce fecal mass and alter its consistency, making elimination more difficult. Finally, the act of defecation itself may become such a negative (unpleasant) experience that powerful avoidance behaviors develop.[1,6] The patient may be strongly deterred from regular defecation by the awkward, ineffective (unphysiologic) positions necessary for the use of a bedpan or other device, as well as by a lack of privacy and the resultant embarrassment. Over time, the avoidance of defecation can actually desensitize the reflex mechanisms that make it possible.

Constipation usually results, accompanied by manifestations such as headache, anorexia, distension, malaise, vertigo, and pain in the buttocks and sacrum.[1,6] **Fecal impaction can then develop** as a consequence of prolonged retention of fecal material in the rectum or colon. During such retention, water is continually extracted making the material drier and harder and hence more difficult for the rectum to expel. **Impaction can ultimately culminate in partial or complete bowel obstruction, which is a serious medical problem.** With this blockage, there is an interruption of intestinal propulsion and absorption of liquid and gas. Stasis of fluid within the intestine produces distention and increased intraluminal pressure. With the expansion of the intestinal wall, the mesenteric vessels may be stretched to the point of occlusion, impairing regional circulation.[6] Intestinal function becomes depressed, dehydration occurs, and absorption ceases, contributing to fluid and electrolyte imbalance. The distention produces pain and discomfort for the patient. Respiration may become difficult as the elevated intra-abdominal pressure interferes with the descent of the diaphragm.[6] The increased pressure on the large veins of the abdomen may retard venous return from the legs and contribute to the formation of thrombi in the veins of the lower extremities. Frequently, liquid material may be forced past an impaction producing a "spurious" diarrhea. This may further disrupt fluid balance and may be treated with antidiarrheals that aggravate the underlying constipation. Manual removals of impactions or finally surgical intervention may be required. Autonomic hyperreflexia can be precipitated by fecal impaction and necessitates close monitoring of vital signs and blood pressure during release of the impaction.

Gastrointestinal complications are particularly severe in spinal cord–injured patients, arising during both the acute and chronic phases of injury.[19,21,23,31–33] Gastric dilatation and ileus (intestinal stasis) occur frequently in the acute phase of cervical and high thoracic lesions and can be life-threatening. Gastrointestinal stasis reflects the abrupt change in nervous (autonomic) control of the gut, neuroendocrine responses to stress, or coincidental trauma to abdominal structures. Acute gastric dilatation may be associated with the loss of large amounts of fluid into the stomach and the precipitation of hypovolemic shock. Gastric dilatation may also compromise respiratory function further by limiting diaphragmatic movements, and it may increase the risk of aspiration.

Peptic ulcers (gastroduodenal) and bleeding are important complications in both acutely injured patients and those in the chronic stages of their disability. Often referred to as "stress ulcers," the development of these lesions during the acute period may be promoted by excessive vagal activity and elevated levels of corticosteroids (secondary to stress-induced release or exogenous administration). Declining renal function, immobilization hypercalcemia, the use of anti-inflammatory drugs for relief of spastic muscle aches, and reflux of bile into the stomach all have been implicated in the etiology of peptic ulcers during the chronic stages of spinal cord injury.[19,21,23,31–33] Prolonged supine position, depressed diaphragmatic function, and chronic constipation all may contribute to gastroesophageal reflux in these patients.

Constipation and impaction, with or without spurious diarrhea, are a frequent problem throughout the chronic phase. Treatment and prevention of these complications play major parts in the management of these patients.

RECOMMENDED READINGS

Bader, DL: Pressure Sores. Clinical Practice and Scientific Approach. Macmillan Press, London, 1990.

Bloch, RF and Basbaum, M (eds): Management of Spinal Cord Injuries. Williams & Wilkins, Baltimore, 1986.

Browse, NL: The Physiology and Pathology of Bed Rest. Charles C Thomas, Springfield, IL, 1965.

Coletta, EM and Murphy, JB: The Complications of Immobility in the Elderly Stroke Patient. J Am Board Fam Pract 5:389, 1992.

Delisa, JA and Gans, BM (eds): Rehabilitation Medicine: Principles and Practice. Part 3, ed 2. JB Lippincott, Philadelphia, 1993.

Goodgold, J (ed): Rehabilitation Medicine. CV Mosby, St. Louis, 1988.

Harper, C and Lyles, Y: Physiology and Complications of Bed Rest. J Am Geriatr Soc 36:1047, 1988.

Hoening, H and Rubenstein, L: Hospital Associated Deconditioning and Dysfunction. J Am Geriatr Soc 39(2): 270, 1991.

Judd, M: Mobility: Patient Problems and Nursing Care. Heinemann Nursing, London, 1989.

Lee, BY, et al: The Spinal Cord Injured Patient: Comprehensive Management. Comprehensive Management. WB Saunders, Philadelphia, 1991.

Mobily, PR and Kelly, LS: Iatrogenesis in the Elderly: Factors of Immobility. J Gerontol Nurs 17(9):25, 1991.

Olson, EV: The Hazards of Immobility. Am J Nurs 67:780, 1967.

Sandler, H and Vernikos, J (eds): Inactivity: Physiological Effects. Academic Press, Orlando, 1986.

Selikson, J, Damus, K, and Hamerman, D: Risk Factors Associated with Immobility. J Am Geriatr Soc 36:707, 1986.

Steinberg, FV (ed): Immobilized Patient: Functional Pathology and Management. Plenum Medical Book Company, New York, 1980.

Sugarman, B: Medical Complications of Spinal Cord Injury. Q J Med 54(213):3, 1985.

REFERENCES

1. Milde, FK: Physiological Immobilization. Chapter 5. In Hart, LK, Reese, JL, and Fearing, MO (eds): Concepts Common to Acute Illness. Identification and Management. CV Mosby, St. Louis, 1981.

2. Mobily, PR and Kelly, LS: Iatrogenesis in the Elderly: Factors of Immobility. J Gerontol Nurs 17(9):25, 1991.

3. Harper, C and Lyles, Y: Physiology and Complications of Bed Rest. J Am Geriatr Soc 36:1047, 1988.

4. Halar, EM and Bell, KR: Rehabilitation's Relationship to Inactivity. Chapter 52. In Kottke, FJ and Lehmann, JF (eds): Krusen's Handbook of Physical Medicine and Rehabilitation, ed 4. WB Saunders, Philadelphia, 1990.

5. Vallbona, C: Bodily Responses to Immobilization. Chapter 52. In Kottke, FJ, Stillwell, GK, and Lehmann, JF (eds): Krusen's Handbook of Physical Medicine and Rehabilitation, ed 3. WB Saunders, Philadelphia, 1982.

6. Olson, EV: The Hazards of Immobility. Am J Nurs 67:780, 1967.

7. Sandler, H and Vernikos, J (eds): Inactivity: Physiologic Effects. Academic Press, Orlando, 1986.

8. Steinberg, FU (ed): Immobilized Patient: Functional Pathology and Management. Plenum Medical Book Company, New York, 1980.

9. Morgan, MDL, Silver, JR, and Williams, JJ: The Respiratory System of the Spinal Cord Patient. Chapter 3. In Bloch, RF and Basbaum, M (eds): Management of Spinal Cord Injuries. Williams & Wilkins, Baltimore, 1986.

10. Halar, EM and Bell, KR: Contracture and Other Deleterious Effects of Immobility. Chapter 33. In Delisa, JA and Gans, BM (eds): Rehabilitation Medicine: Principles and Practice, ed 2. JB Lippincott, Philadelphia, 1993.

11. Schneider, FJ: Traumatic Spinal Cord Injury. Chapter 15. In Umphred, DA: Neurological Rehabilitation, ed 2. CV Mosby, St. Louis, 1990.

12. Peterson, P: Pulmonary Physiology and Medical Management. In Whiteneck, et al (eds): The Management of High Quadriplegia. Demos Publishing, New York, 1989.

13. Winslow, EH: Cardiovascular Consequences of Bed Rest. Rev Cardiol 14(3): 236, 1985.

14. Convertino, VA: Exercise Response After Inactivity. Chapter 7. In Sandler, H and Vernikos, J: Inactivity: Physiological Effects. Academic Press, Orlando, 1986.

15. Bloch, RF: Autonomic Dysfunction. Chapter 6. In Bloch, RF and Basbaum, M. (eds): Management of Spinal Cord Injuries. Williams & Wilkins, Baltimore, 1986.

16. Turpie, AGG: Thrombosis Prevention and Treatment in Spinal Cord Injured Patients. Chapter 9. In Bloch, RF and Basbaum, M (eds): Management of Spinal Cord Injuries. Williams & Wilkins, Baltimore, 1986.

17. Wittert, D and Barden, R: Deep Vein Thrombosis, Pulmonary Embolism, and Prophylaxis in Orthopaedic Patients. Orthop Nurs 5(4):27, 1985.

18. Lee, BY: Deep Venous Thrombosis in Spinal Cord Injured Patients. Chapter 2. In Lee, BY, et al (eds): The Spinal Cord Injured Patient: Comprehensive Management. WB Saunders, Philadelphia. 1991.

19. Sugarman, B: Medical Complications of Spinal Cord Injury. Quart J Med 54(213):3, 1985.

20. Yalla, SV and Fam, BA: Spinal Cord Injury. Chapter 19. In Krane, RJ and Siroky, MB: Clinical Neuro-Urology. Little, Brown & Company, Boston, 1991.

21. Perkesh, I: Management of Neurogenic Dysfunction of the Bladder and Bowel. Chapter 38. In Kottke, FJ and Lehman, JF (eds): In Krusen's Handbook of Physical Medicine and Rehabilitation, ed 4. WB Saunders, Philadelphia, 1990.

22. Morales, P: Urologic Management of the Spinal Cord Injury Patient. Chapter 12. In Goodgold, J (ed): Rehabilitation Medicine. CV Mosby, St. Louis, 1988.

23. Cole, JD: The Pathophysiology of the Autonomic Nervous System in Spinal Cord Injury. Chapter 9. In Illis, LS (ed): Spinal Cord Dysfunction. Oxford University Press, Oxford, 1988.

24. Bader, DL (ed): Pressure Sores: Clinical Practice and Scientific Approach. Macmillan Press, London, 1990.

25. Cherry, GW and Ryan, TJ: Pathophysiology. Chapter 3. In Parish, LC, Witkowski, JA, and Crissey, JT: The Decubitus Ulcer. Masson Publishing, New York, 1983.

26. Lindan, O, Greenway, RM, and Piazza, JM: Pressure Distribution on the Surface of the Body. Arch Phys Med Rehabil 46:378, 1965.

27. Kelly, LS and Mobily, PR: Iatrogenesis in the Elderly: Impaired Skin Integrity. J Gerontol Nurs 17(9):26, 1991.

28. Colen, SR: Pressure Sores. Chapter 11. In Goodgold, J (ed): Rehabilitation Medicine. CV Mosby, St. Louis, 1988.

29. Kosiak, M and Kottke, FJ: Prevention and Rehabilitation of Ischemic Ulcers. Chapter 46. In Kottke, FJ and Lehmann, JF (eds): Krusen's Handbook of Physical Medicine and Rehabilitation, ed 4. WB Saunders, Philadelphia, 1990.

30. Donovan, WH, et al: Pressure Ulcers. Chapter 35. In Delisa, JA and Gans, BM (eds). Rehabilitation Medicine: Principles and Practice, ed 2. JB Lippincott, Philadelphia, 1993.

31. Seaton, T and Hollingsworth, R: Gastrointestinal Complications in Spinal Cord Injuries. Chapter 5. In Bloch, RF and Basbaum, M (eds): Management of Spinal Cord Injuries. Williams & Wilkins, Baltimore, 1986.

32. Gore, RM, Mintzer, RA, and Calenoff, L: Gastrointestinal Complications of Spinal Cord Injury. Spine 6(6):538, 1981.

33. Staas, WE, Jr, et al: Rehabilitation of the Spinal Cord-Injured Patient. Chapter 42. In Delisa, JA and Gans, BM (eds): Rehabilitation Medicine: Principles and Practice, ed 2. JB Lippincott, Philadelphia, 1993.

Index

An "f" page number indicates a figure; a "t" following a page number indicates a table.

necrotizing, 319
rhabdomyolysis, 319
Drug-induced neuropathies, 368
Drugs, excitable cells and, 27–28
Duchenne's muscular dystrophy, 298–301
  features, 297t
  fiber loss in, 295f
Dura mater anatomy, 469f
Dying back (axonal degeneration), 354, 354f
Dynamical systems theory of motor control, 230–234,
    232f, 233f, 233t
  assumptions, 231–234
  clinical applications, 234
  constraining complexity into simplicity, 231
  nonlinear development within subsystems, 231–232
  phase shifts, 232–234, 233f, 233t
  self-organization within subsystems, 231, 232f, 233t
  summary, 235t
Dysarthria, 447
  in multiple sclerosis, 518
  traumatic brain injury and, 478, 482t
Dysdiadochokinesia, 280, 452
Dysesthesias, 267–268, 268t
  in peripheral neuropathies, 361
Dysmetria, 280, 447, 452
Dysmyelinating diseases, 515, 531–532
  cerebellar, 464
Dysphagia, traumatic brain injury and, 478
Dysraphism, 414
Dyssynergia, 280
Dystonia, 277, 278t
  focal, 440, 441f, 441t
  general, 440
Dystonic adductor dysphonia, 441t
Dystonic kyphoscoliosis, 279f
Dystrophin, 298, 301
Dystrophy. *See* Muscular dystrophies; Myotonic
    dystrophy

Eccentric contractions, 42
Efferent connections, cerebellar, 187
Efferent fibers, spinal gray matter, 113
Efferent neuron, 18, 18t
Ejaculatory dysfunction, spinal cord disorders
    and, 408
Electrical synapses, 20, 21f, 222
Electricity, neuronopathies from, 389
Embolic ischemic strokes, 488, 490, 490t
  clinical picture, 493t
Embryogenesis, motor neurons and, 74
Emotion
  cerebellum and, 199–200
  limbic cortex and, 174
Emotional lability, traumatic brain injury and, 483t
Encephalomyelitis, acute disseminated (ADEM), 529f,
    529–530
Endocrine myopathies, 294t, 314t, 314–318
  adrenal dysfunction, 314t, 314–315
  metabolic bone disease (osteomalacia), 314t,
    317–318
  parathyroid dysfunction, 314t, 317–318
  pituitary dysfunction, 314t, 317
  steroids, 314t, 314–315
  thyroid dysfunction, 314t, 315–317, 316f
Endomysium, 31, 31f

Endoneurium, 350
Endurance, decreased, 275
  strokes and, 496f, 496–497
  traumatic brain injury and, 478–479
Enteroviruses, and poliomyelitis, 384
Environmental contaminants, neuronopathies from,
    388–389
Epidural hemorrhage, 470, 471t
Epimysium, 30, 31f
Epineurium, 350
EPSP. *See* Excitatory postsynaptic potential
Epstein-Barr virus myelitis, 417
Equilibrium, cerebellum and, 194–195
  disorders of, 449
Erectile dysfunction, spinal cord disorders and, 408
Excessive rebound, 448
Excitability, 13–14
  absolute refractory period, 13
  disturbances, 26–28
  neuromuscular junction transmission, 66–72. *See
    also* Acetylcholine
    pharmacologic modification, 72f, 72–74
  relative refractory period, 13
  supernormal period, 13
Excitable cells, 3–28
  action potentials, 11f, 11–16, 12f
    excitability, 13–14
    propagation, 14–16, 15f
  basic membrane properties, 3–5
  cell-to-cell communication, 20–26. *See also* Synapses
  defined, 3
  disturbances of excitability, 26–28
  drugs and, 27–28
  electrical properties of, 8–16
  graded potentials, 9f, 9–11
    decremental conduction, 9–10, 10f
    temporal and spatial summation, 10–11, 11f
  hypoxia and, 27
  membrane potential, 6–8, 7f
  morphology, 16–20
  pH and, 27
  selective permeability, 4, 4f
  synaptic transmission disturbances, 26–28
  transport proteins, 4–5, 5f, 6f
Excitation-contraction coupling, 37–41
  feet, 38
  sarcoplasmic reticulum, 38–39, 39f, 41
  terminal cisternae, 38
Excitatory postsynaptic potential (EPSP), 24, 26, 114
Exercise
  intolerance, immobilization and, 555–556
  muscle fiber transformation in, 56, 56f
  reversibility of effects, 57
Exocytosis, 22
Extensor synergy, 276t
External tension, 42, 43f
Exteroceptors, 86, 86t
Extrafusal fibers of muscle spindles, 98, 98f
Eye movement control, 212–213

Facial (seventh cranial) nerve, 150t, 151t,
    152, 152f
Facilitated diffusion, 5
F-actin, 34, 34f
Faded schedule, 243